Cognitive–Behavioral Treatment of Borderline Personality Disorder

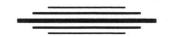

Marsha M. Linehan, Ph.D.
University of Washington

THE GUILFORD PRESS
New York   London

©1993 The Guilford Press
A Division of Guilford Publications, Inc.
72 Spring Street, New York, NY 10012

Printed in the United States of America

This book is printed on acid-free paper.

Last digit is print number: 9   8   7

Library of Congress Cataloging-in-Publication Data

Linehan, Marsha.
   Cognitive-behavioral treatment of borderline personality disorder
/ Marsha M. Linehan.
     p. cm.—(Diagnosis and treatment of mental disorders)
   Includes bibliographical references and index.
   ISBN 0-89862-183-6
   1. Borderline personality disorder—Treatment.   2. Cognitive
therapy.   I. Title.   II. Series.
   [DNLM: 1. Borderline Personality Disorder—therapy.   2. Cognitive
Therapy.   3. Behavior Therapy.   WM 190 L754c 1993]
RC569.5.B67L56   1993
616.85'8520651—dc20
DNLM/DLC
for Library of Congress   93-20483
                                                   CIP

To
John O'Brien,
Al Leventhal,
and
Dick Gode.
Most of the really good strategies in this book
I learned from them.

DIAGNOSIS AND TREATMENT OF MENTAL DISORDERS
Allen Frances, MD, *Series Editor*

THE FATE OF BORDERLINE PATIENTS:
SUCCESSFUL OUTCOME AND PSYCHIATRIC PRACTICE
Michael H. Stone

PREMENSTRUAL SYNDROME: A CLINICIAN'S GUIDE
Sally K. Severino and Margaret L. Moline

SUPPORTIVE THERAPY FOR BORDERLINE PATIENTS:
A PSYCHODYNAMIC APPROACH
Lawrence H. Rockland

COGNITIVE BEHAVIORAL TREATMENT OF
BORDERLINE PERSONALITY DISORDER
Marsha M. Linehan

SKILLS TRAINING MANUAL FOR TREATING
BORDERLINE PERSONALITY DISORDER
Marsha M. Linehan

Foreword

Every once in a very long while in our field, a clinical innovation is introduced that profoundly improves patient care. Marsha Linehan's development of a cognitive–behavioral approach to borderline personality disorder is such a rare innovation. I first discovered Dr. Linehan's work almost ten years ago around the time that she was beginning a series of systematic research studies to determine its efficacy. Even before the positive results were in, I felt sure that Dr. Linehan was on to something important. It has been my pleasure to observe as Dr. Linehan refined her techniques, making them increasingly comprehensive, specific, practical, and applicable to general mental health practice.

The problem Dr. Linehan is addressing—borderline personality disorder—is an important and prevalent one that represents a great clinical puzzle. These individuals suffer and cause suffering, often in the most poignant and dramatic fashion. They constitute the most frequent personality disorder encountered in clinical practice and have the highest rate of completed suicide and of suicide attempts. Individuals meeting diagnostic criteria for borderline personality disorder present a great treatment challenge. They are often recalcitrant, unpredictable, and get too close or stray too far in the therapeutic relationship. They provoke strong countertransferences in the therapist who may become too seductive or too rejecting, or more likely may oscillate between these extremes. "Borderline" (what a terrible term, but we have failed to find a suitable replacement) individuals are also the most likely to have bad responses to treatment. They present, not infrequently, with a suicide attempt or self-mutilation made in response to a real or imagined rejection from their therapist (a vacation perhaps being the most common precipitant). They often tie the therapist in therapeutic knots so that every intervention feels wrongheaded and cruel hearted. The treatments typically end in a huff, and not infrequently in a hospitalization.

Clinicians are most likely to feel bewildered and deskilled by the borderline individuals in their practice, and search for ways of dealing with them.

For some clinicians, the major hope has been the discovery of an effective pharmacological intervention. The results to date have been decidedly mixed. There is no specific pharmacological treatment for the instability of border-line patients, and even the medications (neuroleptics, antidepressants, lith-ium, carbomezapine) most effective for accompanying target symptoms have their own side-effects and complications. Other clinicians have turned to psy-chotherapeutic (particularly psychodynamic) strategies developed for border-line individuals. But here, too, the results are quite mixed and the treatments have many side-effects and complications of their own (particularly the trans-ference/countertransference reenactments described above). It is probably fair to say that individuals with borderline personality disorder constitute the toughest and most insoluble problem for the average clinician and the aver-age clinic or inpatient facility. Everyone talks about borderline personality disorder but it usually seems that no one knows quite what to do about it.

Until Dr. Linehan that is. She combines an unusually empathic under-standing of the internal experience of borderline individuals with the techni-cal tools of a cognitive/behavioral therapist. Dr. Linehan is a creative clinical innovator. She has analyzed the aspects of borderline behavior into their com-ponent parts and has developed a systematized and integrated approach to each of them. Her techniques are clear, teachable, and learnable, and make good common sense to the therapist and to the patient. Dr. Linehan's methods have greatly improved my treatment of borderline individuals and my teach-ing of others in how best to understand and treat these patients. I have no doubt that this book will change your practice and make you much more effective with these most troubled and needful individuals.

ALLEN FRANCES, M.D.

Acknowledgments

This book and this form of treatment, dialectical behavior therapy (DBT), are the products of many minds and hearts. I have been influenced by most of my colleagues, students, and patients, and have appropriated the ideas of many. It would be impossible to cite everyone who has contributed, but I do want to acknowledge several whose influence has been enormous.

First, I learned many of the most important elements of DBT from individuals who were my own therapists and consultants. The people to whom I have dedicated the book—Richard Gode, M.D., Allan Leventhal, Ph.D., and John O'Brien, M.D.—fall into this category, as does Helen McLean. I was fortunate indeed to find people so able to care so skillfully. Gerald Davison, Ph.D., and Marvin Goldfried, Ph.D., were my first clinical teachers in behavior therapy. They taught me most of what I know about clinical behavior change, and their ideas and influence pervade this book. My early training at the Buffalo Suicide Prevention and Crisis Service, Inc., has also had a strong influence; there, out of thin air, Gene Brockopp, Ph.D., created an internship for me when everyone else had turned me down. The therapy I have developed is in most respects an integration of my background in suicide prevention and behavior therapy with my experience as a Zen student. My teacher, Willigis Jäger, O.S.B. (Ko-un Roshi), a Zen master who is also a Benedictine monk, taught me, and still teaches me, most of what I know about acceptance.

Much of the theoretical scaffolding of my approach to psychotherapy and borderline personality disorder (BPD) is a product of the swirl of ideas constantly circulating in the psychology department at the University of Washington. It is no accident that many of us here are arriving at similar points in quite diverse areas. I have been most influenced by the ideas of our resident radical behaviorist, Robert Kohlenberg, Ph.D.; the relapse prevention work of Alan Marlatt, Ph.D., and Judith Gordon, Ph.D.; and the developmental theories and clinical perspectives of Geraldine Dawson, Ph.D., John Gottman, Ph.D., and Mark Greenberg, Ph.D. Neil Jacobson, Ph.D., has also been expanding many of the ideas in DBT, especially those concerning acceptance versus change, and applying them in the context of marital therapy. In a circular fashion, his creative ideas, especially his contextualizing of acceptance within a radical behavioral framework, have come back to influence the further development of DBT.

No professor can succeed, however, without an army of very bright and capable students prodding, arguing, critiquing, and offering new ideas and suggestions. Certainly that is true for me. Kelly Egan, Ph.D., my first doctoral student at the University of Washington, contributed many creative ideas to this therapy and shot down many of my less creative ones. I have had the joy of working with and supervising the clinical work of perhaps one of the finest groups of clinical graduate students to be found anywhere: Michael Addis, Beatriz Aramburu, Ph.D., Alan Furzzetti, Ph.D., Barbara Graham, Ph.D., Kelly Koerner, Edward Shearin, Ph.D., Amy Wagner, Jennifer Waltz, and Elizabeth Wasson. Jason McClurg, M.D., and Jeanne Blache, R.N., joined them in the clinical supervision seminar; because they came to the therapeutic enterprise from medical rather than psychological backgrounds, they were able to add to and clarify the assumptions underlying DBT. Although I was ostensibly teaching all of these individuals DBT, in reality I was learning much of it from them.

When I began the field trials of this form of treatment, some aspects of the approach were quite controversial. My collaborator, Hugh Armstrong, Ph.D., ran interference. His immense personal and clinical respect in Seattle persuaded the clinical community to give us a chance. My research therapists—Douglas Allmon, Ph.D., Steve Clancy, Ph.D., Decky Fiedler, Ph.D., Charles Huffine, M.D., Karen Lindner, Ph.D., and Alejandra Suarez, Ph.D.—both demonstrated the effectiveness of DBT and found many of the flaws in the original manual. As a group, they embodied the spirit of a dialectical strategy. The success of the clinical trial was due in large part to their ability to remain compassionate, level-headed, and close enough to the treatment manual in the midst of exceptional stress. My research team and colleagues over the years—John Chiles, M.D., Heidi Heard, Andre Ivanoff, Ph.D., Connie Kehrer, Joan Lockard, Ph.D., Steve McCutcheon, Ph.D., Evelyn Mercier, Steve Nielsen, Ph.D., Kirk Strosahl, Ph.D., and Darren Tutek—have been invaluable in providing the support and many of the ideas that have nourished the development of a empirically grounded treatment for BPD. I do not believe I would have written this book if I had not had empirical data to back up the effectiveness of the treatment. I would never have gotten those data without a first-class research team.

My own patients often wonder what new treatment idea I am going to try out on them next. Over the years, they have shown marvelous patience as I fumbled around trying to develop this treatment. I have been encouraged by their courage and tenacity. In circumstances where many others would have quit long ago, not one of them has given up. They have been most gracious in pointing out many of my errors, noting the successes, and giving feedback about how I could improve the treatment. The great thing about treating borderline patients is that it is like having a supervisor always in the room. My patients have been very good and supportive supervisors indeed.

I have many friends who are psychodynamic rather than cognitive–behavioral therapists. A number have contributed to my thinking and to this book. Charles Swenson, M.D., a psychiatrist at Cornell Medical Center/New York Hospital at White Plains, had the courage to try to implement DBT in an inpatient unit at a wholly psychodynamic hospital. We have spent countless hours discussing how to do it and how to overcome or circumvent problems. Out of those hours came a much sharper conceptualization of the treatment. John Clarkin, Ph.D., and Otto Kernberg, M.D., have compared and contrasted this treatment with Kernberg's over many discussions, and in the process nudged my thinking in directions I had perhaps resisted and helped clarify my stance in other ways. Sally Parks, M.A., a Jungian analyst and friend, has debated Jungian versus behavioral ideas with me for years, and much of my thinking about therapy evolved out of these debates. Finally, my good friend Sebern Fisher, M.A., one of the best therapists I know, has listened and shared her insights with me about the problems of borderline patients.

The final draft of the book was written while I was on sabbatical in England at the Medical Research Council Applied Psychology Research Unit, Cambridge University. My colleagues there—J. Mark Williams, Ph.D., John Teasdale, Ph.D., Philip Barnard, Ph.D., and Edna Foa, Ph.D.—critiqued many of my ideas and gave me new ones. Caroline Muncey saved my sanity by typing and retyping draft after draft. Leslie Horton, my secretary on the treatment research project, also deserves much of the credit of organizing me and the materials that later became this book.

I must thank my series editor, Allen Frances, M.D., for his sharp editing and insistence that I stay practical whenever possible. He provided the dialectical opposition to the "ivory tower" that I sometimes work within. The interest in this therapy has been largely generated by his enthusiastic support over the years. My brother, W. Marston Linehan, M.D., who is also a researcher, has never tired of helping me "keep my eye on the prize" so that I could get this book written. He and his wife, Tracey Rouault, M.D., and my sister, Aline Haynes, have been wonderfully supportive over the years.

Development and writing of this volume were partially supported by Grant No. MH34486 from the National Institute of Mental Health. Morris Parloff, Ph.D., Irene Elkin, Ph.D., Barry Wolfe, Ph.D., and Tracie Shea, Ph.D. nurtured and fought for this work from the beginning, and deserve much of the credit for the success of the research on which this treatment approach is based.

Last, but certainly not least, I want to thank my copy editor, Marie Sprayberry. She worked miracles on the organization and clarity of this book, and with marvelous patience waited for me to come around to her better point of view on many matters of controversy.

Contents

PART I. THEORY AND CONCEPTS

1. Borderline Personality Disorder: **3**
Concepts, Controversies, and Definitions

The Concept of Borderline Personality Disorder / 5
The Concept of Parasuicidal Behaviors / 13
The Overlap Between Borderline Personality Disorder
    and Parasuicidal Behavior / 15
Therapy for Borderline Personality Disorder: A Preview / 19
Concluding Comments / 25
Notes / 26

2. Dialectical and Biosocial Underpinnings of Treatment   **28**

Dialectics / 28
Borderline Personality Disorder as Dialectical Failure / 35
Case Conceptualization: A Dialectical
    Cognitive–Behavioral Approach /37
Biosocial Theory: A Dialectical Theory of Borderline
    Personality Disorder Development / 42
Implications of the Biosocial Theory for Therapy
    with Borderline Patients / 62
Concluding Comments / 64
Notes / 65

3. Behavioral Patterns: Dialectical Dilemmas   **66**
in the Treatment of Borderline Patients

Emotional Vulnerability versus Self-Invalidation / 67
Active Passivity versus Apparent Competence / 78
Unrelenting Crises versus Inhibited Grieving / 85
Concluding Comments / 93
Notes / 94

PART II. TREATMENT OVERVIEW AND GOALS

4. Overview of Treatment: Targets, Strategies,   **97**
and Assumptions in a Nutshell

Crucial Steps in Treatment / 97
Setting the Stage: Getting the Patient's Attention 97 / Staying Dialectical 98 / Applying Core Strategies: Validation and Problem Solving 99 / Balancing Interpersonal Communication Styles 100 / Combining Consultation-to-the-Patient Strategies with Interventions in the Environment 101 / Treating the Therapist 101

Modes of Treatment / 101
Individual Outpatient Psychotherapy 102 / Skills Training 103 / Supportive Process Group Therapy 103 / Telephone Consultation 104 / Case Consultation Meetings for Therapists 104 / Ancillary Treatments 105

Assumptions About Borderline Patients and Therapy / 106
1. Patients Are Doing the Best They Can 106 / 2. Patients Want to Improve 106 / 3. Patients Need to Do Better, Try Harder, and Be More Motivated to Change 106 / 4. Patients May Not Have Caused All of Their Own Problems, but They Have to Solve Them Anyway 107 / 5. The Lives of Suicidal, Borderline Individuals Are Unbearable as They Are Currently Being Lived 107 / 6. Patients Must Learn New Behaviors in All Relevant Contexts 107 / 7. Patients Cannot Fail in Therapy 108 / 8. Therapists Treating Borderline Patients Need Support 108

Therapist Characteristics and Skills / 108
Stance of Acceptance versus Change 109 / Stance of Unwavering Centeredness versus Compassionate Flexibility 110 / Stance of Nurturing versus Benevolent Demanding 111

Agreements of Patients and Therapists / 112
Patient Agreements 112 / Therapist Agreements 115

Therapist Consultation Agreements / 117
Dialectical Agreement 117 / Consultation-to-the-Patient Agreement 117 / Consistency Agreement 117 / Observing-Limits Agreement 118 / Phenomenological Empathy Agreement 118 / Fallibility Agreement 118

Concluding Comments / 119
Note / 119

5. Behavioral Targets in Treatment: **120**
Behaviors to Increase and Decrease

The Overall Goal: Increasing Dialectical Behavior Patterns / 120
Dialectical Thinking 120 / Dialectical Thinking and Cognitive Therapy 123 / Dialectical Behavior Patterns: Balanced Lifestyle 124

Primary Behavioral Targets / 124
Decreasing Suicidal Behaviors 124 / Decreasing Therapy-Interfering Behaviors 129 / Decreasing Behaviors That Interfere with Quality of Life 141 / Increasing Behavioral Skills 143 / Decreasing Behaviors Related to Posttraumatic Stress 155 / Increasing Respect for Self 160

Secondary Behavioral Targets / 160
Increasing Emotion Modulation; Decreasing Emotional Reactivity 161 / Increasing Self-Validation; Decreasing Self-Invalidation 161 / Increasing Realistic Decision Making and Judgment; Decreasing Crisis-Generating Behaviors 162 / Increasing Emotional Experiencing; Decreasing Inhibited Grieving 162 / Increasing Active Problem Solving; Decreasing Active-Passivity Behaviors 162 / Increasing Accurate Communication of Emotions and Competencies; Decreasing Mood Dependency of Behavior 163

Concluding Comments / 164
Note / 164

6. Structuring Treatment Around Target Behaviors: 165
Who Treats What and When
The General Theme: Targeting Dialectical Behaviors / 166
The Hierarchy of Primary Targets / 166
Treatment Targets and Session Agenda 167 / Treatment Targets and Modes of Therapy 167 / The Primary Therapist and Responsibility for Meeting Targets 168
Progress Toward Targets Over Time / 168
Pretreatment Stage: Orientation and Commitment 169 / Stage 1: Attaining Basic Capacities 169 / Stage 2: Reducing Posttraumatic Stress 170 / Stage 3: Increasing Self-Respect and Achieving Individual Goals 172
Setting Priorities within Target Classes in Outpatient
Individual Therapy / 173
Decreasing Suicidal Behaviors 174 / Decreasing Therapy-Interfering Behaviors 175 / Decreasing Quality-of-Life-Interfering Behaviors 177 / Increasing Behavioral Skills 178 / Reducing Posttraumatic Stress 179 / Increasing Self-Respect and Achieving Individual Goals 179 / Using Target Priorities to Organize Sessions 180 / Patient and Therapist Resistance to Discussing Target Behaviors 181 / Individual Therapy Targets and Diary Cards 184
Skills Training: Hierarchy of Targets / 186
Supportive Process Groups: Hierarchy of Targets / 187
Telephone Calls: Hierarchy of Targets / 188
Calls to the Primary Therapist 188 / Calls to Skills Trainers and Other Therapists 190
Target Behaviors and Session Focus: Who Is in Control? / 190
Modification of Target Hierarchies in Other Settings / 191
Responsibility for Decreasing Suicidal Behaviors 192 / Responsibility for Other Targets 193 / Specifying Targets for Other Modes of Treatment 193
Turf Conflicts with Respect to Target Responsibilities / 194
Concluding Comments / 195

PART III. BASIC TREATMENT STRATEGIES

7. Dialectical Treatment Strategies 199
Defining Dialectical Strategies /201
BALANCING TREATMENT STRATEGIES: DIALECTICS
OF THE THERAPEUTIC RELATIONSHIP / 202
TEACHING DIALECTICAL BEHAVIOR PATTERNS / 204
SPECIFIC DIALECTICAL STRATEGIES / 205
1. ENTERING THE PARADOX 205 / 2. THE USE OF METAPHOR 209 / 3. THE DEVIL'S ADVOCATE TECHNIQUE 212 / 4. EXTENDING 213 / 5. ACTIVATING "WISE MIND" 214 / 6. MAKING LEMONADE OUT OF LEMONS 216 / 7. ALLOWING NATURAL CHANGE 217 / 8. DIALECTICAL ASSESSMENT 218
Concluding Comments / 219
Notes / 220

8. Core Strategies: Part I. Validation 221
Defining Validation / 222
Why Validate? / 225
EMOTIONAL VALIDATION STRATEGIES / 226
1. PROVIDING OPPORTUNITIES FOR EMOTIONAL EXPRESSION 228 / 2. TEACHING EMOTION OBSERVATION AND LABELING SKILLS 230 / 3. READING EMOTIONS 231 / 4. COMMUNICATING THE VALIDITY OF EMOTIONS 234

BEHAVIORAL VALIDATION STRATEGIES / 235
1. TEACHING BEHAVIOR OBSERVATION AND LABELING SKILLS 235 /
2. IDENTIFYING THE "SHOULD" 237 / 3. COUNTERING THE "SHOULD"
237 / 4. ACCEPTING THE "SHOULD" 238 / 5. MOVING TO DISAPPOINT-
MENT 239
COGNITIVE VALIDATION STRATEGIES / 239
1. ELICITING AND REFLECTING THOUGHTS AND ASSUMPTIONS 240
/ 2. DISCRIMINATING FACTS FROM INTERPRETATIONS 240 / 3. FIND-
ING THE "KERNEL OF TRUTH" 241 / 4. ACKNOWLEDGING "WISE MIND"
242 / 5. RESPECTING DIFFERING VALUES 242
CHEERLEADING STRATEGIES / 242
1. ASSUMING THE BEST 244 / 2. PROVIDING ENCOURAGEMENT 245
/ 3. FOCUSING ON THE PATIENT'S CAPABILITIES 246 / 4. CONTRADICT-
ING/MODULATING EXTERNAL CRITICISM 247 / 5. PROVIDING PRAISE
AND REASSURANCE 247 / 6. BEING REALISTIC, BUT DEALING DIRECT-
LY WITH FEARS OF INSINCERITY 248 / 7. STAYING NEAR 249
Concluding Comments / 249

9. Core Strategies: Part II. Problem Solving   250
Levels of Problem Solving / 250
First Level 250 / Second Level 250 / Third Level 251
Mood and Problem Solving / 251
Overview of Problem-Solving Strategies / 253
BEHAVIORAL ANALYSIS STRATEGIES / 254
1. DEFINING THE PROBLEM BEHAVIOR 255 / 2. CONDUCTING A CHAIN
ANALYSIS 258 / 3. GENERATING HYPOTHESES ABOUT FACTORS CON-
TROLLING BEHAVIOR 264
INSIGHT (INTERPRETATION) STRATEGIES /265
What and How to Interpret: Guidelines for Insight 266 / 1. HIGHLIGHTING
270 / 2. OBSERVING AND DESCRIBING RECURRENT PATTERNS 271 /
3. COMMENTING ON IMPLICATIONS OF BEHAVIOR 271 / 4. ASSESSING
DIFFICULTIES IN ACCEPTING OR REJECTING HYPOTHESES 271
DIDACTIC STRATEGIES / 272
1. PROVIDING INFORMATION 273 / 2. GIVING READING MATERIALS
274 / 3. GIVING INFORMATION TO FAMILY MEMBERS 274
SOLUTION ANALYSIS STRATEGIES / 275
1. IDENTIFYING GOALS, NEEDS, AND DESIRES 276 / 2. GENERATING
SOLUTIONS 278 / 3. EVALUATING SOLUTIONS 279 / 4. CHOOSING A
SOLUTION TO IMPLEMENT 281 / 5. TROUBLESHOOTING THE SOLU-
TION 281
ORIENTING STRATEGIES / 281
1. PROVIDING ROLE INDUCTION 282 / 2. REHEARSING NEW EXPEC-
TATIONS 283
COMMITMENT STRATEGIES / 284
Levels of Commitment 284 / Commitment and Recommitment 285 / The Need
for Flexibility 286 / 1. SELLING COMMITMENT: EVALUATING THE PROS
AND CONS 286 / 2. PLAYING THE DEVIL'S ADVOCATE 286 / 3. "FOOT-
IN-THE-DOOR" AND "DOOR-IN-THE-FACE" TECHNIQUES 288 / 4. CON-
NECTING PRESENT COMMITMENTS TO PRIOR COMMITMENTS 289
/ 5. HIGHLIGHTING FREEDOM TO CHOOSE AND ABSENCE OF ALTER-
NATIVES 289 / 6. USING PRINCIPLES OF SHAPING 290 / 7. GENERAT-
ING HOPE: CHEERLEADING 290 / 8. AGREEING ON HOMEWORK 291
Concluding Comments / 291

10. Change Procedures: Part I. Contingency Procedures   **292**
(Managing Contingencies and Observing Limits)

The Rationale for Contingency Procedures / 294
The Distinction Between Managing Contingencies and Observing Limits 295 /
The Therapeutic Relationship as Contingency 296

CONTINGENCY MANAGEMENT PROCEDURES / 297
Orienting to Contingency Mangement: Task Overview 297 / 1. REINFORCING
TARGET-RELEVANT ADAPTIVE BEHAVIORS 301 / 2. EXTINGUISHING
TARGET-RELEVANT MALADAPTIVE BEHAVIORS 302 / 3. USING AVER-
SIVE CONSEQUENCES . . . WITH CARE 306 / Determining the Potency of
Consequences 314 / Using Natural Over Arbitrary Consequences 317 / Princi-
ples of Shaping 318

OBSERVING-LIMITS PROCEDURES / 319
Rationale for Observing Limits 320 / Natural versus Arbitrary Limits 321 / 1.
MONITORING LIMITS 322 / 2. BEING HONEST ABOUT LIMITS 323 / 3.
TEMPORARILY EXTENDING LIMITS WHEN NEEDED 325 / 4. BEING
CONSISTENTLY FIRM 325 / 5. COMBINING SOOTHING, VALIDATING,
AND PROBLEM SOLVING WITH OBSERVING LIMITS 326 / Difficult Areas
for Observing Limits with Borderline Patients 326

Concluding Comments / 327

11. Change Procedures: Part II. Skills Training, Exposure,   **329**
Cognitive Modification

SKILLS TRAINING PROCEDURES / 329
Orienting and Committing to Skills Training: Task Overview 330 / SKILL AC-
QUISITION PROCEDURES 331 / SKILL STRENGTHENING PROCEDURES
334 / SKILL GENERALIZATION PROCEDURES 337

EXPOSURE-BASED PROCEDURES / 343
Orienting and Commitment to Exposure: Task Overview 345 / 1. PROVIDING
NONREINFORCED EXPOSURE 347 / 2. BLOCKING ACTION TENDEN-
CIES ASSOCIATED WITH PROBLEM EMOTIONS 354 / 3. BLOCKING EX-
PRESSIVE TENDENCIES ASSOCIATED WITH PROBLEM EMOTIONS 356
/ 4. ENHANCING CONTROL OVER AVERSIVE EVENTS 357 / Structured
Exposure Procedures 358

COGNITIVE MODIFICATION PROCEDURES / 358
Orienting to Cognitive Modification Procedures 360 / CONTINGENCY CLARIFI-
CATION PROCEDURES 361 / COGNITIVE RESTRUCTURING PROCE-
DURES 364

Concluding Comments / 370
Note / 370

12. Stylistic Strategies: Balancing Communication   **371**

RECIPROCAL COMMUNICATION STRATEGIES / 372
Power and Psychotherapy: Who Makes the Rules? 372 / 1. RESPONSIVENESS
373 / 2. SELF-DISCLOSURE 376 / 3. WARM ENGAGEMENT 383 / 4.
GENUINENESS 388 / The Need for Therapist Invulnerability 390

IRREVERENT COMMUNICATION STRATEGIES / 393
Dialectical Strategies and Irreverence 393 / 1. REFRAMING IN AN UNORTHO-
DOX MANNER 394 / 2. PLUNGING IN WHERE ANGELS FEAR TO TREAD
395 / 3. USING A CONFRONTATIONAL TONE 396 / 4. CALLING THE PA-
TIENT'S BLUFF 396 / 5. OSCILLATING INTENSITY AND USING SILENCE
396 / 6. EXPRESSING OMNIPOTENCE AND IMPOTENCE 397

Concluding Comments / 397
Note / 398

13. **Case Management Strategies: Interacting**   **399**
with the Community
ENVIRONMENTAL INTERVENTION STRATEGIES / 401
Case Management and Observing Limits 401 / Conditions Mandating Environ-
mental Intervention 402 / 1. PROVIDING INFORMATION INDEPENDENT-
LY OF THE PATIENT 404 / 2. PATIENT ADVOCACY 404 / 3. ENTERING
THE PATIENT'S ENVIRONMENT TO GIVE HER ASSISTANCE 405
CONSULTATION-TO-THE-PATIENT STRATEGIES / 406
Rationale and Spirit of Consultation to the Patient 407 / The "Treatment Team"
versus "Everyone Else" 408 / 1. ORIENTING THE PATIENT AND THE NET-
WORK TO THE APPROACH 409 / 2. CONSULTATION TO THE PATIENT
ABOUT HOW TO MANAGE OTHER PROFESSIONALS 411 / 3. CONSUL-
TATION TO THE PATIENT ABOUT HOW TO HANDLE FAMILY AND
FRIENDS 419 / Arguments Against the Consultation Approach 421
THERAPIST SUPERVISION/CONSULTATION STRATEGIES / 423
The Need for Supervision/Consultation 424 / 1. MEETING TO CONFER ON
TREATMENT 426 / 2. KEEPING SUPERVISION/CONSULTATION AGREE-
MENTS 428 / 3. CHEERLEADING 429 / 4. PROVIDING DIALECTICAL
BALANCE 430 / Working Out Problems of "Staff Splitting" 431 / Dealing with
Unethical or Destructive Therapist Behavior 433 / Keeping Information Confiden-
tial 434
Concluding Comments / 434

PART IV. STRATEGIES FOR SPECIFIC TASKS

14. **Structural Strategies**   **437**
CONTRACTING STRATEGIES: STARTING TREATMENT / 438
1. CONDUCTING A DIAGNOSTIC ASSESSMENT 438 / 2. PRESENTING
THE BIOSOCIAL THEORY OF BORDERLINE BEHAVIOR 440 / 3. ORIENT-
ING THE PATIENT TO TREATMENT 442 / 4. ORIENTING THE NETWORK
TO TREATMENT 443 / 5. REVIEWING TREATMENT AGREEMENTS AND
LIMITS 444 / 6. COMMITTING TO THERAPY 444 / 7. CONDUCTING
ANALYSES OF MAJOR TARGET BEHAVIORS 446 / 8. BEGINNING TO DE-
VELOP THE THERAPEUTIC RELATIONSHIP 446 / Caveats in the Real World
447
SESSION-BEGINNING STRATEGIES / 448
1. GREETING THE PATIENT 449 / 2. RECOGNIZING THE PATIENT'S CUR-
RENT EMOTIONAL STATE 449 / 3. REPAIRING THE RELATIONSHIP 450
TARGETING STRATEGIES / 450
1. REVIEWING TARGET BEHAVIORS SINCE THE LAST SESSION 452 / 2.
USING TARGET PRIORITIES TO ORGANIZE SESSIONS 453 / 3. ATTEND-
ING TO STAGES OF THERAPY 453 / 4. CHECKING PROGRESS IN OTHER
MODES OF THERAPY 453
SESSION-ENDING STRATEGIES / 454
1. PROVIDING SUFFICIENT TIME FOR CLOSURE 454 / 2. AGREEING ON
HOMEWORK FOR THE COMING WEEK 454 / 3. SUMMARIZING THE
SESSION 455 / 4. GIVING THE PATIENT A TAPE OF THE SESSION 455
/ 5. CHEERLEADING 456 / 6. SOOTHING AND REASSURING THE PA-
TIENT 456 / 7. TROUBLESHOOTING 457 / 8. DEVELOPING ENDING
RITUALS 457
TERMINATING STRATEGIES / 457
1. BEGINNING DISCUSSION OF TERMINATING: TAPERING OFF SESSIONS
457 / 2. GENERALIZING INTERPERSONAL RELIANCE TO THE SOCIAL
NETWORK 458 / 3. ACTIVELY PLANNING FOR TERMINATION 459 / 4.
MAKING APPROPRIATE REFERRALS 460
Concluding Comments / 461

15. Special Treatment Strategies   462

CRISIS STRATEGIES / 462

1. PAYING ATTENTION TO AFFECT RATHER THAN CONTENT 463 / 2. EXPLORING THE PROBLEM NOW 463 / 3. FOCUSING ON PROBLEM SOLVING 465 / 4. FOCUSING ON AFFECT TOLERANCE 467 / 5. OBTAINING COMMITMENT TO A PLAN OF ACTION 468 / 6. ASSESSING SUICIDE POTENTIAL 468 / 7. ANTICIPATING A RECURRENCE OF THE CRISIS RESPONSE 468

SUICIDAL BEHAVIOR STRATEGIES / 468

The Therapeutic Task 469 / PREVIOUS SUICIDAL BEHAVIORS: PROTOCOL FOR THE PRIMARY THERAPIST 469 / THREATS OF IMMINENT SUICIDE OR PARASUICIDE: PROTOCOL FOR THE PRIMARY THERAPIST 476 / ONGOING PARASUICIDAL ACT: PROTOCOL FOR THE PRIMARY THERAPIST 490 / SUICIDAL BEHAVIORS: PROTOCOL FOR COLLATERAL THERAPISTS 492 / Principles of Risk Management with Suicidal Patients 493

THERAPY-INTERFERING BEHAVIOR STRATEGIES / 495

1. DEFINING THE INTERFERING BEHAVIOR 495 / 2. CONDUCTING A CHAIN ANALYSIS OF THE BEHAVIOR 495 / 3. ADOPTING A PROBLEM-SOLVING PLAN 496 / 4. RESPONDING TO THE PATIENT WHO REFUSES TO MODIFY INTERFERING BEHAVIOR 497

TELEPHONE STRATEGIES / 497

1. ACCEPTING PATIENT-INITIATED PHONE CALLS UNDER CERTAIN CONDITIONS 498 / 2. SCHEDULING PATIENT-INITIATED PHONE CALLS 502 / 3. INITIATING THERAPIST PHONE CONTACTS 502 / 4. GIVING FEEDBACK ABOUT PHONE CALL BEHAVIOR DURING SESSIONS 502 / Therapist Availability and Management of Suicidal Risk 503

ANCILLARY TREATMENT STRATEGIES / 504

1. RECOMMENDING ANCILLARY TREATMENT WHEN NEEDED 504 / 2. RECOMMENDING OUTSIDE CONSULTATION FOR THE PATIENT 505 / MEDICATION PROTOCOL 507 / HOSPITAL PROTOCOL 510

RELATIONSHIP STRATEGIES / 514

1. RELATIONSHIP ACCEPTANCE 515 / 2. RELATIONSHIP PROBLEM SOLVING 517 / 3. RELATIONSHIP GENERALIZATION 519

Concluding Comments / 519

Appendix 15.1 Scale Points for Lethality Assessment / 519

Note / 523

Appendix: Suggested Reading   524

References   527

Index   547

Theory and Concepts

1

Borderline Personality Disorder: Concepts, Controversies, and Definitions

In recent years, interest in borderline personality disorder (BPD) has exploded. This interest is related to at least two factors. First, individuals meeting criteria for BPD are flooding mental health centers and practitioners' offices. Eleven percent of all psychiatric outpatients and 19% of psychiatric inpatients are estimated to meet criteria for BPD; of patients[1] with some form of a personality disorder, 33% of outpatients and 63% of inpatients appear to meet BPD criteria (see Widiger & Frances, 1989, for a review). Second, available treatment modalities appear to be woefully inadequate. Follow-up studies suggest that the initial dysfunction of these patients may be extreme; that significant clinical improvement is slow, taking many years; and that improvement is marginal for many years after initial assessment (Carpenter, Gunderson, & Strauss, 1977; Pope, Jonas, Hudson, Cohen, & Gunderson, 1983; McGlashan, 1986a, 1986b, 1987). Borderline patients are so numerous that most practitioners must treat at least one. They present with severe problems and intense misery. They are difficult to treat successfully. It is no wonder that many mental health clinicians are feeling overwhelmed and inadequate, and are in search of a treatment that promises some relief.

Interestingly, the behavior pattern most frequently associated with the BPD diagnosis—a pattern of intentional self-damaging acts and suicide attempts—has been comparatively ignored as a target of treatment efforts. Gunderson (1984) has suggested that this behavior may come closest to representing the "behavioral specialty" of the borderline patient. The empirical data bear him out: From 70% to 75% of borderline patients have a history of a least one self-injurious act (Clarkin, Widiger, Frances, Hurt, & Gilmore, 1983; Cowdry, Pickar, & Davis; 1985). These acts can vary in in-

3

tensity from ones requiring no medical treatment (e.g., slight scratches, head banging, and cigarette burns) to ones requiring care on an intensive care unit (e.g., overdoses, self-stabbings, and asphyxiations). Nor is the suicidal behavior of borderline patients always nonfatal. Estimates of suicide rates among BPD patients vary, but tend to be about 9% (Stone, 1989; Paris, Brown, & Nowlis, 1987; Kroll, Carey, & Sines, 1985). In a series of BPD inpatients followed from 10 to 23 years after discharge (Stone, 1989), patients exhibiting all eight DSM-III criteria for BPD at the index admission had a suicide rate of 36%, compared to a rate of 7% for individuals who met five to seven criteria. In the same study, individuals with BPD and a history of previous parasuicide had suicide rates that were double the rates of individuals without previous parasuicide. Although there are substantial literatures both on suicidal and self-injurious behavior and on BPD, there is virtually no communication between the two areas of study.

Individuals who intentionally injure or try to kill themselves and the BPD population have a number of overlapping characteristics, which I describe later in this chapter. One overlap, however, is particularly noteworthy: Most individuals who engage in nonfatal self-injurious behavior and most individuals who meet criteria for BPD are women. Widiger and Frances (1989) reviewed 38 studies reporting the gender of patients meeting criteria for BPD; women comprised 74% of this population. Similarly, intentional self-injuries, including suicide attempts, are more frequent among women than among men (Bancroft & Marsack, 1977; Bogard, 1970; Greer, Gunn, & Kolller, 1966; Hankoff, 1979; Paerregaard, 1975; Shneidman, Faberow, & Litman, 1970). A further demographic parallel of note is the relationship of age both to BPD and to nonfatal self-injurious behaviors. Approximately 75% of instances of self-injurious behavior involve persons between the ages of 18 and 45 years (Greer & Lee, 1967; Paerregaard, 1975; Tuckman & Youngman, 1968). Borderline patients also tend to be younger (Akhtar, Byrne, & Doghramji, 1986), and BPD characteristics decrease in severity and prevalence into middle age (Paris et al, 1987). These demographic similarities, together with others discussed later, raise the interesting possibility that the research studies conducted on these two populations, although carried out separately, have in fact been studies of essentially overlapping populations. Unfortunately, most studies of suicidal behaviors do not report Axis II diagnoses.

The treatment described in this book is an integrative cognitive–behavioral treatment, dialectical behavior therapy (DBT), developed and evaluated with women who not only met criteria for BPD but also had histories of multiple nonfatal suicidal behaviors. The theory I have constructed may be valid, and the treatment program described in this book and the companion manual may be effective, for men as well as for nonsuicidal borderline patients. However, from the outset, it is important for the reader to realize that the empirical base demonstrating the effectiveness of the treatment program described here is limited to BPD women with a history of chronic parasuicidal behavior (intentional self-injury, including suicide attempts). (In keeping with this, I use the pronouns "she" and "her" throughout this book to refer to a typical patient.) This group is perhaps the most disturbed portion of the borderline population; certainly it constitutes the majority. The treatment is designed flexibly, such that as a patient progresses, changes are made in the treatment application. Thus, it is not unlikely that the treatment program would also be effective with less severely disturbed individuals. But at the moment such an extension would be based on speculation, not well-controlled empirical treatment studies.

The Concept of Borderline Personality Disorder

Definitions: Four Approaches

The formal concept of BPD is relatively new in the field of psychopathology. It did not appear in the *Diagnostic and Statistical Manual of Mental Disorders* (DSM) published by the American Psychiatric Association until the [*1980*] publication of DSM-III in 1980. Although the particular constellation of traits comprising the diagnostic entity was recognized much earlier, much of the current interest in this population has resulted from its recently gained official status. That status was not achieved without much controversy and dispute. The "official" nomenclature and diagnostic criteria have been arrived at both through political compromise and through attention to empirical data.

Perhaps most controversial was the decision to use the word "borderline" in the official designation of the disorder. The term itself has been popular for many years in the psychoanalytic community. It was first used by Adolf Stern in 1938 to describe a group of outpatients who did not profit from classical psychoanalysis and who did not seem to fit into the then-standard "neurotic" or "psychotic" psychiatric categories. Psychopathology at that time was conceptualized as occurring on a continuum from "normal" to "neurotic" to "psychotic." Stern labeled his group of outpatients as suffering from a "borderline group of neuroses." For many years thereafter, the term was used colloquially among psychoanalysts to describe patients who, although they had severe problems in functioning, did not fit into other diagnostic categories and were difficult to treat with conventional analytic methods. Different theorists have viewed borderline patients as being on the borderline between neurosis and psychosis (Stern, 1938; Schmideberg, 1947; Knight, 1954; Kernberg, 1975), schizophrenia and nonschizophrenia (Noble, 1951; Ekstein, 1955), and the normal and the abnormal (Rado, 1956). Table 1.1 provides a sampling of early definitions of the term. Over the years, the term "borderline" generally evolved in the psychoanalytic community to refer both to a particular structure of personality organization and to an intermediate level of severity of personality functioning. The term clearly conveys this latter notion.

TABLE 1.1. Borderline Conditions: Early Definitions and Interrelationships

Stern (1938)

1. Narcissism—Simultaneous idealization and contemptuous devaluation of the analyst, as well as of other important persons earlier in life.
2. Psychic bleeding—Paralysis in the face of crises; lethargy; tendency to give up.
3. Inordinate hypersensitivity—Overreaction to mild criticism or rejection, so gross that it suggests paranoia, but falling short of outright delusion.
4. Psychic and body rigidity—A state of tension and stiffness of posture readily apparent to a casual observer.
5. Negative therapeutic reaction—Certain interpretations by analyst, meant to be helpful, are experienced as discouraging or as manifestations of lack of love and appreciation. Depression or rage outbursts may ensue; at times, suicidal gestures.
6. Constitutional feeling of inferiority—Some exhibit melancholia, others an infantile personality.
7. Masochism, often accompanied by severe depression.
8. Organic insecurity—Apparently a constitutional incapacity to tolerate much stress, especially in the interpersonal field.
9. Projective mechanisms—A strong tendency to externalize, at times carrying patients close to delusory ideation.
10. Difficulties in reality testing—Faulty empathic machinery in relation to others. Impaired capacity to fuse partial object representations of another person into appropriate and realistic perceptions of the whole person.

Deutsch (1942)

1. Depersonalization that is not ego-alien or disturbing to the patient.
2. Narcissistic identifications with others, which are not assimilated into the self but repeatedly acted out.
3. A fully maintained grasp on reality.
4. Poverty of object relations, with a tendency to adopt the qualities of the other person as a means of retaining love.
5. A masking of all aggressive tendencies by passivity, lending an air of mild amiability, which is readily convertible to evil.
6. Inner emptiness, which the patient seeks to remedy by attaching himself or herself to one after the other social or religious group, no matter whether the tenets of this year's group agree with those of last year's or not.

Schmideberg (1947)

1. Unable to tolerate routine and regularity.
2. Tends to break many rules of social convention.
3. Often late for appointments and unreliable about payment.
4. Unable to reassociate during sessions.
5. Poorly motivated for treatment.
6. Fails to develop meaningful insight.
7. Leads a chaotic life in which something dreadful is always happening.
8. Engages in petty criminal acts, unless wealthy.
9. Cannot easily establish emotional contact.

Rado (1956) ("extractive disorder")

1. Impatience and intolerence of frustration.
2. Rage outbursts.
3. Irresponsibility.
4. Excitability.
5. Parasitism.
6. Hedonism
7. Depressive spells.
8. Affect hunger.

(cont)

TABLE 1.1 (*cont.*)

<hr>

Esser and Lesser (1965) ("hysteroid disorder")

1. Irresponsibility.
2. Erratic work history.
3. Chaotic and unfulfilling relationships that never become profound or lasting.
4. Early childhood history of emotional problems and disturbed habit patterns (enuresis at a late age, for example).
5. Chaotic sexuality, often with frigid and promiscuity combined.

Grinker, Werble, and Drye (1968)

Common characteristics of all borderlines:

1. Anger as main or only affect.
2. Defect in affectional (interpersonal) relations.
3. Absence of consistent self-identity.
4. Depression as characteristic of life.
    Subtype I: The psychotic border
      Behavior inappropriate, nonadaptive.
      Self-identity and reality sense deficient.
      Negative behavior and anger expressed.
      Depression.
    Subtype II: The core borderline syndrome
      Vacillating involvement with others.
      Anger acted out.
      Depression.
      Self-identity not consistent.
    Subtype III: The adaptive, affectless, defended, "as if"
      Behavior adaptive, appropriate.
      Complementary relationships.
      Little affect; spontaneity lacking.
      Defenses of withdrawal and intellectualization.
    Subtype IV: The border with the neuroses
      Anaclitic depression.
      Anxiety.
      Resemblance to neurotic, narcissistic character.

<hr>

Note. Adapted from *The Borderline Syndromes: Constitution, Personality, and Adaptation,* by M. H. Stone, 1980, New York: McGraw-Hill. Copyright © 1980 by McGraw-Hill. Adapted by permission.

Gunderson (1984) has summarized four relatively distinct clinical phenomena responsible for the continued psychoanalytic interest over the years in the borderline population. First, certain patients who apparently functioned well, especially on structured psychological tests, nonetheless were scored as demonstrating dysfunctional thinking styles ("primitive thinking" in psychoanalytic terms) on unstructured tests. Second, a sizeable group of individuals who initially appeared suitable for psychoanalysis tended to do very poorly in treatment and often required termination of the analysis and hospitalization.[3] Third, a group of patients were identified who, in contrast to most other patients, tended to deteriorate behaviorally within supportive, inpatient treatment programs. Finally, these individuals characteristically engendered intense anger and helplessness on the part of the treatment personnel dealing with them. Taken together, these four observations suggested the existence of a group of individuals who did not do well in traditional forms of treatment, despite positive prognostic indicators. The emotional state of both the patients and the therapists seemed to deteriorate when these individuals entered psychotherapy.

The heterogeneity of the population referred to as "borderline" has led to a number of other conceptual systems for organizing behavioral syndromes and etiological theories associated with the term. In contrast to the single continuum proposed in psychoanalytic thought, biologically oriented theorists have conceptualized BPD along several continua. From their viewpoint, the disorder represents a set of clinical syndromes, each with its own etiology, course, and outcome. Stone (1980, 1981) has reviewed this literature extensively and concludes that the disorder is related to several of the major Axis I disorders in terms of clinical characteristics, family history, treatment response, and biological markers. For example, he suggests three borderline subtypes: one related to schizophrenia, one related to affective disorder, and a third related to organic brain disorders. Each subtype occurs on a spectrum ranging from "unequivocal" or "core" cases of the subtype to milder, less easily identifiable forms. These latter cases are the ones to which the term "borderline" is applied (Stone, 1980). In recent years, the tendency in the theoretical and research literature has been toward conceiving of the borderline syndrome as located primarily on the affective disorders continuum (Gunderson & Elliott, 1985), although accumulating empirical data cast doubt on this position.

A third approach to understanding borderline phenomena has been labeled the "eclectic–descriptive" approach by Chatham (1985). This approach, embodied primarily at present in the forthcoming DSM-IV (American Psychiatric Association, 1991) and Gunderson's (1984) work, rests on a definitional use of borderline criteria sets. The defining characteristics have been derived largely by consensus, although empirical data are now being used to some extent to refine the definitions. For example, Gunderson's criteria (Gunderson & Kolb, 1978; Gunderson, Kolb, & Austin, 1981) were originally developed through a review of the literature and distillation of six features that most theorists described as characteristic of borderline patients. Zanarini, Gunderson, Frankenburg, and Chauncey (1989) have recently revised their BPD criteria to achieve better empirical discrimination between BPD and other Axis II diagnoses. However, even in this latest version, the methods of selecting new criteria are not made clear; they appear to be based on clinical criteria rather than empirical derivation. Similarly, the criteria for BPD listed in DSM-III, DSM-III-R, and the new DSM-IV were defined by consensus of committees formed by the American Psychiatric Association, and were based on the combined theoretical orientations of the committee members, data on how psychiatrists in practice use the term, and empirical data collected to date. The most recent criteria used to define BPD, the DSM-IV and Diagnostic

TABLE 1.2. Diagnostic Criteria for BPD

DSM-IV[a]

1. Frantic efforts to avoid real or imagined abandonment (do not include suicidal or self-mutilating behavior covered in criterion 5).

2. A pattern of unstable and intense interpersonal relationships characterized by alternating between extremes of idealization and devaluation.

3. Identity disturbance: persistent and markedly disturbed, distorted, or unstable self-image or sense of self (e.g., feeling like one does not exist or embodies evil).

4. Impulsiveness in at least two areas that are potentially self-damaging (e.g., spending, sex, substance abuse, shoplifting, reckless driving, binge eating—do not include suicide or self-mutilating behavior covered in criterion 5).

5. Recurrent suicidal threats, gestures, or behavior, or self-mutilating behavior.

6. Affective instability: marked reactivity of mood (e.g., intense episodic dysphoria, irritability, or anxiety) usually lasting a few hours and only rarely more than a few days.

7. Chronic feelings of emptiness.

8. Inappropriate, intense anger or lack of control of anger (e.g., frequent displays of temper, constant anger, recurrent physical fights).

9. Transient, stress-related severe dissociative symptoms or paranoid ideation.

Diagnostic Interview for Borderlines—Revised (DIB-R)[b]

Affect section
1. Chronic/major depression
2. Chronic helplessness/hopelessness/worthlessness/guilt
3. Chronic anger/frequent angry acts
4. Chronic anxiety
5. Chronic loneliness/boredom/emptiness

Cognition section
6. Odd thinking/unusual perceptual experiences
7. Nondelusional paranoid experiences
8. Quasi-psychotic experiences

Impulse Action Patterns section
9. Substance abuse/dependence
10. Sexual deviance
11. Self-mutilation
12. Manipulative suicide efforts
13. Other impulsive patterns

Interpersonal Relationships section
14. Intolerance of aloneness
15. Abandonment/engulfment/annihilation concerns
16. Counterdependency/serious conflict over help or care
17. Stormy relationships
18. Dependency/masochism
19. Devaluation/manipulation/sadism
20. Demandingness/entitlement
21. Treatment regressions
22. Countertransference problems/"special" treatment relationships

[a] From *DSM-IV Options Book: Work in Progress 9/1/91* by the Task Force on DSM-IV, American Psychiatric Association, 1991, Washington, DC. Copyright 1991 by the American Psychiatric Association. Reprinted by permission.
[b] From "The Revised Diagnostic Interview for Borderlines: Discriminating BPD from Other Axis II Disorders" by M. C. Zanarini, J. G. Gunderson, F. R. Frankenburg, and D. L. Chauncey, 1989, *Journal of Personality Disorders, 3*(1), 10–18. Copyright 1989 by Guilford Publications, Inc. Reprinted by permission.

Interview for Borderlines—Revised (DIB-R) criteria, are listed in Table 1.2.

A fourth approach to understanding borderline phenomena, based on a biosocial learning theory, has been proposed by Millon (1981, 1987a). Millon is one of the most articulate dissenters from the use of the term "borderline" to describe this personality disorder. Instead, Millon has suggested the term "cycloid personality" to highlight the behavioral and mood instability that he views as central to the disorder. From Millon's perspective, the borderline personality pattern results from a deterioration of previous, less severe personality patterns. Millon stresses the divergent background histories found among borderline individuals, and suggests that BPD can be reached via a number of pathways.

The theory I present in this book is based on a biosocial theory, and in many ways is similar to that of Millon. Both of us stress the reciprocal interaction of biological and social learning influences in the etiology of the disorder. In contrast to Millon, I have not developed an independent definition of BPD. I have, however, organized a number of behavioral patterns associated with a subset of borderline individuals—those with histories of multiple attempts to injure, mutilate, or kill themselves. These patterns are discussed in detail in Chapter 3; for illustrative purposes, they are outlined in Table 1.3.

TABLE 1.3. Behavioral Patterns in BPD

---

1. *Emotional vulnerability:* A pattern of pervasive difficulties in regulating negative emotions, including high sensitivity to negative emotional stimuli, high emotional intensity, and slow return to emotional baseline, as well as awareness and experience of emotional vulnerability. May include a tendency to blame the social environment for unrealistic expectations and demands.

2. *Self-invalidation:* Tendency to invalidate or fail to recognize one's own emotional responses, thoughts, beliefs, and behaviors. Unrealistically high standards and expectations for self. May include intense shame, self-hate, and self-directed anger.

3. *Unrelenting crises:* Pattern of frequent, stressful, negative environmental events, disruptions, and roadblocks—some caused by the individual's dysfunctional lifestyle, others by an inadequate social milieu, and many by fate or chance.

4. *Inhibited grieving:* Tendency to inhibit and overcontrol negative emotional responses, especially those associated with grief and loss, including sadness, anger, guilt, shame, anxiety, and panic.

5. *Active passivity:* Tendency to passive interpersonal problem-solving style, involving failure to engage actively in solving of own life problems, often together with active attempts to solicit problem solving from others in the environment; learned helplessness, hopelessness.

6. *Apparent competence:* Tendency for the individual to appear deceptively more competent than she actually is; usually due to failure of competencies to generalize across expected moods, situations, and time, and to failure to display adequate nonverbal cues of emotional distress.

In general, neither behavioral nor cognitive theorists have proposed definitional or diagnostic categories of dysfunctional behaviors comparable to the others described here. This is primarily a result of behaviorists' concerns about inferential theories of personality and personality organization as well as their preference for understanding and treating behavioral, cognitive, and affective phenomena associated with various disorders rather than "disorders" per se. Cognitive theorists, however, have developed etiological formulations of borderline behavioral patterns. These theorisits view BPD as a result of dysfunctional cognitive schemas developed early in life. Purely cognitive theories are, in many respects, similar to more cognitively oriented psychoanalytic theories. The various orientations to borderline phenomenology described here are outlined in Table 1.4.

Diagnostic Criteria: A Reorganization

The criteria for BPD, as currently defined, reflect a pattern of behavioral, emotional, and cognitive instability and dysregulation. These difficulties can be summarized in the five categories listed in Table 1.5. I have reorganized the usual criteria somewhat, but a comparison of the five categories I discuss below with the DSM-IV and DIB-R criteria in Table 1.2 shows that I have reorganized but not redefined the criteria.

First, borderline individuals generally experience emotional dysregulation. Emotional responses are highly reactive, and the individual generally has difficulties with episodic depression, anxiety, and irritability, as well as problems with anger and anger expression. Second, borderline individuals often experience interpersonal dysregulation. Their relationships may be chaotic, intense, and marked with difficulties. Despite these problems, borderline individuals often find it extremely hard to let go of relationships; instead, they may engage in intense and frantic efforts to keep significant individuals from leaving them. In my experience, borderline individuals, more so than most, seem to do well when in stable, positive relationships and to do poorly when not in such relationships.

Third, borderline individuals have patterns of behavioral dysregulation, as evidenced by extreme and problematic impulsive behaviors as well as suicidal behaviors. Attempts to injure, mutilate, or kill themselves are common in this population. Fourth, borderline individuals are at times cognitively dysregulated. Brief, nonpsychotic forms of thought dysregulation, including depersonalization, dissociation, and delusions, are at times brought on by stressful situations and usually clear up when the stress is ameliorated. Finally, dysregulation of the sense of self is common. It is not unusual for a borderline individual to report that she has no sense of a self at all, feels empty, and does not know who she is. In fact, one can consider BPD a pervasive disorder of both the regulation and experience of the self—a notion also proposed by Grotstein (1987).

This reorganization is supported by interesting data collected by Stephen

TABLE 1.4. Major Orientations to BPD

Dimensions	Psychoanalytic	Biological	Eclectic	Biosocial	Cognitive
1. Major theorists	Adler, Kernberg Masterson, Meissner, Rinsley	Akiskal, Adrulonis, Cowdry, Gardner, Hoch, Kasanin, D. Klein, Kety, Polatin, Soloff, Stone, Wender	Frances; Grinker; Gunderson; Spitzer's DSM-III, DSM-III-R, DSM-IV	Linehan, Millon, Turner	Beck, Pretzer, Young
2. What is meant by "borderline"	Psychostructural level or psycho-dynamic conflict	Mild varient of one of the major disorders	A specific personality disorder	A specific personality disorder	A specific personality disorder
3. Data on which diagnosis is based	Symptoms, inferred intrapsychic structures, transference	Clinical symptoms, familial–genetic history, treatment response, and biological markers	Combination of symptoms and behavioral observations, psycho-dynamics and psycho-logical test data (WAIS, Rorschach)	Behavioral observation, structured interviews, behaviorally anchored test data	Behavioral observation, structured interviews, behaviorally anchored test data
4. Etiology of disorder	Nurture, nature, fate[a]	Nature[b]	Unspecified	Nature, nurture	Nurture
5. Composition of borderline population	Homogeneous: intrapsychic structure Heterogeneous: descriptive symptoms	Heterogeneous: total sample Homogeneous: each subtype	Heterogeneous	Heterogeneous	Unspecified
6. Importance of diagnostic subtyping	Not important, except Meissner	Important	Somewhat important	Important	Unspecified
7. Basis on which subtyping made	–	Etiology	Grinker and Gunderson: clinical; DSM: clinical and etiological	Behavioral patterns	Unspecified
8. Recommended treatment	Modified psychoanalysis, confrontive psychotherapy	Chemotherapy	Unspecified	Modified behavior/cognitive–behavior therapy	Modified cognitive therapy

Note. Adapted from *Treatment of the Borderline Personality* by P. M. Chatham, 1985, New York: Jason Aronson. Copyright 1985 by Jason Aronson, Inc. Adapted by permission.
[a] Cognitive components can play a role, as can fate; most theorists except Kernberg consider nurture a major cause.
[b] Stone (1981) believes that 10–15% of all cases of BPD in adults are purely psychogenic in origin.

Hurt, John Clarkin, and their colleagues (Hurt et al., 1990; Clarkin, Hurt, & Hull, 1991; see Hurt, Clarkin, Munroe-Blum, & Marziali, 1992, for a review). Using hierarchical cluster analysis of the eight DSM-III criteria, they found three clusters of criteria: an Identity cluster (chronic feelings of emptiness or boredom, identity disturbance, intolerance of being alone); an Affective cluster (labile affect, unstable interpersonal relations, intense and inappropriate anger); and

TABLE 1.5. Comparison of BPD and Parasuicide Characteristics

BPD	Parasuicide
Emotional dysregulation	
1. Emotional instability	1. Chronic, aversive affect
2. Problems with anger	2. Anger, hostility, irritability
Interpersonal dysregulation	
3. Unstable relationships	3. Conflictual relationships
4. Efforts to avoid loss	4. Weak social support
	5. Interpersonal problems paramount
	6. Passive interpersonal problem solving
Behavioral dysregulation	
5. Suicide threats, parasuicide	7. Suicide threats, parasuicide
6. Self-damaging, impulsive behaviors, including alcohol and drug abuse	8. Alcohol, drug abuse, promiscuity
Cognitive dysregulation	
7. Cognitive disturbances	9. Cognitive rigidity, dichotomous thinking
Self dysfunction	
8. Unstable self, self-image	10. Low self-esteem
9. Chronic emptiness	

an Impulse cluster (self-damaging acts and impulsivity). Cognitive dysregulation did not show up in the results because the cluster analysis was based on DSM-III criteria, which did not include cognitive instability as a criterion for BPD.

There are a number of diagnostic instruments for BPD. The research tool that has been used most often is the original DIB, which was developed by Gunderson et al. (1981); it was recently revised by Zanarini et al. (1989), as noted earlier. The criteria most commonly used for clinical diagnosis are those listed in the various versions of the *Diagnostic and Statistical Manual,* most recently DSM-IV. As Table 1.2 has shown, there is a substantial overlap between the DIB-R and the DSM-IV. This should come as no surprise, since Gunderson both developed the original DIB and was chair of the Axis II work group for DSM-IV. There are also a number of self-report instruments that are suitable for screening patients (Millon, 1987b; see Reich, 1992, for a review).

The Concept of Parasuicidal Behaviors

Much controversy has surrounded the labeling of nonfatal self-harm. Disagreements generally revolve around the degree and kind of intent required (Linehan, 1986; Linehan & Shearin, 1988). In 1977, Kreitman introduced the term "parasuicide" as a label for (1) nonfatal, intentional self-injurious behavior resulting in actual tissue damage, illness, or risk of death; or (2) any ingestion of drugs or other substances not prescribed or in excess of prescription with clear intent to cause bodily harm or death. Parasuicide, as defined by Kreitman, includes both actual suicide attempts and self-injuries (including self-mutilation and self-inflicted burns) with little or no intent to cause death.[3] It does *not* include the taking of nonprescribed drugs to get high, to get a normal night of sleep, or to self-medicate. It is also distinguished from suicide, where intentional, self-inflicted death occurs: suicide threats, where the individual says she is going to kill or harm herself but has yet to act on the statement; almost suicidal behaviors, where the individual puts herself at risk but does not complete the act (e.g., dangling from a bridge or putting pills in her mouth but not swallowing them); and suicide ideation.

Parasuicide includes behaviors commonly labelled "suicide gestures" and "manipulative suicide attempts." The term "parasuicide" is preferred over other terms for two reasons. First, it does not confound a motivational hypothesis with a descriptive statement. Terms such as "gesture," "manipulative," and "suicide attempt" assume that the parasuicide is motivated by an attempt to communicate, to influence others covertly, or to try to commit suicide, respectively. There are other possible motivations for parasuicide, however, such as mood regulation (e.g., reduction of anxiety). In each case, careful assessment is needed—a necessity obscured by the use of descriptions assuming that such an assessment has already been conducted. Second, parasuicide is a less pejorative term. It is difficult to like a person who has been labeled a "manipulator." The difficulties in treating these individuals make it particularly easy to "blame the victims" and consequently to dislike them. Yet liking borderline patients is correlated with helping them (Woollcott, 1985). This is a particularly salient issue, and I discuss it further in a moment.

Research studies of parasuicide have typically employed a design in which individuals with a history of parasuicidal behaviors are compared to other individuals without such a history. Comparison groups might be other suicidal groups, such as suicide completers or ideators; other, nonsuicidal psychiatric patients; or nonpsychiatric control individuals. Although at times Axis I diagnoses are held constant, such a strategy is not the norm. Indeed, one of the goals of the research has been to determine which diagnostic categories are most frequently associated with the behavior. In only very recent data, and rarely at that, are Axis II diagnoses held constant or even reported. Nevertheless, in reviewing the parasuicide literature, one cannot help being struck by the similarities between the characteristics attributed to parasuicidal individuals and those attributed to borderline individuals.

The emotional picture of parasuicidal individuals is one of chronic, aversive emotional dysregulation. They appear to be more angry, hostile, and irritable (Crook, Raskin, & Davis, 1975; Nelson, Nielsen, & Checketts, 1977; Richman & Charles, 1976; Weissman, Fox, & Klerman, 1973) than nonsuicidal psychiatric and nonpsychiatric individuals and more depressed than both suicide completers (Maris, 1981) and other psychiatric and nonpsychiatric

groups (Weissman, 1974). Interpersonal dysregulation is evidenced by rela-
tionships that are characterized by hostility, demandingness, and conflict
(Weissman, 1974; Miller, Chiles, & Barnes, 1982; Greer et al., 1966; Adam,
Bouckoms, & Scarr, 1980; Taylor & Stansfeld, 1984). Relative to others, parasuicidal individuals have weak social support systems (Weissman, 1974; Slater
& Depue, 1981). When asked, they report interpersonal situations as their
chief problems in living (Linehan, Camper, Chiles, Strosahl, & Shearin, 1987;
Maris, 1981). Patterns of behavioral dysregulation, such as substance abuse,
sexual promiscuity, and previous parasuicidal acts are frequent (see Linehan,
1981, for a review; see also Maris, 1981). Generally, these individuals are unlikely to have the cognitive skills required to cope effectively with their emotional, interpersonal, and behavioral stresses.

Cognitive difficulties consist of cognitive rigidity (Levenson, 1972; Neuringer, 1964; Patsiokas, Clum, & Luscomb, 1979; Vinoda, 1966), dichotomous thinking (Neuringer, 1961), and poor abstract and interpersonal problem
solving (Goodstein, 1982; Levenson & Neuringer, 1971; Schotte & Clum,
1982). Impairments in problem solving may be related to deficits in specific
(as compared to general) episodic memory capabilities (Williams, 1991), which
have been found to characterize parasuicidal patients when compared to other
psychiatric patients. My colleagues and I have found that parasuicidal individuals exhibit a more passive (or dependent) interpersonal problem-solving style
(Linehan et al., 1987). In the face of their emotional and interpersonal difficulties, many of these individuals report that their behavior is designed to
provide an escape from what, to them, seems like an intolerable and unsolvable life. A comparison of borderline and parasuicidal individual characteristics is shown in Table 1.5.

The Overlap Between Borderline Personality Disorder and Parasuicidal Behavior

As I have noted earlier, much of my treatment research and clinical work has
been with the chronically parasuicidal individual who also meets criteria for
BPD. From my vantage point, these particular individuals meet the criteria
for BPD in a unique way. They seem more depressed than one might expect
from DSM-IV criteria. They also often exhibit overcontrol and inhibition of
anger, which are not discussed in either DSM-IV or the DIB-R. I do not view
these patients in the pejorative terms suggested by both DSM-IV and the DIB-
R. My clinical experience and reasoning on each of these issues are as follows.

Emotion Dysregulation: Depression

"Affective instability" in DSM-IV refers to marked reactivity of mood causing episodic depression, irritability, or anxiety, usually lasting a few hours
and only rarely more than a few days. The implication here is that the base-

line mood is not particularly negative or depressed. In my experience with parasuicidal borderline individuals, however, their baseline affective state is generally extremely negative, at least with respect to depression. For example, in a sample of 41 women at my clinic who met criteria for both BPD and recent parasuicidal behavior, 71% met criteria for major affective disorder and 24% met criteria for dysthymia. In our most recent treatment study (Linehan, Armstrong, Suarez, Allman, & Heard, 1991), my colleagues and I were amazed at the apparent stability over a 1-year period of self-reports of depression and hopelessness. Thus, the DIB-R with its emphasis on chronic depression, hopelessness, worthlessness, guilt, and helplessness, seems to characterize parasuicidal borderline individuals better than the DSM-IV does.

Emotion Dysregulation: Anger

Both the DSM-IV and the DIB-R emphasize problems with anger dyscontrol in borderline functioning. Frequent, intense anger and angry acts are included in both sets of criteria. Our clinic of parasuicidal borderline patients certainly includes a number of individuals who meet this requirement. However, it also includes a number of other individuals who are characterized by overcontrol of angry feelings. These individuals rarely if ever display anger; indeed, they display a pattern of passive and submissive behaviors when anger, or at least assertive behavior, would be appropriate. Both groups have trouble with anger expression, but one group overexpresses anger and one group underexpresses it. In the latter case, underexpression is at times related to a history of previous overexpression of anger. In almost all cases, the underexpressive borderline individuals have marked fear and anxiety about anger expression; at times they fear that they will lose control if they express even the slightest anger, and at other times they fear that targets of even minor anger expression will retaliate.

Manipulation and Other Pejorative Descriptors

Both the DIB-R and the DSM-IV stress so-called "manipulative" behavior as part of the borderline syndrome. Unfortunately, in neither set of criteria is it particularly clear how one would operationally define such behavior. The verb "manipulate" is defined as "to influence or manage shrewdly or deviously" in the *American Heritage Dictionary* (Morris, 1979, p. 794) and as "to manage or control artfully or by shrewd use of influence, often in an unfair or fraudulent way" by *Webster's New World Dictionary* (Guralnik, 1980, p. 863). Both definitions suggest that the manipulating individual intends to influence another person by indirect, insidious, or devious means.

Is this typical behavior of borderline individuals? In my own experience, it has not been. Indeed, when they are trying to influence someone, borderline individuals are typically direct, forceful, and, if anything, unartful. It is surely the case that borderline individuals do influence others. Often the most influential behavior is parasuicide or the threat of impending suicide; at other times, the behaviors that have the most influence are communications of intense pain and agony, or current crises that the individuals cannot solve themself. Such behaviors and communications, of course, are not by themselves evidence of manipulation. Otherwise, we would have to say that people in pain or crises are "manipulating" us if we respond to their communications of distress. The central question is whether or not borderline individuals purposely use these behaviors or communications to influence others artfully, shrewdly, and fraudulently. Such an interpretation is rarely in accord with borderline individuals' own self-perceptions of their intent. Since behavioral intent can only be measured by self-report, to maintain that the intent is present in spite of the individuals' denial would require us either to view borderline individuals as chronic liars or to construct a notion of unconscious behavioral intent.

It is difficult to answer contentions by some theorists that borderline individuals frequently lie. With one exception, that has not been my experience. The exception has to do with use of illicit and prescription drugs in an environment that is highly controlling of drugs, a topic that is discussed later in Chapter 15. My own experience in working with suicidal borderline patients has been that the frequent interpretation of their suicidal behavior as "manipulative" is a major source of their feelings of invalidation and of being misunderstood. From their own point of view, suicidal behavior is a reflection of serious and at times frantic suicide ideation and ambivalence over whether to continue life or not. Although the patients' communication of extreme ideas or enactment of extreme behaviors may be accompanied by the desire to be helped or rescued by the persons they are communicating with, this does not necessarily mean that they are acting in this manner in order to get help.

These individuals' numerous suicidal behaviors and suicide threats, extreme reactions to criticism and rejection, and frequent inability to articulate which of a number of factors are directly influencing their own behavior do at times make other people feel manipulated. However, inferring behavioral intent from one or more of the effects of the behavior—in this case, making others feel manipulated—is simply an error in logic. The fact that a behavior is influenced by its effects on the environment ("operant behavior," in behavioral terms) says little if anything about an individual's intent with respect to that behavior. Function does not prove intention. For example, a person may quite predictably threaten suicide whenever criticized. If the criticism then always turns to reassurance, we can be quite confident that the relationship between criticism and suicide threats will grow. However, the fact of the correlation in no way implies that the person is trying or intending to change the criticizer's behavior with threats, or is even aware of the correlation. Thus, the behavior is not manipulative in any standard use of the term. To say then that the "manipulation" is unconscious is a tautology based on clinical inference. Both the pejorative nature of such inferences and the low reliability of clinical inferences in general (see Mischel, 1968, for a review) make such a practice unwarranted in most cases.

There are a number of other uses of pejorative terminology in both the DIB-R and the DSM-IV. For example, one proposed criterion of unstable self-image for the DSM-IV included the following sentence: "Typically this involves the shift from being a needy supplicant for help to being a righteous and vengeful victim." Let us take first the term "righteous and vengeful victim." Use of such a term suggests that such a stance is somehow dysfunctional or pathological. However, the recent evidence that up to 76% of women meeting criteria for BPD are indeed victims of sexual abuse during childhood, together with the evidence for neglect and physical abuse suffered by these individuals (see Chapter 2 for reviews of these data), suggests that such a stance is isomorphic with reality.

Or let us examine the term "needy." It does not seem unreasonable for a person in intense pain to present as a "needy supplicant." Indeed, such a stance may be essential if the person is to get what is needed to ameliorate the current painful condition. This is especially the case when resources are scarce in general, or when the applicant for help does not have sufficient resources to "buy" the needed help—both of which are often true of borderline individuals. We in the mental health community have few resources to help them. What little help we can give them is limited by other obligations and demands on our time and lives as individual caregivers. Often, what borderline patients want the most—our time, attention, and care—are available only in brief, rationed hours of the week. Nor do borderline individuals have the interpersonal skills to find, develop, and maintain other interpersonal relationships where they might get more of what they need. To say that needing more than others can reasonably give is being too "needy" seems to cut too wide a swath. When burn or cancer patients in extreme pain act in a similar manner, we do not usually call them "needy supplicants." My guess is that if we withheld pain medicine from them, they would vacillate in exactly the same manner as borderline individuals.

The case can be made that in the minds of professional caregivers, these terms are not pejorative; indeed, that might be true. However, it seems to me that such pejorative terms do not themselves increase compassion, understanding, and a caring attitude for borderline patients. Instead, for many therapists such terms create emotional distance from and anger at borderline individuals. At other times, such terms reflect already rising emotional distance, anger, and frustration. One of the main goals of my theoretical endeavors has been to develop a theory of BPD that is both scientifically sound and nonjudgmental and nonpejorative in tone. The idea here is that such a theory should lead to effective treatment techniques as well as to a compassionate attitude. Such an attitude is needed, especially with this population: Our tools to help them are limited; their misery is intense and vocal; and the success or failure of our attempts to help can have extreme outcomes.

Therapy for Borderline Personality Disorder: A Preview

The treatment program I have developed—dialectical behavior therapy or DBT—is, for the most part, the application of a broad array of cognitive and behavior therapy strategies to the problems of BPD, including suicidal behaviors. The emphasis on assessment; data collection on current behaviors; precise operational definition of treatment targets; a collaborative working relationship between therapist and patient, including attention to orienting the patient to the therapy program and mutual commitment to treatment goals; and application of standard cognitive and behavior therapy techniques all suggest a standard cognitive–behavioral therapy program. The core treatment procedures of problem solving, exposure techniques, skill training, contingency management, and cognitive modification have been prominent in cognitive and behavior therapy for years. Each set of procedures has an enormous empirical and theoretical literature.

DBT also has a number of distinctive defining characteristics. As its name suggests, its overriding characteristic is an emphasis on "dialectics"—that is, the reconciliation of opposites in a continual process of synthesis. The most fundamental dialectic is the necessity of accepting patients just as they are within a context of trying to teach them to change. The tension between patients' alternating, excessively high and low aspirations and expectations relative to their own capabilities offers a formidable challenge to therapists; it requires moment-to-moment changes in the use of supportive acceptance versus confrontation and change strategies. This emphasis on acceptance as a balance to change flows directly from the integration of a perspective drawn from Eastern (Zen) practice with Western psychological practice. The term dialectics also suggests the necessity of dialectical thinking on the part of the therapist, as well as of targeting for change nondialectical, dichotomous, and rigid thinking on the part of the patient. Stylistically, DBT blends a matter-of-fact, somewhat irreverent, and at times outrageous attitude about current and previous parasuicidal and other dysfunctional behaviors with therapist warmth, flexibility, responsiveness to the patient, and strategic self-disclosure. The continuing efforts in DBT to "reframe" suicidal and other dysfunctional behaviors as part of the patient's learned problem-solving repertoire, and to focus therapy on active problem solving, are balanced by a corresponding emphasis on validating the patient's current emotional, cognitive, and behavioral responses just as they are. The problem-solving focus requires that the therapist address all problematic patient behaviors (in and out of sessions) and therapy situations in a systematic manner, including conducting a collaborative behavioral analysis, formulating hypotheses about possible variables influencing the problem, generating possible changes (behavioral solutions), and trying out and evaluating the solutions.

Emotion regulation, interpersonal effectiveness, distress tolerance, core mindfulness, and self-management skills are actively taught. In all modes of treatment, the application of these skills is encouraged and coached. The use of contingencies operating within the therapeutic environment requires the therapist to pay close attention to the reciprocal influence that each participant, therapist and patient, has on the other. Although natural contingencies are highlighted as a means of influencing patient behavior, the therapist is not prohibited from using arbitrary reinforcers as well as aversive contingencies when the behavior in question is lethal or the behavior required of the patient is not readily produced under ordinary therapeutic conditions. The tendency of borderline patients to actively avoid threatening situations is a continuing focus of DBT. Both in-session and *in vivo* exposure to fear-eliciting stimuli are arranged and encouraged. The emphasis on cognitive modification is less systematic than in pure cognitive therapy, but such modification in encouraged both in ongoing behavioral analysis and in the prompting of change.

The focus on validating requires that the DBT therapist search for the grain of wisdom or truth inherent in each of the patient's responses and communicate that wisdom to the patient. A belief in the patient's essential desire to grow and progress, as well as a belief in her inherent capability to change, underpins the treatment. Validation also involves frequent, sympathetic acknowledgment of the patient's sense of emotional desperation. Throughout treatment, the emphasis is on building and maintaining a positive, interpersonal, collaborative relationship between patient and therapist. A major characteristic of the therapeutic relationship is that the primary role of the therapist is as consultant to the patient, not as consultant to other individuals.

Differences Between This Approach and Standard Cognitive and Behavior Therapies

A number of aspects of DBT set it off from "usual" cognitive and behavior therapy: (1) the focus on acceptance and validation of behavior as it is in the moment; (2) the emphasis on treating therapy-interfering behaviors; (3) the emphasis on the therapeutic relationship as essential to the treatment; and (4) the focus on dialectical processes. First, DBT emphasizes acceptance of behavior and reality as it is more than do most cognitive and behavior therapies. To a great extent, in fact, standard cognitive–behavioral therapy can be thought of as a technology of change. It derives many of its techniques from the field of learning, which is the study of behavioral change through experience. In contrast, DBT emphasizes the importance of balancing change with acceptance. Although acceptance of patients as they are is crucial to any good therapy, DBT goes a step further than standard cognitive–behavioral therapy in emphasizing the necessity of teaching patients to accept themselves and their world as it is in the moment. Thus, a technology of acceptance is as important as the technology of change.

This emphasis in DBT on a balance of acceptance and change owes much to my experiences in studying meditation and Eastern spirituality. The DBT tenets of observing, mindfulness, and avoidance of judgment are all derived from the study and practice of Zen meditation. The behavioral treatment most similar to DBT in this respect is Hayes's (1987) contextual psychotherapy. Hayes is a radical behavior therapist who also emphasizes the necessity of behavioral acceptance. A number of other theorists are applying these principles to specific problem areas and have influenced the development of DBT. Marlatt and Gordon (1985), for example, teach mindfulness to alcoholics, and Jacobson (1991) has recently begun to systematically teach acceptance to distressed marital couples.

The emphasis in DBT on therapy-interfering behaviors is more similar to the psychodynamic emphasis on "transference" behaviors than it is to any aspect of standard cognitive–behavioral therapies. Generally, behavior therapists have given little empirical attention to the treatment of behaviors that interfere with the therapy. The exception here is the large literature on treatment compliance behaviors (e.g., Shelton & Levy, 1981). Other approaches to the problem have been generally handled under the rubric of "shaping," which has received a fair amount of attention in the treatment of children, chronic psychiatric inpatients, and the mentally retarded (see Masters, Burish, Hollon, & Rimm, 1987). This is not to say that the problem has been ignored completely. Chamberlain and her colleagues (Chamberlain, Patterson, Reid, Kavanagh, & Forgatch, 1984) have even developed a measure of treatment resistance for use with families undergoing her behavioral family interventions.

My emphasis on the therapeutic relationship as crucial to progress in DBT comes primarily from my work in interventions with suicidal individuals. At times, this relationship is the only thing that keeps them alive. Behavior therapists attend to the therapeutic relationship (see Linehan, 1988, for a review of this literature), but have not historically given it the prominence that I give it in DBT. Kohlenberg and Tsai (1991) have recently developed an integrated behavioral therapy in which the vehicle of change is the relationship between therapist and patient; their thinking has influenced the development of DBT. Cognitive therapists, while always noting its importance, have written little about how to achieve the collaborative relationship viewed as necessary to the therapy. An exception here is the recent book by Safran and Segal (1990).

Finally, the focus on dialectical processes (which I discuss in detail in Chapter 2) sets DBT off from standard cognitive–behavioral therapy, but not as much as it appears at first glance. Similar to behavior therapy, dialectics stresses process over structure. Recent advances in radical behaviorism and contextual theories and the approaches to behavior therapy they have generated (e.g., Hayes, 1987; Kohlenberg & Tsai, 1992; Jacobson, 1992) share many characteristics of dialectics. The newer information-processing approaches to cognitive therapy (e.g., Williams, in press) also emphasize process over structure. DBT, however, takes the application of dialectics substantially further than do many standard cognitive and behavior therapies. The force of the dialectical tone in determining therapeutic strategies at any given moment is substantial. The emphasis on dialectics in DBT is most similar to the therapeutic emphasis in Gestalt therapy, which also springs from a wholistic, systems theory and focuses on ideas such as synthesis. Interestingly, the newer cognitive therapy approaches to BPD developed by Beck and his colleagues (Beck, Freeman, & Associates, 1990; Young, 1988) explicitly incorporate Gestalt techniques.

Whether these differences are fundamentally important is, of course, an empirical question. Certainly, when all is said and done, the standard cognitive–behavioral components may be the ones most responsible for the effectiveness of DBT. Or, as cognitive and behavior therapies expand their scope, we may find that the differences between DBT and more standard applications are not as sharp as I suggest.

Is the Treatment Effective?: The Empirical Data

At this writing, DBT is one of the few psychosocial interventions for BPD that have controlled, empirical data supporting its actual effectiveness. Given the immense difficulties in treating these patients, the literature on how to treat them, and the widespread interest in the topic, this is rather surprising. I have been able to find only two other treatments that have been subjected to a controlled clinical trial. Marziali and Munroe-Blum (1987; Munroe-Blum & Marziali, 1987, 1989; Clarkin, Marziali, & Munroe-Blum, 1991) compared a psychodynamic group therapy for BPD (Relationship Management Psychotherapy, RMP) to individual-treatment-as-usual in the community. They found no differences in treatment outcome although RMP was somewhat more successful in keeping patients in therapy. Turner (1992) has recently completed a randomized controlled trial of a structured, multimodal treatment consisting of pharmacotherapy combined with an integrative dynamic/cognitive–behavioral treatment, quite similar to DBT. Preliminary results indicate promising outcomes, with gradual reductions reported in problematic cognitions and behaviors, anxiety, and depression.

Two clinical trials have been conducted on DBT. In both, chronically parasuicidal women meeting criteria for BPD were randomly assigned to DBT or to a community treatment-as-usual control condition. Therapists included myself as well as other psychologists, psychiatrists, and mental health professionals trained and supervised by me in DBT. The research treatment lasted for 1 year. Assessments were conducted every 4 months until posttreatment. Following treatment, two assessments were conducted at 6-month intervals.

Study 1

In the first study, 24 subjects were assigned to DBT and 23 were assigned to treatment-as-usual. Except when looking at treatment drop-out rates, only those DBT subjects who stayed in treatment for four or more sessions ($n =$

22) were included in analyses. One treatment-as-usual subject never came back for assessments. Results favoring DBT were found in each target area.

1. Compared to treatment-as-usual subjects, subjects assigned to DBT were significantly less likely to engage in parasuicide at all during the treatment year, reported fewer parasuicide episodes at each assessment point, and had less medically severe parasuicides over the year. These results obtained in spite of the fact that DBT was no better than treatment-as-usual at improving self-reports of hopelessness, suicide ideation, or reasons for living. Similar reductions in frequency of parasuicide episodes were found by Barley et al. (in press) when they instituted DBT on a psychiatric inpatient unit.

2. DBT was more effective than treatment-as-usual at limiting treatment dropout, the most serious therapy-interfering behavior. At one year, only 16.4% had dropped out, considerably fewer than the 50–55% who drop out of other treatments by that time (see Koenigsberg, Clarkin, Kernberg, Yeomans, & Gutfreund, in press).

3. Subjects assigned to DBT had a tendency to enter psychiatric units less often and had fewer inpatient psychiatric days per patient. Those in DBT had an average of 8.46 psychiatric inpatient days over the year compared to 38.86 for subjects assigned to treatment-as-usual.

In many clinical treatment studies, subjects who either attempt suicide or are hospitalized for psychiatric reasons are dropped from the clinical trial. Thus, I was particularly interested in looking at these two outcomes jointly. A system was developed to categorize psychological functioning on a continuum from poor to good as follows: Subjects who had no psychiatric hospitalization and no parasuicide episodes during the last four months of their treatment were labeled "good." Those with either a hospitalization or a parasuicide episode were labeled "moderate," and those with both a hospitalization and a parasuicide episode during the last four months of treatment, as well as the one subject who suicided, were labeled poor. Using this system, 13 DBT subjects had good outcomes, 6 had moderate outcomes, and 3 had poor outcomes. In the treatment-as-usual condition, there were 6 each with good and with poor outcomes and 10 with moderate outcomes. The difference in outcome was significant at the $p < .02$ level.

4. At termination of treatment, DBT subjects, compared to subjects in treatment-as-usual, were rated higher on global adjustment by an interviewer and rated themselves higher on a measure of general role (work, school, household) performance. These results, combined with DBT's success at reducing inpatient psychiatric days, suggest that DBT was somewhat effective at improving life interfering behaviors.

5. DBT's effectiveness at enhancing the behavioral skills targeted was mixed. With respect to emotion regulation, DBT subjects, more so than treatment-as-usual subjects, tended to rate themselves more successful in changing their emotions and improving general emotional control. They also had significantly lower scores on self-report measures of trait anger and

anxious rumination. However, there were no differences between groups in self-reported depression even though all subjects improved. With respect to interpersonal skills, subjects receiving DBT, compared to those receiving treatment-as-usual, rated themselves better on interpersonal effectiveness and interpersonal problem-solving, and were higher on both self-report and interviewer-rated measures of social adjustment. DBT was not more effective, relative to the treatment-as-usual condition, in raising subjects' ratings of their own success in accepting and tolerating both themselves and reality. However, the greater reduction in parasuicidal behavior, inpatient psychiatric days, and anger among DBT patients, in spite of no differential improvement in depression, hopelessness, suicide ideation, or reasons for living, suggests that distress tolerance, at least as manifested by behavioral and emotional responses, did improve among those receiving DBT.

Treatment superiority of DBT was maintained when DBT subjects were compared to only those treatment-as-usual subjects who received stable individual psychotherapy during the treatment year. This suggests that the effectiveness of DBT is not simply a result of providing individual, stable psychotherapy. These results are presented more fully elsewhere (Linehan et al., 1991; Linehan & Heard, 1993; Linehan, Tutek, & Heard, 1992).

We located 37 subjects for 18-month follow-up interviews and 35 for 24-month follow-ups. (Linehan, Heard, & Armstrong, in press). Many were unwilling to complete the entire assessment battery, but were willing to do an abbreviated interview covering essential outcome data. The superiority of DBT over treatment-as-usual achieved during the treatment year was generally maintained during the year following treatment. At each follow-up point, those receiving DBT were doing better than those in treatment-as-usual on measures of global adjustment, social adjustment, and work performance. In every area where DBT was superior to treatment-as-usual at posttreatment, there was maintenance of DBT gains during follow-up for at least 6 months. DBT superiority was stronger during the first 6 months of follow-up for measures of parasuicidal behavior and anger, and was stronger during the latter 6 months in reducing psychiatric inpatient days.

It is important to keep a number of things in mind when considering the research bases of DBT's effectiveness. First, although there were very significant gains over one year, most of which were maintained over a year of follow-up, our data do not support a claim that 1 year of treatment is sufficient for these patients. Our subjects were still scoring in the clinical range on almost all measures. Second, one study is a very slim basis for deciding that a treatment is effective. Although our outcomes have been replicated by Barley et al. (in press), much more research is needed. Third, there are few or no data to indicate that other treatments are *not* effective. With the two exceptions I noted above, no other treatments have ever been evaluated in a controlled clinical trial.

Study 2

In the second study (Linehan, Heard, & Armstrong, 1993), we addressed the following question: If a borderline patient is in individual, non-DBT psychotherapy, will treatment effectiveness be improved if DBT group skills training is added to the therapy? Eleven subjects were randomly assigned to DBT group skills training, and 8 were assigned to a no-skills-training control condition. All subjects were already receiving individual, continuing therapy in the community and were referred for group skills training by their individual therapists. Subjects were matched and randomly assigned to conditions. Other than their therapy status, there were no significant differences between subjects in this study and those in the first study described above. With the exception of the fact that we retained subjects in skills training reasonably well over the year (73%), the results suggested that DBT group skills training may have little if anything to recommend it as an additive treatment to ongoing individual (non-DBT) psychotherapy. At posttreatment, there were no significant between-group differences on any variable, nor did means suggest that the failure to find such differences was a result of the small sample size.

We next conducted a post hoc comparison of all Study 2 patients in stable individual psychotherapy ($n=18$) with Study 1 patients who were stable in standard DBT ($n=21$). This allowed us to compare DBT to other individual psychotherapy where the therapist was as committed to the patient as in DBT. The Study 1 patients getting standard DBT did better in all target areas. Patients in stable individual treatment-as-usual, whether or not they received DBT group skills training, did not do any better (or worse) than the 22 subjects in Study 1 who were assigned to treatment-as-usual. What can we conclude from these findings? First, the second study strengthens the findings of the first study: Standard DBT (that is, the psychotherapy plus skills training) is more effective than general treatment-as-usual. We cannot conclude, however, that DBT group skills training is ineffective or unimportant when offered within the standard DBT format. Nor is it clear whether DBT skills training would be effective if offered alone, without concomitant non-DBT individual psychotherapy. In standard DBT, the skills training is integrated within individual DBT. The individual therapy provides an enormous amount of skills coaching, feedback, and reinforcement. This integration of both types of treatment, including the individual help in applying new behavioral skills, may be critical to the success of standard DBT. Furthermore, combining non-DBT individual therapy with DBT skills training might create a conflict for the patient that adversely affects outcome. We are currently studying these issues.

Concluding Comments

Although there is a fair amount of research on BPD, there is still some controversy about whether the diagnostic entity is useful and valid. The prejudice against individuals labeled as "borderline" has led many to protest the diagnostic label. The term has been associated with so much blaming of the victims that some believe it should be discarded altogether. Some, pointing to the relationship between the diagnoses and childhood sexual abuse (see Chapter 2 for a review of this literature), believe that these individuals should carry a diagnosis that highlights this association, such as "posttraumatic syndrome." The idea seems to be that if a label suggests that problem behavior is a result of abuse (rather than a fault of the individual), prejudice will be reduced.

Although I am no fan of the term "borderline," I do not believe that we will reduce prejudice against these difficult-to-treat individuals by changing labels. Instead, I believe that the solution has to be the development of a theory that is based on sound scientific principles, highlighting the basis of the disordered "borderline" behaviors in "normal" responses to dysfunctional biological, psychological, and environmental events. It is by making these individuals different in principle from ourselves that we can demean them. And perhaps, at times, we demean them to make them different. Once we see, however, that the principles of behavior influencing normal behavior (including our own) are the same principles influencing borderline behavior, we will more easily empathize and respond compassionately to the difficulties they present us with. The theoretical position described in the next two chapters attempts to meet this need.

NOTES

1 Psychotherapists usually use either the word "patient" or the word "client" to refer to an individual receiving psychotherapy. In this book, I use the term "patient" consistently; in the companion skills training manual, I use the term "client." A reasonable case can be made for using either term. The case for using the term "patient" can be found in the first definition of the term (as a noun) given by the *Original Oxford English Dictionary on Compact Disc* (1987): "A sufferer; one who suffers patiently." Although now rare, the definition nonetheless fits perfectly the borderline individuals I see for psychotherapy. The more common meanings of the term— "One who is under medical treatment for the cure of some disease or wound," or "A person or thing that undergoes some action, or to whom or which something is done" — are less applicable, since DBT is not based solely on a disease model, nor does it view the patient as passive or one to whom things are done.

2. It is interesting to note that within both the psychoanalytic and the cognitive–behavioral communities, attention to BPD started during the third decade of the therapeutic discipline, and for the very same reasons. Treatment techniques that are otherwise very effective are less effective when the patient meets criteria for BPD.

3. Diekstra has been developing a new set of definitions of nonfatal suicidal behaviors for inclusion in the 10th revision of the *International Classification of Diseases* (Diekstra, 1988, cited in Van Egmond & Diekstra, 1989). In this new system, attempted suicide is distinguished from parasuicide. The definitions are as follows:

Attempted suicide:
  (a) A non-habitual act with non-fatal outcome;
  (b) that is deliberately initiated and performed by the individual involved;
  (c) that causes self-harm or without intervention by others will do so or consists of ingesting a substance in excess of its generally recognized therapeutic dosage.

Parasuicide:
  (a) A non-habitual act with non-fatal outcome;
  (b) that is deliberately initiated and performed by the individual involved in expectation of such an outcome;
  (c) that causes self-harm or without intervention from others will do so or consists of ingesting a substance in excess of its generally recognized therapeutic dosage;
  (d) the outcome being considered by the actor as instrumental in bringing about desired changes in consciousness and/or social condition" (Van Egmond & Diekstra, 1989, p. 53–54).

2

Dialectical and Biosocial Underpinnings of Treatment

Dialectics

Every theory of personality functioning and of its disorders is based on some fundamental world view. Often this world view is left unspoken, and one has to read between the lines to figure it out. For example, Rogers's client-centered theory and therapy are based on the assumptions that people are fundamentally good and that they have an innate drive toward self-actualization. Freud assumed that individuals seek pleasure and avoid pain. He further assumed that all behavior is psychologically determined, and that there is no accidental behavior (behavior determined by accidental events of one's environment).

Similarly, DBT is based on a specific world view, that of dialectics. In this section, I provide an overview of what I mean by "dialectics." I hope to show you that understanding this point of view is important and can enhance the ways of thinking about and interacting with borderline patients. I am not going to give a philosophical lecture on the meaning and history of the term, nor an in-depth coverage of current philosophical thinking in this area. Suffice it to say that dialectics is alive and well. Most people are aware of dialectics through the socioeconomic theory of Marx and Engels (1970). As a world view, however, dialectics also figures in theories of the development of science (Kuhn, 1970), biological evolution (Levins & Lewontin, 1985), sexual relations (Firestone, 1970), and more recently the development of thinking in adults (Basseches, 1984). Wells (1972, cited in Kegan, 1982) has documented a shift toward dialectical approaches in almost every social and natural science during the last 150 years.

Why Dialectics?

The application of dialectics to my treatment approach began in the early 1980s with a series of therapy observations and discussions by my clinical research team. The team observed me in weekly therapy sessions while I attempted to apply to parasuicidal patients the cognitive–behavioral therapy I had learned at the State University of New York at Stony Brook under Gerald Davison and Marvin Goldfried. After each session, we would discuss both my behavior and that of the patient. At that time, the aims were to identify helpful techniques or, at a minimum, those that did not hamper therapeutic change and a positive working relationship. I was then to try to apply them in a consistent manner in future sessions. Subsequent discussions were aimed at keeping what was useful, discarding what was not, and developing behaviorally anchored descriptions of what exactly I as the therapist was doing.

A number of things happened during the course of treatment development. First, we verified that I could apply cognitive–behavioral therapy with this population; that was reassuring, since that was the primary intent of the project. However, as we observed what I was doing, it seemed that I was also applying a number of other procedures not traditionally associated with cognitive or behavior therapy. These techniques were things such as matter-of-fact exaggerations of the implications of events, similar to Whitaker's (1975, pp. 12–13); encouraging the acceptance rather than change of feelings and situations, in the tradition of Zen Buddhism (e.g., Watts, 1961); and double-bind statements such as those of the Bateson project directed at pathological behavior (Watzlawick, 1978). These techniques are more closely aligned with paradoxical therapy approaches than with standard cognitive and behavioral therapy. In addition, the pace of therapy seemed to include rapid changes in verbal style between, on the one hand, warm acceptance and empathetic reflection reminiscent of client-centered therapy, and, on the other hand, blunt, irreverent, confrontational comments. Movement and timing seemed as important as context and technique.

Although a colleague and I subsequently developed the relationship between DBT and paradoxical treatment strategies (Shearin & Linehan, 1989), when I was originally explicating the treatment I was reluctant to identify the approach with paradoxical procedures, because I was afraid that inexperienced therapists might overgeneralize from the "paradoxical" label and prescribe suicidal behavior itself; this was and is explicitly not done in the therapy. But I needed a label for the therapy. Clearly, it was not only standard cognitive–behavioral therapy. The emphasis at that time in cognitive therapy on rationality as the criterion of healthy thought seemed incompatible with my attention to intuitive and nonrational thought as equally advantageous. I was also becoming convinced that the problems of these patients did not result primarily from cognitive distortions of themselves and their environment, even though distortions seemed to play an important role in maintaining problems once they began. My focus in much of treatment on accepting painful emotional states and problematic environmental events seemed different from the usual cognitive–behavioral approach of trying to change or modify painful emotional states or act on environments to change them.

I began to think of "dialectical" as a descriptor of the therapy because of my intuitive experience in conducting therapy with this population of severely disturbed, chronically suicidal patients. The experience can best be described in terms of an image. It is as if the patient and I are on opposite ends of a teeter-totter; we are connected to each other by the board of the teeter-totter. Therapy is the process of going up and down, each of us sliding back and forth on the teeter-totter, trying to balance it so that we can get to the middle together and climb up to a higher level, so to speak. This higher level, representing growth and development, can be thought of as a synthesis of the preceding level. Then the process begins again. We are on a new teeter-totter trying to get to the middle in an effort to move to the next level, and so on. In the process, as the patient is continually moving back and forth on the teeter-totter, from the end toward the middle and from the middle back toward the end, I move also, trying to maintain a balance.

The difficulty in treating a suicidal borderline patient is that instead of on a teeter-totter, we are actually balanced on a bamboo pole perched precariously on a high wire stretched over the Grand Canyon. Thus, when the patient moves backward on the pole, if I move backward to gain balance, and then the patient moves backward again to regain balance, and so forth, we are in danger of falling into the canyon. (The pole is not infinitely long.) Thus, it seems that my task as the therapist is not only to maintain the balance, but to maintain it in such a way that both of us move to the middle rather than back off the ends of the pole. Very rapid movement and countermovement of the therapist seem to constitute a central part of the treatment.

The tensions that I experienced during therapy; the need to move to balance or synthesis with this patient population; and the treatment strategies reminiscent of paradoxical techniques that seemed a necessary adjunct to standard behavioral techniques — all these led me to the study of dialectical philosophy as a possible organizing theory or point of view.[1] Dialectically speaking, the ends of the teeter-totter represent the opposites ("thesis" and "antithesis"); moving to the middle and up to the next level of the teeter-totter represents the integration or "synthesis" of these opposites, which immediately dissolves into opposites once again. This psychotherapeutic relationship between the opposites embodied in the term "dialectics" has been regularly pointed out since the early writings of Freud (Seltzer, 1986).

However serendipitous the original choice of a label was, the movement to a dialectical view subsequently guided the therapy development in a much broader fashion than would have been possible with just a paradoxical twist to techniques. Consequently, the treatment has evolved into its form of the past few years as an interaction between therapy process and dialectical theory. Over time, the term "dialectics" as applied to behavior therapy has come to imply two contexts of usage: that of the fundamental nature of reality and that of persuasive dialogue and relationship. As a world view or philosophical position, dialectics forms the basis of the therapeutic approach presented in this book. Alternatively, as a form of dialogue and relationship, dialectics refers to the treatment approach or strategies used by the therapist to effect change. Thus, central to DBT are a number of therapeutic dialectical strategies; these are described in Chapter 8.

Dialectical World View

A dialectical perspective on the nature of reality and human behavior has three primary characteristics.

The Principle of Interrelatedness and Wholeness

First, dialectics stresses interrelatedness and wholeness. Dialectics assumes a systems perspective on reality. The analysis of parts of a system is of limited value unless the analysis clearly relates the part to the whole. Thus. identity itself is relational, and boundaries between parts are temporary and exist only in relation to the whole; indeed, it is the whole that determines the boundaries. Levins and Lewontin (1985) state this well:

> Parts and wholes evolve in consequence of their relationship, and the relationship itself evolves. These are the properties of things that we call dialectical: that one thing cannot exist without the other, that one acquires its properties from its relation to the other, that the properties of both evolve as a consequence of their interpretation. (p. 3)

This holistic view is compatible with both feminist and contextual views of psychopathology. Such a perspective, when applied to treatment of BPD made me question the importance given to separation, differentiation, individuation, and independence in Western cultural thought. Notions of the individual as unitary and separate have only gradually emerged over the last several hundred years (Baumeister, 1987; Sampson, 1988). Since women receive the diagnosis of BPD much more frequently than men, the influence of gender on notions of self and appropriate interpersonal boundaries is of particular interest in our thinking about the disorder.

Both gender and social class significantly influence how one defines and experiences the self. Women, as well as other individuals with less social power, are more likely to have a relational or social self (a self that includes the group) as opposed to an individuated self (one that excludes the group) (McGuire & McGuire, 1982; Pratt, Pancer, Hunsberger, & Manchester, 1990). The importance of a relational or social self among women has been highlighted by many feminist writers, the best-known of whom is Gilligan (1982). Lykes (1985) has perhaps argued the feminist position most cogently in defining "the self as an ensemble of social relations" (p. 364). It is very important to note that Lykes and others do not speak simply of the value of interdependence among autonomous selves. Rather, they describe a social or relational self that is itself "a coacting network of relationships embedded in an intricate system of social exchanges and obligations" (Lykes, 1985, p. 362). When the self is defined as "in relation," inclusive of others in its very definition, no fully separate self exists—that is, no self separated from the whole. Such a relational self, or "ensembled individualism" in Sampson's terms, characterizes the majority of societies, both historically and cross-culturally (Sampson, 1988).

Attention to these contextual factors is particularly essential when a cultural construct such as "self" is employed to explain and describe another cultural construct such as "mental health." While the traditional definition of self may generally prove adaptive for some individuals in Western society, one must consider that our definitions and theories are not universal but are products of Western society, and thus may prove inappropriate for many individuals. As Heidi Heard and I have argued elsewhere (Heard & Linehan, 1993), and as I discuss later in this chapter and in Chapter 3, the problems encountered by the borderline individual may result in part from the collision of a relational self with a society that recognizes and rewards only the individuated self.

The Principle of Polarity

Second, reality is not static, but is comprised of internal opposing forces ("thesis" and "antithesis"), out of whose integration ("synthesis") evolves a new set of opposing forces. Although dialectics focuses on the whole, it also emphasizes the complexity of any whole. Thus, within each one thing or system, no matter how small, there is polarity. In physics, for example, no matter how hard physicists try to find the single particle or element that is the basis of all existence, they always end up with an element that can be further reduced. In the single atom there is a negative and a positive charge; for each force, there is a counterforce; even the smallest element of matter is balanced by anti-matter.

A very important dialectical idea is that all propositions contain within them their own oppositions. Or, as Goldberg (1980) put it,

> I assume that truth is paradoxical, that each article of wisdom contains within it its own contradictions, that truths stand side by side. Contradictory truths do not necessarily cancel each other out or dominate each other, but stand side by side, inviting participation and experimentation. (pp. 295–296)

If you take this idea seriously, it can have a rather profound impact on your clinical practice. For example, in most descriptions of BPD, the emphasis is on identifying the pathology that sets the individual apart from others. Treatment is then designed to ferret out the pathology and create conditions for change. A dialectical perspective, however, suggests that within dysfunction there is also function; that within distortion there is accuracy; and that within destruction one can find construction. It was turning this idea around—"contradictions within wisdom" to "wisdom within contradictions"—that led me to a number of decisions about the form of DBT. Instead of searching for the validity of the patient's current behavior in the learning of the past, I began to search for and find it in the current moment. Thus, the idea took me a step beyond simply empathizing with the patient. Validation is now a crucial part of DBT.

The same idea led me to the construct of "wise mind," which is a focus on the inherent wisdom of patients. DBT assumes that each individual is capable of wisdom with respect to her own life, although this capability is not always obvious or even accessible. Thus, the DBT therapist trusts that the patient has within herself all of the potential that is necessary for change. The essential elements for growth are already present in the current situation. The acorn is the tree. Within the DBT case consultation team, the idea led to the emphases on finding the value in each person's point of view, rather than defending the value of one's own position.

Thesis, Antithesis, Synthesis: The Principle of Continuous Change

Finally, the interconnected, oppositional, and nonreducible nature of reality leads to a wholeness continually in the process of change. It is the tension between the thesis and antithesis forces within each system (positive and negative, good and bad, children and parents, patient and therapist, person and environment, etc.) that produces change. The new state following change (the synthesis), however, is also comprised of polar forces; and, thus, change is continuous. The principle of dialectical change is important to keep in mind, even though I use these terms ("thesis," "antithesis," "synthesis") rarely.

Change, then (or "process," if you will), rather than structure or content, is the essential nature of life. Robert Kegan (1982) captures this point of view in his description of the evolution of self as a process of transformations over one's lifespan, generated by tensions between self-preservation and self-transformation within the person and within the person-environment system punctuated by temporary truces or developmental balances. He writes:

> As it is to understand the way the person creates the world, we must also understand the way the world creates the person. In considering where a person is in his or her evolutionary balancing we are looking not only at how meaning is made; we are looking too, at the possibility of the person losing this balance. We are looking, in each balance, at a new sense of what is ultimate and what is ultimately at stake. We are looking, in each new balance, at a new vulnerability. Each balance suggests how the person is composed, but each suggests, too, a new way for the person to lose her composure. (p. 114)

A dialectical point of view is quite compatible with psychodynamic theory, which stresses the inherent role of conflict and opposition in the process of growth and change. It is also compatible with a behavioral perspective which stresses the inherent wholeness of the environment and individual, and the interrelatedness of each in producing change. Dialectics as a theory of change is somewhat different from the self-actualizing notion of development assumed by client-centered therapy. In that perspective, each thing has within it a potentiality that will unfold naturally throughout its lifetime. "Unfolding" does not imply the tension inherent in dialectical growth. It is this tension that produces gradual change, punctuated by spurts of sudden shifts and dramatic movement.

In DBT, the therapist channels change in the patient, while at the same time recognizing that the change engendered is also transforming the therapy and the therapist. Thus, there is an ever-present dialectical tension within therapy itself between the process of change and the outcome of change. At each moment, there is a temporary balance between the patient's attempts to maintain herself as she is without changing, and her attempts to change herself regardless of the constraints of her history and current situation. The transition to each new temporary stability is often experienced as a painful crisis. "Any real resolution of the crisis must ultimately involve a new way of being in the world. Yet the resistance to doing so is great, and will not occur in the absence of repeated and varied encounters in natural experience" (Kegan, 1982, p. 41). The therapist helps the patient resolve crises by supporting simultaneously her attempts at self-preservation and at self-transformation. Control and direction channel the patient toward increased self-control and self-direction. Nurturing stands side by side with teaching the patient to care for herself.

Dialectical Persuasion

From the point of view of dialogue and relationship, "dialectics" refers to change by persuasion and by making use of the oppositions inherent in the therapeutic relationship, rather than by formal impersonal logic. Thus, unlike analytical thinking, dialectics is personal, taking into account and affecting the total person. It is an approach to engaging a person in dialogue so that movement can be made. Through the therapeutic opposition of contradictory positions, both patient and therapist can arrive at new meanings within old meanings, moving closer to the essence of the subject under consideration.

As noted above, the synthesis in a dialectic contains elements of both the thesis and antithesis, so that neither of the original positions can be regarded as "absolutely true." The synthesis, however, always suggests a new antithesis and thus acts as a new thesis. Truth, therefore, is neither absolute nor relative; rather, it evolves, develops, and is constructed over time. From the dialectical perspective, nothing is self-evident, and nothing stands apart from anything else as unrelated knowledge. The spirit of a dialectical point of view is never to accept a final truth or an undisputable fact. Thus, the question addressed by both patient and therapist is "What is being left out of our understanding?"

I do not mean to imply that a sentence such as "It is raining and it is not raining" embodies a dialectic. Nor am I suggesting that a statement cannot be wrong, or not factual in a particular context. False dichotomies and false dialectics can occur. However, in these cases the thesis and/or antithesis has been misidentified, and thus one does not have a genuine antagonism. For example, a common statement during the Vietnam War, "Love it or leave it," was a classic case of a misidentification of the dialectic.

As I discuss in Chapters 4 and 13, dialectical dialogue is also very important in therapy team meetings. Perhaps more than any other factor, attention to dialectics can reduce the chances of staff splitting in treating borderline patients. Splitting among staff members almost always results from a conclusion by one or more factions within the staff that they (and sometimes they alone) have a "lock" on the truth about a particular patient or clinical problem.

Borderline Personality Disorder as Dialectical Failure

In some ways, borderline behaviors can be viewed as results of dialectical failures.

Borderline "Splitting"

As discussed in Chapter 1, borderline and suicidal individuals frequently vacillate between rigidly held yet contradictory points of view, and are unable to move forward to a synthesis of the two positions. They tend to see reality in polarized categories of "either–or," rather than "all," and within a very fixed frame of reference. For example, it is not uncommon for a such individuals to believe that the smallest fault makes it impossible for a person to be "good" inside. Their rigid cognitive style further limits their ability to entertain ideas of future change and transition, resulting in feelings of being in an interminable painful situation. Things once defined do not change. Once a person is "flawed," for instance, that person will remain flawed forever.

Such thinking among borderline individuals has been labeled "splitting" by psychoanalysts, and it forms an important part of psychoanalytic theory on BPD (Kernberg, 1984). Dichotomous thinking or splitting can be viewed as the tendency to get stuck in either the thesis or the antithesis, unable to move toward synthesis. An inability to believe that both a proposition (e.g., "I want to live") and its opposite ("I want to die") can be simultaneously true characterizes the suicidal and borderline individual. Splitting, from a psychodynamic point of view, is a product of the irresolvable conflict between intense negative and positive emotions.

From the dialectical perspective, however, conflict that is maintained is a dialectical failure. Instead of synthesis and transcendence, in the conflict typical of borderline individuals there is opposition between firmly rooted but contradictory positions, wishes, points of view, and so on. The resolution of conflict requires first the recognition of the polarities and then the ability to rise above them, so to speak, seeing the apparently paradoxical reality of both and neither. At the level of synthesis and integration that occurs when polarity is transcended, the seeming paradox resolves itself.

Difficulties with Self and Identity

Borderline individuals are frequently confused about their own identity, and tend to scan the environment for guidelines on how to be and what to think and feel. Such confusion can arise from a failure to experience their essential relatedness with other people, as well as the relationship of this moment to other moments in time. They are forever on the edge of the abyss, so to speak. Without these relational experiences, identity becomes defined in terms of each current moment and interaction experienced in isolation, and thus is variable and unpredictable rather than stable. In addition, there is no other moment in time to modulate the impact of the current moment. For a borderline patient, another person's anger at her in a particular interaction is not buffered by either other relationships where people are not angry or other points in time when this person is not angry at her. "You are angry at me" becomes infinite reality. The part becomes the whole. A number of other theorists have pointed out the important role of memory for affective events (Lumsden, 1991), especially interpersonal events (Adler, 1985), in the development and maintenance of BPD. Mark Williams (1991) has made a similar argument with respect to failures in autobiographical memory. Clearly, prior events and relationships must be available to memory if they are to buffer and be integrated within the present.

Interpersonal Isolation and Alienation

The dialectical perspective on unity presupposes that individuals are not separate from their environment. Isolation, alienation, feelings of being out of contact or not fitting in—all characteristic feelings of borderline individuals—are dialectical failures coming from the individuals setting up of a self-other opposition. Such an opposition can occur even in the absence of an adequate sense of self-identity. Often among borderline individuals, a sense of unity and integration is sought by suppression and/or nondevelopment of self-identity (beliefs, likes, desires, attitudes, independent skills, etc.), rather than by the dialectical strategy of synthesis and transcendence. The paradox that one can be different but at the same time part of the whole is not grasped. The opposition between person (part) and environment (whole) is maintained.

Case Conceptualization:
A Dialectical Cognitive–Behavioral Approach

Case conceptualization in DBT is guided both by dialectics and by the assumptions of cognitive–behavioral theory. In this section, I review several characteristics of cognitive–behavioral theory that are important to DBT; I also suggest how a dialectical cognitive–behavioral approach differs somewhat from more traditional cognitive, behavioral, and biological theories. More specific theoretical points are reviewed as they relate to the specific DBT intervention strategies.

The Definition of "Behavior"

"Behavior," as used by cognitive–behavioral therapists, is a very broad term. It includes any activity, functioning, or reaction of the person—that is, "anything that an organism does involving action and response to stimulation" (*Merriam–Webster Dictionary,* 1977, p. 100). Physicists are using the term similarly when they speak of the behavior of a molecule; likewise systems analysts speak of the behavior of a system. Human behavior can be overt, (i.e., public and observable to others) or covert (i.e., private and observable only to the person behaving). In turn, covert behaviors may occur inside the person's body (e.g., stomach muscles tightening) or outside the body but nonetheless private, (e.g., behavior when a person is alone).[2]

The Three Modes of Behavior

Contemporary cognitive–behavioral therapists typically categorize behavior into one of three modes: motoric, cognitive–verbal, and physiological. Motor behaviors are what most people think of as behavior; they include overt and covert actions and movements of the skeletal muscular system. Cognitive–verbal behavior includes such activities as thinking, problem solving, perceiving, imaging, speaking, writing, and gestural communication, as well as observational behavior (e.g., attending, orienting, recalling, and reviewing). Physiological behaviors include activities of the nervous system, glands, and smooth muscles. Although usually covert (e.g., heartbeat), physiological behaviors can also be overt (e.g., blushing and crying).

A number of things are important to note here. First, dividing behaviors into categories or modes is intrinsically arbitrary and is done for the convenience of the observer. Human functioning is continuous, and any response involves the total human system. Even partially independent behavioral subsystems share neural circuits and interconnecting neural pathways. However, behavioral systems that in nature do not occur separately are nonetheless often distinguished conceptually, because the distinction provides some increase in our ability to analyze the processes in question.

Emotions as Full-System Responses[3]

Emotions, from the present perspective, are integrated responses of the total system. Generally, the form of the integration is automatic, either because of biological hard-wiring (the basic emotions) or because of repeated experiences (learned emotions). That is, an emotion typically comprises behaviors from each of the three subsystems. For example, basic researchers define emotions as comprised of phenomenological experience (cognitive system), biochemical changes (physiological system), and expressive and action tendencies (physiological plus motor systems). Complex emotions might also include one or more appraisal activities (cognitive system). Emotions, in turn, usually have important consequences for subsequent cognitive, physiological, and motor behavior. Thus, emotions not only are full-system behavioral responses, but themselves affect the full system. The complex, systemic nature of emotions makes it unlikely that any unique precursor of emotion dysregulation, either in general or with particular respect to BPD, will be found. There are many roads to Rome.

Intrinsic Equality of Behavioral Modes as Causes of Functioning

In contrast to biological psychiatry and cognitive psychology, the position taken here is that no mode of behavior is intrinsically more important than the others as a cause of human functioning. Thus, in contrast to cognitive theories (e.g., Beck, 1976, Beck et al., 1973, 1990), DBT does not view behavioral dysfunction, including emotion dysregulation, as necessarily resulting from dysfunctional cognitive processes. This is not to say that under some conditions cognitive activities do not influence motor and physiological behaviors, as well as the activation of emotional behaviors; in fact, a wealth of data suggests that the opposite is the case. Close to the topic of this book, for example, are the repeated findings of Aaron Beck and his colleagues (Beck, Brown, & Steer, 1989; Beck, Steer, Kovacs, & Garrison, 1985) that hopeless expectations about the future predict subsequent suicidal behaviors.

Moreover, in contrast to biological psychology and psychiatry, DBT does not view neurophysiological dysfunctions as intrinsically more important influences on behavior than other avenues of influence. Thus, from my perspective, although behavior–behavior or response system–response system relationships and causal pathways are important in human functioning, they are not more influential than any other pathways. The crucial question becomes this: Under what conditions does one behavior or behavioral pattern occur and influence another (Hayes, Kohlenberg, & Melancon, 1989)? Ultimately, however, from a dialectical framework, simple linear causal patterns of behavioral influence are not sought. Rather, the important question is more like that suggested by Manicas and Secord (1983): What is the nature of a given organism or process under prevailing circumstances? From this perspective, events, including behavioral events, are always the outcome of complex causal configurations at the same and at many different levels.

The Individual–Environment System:
A Transactional Mode

A number of etiological models of psychopathology have been offered in the literature. Most current theories are based on some version of an interaction model, in which characteristics of the individual interact with characteristics of the environment to produce an effect—in this case, psychological disorder. The "diathesis–stress model" is by far the most general and ubiquitous interactive model. This model suggests that a psychological disorder is the result of a disorder-specific predisposition toward disease (the diathesis), which is expressed under conditions of general or specific environmental stress. The term "diathesis" generally refers to a constitutional or biological predisposition, but more modern usage includes any individual characteristic that increases a person's chance of developing a disorder. Given a certain amount of stress (i.e., noxious or unpleasant environmental stimuli), the individual develops the diathesis-linked disorder. The person is not equipped to cope with such stress, and thus behavioral functioning disintegrates.

In contrast, a dialectical or transactional model assumes that individual functioning and environmental conditions are mutually and continuously interactive, reciprocal, and interdependent. Within social learning theory, this is the principle of "reciprocal determinism": The environment and the individual adapt to and influence each other. Although the individual is surely affected by the environment, the environment is also affected by the individual. It is conceptually convenient to distinguish the environment from the individual person, but in reality they cannot be distinguished. The individual–environment is a whole system, defined by and defining the constituent parts. Because influence is reciprocal, it is transactional rather than interactional.

Chess and Thomas (1986) have written extensively about this pattern of reciprocal influence with respect to the effects of different temperamental characteristics of children on their family environments, and vice versa. Their notion of "poorness of fit" as an important factor in the etiology of psychological dysfunction has heavily influenced the theory proposed here. I discuss these ideas more fully later in the chapter.

Besides focusing on reciprocal influence, a transactional view also highlights the constant state of flux and change of the individual-environment system. Thomas and Chess (1985) have labeled such a model "homeodynamic," in contrast to interactive models that conceptualize the end state of individuals and environments as some sort of "homeostatic" equilibrium. A homeodynamic model is also dialectical. They quote from Sameroff (1975, p. 290), who makes this point very well:

> [The interactive model] is insufficient to facilitate our understanding of the actual mechanisms leading to later outcomes. The major reason behind the inadequacy of this model is that neither constitution nor environment are necessarily constant over time. At each moment, month, or year the characteristics of both the child and his [sic] environment change in important ways. Moreover, these differences are interdependent and change as a function of their mutual influence on one another.

Millon (1987a) has made much the same point in discussing the etiology of BPD and the futility of attempting to locate the "cause" of the disorder in any single event or time period.

A transactional model highlights a number of points that are easy to overlook in a diathesis–stress model. For example, people in a particular environment may act in a manner that is stressful to an individual in it only because the environment itself was exposed to the stress that this individual placed on it. Examples of such individuals include the child who, due to sickness, requires expenditure of much of the family's financial resources, or the psychiatric patient who uses up much of the inpatient nursing resources because of the need for constant suicide precautions. Both of these individuals' environments are stretched in their ability to respond well to further stress; other people in both environments may invalidate or temporarily blame the victim if any further demand on the system is made. Although the system (e.g., the child's family) may have been predisposed to respond dysfunctionally in any case, it may have avoided such responses if it had not been exposed to the stress of that particular individual.

A transactional model does not assume necessarily equal power of influence on both sides of the equation. For example, some genetic influences can be powerful enough to overwhelm a benign or even a healing environment. Current research suggests a much greater influence of genetic heritage on even normal adult personality characteristics than was previously believed (Scarr & McCartney, 1983; Tellegen et al., 1988). Nor can we discount the influence of a powerful situation on the behavior of most individuals exposed to the situation, despite large, pre-existing individual personality differences (Milgram, 1963, 1964). Any person, no matter how hardy, who is exposed repeatedly to violent sexual or physical abuse will be harmed.

A Visual Representation of an Environment–Person System

A visual representation of an environment–person system is shown in Figure 2.1. I developed the particular model shown here a number of years ago to capture the data on suicidal and parasuicidal behavior. To the left is a box representing the environmental subsystem. Although in this scheme the environment is represented as four-cornered, this is done only for theoretical purposes relevant to suicidal behavior. Depending on the particular environmental factors believed to be important in an event or behavior pattern under study, one could represent the environment with as many sides as there are factors in the theory.

The person is subdivided into two separate subsystems. The behavioral subsystem is a triangle representing the three modes of behavior described above. The circular arrows at each point of the triangle indicate that responses within each behavioral mode are self-regulatory, in that changes in one response effect changes in another. Interestingly, although this aspect of behavior is well studied for physiological responses, corresponding attention

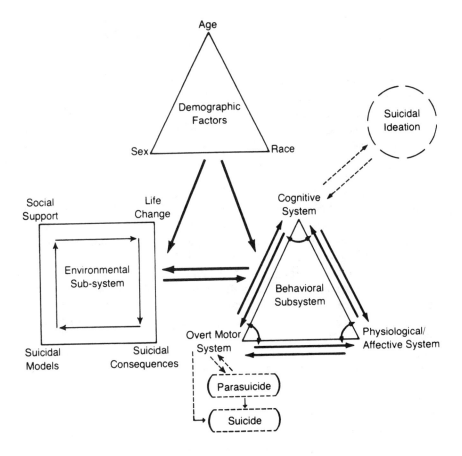

FIGURE 2.1. Social–behavioral model of suicidal behavior: An environment–person system. From Linehan (1981), p. 252. Copyright 1981 by Garland Publishing, New York. Reprinted by permission.

has not been paid to how the motor–behavioral and the cognitive–verbal response modes self-regulate.

The second triangle represents stable, organismic characteristics of the person that are not typically influenced by either the individual's behavior or the environment. These stable characteristics can, however, have important influences on both the environment and the behavior of the individual. In the model represented here, the triangular points represent gender, race, and age. As with the environmental square, however, these points are simply conceptually convenient. Gender, race, and age are related in important ways to suicidal behaviors. Other disorders will require representation of different organismic variables. For example, in the study of schizophrenia, one might want an organismic point representing genetic makeup.

Biosocial Theory: A Dialectical Theory of Borderline Personality Disorder Development

Overview

DBT is based on a biosocial theory of personality functioning. The major premise is that BPD is primarily a dysfunction of the emotion regulation system; it results from biological irregularities combined with certain dysfunctional environments, as well as from their interaction and transaction over time. The characteristics associated with BPD (see Chapter 1, especially Tables 1.2 and 1.5) are sequelae of, and thus secondary to, this fundamental emotion dysregulation. Moreover, these same patterns cause further deregulation. Invalidating environments during childhood contribute to the development of emotion dysregulation; they also fail to teach the child how to label and regulate arousal, how to tolerate emotional distress, and when to trust her own emotional responses as reflections of valid interpretations of events.

As adults, borderline individuals adopt the characteristics of the invalidating environment. Thus, they tend to invalidate their own emotional experiences, look to others for accurate reflections of external reality, and oversimplify the ease of solving life's problems. This oversimplification leads inevitably to unrealistic goals, an inability to use reward instead of punishment for small steps toward final goals, and self-hate following failure to achieve these goals. The shame reaction—a characteristic response to uncontrollable and negative emotions among borderline individuals—is a natural result of a social environment that "shames" those who express emotional vulnerability.

As noted in Chapter 1 in a slightly different context, the formulation proposed here is similar to that of Grotstein et al. (1987), who have proposed that BPD is a disorder of self-regulation. By this they mean that the disorder represents a primary breakdown of the regulation of states of self, such as arousal, attention, sleep, wakefulness, self-esteem, affects, and needs, together with the secondary sequelae of such a breakdown. As Grotstein et al. have noted, few theories of BPD have integrated biological and psychological factors into a coherent theory. To date, most theories have been either squarely psychological, whether psychoanalytic (e.g., Adler, 1985; Masterson, 1972, 1976; Kernberg, 1975, 1976; Rinsley, 1980a, 1980b; Meissner, 1984) or cognitive–behavioral (e.g., Beck et al., 1990; Young, 1987; Pretzer, in press); or they have been products of biological psychiatry (e.g., Klein, 1977; Cowdry & Gardner, 1988; Akiskal, 1981, 1983; Wender & Klein, 1981). Grotstein's (1987) formulation is a wedding of biological psychiatry and psychoanalytically informed psychological theory. Stone (1987) has suggested a similar integration. He nicely describes the difficulty of becoming well versed in the two broad areas of psychology and biology and integrating them into a theoretical position on BPD as approximating "in complexity the task of translating a text composed, perversely, of Arabic words alternating with Chinese" (pp. 253–254).

The biosocial formulation presented here is based primarily on the experimental literature in psychology. What I have found in perusing this literature is that there is a wealth of basic empirical data on such diverse topics as personality and behavioral functioning, genetic and physiological bases of behavior and personality, temperament, basic emotional functioning, and environmental effects on behavior; however, with only a few exceptions (e.g., Costa and McCrae, 1986), there has been little attempt to apply this basic research literature in psychology to the understanding of personality disorders. This state of affairs probably exists because, until very recently, the empirical study of personality disorders has been done primarily by psychiatrists, whereas the empirical study of behavior per se (including the study of biological bases of behavior) has been the domain of psychologists. The gulf between these two fields has been large, with members of neither reading much of the literature in the other. Empirically based clinical psychology, which one could consider the natural bridge between the two disciplines, has until recently shown little or no interest in personality disorders.

Borderline Personality Disorder and Emotion Dysregulation

As I stated above, the biosocial theory is that BPD is primarily a disorder of the emotion regulation system. Emotion dysregulation, in turn, is due to high emotional vulnerability plus an inability to regulate emotions.[4] The more emotionally vulnerable the individual is, the greater the need for emotion modulation. The thesis here is that borderline individuals are emotionally vulnerable as well as deficient in emotion modulation skills, and that these difficulties have their roots in biological predispositions, which are exacerbated by specific environmental experiences.

The premise of excessive emotional vulnerability fits empirical descriptions, developed in entirely separate research traditions, of both parasuicidal and borderline populations. I have reviewed this literature in Chapter 1. In summary, the emotional picture of both parasuicidal and borderline individuals is one of chronic, aversive affective experiences. Failures to inhibit maladaptive, mood-dependent actions are by definition part of the borderline syndrome. Discussions of affect dysregulation with respect to BPD usually concentrate on the depression–mania continuum (e.g., Gunderson & Zanarini, 1989). In contrast, I am using "affect" here in a much more global sense, and suggest that borderline individuals have regulation difficulties across several (if not all) emotional response systems. Although it is likely that emotion dysregulation is most pronounced in negative emotions, borderline individuals also seem to have difficulty regulating positive emotions and their sequelae.

Emotional Vulnerability

Characteristics of emotional vulnerability include high sensitivity to emotional stimuli, emotional intensity, and slow return to emotional baseline. "High sensitivity" means that the individual reacts quickly and has a low threshold for an emotional reaction; that is, it does not take much to provoke an emotional reaction. Events that might not bother many people are likely to bother the emotionally vulnerable person. The sensitive child reacts emotionally to even slight frustration or disapproval. At the adult level, the therapist's leaving town for the weekend may elicit an emotional response from the borderline patient, but not from most other patients. The implications for psychotherapy are, I suspect, obvious. The feeling, noted frequently by therapists and families of borderline individuals, of having to "walk on eggs" is a result of this sensitivity.

"Emotional intensity" means that emotional reactions are extreme. Emotionally intense individuals are the dramatic people of the world. On the negative side, partings may precipitate very intense and painful grief; what would cause slight embarrassment for another may cause deep humiliation; annoyance may turn to rage; shame may develop from slight guilt; apprehension may escalate to a panic attack or incapaciting terror. On the positive side, emotionally intense individuals may be idealistic and likely to fall in love at the drop of a hat. They may experience joy more easily, and thus may also be more susceptible to spiritual experiences.

A number of investigators have found that increases in emotional arousal and intensity narrow attention, so that emotion-relevant stimuli become more salient and are more closely attended to (Easterbrook, 1959; Bahrick, Fitts, & Rankin, 1952; Bursill, 1958; Callaway & Stone, 1960; Cornsweet, 1969; McNamara & Fisch, 1964). The stronger the arousal and the greater the intensity, the narrower the attention becomes. Clinically, these phenomena seem exceptionally characteristic of borderline individuals. It is an important point to keep in mind, however, that these tendencies are not pathological per se; they are characteristic of any individual during extreme emotional arousal. The relative paucity of theory and research examining the emotions as antecedents of cognitions, compared to the large amount on cognitions as precursors to emotion, may be the consequence of our Western view of individual behavior as a product of the rational mind (Lewis, Wolan-Sullivan, & Michalson, 1984).

"Slow return to emotional baseline" means that reactions are long-lasting. It is important to note here, however, that all emotions are relatively brief, lasting from seconds to minutes. What makes an emotion feel long-lasting is that emotional arousal, or mood, tends to have a pervasive effect on a number of cognitive processes, which in turn are related to the activation and reactivation of emotional states. Bower and his colleagues (Bower, 1981; Gilligan & Bower, 1984) have reviewed a large number of research studies indicating that emotional states (1) selectively bias the recall of affectively toned material, resulting in superior memory when the emotional state at recall matches the learning state; (2) enhance the learning of mood-congruent material; and (3) can bias interpretations, fantasies, projections, free associations, personal forecasts, and social judgments in a fashion congruent with current mood.

Emotions may also be more self-perpetuating among borderline individuals because of the greater intensity of their emotional responses, as suggested above. With high emotional arousal, the environment (including the therapist's behavior) can be selectively attended to, so that actions and events consistent with the current primary mood are attended to and other aspects are neglected.

The effect of mood on cognitive processes makes sense in view of the theory that emotions are full-system responses. A current emotion integrates the entire system in its favor. In some senses, it is rather surprising that any emotion ever ends, since emotions, once started, are repeatedly refired. A slow return to emotional baseline exacerbates this reactivating effect; it also contributes to high sensitivity to the next emotional stimulus. This characteristic can be very important in treatment. It is not unusual for a borderline patient to say that it takes several days to recover from a psychotherapy session.

Emotion Modulation

The research on emotional behavior suggests that emotion regulation requires two somewhat paradoxical strategies. The individual must first learn to experience and label the discrete emotions that are hard-wired into the neurophysiological, behavioral–expressive, and sensory–feeling systems. Then the individual must learn to reduce emotionally relevant stimuli that serve either to reactivate and augment ongoing negative emotions or to set off secondary dysfunctional emotional responses. Once an intense emotion is activated, the individual must be able to inhibit or interfere with the activation of mood-congruent afterimages, afterthoughts, afterappraisals, afterexpectations, and afteractions, so to speak.

Basic emotions are fleeting and generally adaptive (Ekman, Friesen, & Ellsworth, 1972; Buck, 1984). Constant inhibition or truncating of negative emotions seems to have a number of dysfunctional consequences. First, inhibition can lead to neglect of the problem situation instigating the emotion. An individual who never experiences anger in the face of injustice is less likely to remember unjust situations. Situations that are truly dangerous may not be avoided if fear is never experienced. Apologies may never be given and relationships may be left unrepaired when guilt or shame is always cut off before it can affect a person's behavior within a relationship.

Second, the inhibition or truncating of negative emotions serves to increase emotional avoidance. If the individual has learned a secondary emotional reaction to negative emotions, the inhibition of the original emotion removes any chance of relearning. The paradigm is similar to the escape-learning paradigm. Animals taught to escape from a chamber by having their feet shocked whenever they enter the chamber will cease to enter the chamber; if the shock apparatus is subsequently turned off, the animals will never learn the new contingencies. They must enter the chamber for new learning to occur. The invalidating family (which I describe later) is much like the shock apparatus in the escape-learning paradigm. Borderline individuals learn to avoid negative emotional cues; they become negative-emotion-phobic. Without experiencing the negative emotions, however, the individual fails to learn that she can tolerate the emotions and that punishment will not follow their expression.

Third, we simply do not know the outcomes of emotional inhibition and truncation over the long run. Research is desperately needed here. There is some evidence that emotional experiencing and catharsis lead to less stressful negative emotional states. There is also evidence that emotional catharsis increases emotionality rather than reduces it (see Bandura, 1973, for a review of this research). Under what conditions emotional experiencing enhances versus interferes with therapeutic progress is an important question that has not been adequately addressed.

John Gottman and Lynn Katz (1990) have outlined four emotion modulation activities or abilities. These include the abilities to (1) inhibit inappropriate behavior related to strong negative or positive affect, (2) self-regulate physiological arousal associated with affect, (3) refocus attention in the presence of strong affect, and (4) organize one self for coordinated action in the service of an external, non-mood-dependent goal.

The principle of changing or modulating emotional experiences by changing or resisting emotion-linked behavior is one of the important principles underlying behavior therapy exposure techniques. Besides increasing emotionality directly, inappropriate, mood-dependent behavior usually leads to consequences that elicit other unwanted emotions. Coordinated action in the service of an external goal serves to keep life progressing forward. Thus, such behavior has the long-term potential to enhance positive emotions, decrease stress and thereby reduce vulnerability to emotionality. In addition, such action is the opposite of mood-dependent behavior, and thus is an instance of acting oneself into feeling different. I discuss these principles in some detail in Chapter 11.

Changing emotions by changing physiological arousal is the principle behind a number of therapeutic emotion change strategies, such as relaxation therapies (including desensitization), some medications, and breathing training in the treatment of panic. The ability to modify physiological arousal associated with affect means that the individual is able not only to reduce the high arousal associated with some emotions, such as anger and fear (i.e., to calm down), but to increase the low arousal associated with other emotions, such as sadness and depression (i.e. to "rev up," so to speak). Usually, this will require the ability to force activity, even when the person is not in the mood. For example, one of the basic techniques in cognitive therapy of depression is activity scheduling.

The important role of controlling attention as a way to regulate contact with emotional stimuli has been pointed out by many (e.g., Derryberry & Rothbart, 1984, 1988). Shifting attention toward a positive stimulus can enhance or maintain ongoing positive arousal and emotion; shifting it away from a negative stimulus may attenuate or contain negative arousal and emotion.

Thus, individuals with control over attention focusing and attention shifting — two related but distinct processes (Posner, Walker, Friedrich, & Rafal, 1984) — have an advantage in regulation of emotional responses. In turn, individual differences in attention control are evident from the earliest years of life (Rothbart & Derryberry, 1981) and appear as stable temperamental characteristics in adults (Keele & Hawkins, 1982; Derryberry, 1987; MacLeod, Mathews, & Tata, 1986). This point is particularly interesting, in light of data reviewed by Nolen-Hoeksema (1987) suggesting gender differences in attentional response sets under stress. She concludes that, at least when depressed, women have a more ruminative response set than men. Rumination about one's current depressed mood, in turn, generates depressing explanations that increase depression further and lead to greater helplessness on future tasks (Diener & Dweck, 1978). In contrast, men are more likely to engage in distracting behaviors that dampen depressed mood. It seems reasonable to hypothesize that an inability to distract oneself from negative, emotionally sensitive stimuli may be an important part of the emotion dysregulation found among borderline individuals.

Biological Underpinnings

The mechanisms of emotion dysregulation in BPD are unclear, but difficulties in limbic system reactivity and attention control may be important. The emotion regulation system is a complex one, and there is no *a priori* reason to expect that the dysfunction will be the result of a common factor in all borderline individuals. Biological causes could conceivably range from genetic influences to disadvantageous intrauterine events to early childhood environmental effects on development of the brain and nervous system.

Cowdry et al. (1985) report data suggesting that some borderline individuals may have a low threshold for activation of limbic structures, the brain system associated with emotion regulation. In particular, they note the overlap among symptoms of complex partial seizures, episodic dyscontrol, and BPD. Positive benefits among borderline individuals for an anticonvulsant (carbamazepine) whose neurophysiological effects are known to be located in the limbic area lends further support to this notion (Gardner & Cowdry, 1986, 1988).

Other investigators have reported that patients with BPD have significantly more electroencephalographic (EEG) dysrhythmias than their depressed control patients (Snyder & Pitts, 1984; Cowdry et al., 1985). Andrulonis and his colleagues (Andrulonis et al., 1981; Akiskal et al., 1985a, 1985b) have attempted to link neurologically based dysfunctions to BPD. However, they did not employ comparison groups, and thus it is difficult to interpret their findings. In contrast, Cornelius et al. (1989) reviewed a number of studies in which borderline patients were compared with patients exhibiting various other psychiatric disorders. Generally, they reported no EEG differences; no differences in familial mental retardation, epilepsy, or neurological disorders; no differences on a broad battery of tests assessing major areas of cognitive functioning; and no differences in overall neurodevelopmental histories. Interestingly, Cornelius et al. did report data indicating the early onset of borderline-type behavior patterns among borderline patients. For example, childhood temper tantrums and persistent rocking or head banging were more frequent among children later diagnosed as having BPD than among those later diagnosed as depressed or schizophrenic.

Still another research strategy attempting to locate biological influences on behavior is the comparison of various behavioral dysfunctions in family members of the population of interest. Studies of first-degree relatives of borderline patients have found higher prevalences of affective disorder (Akiskal, 1981; Andrulonis et al., 1981; Baron, Gruen, Asnis & Lord, 1985; Loranger, Oldham, & Tulis, 1982; Pope et al., 1983; Schulz et al., 1986; Soloff & Millward, 1983; Stone, 1981), of closely related personality traits such as histrionic and antisocial characteristics (Links, Steiner, & Huxley, 1988; Loranger et al., 1982; Pope et al., 1983; Silverman et al., 1987), and of borderline personality disorder (Zanarini, Gunderson, Marino, Schwartz & Frankenburg, 1988) than among relatives of control groups. However, many other investigators have failed to find similar associations when all relevant characteristics have been controlled (see Dahl, 1990, for a review of this literature). A twin study by Torgersen (1984) supports a psychosocial over a genetic model of transmission. There has been little or no research attempting to link temperamental characteristics of borderline individuals to data on the genetic and biological etiology of those particular temperamental attributes. Such research is sorely needed.

Factors other than genes, however, may be equally important in determining neurophysiological functioning, especially in the emotion regulation system. We know, for example, that characteristics of the intrauterine environment can be crucial in the development of the fetus. Furthermore, these characteristics influence later behavioral patterns of the individual. Just a few examples will make my point here. Fetal alcohol syndrome, characterized by mental retardation and hyperactivity, impulsiveness, distractibility, irritability, delayed development, and sleep disorders, is caused by maternal ingestion of excessive alcohol (Abel, 1981, 1982). Similar dysfunctions are regularly noted in babies of drug-addicted mothers (Howard, 1989). There is accumulating evidence that environmental stress experienced by the mother during pregnancy can have deleterious effects on the later development of the child (Davids & Devault, 1962; Newton, 1988).

Postnatal experiences can also have important biological consequences. It has been well established that radical environmental events and conditions can modify neural structures (Dennenberg, 1981; Greenough, 1977). There is little reason to doubt that neural structures and functions related to emotional behaviors are similarly affected by experiences with the environment (see Malatesta & Izard, 1984 for a review). The relationship of environmental trauma to emotion regulation is particularly salient in the case of BPD given the prevalence of childhood sexual abuse among this population — a topic I discuss later in this chapter.

Borderline Personality Disorder and Invalidating Environments

The temperamental picture of the borderline adult is quite similar to that of the "difficult child" described by Thomas and Chess (1985). From their studies of temperamental characteristics of infants, they identified difficult children as the "group with irregularity in biological functions, negative withdrawal responses to new stimuli, non-adaptability or slow adaptability to change, and intense mood expressions that are frequently negative" (p. 219). In their research, this group comprised approximately 10% of their sample. Clearly, however, not all children with a difficult temperament grow up to meet criteria for BPD. Although the majority (70%) of difficult children studied by Chess and Thomas (1986) had behavior disorders during childhood, most of these children improved or recovered by adolescence. In addition, as Chess and Thomas point out, children who originally do not have a difficult temperament may acquire one as they develop.

Thomas and Chess have suggested that the "goodness of fit" or "poorness of fit" of the child with the environment is crucial for understanding later behavioral functioning. Goodness of fit results when the properties of the child's environment and its expectations and demands are in accord with the individual's own capacities, characteristics, and style of behavior. Optimal development and behavioral functioning are the results. In contrast, poorness of fit results when there are discrepancies and dissonances between environmental opportunities and demands and the capacities and characteristics of the child. In these instances, distorted development and maladaptive functions result (Thomas & Chess, 1977; Chess & Thomas, 1986). It is this notion of "poorness of fit" that I propose as crucial for understanding the development of BPD. But what kind of environment would constitute a "poor fit" leading to this particular disorder? I propose that an "invalidating environment" is most likely to facilitate development of BPD.

Characteristics of Invalidating Environments

An invalidating environment is one in which communication of private experiences is met by erratic, inappropriate, and extreme responses. In other words, the expression of private experiences is not validated; instead, it is often punished, and/or trivialized. The experience of painful emotions, as well as the factors that to the emotional person seem causally related to the emotional distress, are disregarded. The individual's interpretations of her own behavior, including the experience of the intents and motivations associated with behavior, are dismissed.

Invalidation has two primary characteristics. First, it tells the individual that she is wrong in both her description and her analyses of her own experiences, particularly in her views of what is causing her own emotions, beliefs, and actions. Second, it attributes her experiences to socially unacceptable characteristics or personality traits. The environment may insist that the individual feels what she says she does not ("You are angry, but you just won't admit it"), likes or prefers what she says she does not (the proverbial "When she says no, she means yes"), or has done what she said she did not. Negative emotional expressions may be attributed to traits such as overreactivity, oversensitivity, paranoia, a distorted view of events, or failure to adopt a positive attitude. Behaviors that have unintended negative or painful consequences for others may be attributed to hostile or manipulative motives. Failure, or any deviation from socially defined success, is labeled as resulting from lack of motivation, lack of discipline, not trying hard enough, or the like. Positive emotional expressions, beliefs, and action plans may be similarly invalidated by being attributed to lack of discrimination, naiveté, overidealization, or immaturity. In any case, the individual's private experiences and emotional expressions are not viewed as valid responses to events.

Emotionally invalidating environments are generally intolerant of displays of negative affect, at least when such displays are not accompanied by public events supporting the emotion. The attitude communicated is similar to the "you can pull yourself up by the bootstraps" approach; it is the belief that any individual who tries hard enough can make it. Individual mastery and achievement are highly valued, at least with respect to controlling emotional expressiveness and limiting demands on the environment. Invalidating members of such environments are often vigorous in promulgating their point of view and actively communicate frustration with an individual's inability to adhere to a similar point of view. Great value is attached to being happy, or at least grinning in the face of adversity; to believing in one's capacity to achieve any objective, or at least never "giving in" to hopelessness; and, most of all, to the power of a "positive mental attitude" in overcoming any problem. Failures to live up to these expectations lead to disapproval, criticism, and attempts on the part of others to bring about or force a change of attitude. Demands that a person can place on these environments are usually very restricted.

This pattern is very similar to the pattern of high "expressed emotion," found in the families of both depressives and schizophrenics with high relapse rates (Leff & Vaughn, 1985). The work with expressed emotion suggests that such a family constellation can be extremely powerful with the vulnerable individual. "Expressed emotion," in that literature, refers to criticism and overinvolvement. The notion here includes those two aspects, but in addition stresses a nonrecognition of the actual state of the individual. The consequence is that the behaviors of others, including caregivers, in the individual's environment are not only invalidating of the individual's experiences but also nonresponsive to the needs of the individual.

A few clinical examples may provide a better idea of what I mean here. During a family session with a borderline woman who had a history of alcoholism and frequent serious suicide attempts, her son commented that he just didn't understand why she couldn't let problems "roll off her back" as he, his brother, and his father did. A substantial number of patients in my research project were actively dissuaded from going into psychotherapy by their parents. One 18-year-old patient who had been hospitalized several times, had a history of numerous attempts to harm herself, was hyperactive and dyslexic, and was heavily involved in the drug culture was told weekly by her parents after her group therapy sessions that she did not need therapy and that she could just straighten up on her own if she really wanted to. "Talking about problems just makes problems worse," her father said. Another patient was told while growing up that if she cried when she got hurt playing, her mother would give her a "real" reason to cry: If the tears continued, her mother would hit her.

Consequences of Invalidating Environments

The consequences of invalidating environments are as follows. First, by failing to validate emotional expression, an invalidating environment does not teach the child to label private experiences, including emotions, in a manner normative in her larger social community for the same or similar experiences. Nor is the child taught to modulate emotional arousal. Because the problems of the emotionally vulnerable child are not recognized, little effort goes into attempts to solve the problems. The child is told to control her emotions, rather than being taught exactly how to do that. It is a bit like telling a child with no legs to walk without providing artificial legs for her to walk on. The nonacceptance or oversimplification of the original problems precludes the type of attention, support, and diligent training such an individual needs. Thus, the child does not learn to adequately label or control emotional reactions.

Second, by oversimplifying the ease of solving life's problems, the environment does not teach the child to tolerate distress or to form realistic goals and expectations.

Third, within an invalidating environment, extreme emotional displays and/or extreme problems are often necessary to provoke a helpful environmental response. Thus, the social contingencies favor the development of extreme emotional reactions. By erratically punishing communication of negative emotions and intermittently reinforcing displays of extreme or escalated emotions, the environment teaches the child to oscillate between emotional inhibition on the one hand, and extreme emotional states on the other.

Finally, such an environment fails to teach the child when to trust her own emotional and cognitive responses as reflections of valid interpretations of individual and situational events. Instead, the invalidating environment teaches the child to actively invalidate her own experiences and to search her social environment for cues about how to think, feel, and act. A person's ability to trust herself, at least minimally, is crucial; she at least has to trust her decision not to trust herself. Thus, invalidation is ordinarily experienced as aversive. People who are invalidated will usually either leave the invalidating environment, attempt to change their behavior so that it meets the expectations of their environment, or try to prove themselves valid and thereby to reduce the environment's invalidation. The borderline dilemma arises when the individual cannot leave the environment and is unsuccessful at changing either the environment or her own behavior to meet the environment's demands.

It might perhaps seems that such an environment would produce an adult with dependent personality disorder instead of BPD. I suspect that such an outcome would be likely with a less emotionally vulnerable child. But with an emotionally intense child, the invalidating information coming in from the environment is almost always competing with an equally strong message from the child's emotional responses: "You may be telling me that what you did was an act of love, but my hurt feelings, terror, and rage tell me that it wasn't loving. You may be telling me that I can do it; and it's no big deal, but my panic is saying that I cannot and it is."

The emotionally vulnerable, invalidated individual is in a bind similar to that of the overweight individual in our society. The culture (including daily weight reduction ads on TV and radio) and thin family members repeatedly tell the obese person that losing weight is easy; and keeping it off requires just a little will power. A body weight over the cultural ideal is thought to be the mark of a gluttonous, lazy, or undisciplined person. A thousand diets, intense hunger while dieting, herculean efforts to get and stay thin, and a body, that regains weight at the drop of a calorie say otherwise. How does the heavy person respond to this double message? Usually by alternating between dieting and extreme discipline on the one hand, and giving in, relaxing, and refusing to diet on the other. The yo-yo syndrome among dieters is similar to the emotional oscillation among borderline individuals. Neither source of information can be comfortably ignored.

Varieties of Sexism: Prototypic Invalidating Experiences

The prevalence of BPD among women requires that we examine the possible role of sexism in its etiology. Certainly, sexism is an important source of invalidation for all women in our culture; just as certainly, all women do not become borderline. Nor do all women with vulnerable temperaments become borderline, even though all women are exposed to sexism in one form or another. I suspect that the influence of sexism in the etiology of BPD depends on other characteristics of the vulnerable child, as well as on the circumstances of sexism in the family raising the child.

Sexual Abuse. The most extreme form of sexism is, of course, sexual abuse. The risk for sexual abuse is approximately two to three times greater for females than for males (Finkelhor, 1979). The prevalence of childhood sexual abuse in the histories of women meeting criteria for BPD is such that it simply cannot be ignored as an important factor in the etiology of the disorder. Of 12 hospitalized borderline patients assessed by Stone (1981), 9, or 75%, reported a history of incest. Childhood sexual abuse was reported by 86% of borderline inpatients compared, to 34% of other psychiatric inpatients, in a study by Bryer, Nelson, Miller, and Krol (1987). Among borderline outpatients, from 67% to 76% report childhood sexual abuse (Herman, Perry, & van der Kolk, 1989; Wagner, Linehan, & Wasson, 1989), in contrast to a 26% rate among nonborderline patients (Herman et al., 1989). Ogata, Silk, Goodrich, Lohr, and Westen (1989) found that 71% of borderline patients reported a history of sexual abuse, compared to 22% of major depressive control patients.

Although in epidemiological data girls are at no higher risk for physical abuse than boys are, one study found rates of reported childhood physical abuse to be higher among borderline patients (71%) than among nonborderline patients (38%) (Herman et al., 1989). Furthermore, there is a positive association between physical and sexual abuse (Westen, Ludolph, Misle, Ruffin, & Block, 1990), suggesting that those at risk for sexual abuse are at higher risk for physical abuse also. Bryer et al. (1987), however, found that whereas early sexual abuse predicted the diagnosis of BPD, the combination of sexual and physical abuse did not. Ogata et al. (1989) also reported similar rates of physical abuse in borderline and depressed patients. Thus, it may be that sexual abuse, in contrast to other types of abuse, is uniquely associated with BPD. Much more research is needed here to clarify the relationships.

A very similar connection has been found between childhood sexual abuse and suicidal (including parasuicidal) behaviors. Victims of such abuse have higher rates of subsequent suicide attempts than nonvictims do (Edwall, Hoffmann, & Harrison, 1989; Herman & Hirschman, 1981; Briere & Runtz, 1986; Briere, 1988); up to 55% of these victims go on to attempt suicide. Furthermore, sexually abused women engage in more medically serious parasuicidal behavior (Wagner et al., 1989). Bryer et al. (1987) found that childhood abuse (both sexual and physical) predicted adult suicidal behavior. Individuals with suicide ideation or parasuicide were three times more likely to have been abused in childhood than were patients without such behaviors.

Although it is generally viewed as a social stressor, child abuse may play a less obvious role as a cause of physiological vulnerability to emotion dysregulation. Abuse may not only be pathogenic for individuals with vulnerable temperaments; it may "create" emotional vulnerability by affecting changes in the central nervous system. Shearer, Peters, Quaytman, and Ogden (1990) suggest that perpetual trauma may physiologically alter the limbic system. Thus, severe, chronic stress may have permanent adverse effects on arousal, emotional sensitivity, and other factors of temperament.

Sexual abuse, as it occurs in our culture, is perhaps one of the clearest examples of extreme invalidation during childhood. In the typical case scenario of sexual abuse, the victim is told that the molestation or intercourse is "OK" but that she must not tell anyone else. The abuse is seldom acknowledged by other family members, and if the child reports the abuse she risks being disbelieved or blamed (Tsai & Wagner, 1978). It is difficult to imagine a more invalidating experience for the typical child. Similarly, physical abuse is often presented to the child as an act of love or is otherwise normalized by the abusive adult. Some clinicians have suggested that the secrecy of sexual abuse may be the factor most related to subsequent BPD. Jacobson and Herald (1990) reported that of 18 psychiatric inpatients with histories of major childhood sexual abuse, 44% had never revealed the experience to anyone. Feelings of shame are common among sexual abuse victims (Edwall et al., 1989) and may account for this failure to disclose the abuse. We cannot exclude the invalidating component of sexual abuse as contributory to the BPD.

Parental Imitation of Infants. Parents' tendencies to imitate an infant's emotionally expressive behaviors constitute an important factor in optimal emotional development (Malatesta & Haviland, 1982). Failure to imitate or noncongruent imitation—the former of which is failure to validate, and the latter of which is invalidation—are related to less optimal development. Interestingly, with respect to gender differences in the incidence of BPD, mothers tend to show more contingent responding to sons' smiles than to daughters' smiles and imitate sons' expressions more often than daughters' (Malatesta & Haviland, 1982).[5]

Dependence and Independence: Invalidating (and Impossible) Cultural Ideals for Women. The research data are overwhelming in confirming large differences between male and female interpersonal relationship styles. Flaherty and Richman (1989) have reviewed extensive data in the areas of primate behavior and evolution, developmental studies, parenthood, and adult social support and mental health. They conclude that various socialization experiences, beginning at infancy, render women more affectively connected and perceptive in the interpersonal sphere than men. The relationship between receiving social support from others and personal well-being, and, conversely, the relationship between social support distress and somatic complaints, depression, and anxiety are stronger for females than for males. That is, whereas the degree of social support received is not closely related to emotional functioning among men, it is highly correlated to emotional well-being among women. In particular, Flaherty and Richman (1989) found that the intimacy component of social support is most closely associated with well-being among women. In reviewing research on assertion and women, Kelly Egan and I concluded that women's behavior in groups or dyads is consistent with an emphasis on maintaining relationships almost to the exclusion of achieving task objectives, such as solving problems or persuading others (Linehan & Egan, 1979).

Given the prevalence of interpersonal bonding and social support as important (indeed, crucial), dimensions for well-adjusted women, one can ask this question: What happens to women who either are not given the social support they need or are taught that their very need for social support is itself unhealthy? Just such situations seem to exist. Almost without exception, interpersonal independence for both males and females is extolled as the ideal of "healthy" behavior. Feminine characteristics such as interpersonal dependence and relying on others—which, as noted above, are positively related to women's mental health—are generally perceived as mentally "unhealthy" (Widiger & Settle, 1987). We so value independence that we apparently cannot conceive of the possibility that a person could have too much independence. For example, although there is a "dependent personality disorder" in the DSM-IV, there is no in "independent personality disorder."

This emphasis on individual independence as normative behavior is unique to, and pervasive in, Western culture (Miller, 1984; see Sampson, 1977, for a review of this literature). In fact, one can conclude that normative feminine behavior, at least that part having to do with interpersonal relationships, is in a collision with current Western cultural values. It is no wonder that many women come to experience conflict over issues of independence and dependence. Indeed, it appears that there is a "poorness of fit" between women's interpersonal style and Western socialization and cultural values for adult behavior. It is interesting, however, that the pathology is laid on the doorstep of the conflicted women, rather than on that of a society that seems to be moving further and further away from valuing community and interpersonal dependency.

Femininity and Bias. Sexism can be a special problem for those female children whose talents are those generally rewarded in men but often ignored or invalidated in women. For example, mechanical ability, sports achievements, interest in math and science, and logical, task-oriented thinking are valued more in men than in women. Any sense of pride or accomplishment can easily be invalidated in women with such characteristics. An even worse situation occurs when these talents valued in men are not matched by talents and interests valued in women (e.g., interest in appearing attractive, home-oriented skills). In such a situation, the female child is not rewarded for the talents that she does have, and in addition is punished for emitting "unfeminine behaviors" or failing to emit "feminine" behaviors. When the child's behaviors are tied to temperamental characteristics, she is in further trouble. For example, gentleness, softness, affection, responsiveness to others, empathy, nurturance and soothing, and similar characteristics are highly valued "feminine" associated characteristics (Widiger & Settle, 1987; Flaherty & Richman, 1989); however, they are not the characteristics associated with a difficult temperament.

For the female child punished for having characteristics that interfere with her meeting the cultural ideal for women, life must be particularly difficult when she has brothers who are not punished for identical behaviors or sisters who effortlessly meet standards for femininity. The injustice is not to be missed in these situations. The environment outside the home does little in these cases to ameliorate the problem, since the same values are held across the culture. It is difficult to imagine how such a child could not grow up believing that there must be something wrong with her.

In my clinical experience, just this state of affairs seems to be common among borderline patients. We have been struck in our clinic with the number of patients who are talented in areas valued highly in men but little in women, such as mechanical and intellectual pursuits. Our borderline group therapy is entirely female, and a frequent topic of discussion is the difficulties the patients experienced as children because their interests and talents appeared more masculine than feminine. Another common experience seems to have been growing up in families that valued the boys more than the girls, or at least gave them more leeway, more privileges, and less punishment for the behaviors that led the girls to grief. Although sexism is clearly a fact, its relationship to BPD as I have described here is just as clearly speculative. We simply need more research data on this point.

Types of Invalidating Families

My colleagues and I have observed three types of invalidating families among patients in our clinic: the "chaotic" family, the "perfect" family, and, less commonly, the "typical" family.

Chaotic Families. In the chaotic family, there may be problems with substance abuse, financial problems, or parents who are out of the home much of the time; in any case, little time or attention is given to the children. For example, the parents of one of my patients spent almost every afternoon and evening at a local tavern. The children came home from school each day to an empty house and were left to fend for themselves for dinner and structure in the evenings. Often they wandered over to a grandmother's for dinner. When the parents were home, they were volatile; the father was often drunk; and they could tolerate few demands from the children. Needs of the children in such a family are disregarded and consequently invalidated. Millon (1987a) has suggested that the increase in chaotic families may be responsible for the increase in BPD.

Perfect Families. In the "perfect" family, the parents for one reason or another cannot tolerate negative emotional displays from their children. Such a stance may be the result of a number of factors, including other demands on the parents (such as a large number of children or stressful jobs), an inability to tolerate negative affect, self-centeredness, or naive fears of spoiling a child with a difficult temperament. In my experience, when members of such a family are asked directly about their feeling toward the borderline family member, they express a great deal of sympathy. However, without meaning to, these other members often express consistent invalidating attitudes—for example, expressing surprise that the borderline individual can't just "control her feeling." One such family member suggested that his daughter's very serious problems would be cured if she just prayed more.

Typical Families. When I originally observed the invalidating environmental style, I called it the "American way syndrome," since it is so prevalent in American culture. However, when I gave a lecture in Germany, my German colleagues informed me that I could have called it the "German way syndrome." It is most likely a product of Western culture in general. A number of emotion theorists have commented on the tendency in Western societies to emphasize cognitive control of emotions and to focus on achievement and mastery as criteria of success. The individuated self in Western culture is defined by sharp boundaries between self and others. In cultures with this view, the behavior of mature persons is assumed to be controlled by internal rather than external forces. "Self-control," in this context, refers to the people's ability to control their own behavior by utilizing internal cues and resources. To define oneself differently—for example, to define the self in relation to others, or to be field-dependent—is labeled as immature and pathological, or at least inimical to good health and smooth societal functioning (Perloff, 1987). (Although this conception of the individual self pervades Western culture, it is universal neither cross-culturally nor even within Western culture itself.)

A key point must be kept in mind about the invalidating family. Within limits, an invalidating cognitive style is not detrimental for everyone or in all contexts. The emotion control strategies used by such a family may even be useful at times to the person who is temperamentally suited to them and who can learn attitude and emotional control. For example, research by Miller and associates (Efran, Chorney, Ascher, & Lukens, 1981; Lamping, Molinaro, & Stevenson, 1985; Miller, 1979; Miller & Managan, 1983; Phipps & Zinn, 1986) indicates that individuals who tend to psychologically "blunt" threat-relevant cues when faced with the prospect of uncontrollable aversive events show lower and less sustained physiological, subjective, and behavioral arousal than individuals who tend to monitor or attend to such cues. Knussen and Cunningham (1988) have reviewed research indicating that belief in one's own behavioral control over negative outcomes, instead of blaming others (a key belief in the invalidating family), is related to more favorable future outcomes in a variety of areas. Thus, cognitive control of emotion can be quite effective in certain circumstances. Indeed, this approach got the railroad across the United States, built the bomb, got many of us through school, and put up skyscrapers in big cities!

The only problem here is that the approach "only works when it works." That is, telling persons who are capable of affect self-regulation to control their emotions is quite a different proposition from telling this to an individual who does not have this capability. For example, one mother I was working with who had a 14-year-old daughter with a "difficult" temperament and a 5-year-old daughter with an "easy" temperament. The older daughter had difficulty with anger, especially when her little sister was teasing her. I was trying to teach the mother to validate this daughter's emotional reactions. After the 5-year-old pushed a complex puzzle of the 14-year old's onto the floor, the older child screamed at her sister and stormed out of the room, leaving the sister in tears. The mother happily reported that she had "validated" the older daughter's emotions by saying, "Mary, I can understand why you got angry. But in the future, you have got to control your explosions!" It was difficult for the mother to see how she had invalidated the daughter's difficulties in controlling her emotions. In the cases of emotionally reactive and vulnerable persons, invalidating environments vastly oversimplify these person's problems. What other people succeed in doing—controlling emotions and emotional expression—the borderline individual can often succeed at only sporadically.

Emotion Dysregulation and Invalidating Environments: A Transactional Vicious Cycle

A transactional analysis suggests that a system that may originally have consisted of a slightly vulnerable child within a slightly invalidating family can, over time, evolve into one in which the individual and the family environment are highly sensitive to, vulnerable to, and invalidating of each other. Chess and Thomas (1986) describe a number of ways in which the temperamental child, the slow-to-warm-up child, the distractible child, and the persistent child can overwhelm, threaten, and disorganize otherwise nurturing parents. Patterson (1976; Patterson & Stouthamer-Loeber, 1984) has also written extensively on the interactive behaviors of child and family that lead to mutually coercive behavior patterns on the part of all parties in the system. Over time, children and caregivers shape and reinforce extreme and coercive behaviors in each other. In turn, these coercive behaviors further exacerbate the invalidating and coercive system, leading to more, not fewer, dysfunctional behaviors within the entire system. One is reminded of a Biblical quotation: ". . . for anyone who has will be given more; from anyone who has not, even what he thinks he has will be taken away" (Luke 8:18; The Jerusalem Bible, 1966).

There is no question that an emotionally vulnerable child puts demands on the environment. Parents or other caregivers have to be more vigilant, more patient, more understanding and flexible, and more willing to put their own wishes for the child on temporary hold when these wishes exceed the child's capabilities. Unfortunately, what often happens is that the child's response to invalidation actually reinforces the family's invalidating behavior. Telling a child that her feelings are stupid or unwarranted does at times quiet the child down. Many people, including those with emotional vulnerability, sometimes withdraw and appear to feel better when their emotions are made light of. Invalidation is aversive, and thus suppresses the behavior it follows.

The "controlling" environment described by Chess and Thomas (1986) is a variation or extreme example of the invalidating environment described here. The controlling environment constantly shapes the child's behavior to fit the family's preferences and convenience rather than the child's short- and long-term needs. In that situation, of course, the validity of the child's behavior as it exists is not recognized. As the child matures, power struggles are inevitable, with the environment sometimes appeasing and giving in and at other times rigidly holding the line. Depending on the child's initial temperament, the eventual result of appeasement is a child tyrant, a child with negative passivity, or both. The manner of this development is described over and over again in manuals on parenting.

In essence, the error in such a family is twofold. First, the caregivers make an error in shaping. That is, they expect more or different behaviors than the child is capable of emitting. Excessive punishment and insufficient modeling, instructing, coaching, cheerleading, and reinforcement follow. Such a pattern creates an aversive environment for the child, in which needed help is not forthcoming and unavoidable punishment occurs. As a result, the child's negative emotional behaviors increase, including the expressive behaviors that are associated with the emotions. These behaviors function to terminate punishment, usually by creating such aversive consequences for the caregivers that they stop attempts at control.

And here caregivers make the second error: They reinforce the functional value of extreme expressive behaviors, and extinguish the functional value of moderate expressive behaviors. Such a pattern of appeasement following extreme emotional displays can unwittingly create the pattern of behaviors associated with BPD in the adult. When appeasement from others does not occur, or occurs unpredictably, the unavoidability of aversive conditions mimics the learned helplessness paradigm: Passive, helpless behaviors can be expected to increase. If passive or helpless behaviors are in turn punished, the person is faced with an unwinnable dilemma and will probably vacillate between extreme emotionally expressive behaviors and equally extreme passive and helpless behaviors. Such a state of affairs can, without too much difficulty, account for the emergence of many borderline characteristics as the child matures.

Emotion Dysregulation and Borderline Behaviors

Very little in human behavior is not affected by emotional arousal and mood states. Such diverse phenomena as concepts of the self, self-attributions, perceptions of control, learning of tasks and performance, patterns of self-reward, and delay of gratification are affected by emotional states (see Izard, Kagan, & Zajonc, 1984, and Garber & Dodge, 1991, for reviews). The thesis here is that most borderline behaviors are either attempts on the part of the individual to regulate intense affect or outcomes of emotion dysregulation. Emotion dysregulation is both the problem the individual is trying to solve and the source of additional problems. The relationship between borderline behavior patterns and emotion dysregulation is depicted in Figure 2.2.

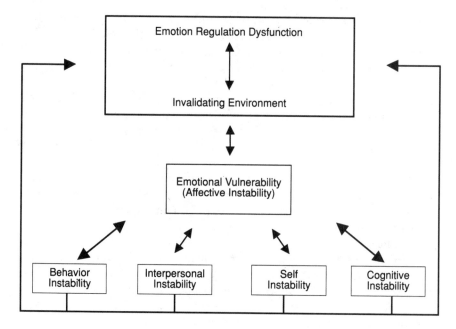

FIGURE 2.2. The relationship between emotion dysregulation and borderline behavior patterns, according to the biosocial theory.

Emotion Dysregulation and Impulsive Behaviors

Suicidal and other impulsive, dysfunctional behaviors are usually maladaptive solution behaviors to the problem of overwhelming, uncontrollable, intensely painful negative affect. Suicide, of course, is the ultimate way to change one's affective state (we presume). Other, less lethal (e.g., parasuicidal) behaviors, however, can also be quite effective. Overdosing, for example, usually leads to long periods of sleep; sleep, in turn, has an important influence on regulating emotional vulnerability. Cutting and burning the body also seem to have important affect-regulating properties. The exact mechanism here is unclear, but it is common for borderline individuals to report substantial relief from anxiety and a variety of other intense negative affective states following cutting themselves (Leinbenluft, Gardner, & Cowdry, 1987).

Suicidal behavior, including suicide threats and parsuicide, is also very effective in eliciting helping behaviors from the environment—help that may be effective in reducing the emotional pain. In many instances, in fact, such behavior is the only way an individual can get others to pay attention to and try to ameliorate her emotional pain. For example, suicidal behavior is a most effective way for a nonpsychotic individual to be admitted to an inpatient psychiatric unit. Many therapists tell their patients that they can or should phone them if they are feeling suicidal. The staff at a psychiatric inpatient unit in my area used to tell one of our patients that she could come right back in if she got "command voices" telling her to commit suicide. In our clinical population of parasuicidal borderline women, a majority report that the intent to change their environment is part of at least one instance of parasuicidal behavior.

Unfortunately, the instrumental character of suicide threats and parasuicide is frequently the most salient one for therapists and theorists working with borderline individuals. Thus, suicide attempts and other intentional self-injurious behaviors are often referred to as "manipulative." The basis of this reference is usually a therapist's own feeling of being manipulated. As I have discussed in Chapter 1, however, it is a logical error to assume that if a behavior has a particular effect, the actor has therefore engaged in the behavior in order to bring about the effect. The labeling of suicidal behavior as manipulative, in the absence of an assessment of the actual intent of the behavior, can have extremely deleterious effects. This issue is discussed further in the Chapter 15 where I describe treatment strategies for suicidal behaviors.

Emotion Dysregulation and Identity Disturbance

Generally, people form a sense of self-identity through their own observations of themselves as well as through others' reactions to them. Emotional consistency and predictability across time and similar situations are prerequisites to this development of identity. All emotions involve some element of preference or approach–avoidance. A sense of identity, among other things, is contingent on preferring or liking something consistently. For example, a person who always enjoys drawing and painting may develop an image of herself that includes aspects of an artist's identity. Others observing this same preference may react to the person as an artist, further developing her image of herself. Unpredictable emotional lability, however, leads to unpredictable behavior and cognitive inconsistency; thus a stable self-concept, or sense of identity, fails to develop.

A tendency of borderline patients to inhibit, or attempt to inhibit, emotional responses may also contribute to an absence of a strong sense of identity. The numbness associated with inhibited affect is often experienced as emptiness, further contributing to an inadequate (and at times completely absent) sense of self. Similarly, if an individual's own sense of events is never "correct" or is unpredictably "correct" — the situation in the invalidating family — then one would expect the individual to develop an overdependence upon others. This overdependence, especially when the dependence relates to preferences, ideas, and opinions, simply exacerbates problems with identity, and a vicious cycle is once again started.

Emotion Dysregulation and Interpersonal Chaos

Effective interpersonal relations are enormously benefited by both a stable sense of self and a capacity for spontaneity in emotional expression. Successful relationships also require a capacity to self-regulate emotions in appropriate ways, to control impulsive behavior, and to tolerate stimuli that produces pain to a certain degree. Without such capabilities, it is understandable that borderline individuals develop chaotic relationships. Difficulties with anger and anger expression, in particular, preclude the maintenance of stable relationships.

In addition, as I discuss further in Chapter 3, the combination of emotional vulnerability with an invalidating environment leads to the development of more intense and more persistent expressions of negative emotions. Essentially, the invalidating environment usually places the individual on an intermittent reinforcement schedule, in which expressions of intensely negative affect or demands for help are reinforced sporadically. Such a schedule is known to create very persistent behavior. When people currently involved with the borderline person also fall into the trap of inconsistently appeasing her—sometimes giving in to and reinforcing high-rate, high-intensity aversive emotional expressions and other times not doing so—they are recreating conditions for the person's learning of relationship-destructive behaviors.

Implications of the Biosocial Theory for Therapy with Borderline Patients

General Aims and Skills Taught

Recognition of these emotion regulation difficulties, originating in both biological makeup and inadequate learning experiences, suggests that treatment should focus on the twin tasks of teaching the borderline patient (1) to modulate extreme emotionality and reduce maladaptive mood-dependent behaviors, and (2) to trust and validate her own emotions, thoughts, and activities. The therapy should focus on skills training and behavior change, as well as on validation of the patient's current capabilities and behaviors.

A major portion of DBT is devoted to teaching just such skills. The skills are broken down into four types: (1) those that increase interpersonal effectiveness in conflict situations, and thus show promise in decreasing environmental stimuli associated with negative emotions; (2) strategies culled from the behavioral treatment literature on affective disorders (depression, anxiety, fear, anger) and posttraumatic stress, which increase self-regulation of unwanted emotions in the face of actual or perceived negative emotional stimuli; (3) skills for tolerating emotional distress until changes are forthcoming; and (4) skills adapted from Eastern (Zen) meditation techniques, such as mindfulness practice, which increase the ability to experience emotions and avoid emotional inhibition.

Avoiding "Blaming the Victim"

The successful extinction of maladaptive, extreme emotional displays is contingent on a number of factors. Most importantly, a validating environment must be created that allows the therapist to extinguish maladaptive behaviors while at the same time soothing, comforting, and cajoling the patient through the experience. The process is tricky and requires an enormous amount of therapist tolerance, willingness to experience emotional pain, and flexibility. Often, however, in conducting therapy, therapists may apply to borderline patients the same expectations as those placed on other patients. When the borderline patients cannot meet these expectations, the therapists may be tolerant for a period. But as the patients' display of negative emotions increases, the therapists' patience or willingness to tolerate the pain they themselves are experiencing runs out, and they then appease, punish, or terminate therapy with these patients. Clinicians experienced in working with borderline patients have perhaps recognized themselves in the earlier descriptions of invalidating, controlling environments and of the families who get caught in the vicious cycle of appeasing and punishing these patients. Such an environment, when recapitulated in therapy, is simply a continuation of the invalidating environment that the patients have experienced throughout their lives.

A most typical form of punishment of borderline patients consists of behaviors that, in sum, are both invalidating of the patients and "blaming the victims." Research in social psychology suggests that a number of factors are important in determining whether observers will blame victims of misfortune for their own misfortune. Relevant to the present topic are findings that in general, females are blamed more for misfortunes than are males in comparable situations (Howard, 1984). In the same research, Howard also found that when a victim is female, observers attribute blame to her character. However, when a victim is male, observers attribute blame to the male's behavior in the situation, not to his character. Other variables are also important: The observer has to care about the misfortune of the victim; the consequences have to be severe (Walster, 1966); and the observer has to feel helpless in controlling the outcome (Sacks & Bugental, 1987). Thus, when people care about what happens to others, they do not want these others to suffer, but they cannot keep misfortune or suffering from happening; they are likely to blame the victims for their own misfortune and suffering.

This is exactly the situation of therapy with most borderline patients. First, the "victims" are primarily women. Usually, their therapists care whether they are suffering. And certainly, few therapies to date have been shown to be particularly effective in stopping that suffering. Even if therapists believe that a particular treatment will be effective in the long run, because it has worked with other patients, helplessness in the face of the borderlines' intense suffering—suffering that causes the therapists reciprocal pain—is the repeated, day-to-day experience of working with these individuals. In the face of this helplessness the therapists may redouble their efforts. When the patients still do not improve, the therapists may begin to say that they are causing their own distress. The patients don't want to improve or change. They are resisting therapy. (After all, it works with almost everyone else.) They are playing games. They are too needy. In short, the therapists make a very fundamental but quite predictable cognitive error: They observe the consequence of behavior (e.g., emotional suffering for the patients or themselves) and attribute that consequence to internal motives on the part of the patients. I refer to this error repeatedly in further discussions of treatment of borderline patients.

"Blaming the victim" has important iatrogenic effects. First, it invalidates an individual's experience of her own problems. What the individual experiences as attempts to end pain are mislabeled as attempts to maintain the pain, to resist improving, or to do something else that the individual is not aware of. Thus, the individual learns to mistrust her own experience of herself. After some time, it is not unusual for the person to learn the point of view of the therapist, both because she does not trust her own self-observations and because doing so leads to more reinforcing outcomes. I once had a patient who was having immense trouble managing her homework practice; either she would not practice, or her practice attempts would not be successful. Simultaneously, she was repeatedly entreating me and my group coleader to help her feel better. One week, when I asked her what had interfered with her practicing her homework, she said with great conviction that she obviously did not want to be happy. If she did, she would have practiced her homework.

A key component of DBT is its insistence that the therapist refrain from blaming the victim for her own problems. This is not a position based on simple naiveté, although I have been accused of that. First, the caregiver's blaming of the victim usually leads to emotional distancing, negative emotions directed at the patient, decreased willingness to help, and punishment of the patient. Thus, the very help that is needed is more difficult to give. The caregiver becomes frustrated and often, but usually very subtly, strikes out at the patient. Because the punishment is not aimed at the actual source of the problem, it simply increases the patient's negative emotionality. A power struggle ensues—one that neither the patient nor the therapist can win.

Concluding Comments

It is important to keep in mind that the dialectical position presented here is a philosophical position. Thus, it can be neither proved nor disproved. For many, however, it is a difficult position to grasp. You may not see the need for it at first. Certainly, you can adopt some of DBT without necessarily embracing (or understanding) dialectics. If you are like me and my students, however, the idea will become more appealing over time and will subtly change your conceptualization of therapy issues. For me, it has had a profound effect on the way I conduct psychotherapy and the way I organize my treatment unit. DBT has been growing and changing continuously; the emerging implications of a dialectical perspective have been a source of much of the growth.

The biosocial theory I am presenting here is speculative. There has been little prospective research to document the application of this approach to the etiology of BPD. Although the theory is in accord with the known literature on BPD, no research has been mounted so far to test the theory prospectively. Thus, the reader should keep in mind that the logic of the biosocial formulation of BPD described in this chapter is based largely on clinical observation and speculation rather than on firm empirical experimentation. Caution is recommended.

Notes

1. My assistant at the time, Elizabeth Trias actually first pointed out the relationship of my experience to dialectics. Her husband was a student of Marxist philosophy.

2. Behaviors can also occur with or without awareness or attention and subsequently may be verbally reportable or unreportable by the individual. In more common parlance, they may or may not be available to consciousness. (See Greenwald, 1992, for a discussion of the emerging respectability of unconscious cognition in experimental psychology.)

3. There are a number of good reviews of research on basic emotional functioning. The reader is refered to the following: Barlow (1988), Buck (1984), Garber and Dodge (1991), Ekman, Levenson, and Friesen (1983), Izard, Kagan, and Zajonc (1984), Izard and Kobak (1991), Lang (1984), Lazarus (1991), Malatesta (1990), Schwartz (1982), and Tomkins (1982) for further reviews of this literature.

4. Kelly Koerner first pointed out that emotion dysregulation could be considered as the product of vulnerability plus the inability to modulate emotions.

5. Gerry Dawson and Mark Greenberg brought this finding and its relevance to invalidation to my attention.

3

Behavioral Patterns: Dialectical Dilemmas in the Treatment of Borderline Patients

Describing behavioral characteristics associated with BPD is a time-honored tradition. As Chapter 1 indicates, innumerable lists of borderline characteristics have been proposed over the years; thus, it is with some trepidation that I present yet another such list. The behavioral patterns discussed in this chapter, however, are not presented as diagnostic or definitional for BPD, nor are they a complete summary of important borderline characteristics. My views on these patterns evolved over a period of years while I struggled to get behavior therapy to work effectively for chronically parasuicidal and borderline patients. As I struggled, I felt that I was repeatedly being tripped up by the same sets of patient characteristics. Through the years, by a reciprocal process of observing (both in the clinic and the research literature) and constructing, I developed a picture of dialectical dilemmas posed by the borderline patient. The behavioral patterns associated with these dilemmas constitute the topic of this chapter.

Although these patterns are common, they are by no means universal among patients meeting criteria for BPD; thus, it is extremely important that their presence in a given case be assessed, not assumed. Given this caveat, I have found it useful for both myself and the patients to be aware of the influence on therapy of these particular patterns. Generally, their description strikes a resonant chord with the patients I treat and helps them achieve a better organization and understanding of their own behaviors. Since the seemingly inexplicable nature of their behavior (especially repetitive self-injuries) is often an important issue, this is no small achievement. Furthermore, the patterns and their interrelationships can have heuristic value in clarifying the development of the patients' problems.

These dilemmas are best viewed as a group of three dimensions defined by their opposite poles. These dialectical dimensions, illustrated in Figure 3.1 are as follows: (1) emotional vulnerability versus self-invalidation; (2) active passivity versus apparent competence; and (3) unrelenting crises versus inhibited grieving. If each dimension is conceptually divided at its midpoint, the characteristics above the midpoint—emotional vulnerability, active passivity, and unrelenting crises—are the ones that have been more influenced during development by the biological substrata for emotion regulation. Correspondingly, the characteristics below the midpoint—self-invalidation, apparent competence, and inhibited grieving—have been more influenced by the social consequences of emotional expression. A key point about these patterns is that the discomfort of the extreme points on each of these dimensions insures that borderline individuals vacillate back and forth between the polarities. Their inability to move to a balanced position representing a synthesis is the central dilemma of therapy.

Emotional Vulnerability versus Self-Invalidation

Emotional Vulnerability

General Characteristics

In Chapter 2, I have discussed the emotional vulnerability of individuals meeting criteria for BPD as a major component of emotion dysregulation, which acts as the person variable in a transactional development of borderline charac-

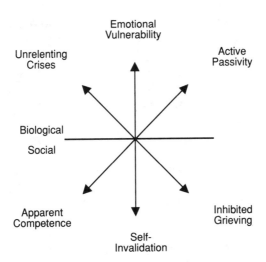

FIGURE 3.1. Borderline behavioral patterns: The three dialectical dimensions.

teristics. One of these borderline characteristics is *continuing* emotional vulnerability—that is, continuing emotional sensitivity, emotional intensity, and tenacity of negative emotional responses. Such vulnerability is, from my perspective, a core characteristic of BPD. When I discuss emotional vulnerability at this level, I am referring both to the individual's actual vulnerability and to her own simultaneous awareness and experience of that vulnerability.

There are four normal characteristics of frequent, high emotional arousal that make matters particularly difficult for the borderline individual. First, one must keep in mind that emotions are not simply internal physiological events, although physiological arousal certainly forms an important part of emotions. As I discussed more fully in Chapter 2, emotions are full-system responses. That is, they are integrated pattern of experiential, cognitive, and expressive, as well as physiological, responses. One component of a complex emotional response is not necessarily more basic than another. Therefore, the problem is not simply that borderline individuals cannot regulate physiological arousal; rather, they often have difficulty regulating the entire pattern of responses associated with particular emotional states. For example, they may not be able to modulate the hostile facial expression, aggressive action patterns, or verbal attacks associated with anger. Or they may not be able to interrupt obsessional worries or to inhibit escape behaviors associated with fear. If this point is kept in mind, then it is easier to understand the complexity of the problem facing borderline patients, as well as their tendency to be at times inexplicably dysfunctional across a wide range of behavioral areas.

Second, intense emotional arousal typically interferes with other ongoing behavioral responses. Thus, regulated, planned, and apparently functional coping behaviors can at times fall apart when interrupted by emotionally related stimuli. The frustration and disillusionment when this happens simply make matters worse. Furthermore, high arousal is associated with dichotomous, either–or thinking; obsessional and perseverative thought; physical distress, complaints, and illness; and avoidance and/or attack behaviors.

Third, high arousal and the inability to regulate it lead to a sense of being out of control and a certain unpredictability about the self. The unpredictability stems from the borderline person's inability to control the onset and offset of internal and external events that influence emotional responses, as well as an inability to modulate her own response to such events. It is made worse by the fact that at unpredictable times the individual does succeed at controlling her emotional responses. The problem here is that the timing and duration of this emotional regulation is unpredictable to the individual (and to others as well). The quality of this experience for the borderline person is that of a nightmare she cannot wake up from.

Finally, this lack of control leads to some specific fears that increase emotional vulnerability still further. First, the borderline person fears situations where she has less control over events (usually new situations, as well as those where previous difficulties have been experienced). The borderline patient's frequent attempts to gain control of the therapeutic situation make perfect sense once this aspect of emotional vulnerability is understood. Second, the patient often has an intense fear of behavioral expectations from individuals she cares about. This fear is reasonable in light of the fact that she experiences dyscontrol not only of private emotional responses, but also of behavior patterns that are contingent on particular emotional states. (For example, studying for an exam requires an ability to concentrate that may be difficult to maintain during periods of high anxiety, overwhelming sadness, or intense anger.) Dyscontrol and unpredictability make environmental expectations fraught with difficulty. The patient can meet expectations at one moment, in one emotional state, that she may not be able to meet at another time.

An important aspect of this particular problem is the association of praise with expectations. Praise, besides communicating approval, also commonly communicates an acknowledgment that the individual *can* emit the praised behavior and an expectation that she can do so again in the future. This is precisely what the borderline individual believes she may not be able to do. Although I have presented the fear of praise here as cognitively mediated, such mediation is not necessary. All that is required is that the individual has past experiences where praise is followed by expectations; expectations are followed by failure to meet the expectations; and disapproval or punishment follows. Just such a sequence of behaviors is typical in the invalidating environment.

The net effect of these emotional difficulties is that borderline individuals are the psychological equivalent of third-degree burn patient. They simply have, so to speak, no emotional skin. Even the slightest touch or movement can create immense suffering. Yet, on the other hand, life is movement. Therapy, at its best, requires both movement and touch. Thus, both the therapist and the process of therapy itself cannot fail to cause intensely painful emotional experiences for the borderline patient. Both the therapist and the patient must have the courage to encounter the pain that arises. It is the experience of their own vulnerability that sometimes leads borderline individuals to extreme behaviors (including suicidal behaviors), both to try to take care of themselves and to alert the environment to take better care of them. Completed suicide among borderline individuals is inevitably an act of final hopelessness that the vulnerability will ever lessen. It is sometimes also a last communication that more care was needed.

Understanding this vulnerability and keeping it in mind are crucial for therapeutic effectiveness. All too often, unfortunately, therapists fail or forget to recognize borderline patients' vulnerability. The problem is that whereas burn victims' sensitivity and the reason for it are apparent to all, borderline individuals' sensitivity is often hidden. For reasons that I discuss later, borderline individuals tend at times to appear to others, including their therapists, deceptively less emotionally vulnerable than they are. One consequence of this state of affairs is that the sensitivity of borderline patient's is far more difficult to comprehend and keep in mind than that of burn victims. We can imagine not having physical skin; it is harder for most of us to imagine what life would be like if we were always emotionally vulnerable or did not have psychological skin ourselves. That is the life of borderline patients.

Anger and Borderline Personality Disorder

Difficulties with anger have been part of the definition of BPD in each edition of the DSM since 1980. In psychoanalytic thought (e.g., Kernberg's theories; see Kernberg, 1984), an excess of hostile affect is viewed as a fundamental etiological factor in the development of BPD. Much of the current treatment of borderline patients is aimed at interpreting behavior in light of its presumed underlying hostility and aggressive intent. A noted psychoanalyst once said to me that all phone calls from patients to therapists at home are acts of aggression. Nearly every time I show a videotape of a therapy session with one of my own patients, someone in the audience interprets a patient's silence, withdrawal, or passive behavior as an aggressive attack on me. Patients in our group therapy often discuss their difficulties in convincing other mental health professionals that their behavior, or at least some of it, is not a reflection of angry and hostile feelings.

Clearly, the experience of anger and hostile/aggressive behaviors play an important role in BPD. However, from my perspective, other negative emotions such as sadness and depression; shame, guilt, and humiliation; and fear, anxiety, and panic are equally important. It stands to reason that a person who is emotionally intense and has generalized difficulty regulating emotions will have specific problems with anger. But whether all or most of borderline behavior is interpreted as associated with anger seems to me to depend largely on who is interpreting the behavior rather than on the actual behavior or its motivation. Often hostile intent is inferred simply on the basis of aversive consequences of the behavior. If the patient's behavior is frustrating or annoying to the therapist, then the patient must mean it to be so — if not consciously, then unconsciously. Although I have no data to back up this point, I sometimes wonder also whether the tendency to infer anger and aggression rather than fear and desperation is not tied to the gender of the observer. One of the few true gender differences is that males are more aggressive than females (Maccoby & Jacklin, 1978); perhaps men are also more likely to see aggressive intent. Theorists who have promulgated anger and coping with hostile motives as essential in the etiology of BPD are, of course, men (e.g., Kernberg, Gunderson, Masterson).[1]

In my experience, much of the borderline behavior that is interpreted as stemming from hostile motives and anger stems in reality from fear, panic, hopelessness, and desperation. (This is similar to Masterson's [1976] position that fear of abandonment underlies much of borderline psychopathology.) The patient who on one of my videotapes is silent and nonresponsive is often struggling to control a panic attack that includes (according to her later descriptions) sensations of choking and fears of dying. Although the panic response itself may stem from the initial, rudimentary experience of anger-related feelings, thoughts, or bodily reactions, this does not mean that the subsequent behavior is aggressive per se or hostile in intent. The overinterpretation of anger and hostile intent, however, can itself generate hostility and anger. Thus, such interpretations create a self-fulfilling prophecy especially when rigidly applied.

Although problems with anger and anger expression may reflect more generalized emotional intensity and dysregulation, they may also be a consequence of other dysregulated negative affective states. Arousal of negative emotions and discomfort of any kind can activate anger-related feelings, action tendencies, and thoughts and memories. Leonard Berkowitz (1983, 1989, 1990) has proposed a cognitive-neoassociationistic model of anger formation. The basic idea is that as a result of various genetic, learned, and situational factors, negative affect and discomfort activate an associative network of initial, rudimentary fear and anger experiences. Subsequent higher order cognitive processing of the initial aversive experience and affect may then give rise to the full development of the anger emotion and experience. According to Berkowitz, therefore, anger and its expression are likely consequences (rather than causes) of more generalized emotional intensity and dysregulation of negative emotional states. He reviews a fair body of data to demonstrate that negative emotional states and discomfort other than anger can produce angry feelings and hostile inclinations. In line with this position, Berkowitz has written that "suffering is seldom ennobling. It is the unusual individual among humanity in general whose character is improved as a result of undergoing painful or even merely unpleasant experiences. . . . When [all] people feel bad, they are all too likely to have angry feelings, hostile thoughts and memories and aggressive inclinations" (Berkowitz, 1990, p. 502).

Unregulated anger and anger expression can, of course, cause any number of other life difficulties. This may be especially the case among women, in whom even mild expressions of anger may be interpreted as aggression. For example, behavior that is labeled as "assertive" in men may be labeled "aggressive" in women (Rose & Tron, 1979). Perceived aggression begets retaliatory aggression, and thus the cycle of interpersonal conflict is born. Depending on one's previous learning history, the emotion of anger itself may also be experienced as so unacceptable that it sets off further emotional reactions of shame and panic. These emotions themselves may contribute to an escalation of the original anger response, increasing distress still further. Or attempts to block direct anger expression and inhibit the emotional response may develop. With time, a pattern of expressive inhibition and overcontrol of anger experiences may become the preferred manner of responding to anger-provoking situations. Passive, helpless behavior may ensue. I take up the topic of the relative merits of direct anger expression versus inhibition later in this chapter.

Self-Invalidation

"Self-invalidation" refers to the adoption by an individual of characteristics of the invalidating environment. Thus, the borderline individual tends to invalidate her own affective experiences, to look to others for accurate reflections of external reality, and to oversimplify the ease of solving life's problems. Invalidation of affective experiences leads to attempts to inhibit emotional experiences and expression. The person's failure to trust her own perceptions of reality prohibits development of a sense of identity or confidence in her own self. Oversimplification of life's difficulties leads inevitably to self-hate following failure to achieve goals.

Outside of clinical observations, empirical support for self-invalidation among borderline individuals is meager. However, a number of problems with emotions can be expected as a result of experiencing an invalidating environment. First, the experience itself of negative emotions can be affected by the invalidating environment. The pressure to inhibit negative emotional expressions interferes with developing the ability to sense postural and muscular expressive (especially facial) changes associated with basic emotions. Such sensing is an integral part of emotional behavior. Second, in such an environment the individual does not learn to label her own negative emotional reactions accurately. Thus, the ability to articulate emotions clearly and to communicate them verbally does not develop. Such inability further increases the emotional invalidation that the environment, and eventually the individual herself, delivers. It is difficult for a person to validate an emotional experience that she does not understand.

A third effect of an invalidating environment, especially when basic emotions such as anger, fear, and sadness are invalidated, is that a person in such an environment does not learn when to trust her own emotional responses as valid reflections of individual and situational events. Thus, she is unable to validate and trust herself. That is, if a child is told that she should not be experiencing particular emotions, then she has to doubt her original observations or interpretations of reality. If communication of negative emotions is punished, as it often is in an invalidating environment, then a response of shame follows experiencing the intense emotion in the first place and expressing it publicly in the second. Thus, a new secondary negative emotion is set in motion. The person learns to respond to her own emotional responses as her environment has modeled—with shame, criticism, and punishment. Compassion for self, and compassionate self-directed behaviors, rarely develop in such an atmosphere. A vicious cycle is set up, since one effective way to reduce the shame following negative emotions is to get the environment to validate the original emotion. Often the borderline individual learns that either an extreme emotional display or presentation of extreme circumstances is necessary to provoke a validating environmental response. In such an environment, the individual learns that both escalation of the original emotional response and exaggerated, but convincing, presentation of negative circumstances elicit validation from the environment. Sometimes other positive responses, such as nurturance and warmth, come along with the validation. The individual thus flips back to the emotionally vulnerable pole of this dimension of borderline experience. The alternative to seeking validation from the environment is simply to change or at least to modulate one's emotional responses in accord with environmental expectations; the inability to regulate affect, however, precludes such a solution for the borderline individual.

In such an environment, it is understandable that the child develops a tendency to scan the environment for what to think and how to feel. The child is punished for relying on private experiences. This pattern of events can account for the problems many borderline patients have in maintaining a point of view in the face of disagreement or criticism, as well as for their frequent tendency to try to extract validation for their point of view from the environment. If relying on private experiences has not been rewarded, and conforming to public experiences has been, an individual has two options: She can try to change the public's experience by persuasive tactics, or she can change her own experience to conform to the public experience. In my experience, borderline patients tend to cycle between these two options.

As the cycle continues, both the original emotional distress and the subsequent shame and self-criticism increase. Breaking into such a cycle can be particularly difficult for the therapist. At one and the same time, the patient is seeking validation for a painful emotion and communicating such intense distress that the therapist empathetically wishes to help reduce the pain as quickly as possible. The most common mistake therapists make in such instances is to move to change the painful original affect (thereby invalidating it), rather than to validate the original emotion and thereby reduce the surrounding shame.

A fourth effect of invalidating environments is that individuals adopt the invalidating behavior change tactics and apply these tactics to themselves. Thus, borderline individuals often set unreasonably high behavioral expectations for themselves. They simply have no concept of the notion of shaping—that is, gradual improvement. Thus, they tend to berate and otherwise punish rather than to reward themselves for approximations to their goal behaviors. Such a self-regulation strategy insures failure and eventual giving up. I have rarely encountered a borderline patient who could spontaneously use reward over punishment as a method of behavior change. Although punishment may be very effective in the short term, it is often ineffective over the long run. Among other negative effects, punishment, especially in the form of self-criticism and blame, elicits guilt. Although moderate guilt may be an efficient way to motivate behavior, excessive guilt, like any intense negative emotion, can disrupt thought and behavior. Often, to reduce the guilt these individuals simply avoid the situation that generate the guilt, thereby avoiding the requisite behavior changes to correct the problem. Persuading borderline patients to forgo punishment and utilize principles of reinforcement is one of the major struggles of behavior therapy with them.

The preference for punishment over reinforcement probably arises from two sources. First, since punishment is the only behavior change tactic she knows, a borderline individual fears that if she does not apply severe punishment to herself, she will slip even further from desired behaviors. The consequence of such slippage is further dyscontrol of her own behavior, and therefore of rewards from the environment. The fear is such that attempts by the therapist to interfere with the punishment cycle sometimes elicit a panic response. Second, an invalidating environment with its emphasis on individual responsibility, teaches that transgressions from desired behavior merit punishment. Borderline patients often find it difficult to believe that they deserve anything other than punishment and pain. Indeed, a number report that they deserve to die.

The Dialectical Dilemma for the Patient

The juxtaposition of an emotionally vulnerable temperament with an invalidating environment presents a number of interesting dilemmas for the borderline patient and has important implications for understanding suicidal behavior in particular, especially as it occurs in psychotherapy. The patient's first dilemma has to do with whom to blame for her predicament. Is she evil, the cause of her own troubles? Or, are other people in the environment or fate to blame? The second, closely related dilemma has to do with who is right. Is the patient really vulnerable and unable to control her own behavior and reactions, as she feels herself to be? Or is she bad, able to control her reactions but unwilling to do so, as the environment tells her? What the borderline individual seems unable to do is to hold both of these contradictory positions in mind at the same time, or to synthesize them. Thus, she vacillates between the two poles. Put simplistically, the borderline patients I see frequently travel between these two opposing orientations to their own behavior. Either they invalidate themselves with a passion and believe that all bad things that happen to them are fair consequences of their own evilness; or they validate their own vulnerability, often simultaneously invalidating fate and the laws of the universe, believing that all of the negative things that happen to them are unfair and should not be happening.

At the first of these extremes, the borderline individual adopts the emotionally invalidating attitude herself, often in an extreme manner, oversimplifying the ease of achieving behavioral goals and emotional goals. The inevitable failure associated with such excessive aspirations is met with shame, extreme self-criticism, and self-punishment, including suicidal behavior. The person deserves to be the way she is. The suffering she has endured is justified because she is so bad. Problems in living are the result of their own willfulness. Failure is attributed to lack of motivation, even in the face of evidence to the contrary. They resemble the powerful person who despises anyone weak, or the terrorist who attacks those who show fear. Rarely have I seen such vengeance as that of borderline individuals' hatred toward themselves. One patient of mine becomes so outraged at herself that in sessions she has clawed her face and legs, leaving long raw scratches. Suicide or parasuicide, from this orientation, is primarily an act of self-directed hostility.

At the other extreme, the borderline individual at times is keenly aware of her emotional and behavioral lack of control. Aspirations are consequently lowered by the individual, but not by the environment. Recognition of the discrepancy between her own capacities for emotional and behavioral control, and excessive demands and criticism on the part of the environment, can lead to both anger and attempts to prove to significant individuals the error of their ways. How better to do that than suicidal behavior or some other form of extreme behavior? Such communication can be essential if the person is to get the help she believes is needed. It is especially likely, of course, when an invalidating interpersonal environment responds in a compassionate and helpful manner only to extreme expressions of distress. Also, the borderline person does not have clear guidelines as to what she should believe when there is a disagreement—her own experience or that of others, particularly the therapist's. Suicidal behavior validates the individual's own sense of vulnerability, reducing the ambiguity of the double messages coming from her own experience versus that of the therapist.

From this orientation, borderline individuals not only validate their own vulnerability, but also invalidate the behavioral and biological laws that have been instrumental in making and keeping them what they are. They are acutely aware of the unfairness of their existence. At times they believe that somehow the universe is capable of being fair, is fair to almost everyone else, should have been fair to them in the first place, and could be fair to them if they simply figure out the right things to do. At other times, however, they are extremely hopeless that they will in fact ever figure out the right things to do. They may experience themselves as good people, or at least wanting to be, with uncontrollable and thereby hopeless flaws. Each behavioral transgression is followed by intense shame, guilt, and remorse. They are vases in a pottery shop that are cracked, broken, and ugly, put on the back shelf where customers do not see them. Although they try their best to find glue to repair themselves, or fresh clay to refashion their shape, their efforts are ultimately not enough to render them acceptable.

In the center of intense emotional pain and vulnerability, the borderline individual frequently believes that others (particularly the therapist) could take away the pain if only they would. (One could almost say that they have trust disorder as opposed to paranoid disorder!) The collision of this firm and sometimes stridently expressed expectation with the therapist's equally intense experience of helplessness anad ineffectiveness sets the stage for one of the most frequent dramas in therapy with borderline patients. In the face of inadequate help, the patient's emotional pain and out-of-control behavior escalate. The patient feels uncared for, deeply hurt, and misunderstood. The therapist feels manipulated and equally misunderstood. Both are poised to withdraw or attack.

Patience, acceptance, and self-compassion, together with gradual attempts at change, self-management, and self-soothing, are both the ingredients and the outcome of synthesis of vulnerability and invalidation. They elude the borderline individual, however. Interestingly, such a pattern of alternating excessive and depressed aspirations has also been found to characterize individuals who have (in a Pavlovian sense) weak, highly reactive nervous systems—that is, who are emotionally vulnerable (Krol, 1977, cited by Strelau, Farley, & Gale, 1986).

The Dialectical Dilemma for the Therapist

These two interrelated patterns may provide us a clue as to why therapy with the borderline patient is sometimes iatrogenic. To the extent that the therapist creates an invalidating environment within the therapy, then the patient may be expected to react strongly. Common instances of invalidation include a therapist's offering or insisting on an interpretation of behavior that is not shared by the patient; setting firm expectations for performance over what the patient can (or believes she can) accomplish; treating the patient as less competent than she actually is; failing to give the patient the help that would be given if the therapist believed the patient's current perspective to be valid; criticizing or otherwise punishing the patient's behavior; ignoring important communications or actions of the patient; and so on. Suffice it to say that in most therapy relationships (even good ones) a fair amount of invalidation is common. In a stressful relationship, such as that with a borderline patient, there is probably even more.

The experience of invalidation is generally aversive, and a borderline patient's emotional reactions to it may vary: anger at the therapist for being so insensitive; a feeling of intense dysphoria at being so misunderstood and alone; anxiety and panic because of the feeling that a therapist who cannot understand and validate the patient's current state cannot help; or shame and humiliation at experiencing and expressing such emotions, thoughts, and behaviors. Behavioral reactions to invalidation can include avoidance behaviors, increased efforts at communication and gaining validation, and attacking the therapist. The most extreme form of avoidance, of course, is suicide. Less drastically, the patients may simply quit therapy or start missing or coming late for sessions. (The high therapy dropout rates among borderline and parasuicidal patients probably result, in part, from difficulties therapists have in validating these patients.) Depersonalization and dissociative phenomena can be other forms of avoidance, as can simply shutting down and verbally withdrawing within therapy sessions. A patient may increase communication efforts by various means, including calling the therapist between sessions, making extra appointments, writing letters, and soliciting friends or other mental health professionals to call the therapist. As I have noted above, suicidal behaviors can at times serve as communication attempts. (It is crucial, however, that the therapist *not* assume that all suicidal behavior is communication behavior.)

Attacks on the therapist are most often verbal: The patient judges and blames, with little empathy for the difficulties the therapist may be experiencing in trying to understand and validate the patient. In my time, I have been called more pejorative names and had my motives attacked more often by borderline patients than by any other group of individuals I can think of. At times, however, attacks on the therapist can be physical; these often consist of attacks on the property of the therapist. For example, patients in our clinic have broken clocks, torn bulletin boards apart, stolen mail, thrown objects, kicked holes in walls, and written graffiti on walls. Such attacks, of course, set up a reciprocal cycle, because the therapist often attacks the patient back. Counterattacks by a therapist are often disguised as therapeutic responses.

The dilemma for the therapist is that attempts at inducing change in the patient and sympathetic understanding of the patient as she is are equally likely to be experienced as invalidating. For example, in reviewing how a particular interaction went wrong or why some goal was not reached, if the therapist in any way implies that the patient could improve her performance the next time, the patient is likely to respond that the therapist must be assuming that the patient has been wrong all along and that the invalidating environment is right. A battle ensues, and attention to behavior change and skill training is diverted. In my experience, many of the day-to-day difficulties in treating this population result from therapists' invalidation of patients' experiences and difficulties. On the other hand, if a therapist uses a non-change oriented tactic—listening to the patient or sympathetically validating the patient's responses—then the patient is likely to panic at the prospect that life will never improve. If she is right, and has been right all along, then this must be the best that can be hoped for. In this case the therapist can expect eventual anger for not being more helpful. Demands for more therapist involvement and concrete suggestions for change ensue. A vicious cycle is begun—one that often wears out both patient and therapist alike.

The experience of this dilemma, perhaps more than anything else, was my primary impetus for developing DBT. Standard behavior therapy (including standard cognitive–behavioral therapy) by itself, at least as I practiced it, invalidated my patients. I was telling them that either their behavior was wrong or their thinking was irrational or problematic in some way. Therapies that failed to teach, however, failed to recognize the very real skill deficits of these individuals. Accepting their pain invalidated it in some senses. It was like being an expert swimmer with a life raft handy, leaving people who couldn't swim to fend for themselves in the middle of the ocean, yelling (in a soothing voice); "You can make it! You can stand it!" The solution, at least in DBT, has been to combine the two treatment strategies. Thus, the treatment calls for a therapist to interact with a patient in a flexible manner that combines keen observation of patient reactions with moment-to-moment changes in the use of supportive acceptance versus confrontation and change strategies.

The dialectical balance that the therapist must strive for is to validate the essential wisdom of each patient's experiences (especially her vulnerabilities and sense of desperation), *and* to teach the patient the requisite capabilities for change to occur. This requires the therapist to combine and juxtapose validation strategies with capability enhancement strategies (skills training). The tension created the patient's alternating excessively between high and low aspirations and expectations relative to her own capabilities offers a formidable challenge to the therapist.

Active Passivity versus Apparent Competence

Active Passivity

The defining characteristic of "active passivity" is the tendency to approach problems passively and helplessly, rather than actively and determinedly, as well as a corresponding tendency under extreme distress to demand from the environment (and often the therapist) solutions to life's problems. Thus, the individual is active in trying to get others to solve her problems or regulate her behavior, but is passive about solving problems on her own. This mode of coping is quite similar to "emotion-focused coping," described by Lazarus and Folkman (1984). Emotion-focused coping consists of responding to stress-provoking situations with efforts to reduce the negative emotional reactions to the situation—for example, by distracting or seeking comfort from others. This contrasts with "problem-focused coping," in which the individual takes direct action to solve the problem. It is this tendency to seek help actively from the environment that differentiates active passivity from learned helplessness. In both cases, the individual is helpless in solving her own problems. However, in learned helplessness, the individual simply gives up and does not even try to get help from the environment. In active passivity, the person continues to try to solicit problem solutions from others, including the therapist.

At times it is this very demand for an immediate problem solution from the therapist, when the therapist does not have one to give, that leads into the cycle of invalidating the patient. Escalating, desperate demands can precipitate a crisis for a therapist. In the face of such helplessness, he or she may begin either to blame or to reject the "victim." Such rejection further exacerbates the problem, leading to further demands, and the vicious cycle is born. Passivity in the face of overwhelming and apparently unsolvable problems with life and self-regulation, of course, does not help remediate such problems, although it may be effective at short-term regulation of the negative affect that accompanies them. The question of whether problems are indeed solvable is, of course, often a bone of contention between patient and therapist. The therapist may believe that the problems can be solved if the patient will just begin to engage actively in coping; by contrast, the patient often views them as hopeless no matter what she does. From the patient's perspective, either there is no solution or there is no problem-solving behavior that the patient believes herself able to produce. The patient's self-efficacy beliefs are discrepant from the therapist's beliefs in the patient's inherent problem-solving ability. Indeed, a passive regulation style, including distraction and problem avoidance, may even be encouraged by the therapist if the therapist also views the problems as unsolvable.

A passive self-regulation style is probably a result of the individual's temperamental disposition as well as the individual's history of failing in attempts to control both negative affects and associated maladaptive behaviors. For example, Bialowas (1976) (cited by Strelau et al., 1986) found a positive relationship between high autonomic reactivity and dependency in a social influence situation. Interesting research by Eliasz (1974, cited by Strelau et al. 1986) suggests that people with high autonomic reactivity, independent of other considerations, will prefer passive self-regulation styles — that is, styles that involve minimal active efforts to improve their own abilities and their environment.

Miller and Mangan (1983) conducted research relevant to this topic on patients' behaviors during medical visits. They found that patients who were alert for and sensitized to the negative or potentially negative aspects of an experience ("high monitors") were more highly concerned with being treated with kindness and respect, getting tests done, getting new prescriptions, getting reassurance about the effects of stress on their health, and wanting more information than were "low monitors." Most important to the points here, they also desired a less active role in their own medical care; in fact, twice as many high monitors as low monitors wanted to play a completely passive role in their own care. Thus, active passivity may not be entirely a result of learning, although a history of failing in efforts to control both themselves and aversive environments is very likely important.

It is easy to see how an active-passivity orientation can be learned. Borderline individuals observe their frequent inability to interact successfully. They are aware of their own unhappiness, hopelessness, and inability to see the world from a positive point of view, as well as their simultaneous inability to maintain an uncracked facade of happiness, hope, and untroubled calm. These observations can lead to a pattern of learned helplessness. The experience of failure despite one's best efforts is often a precursor of such a pattern. In addition, in an environment where difficulties are not recognized, the individual never learns how to deal with problems actively and effectively. Learning such coping strategies requires, at a minimum, the recognition of a problem. In an environment where difficulties are minimized, an individual learns to magnify them so that they will be taken seriously. It is this magnified view of difficulties and incompetence that further characterizes active passivity. The individual balances the failure to recognize inadequacy with extreme inadequacy and passivity.

Empirical support for the active-passivity pattern can be found in work on both parasuicidal and borderline individuals. In my research, inpatients admitted for an immediately preceding parasuicide, compared to both suicide ideators and nonsuicidal psychiatric inpatients, showed markedly lower active interpersonal problem solving and somewhat higher passive problem solving. Active problem solving in this research consisted of an individual's taking actions that led to problem resolution; passive problem solving consisted of getting another person to solve the problems (Linehan et al., 1987). Perry and Cooper (1985) report an association between BPD and low self-efficacy, high dependency, and emotional reliance on others.

The inability to protect themselves from extreme aversive emotions, and the consequent sense of helplessness, hopelessness, and desperation, can be important factors in borderline individuals' frequent interpersonal overdependency. People who cannot solve their own affective and interpersonal problems must either tolerate the aversive conditions or reach out to others for problem resolution. When the psychic pain is extreme and/or distress tolerance is low, this reaching out turns to emotional clinging and demanding behaviors. In turn, this dependency predictably leads to intense emotional responses to the loss or threat of loss of interpersonally significant people. Frantic attempts to avoid abandonment are consistent with this constellation.

The role of cultural gender bias and sex-role stereotypes in inducing active passivity on the part of women cannot be overlooked. In general, females tend to learn interpersonal achievement styles that are effective because they elicit help and protection from others (Hoffman, 1972). Furthermore, women are often restricted by cultural norms and expectations to indirect, personal, and helpless modes of influence (Johnson, 1976). Gender differences show up at an early age. Observation studies of school children, for example, indicates that following criticism boys respond with active efforts, whereas girls tend more to fall into the passive mode of giving up and blaming their own abilities (Dweck & Bush, 1976; Dweck, Davidson, Nelson, & Emde, 1978). Although school-age girls do not, in general, have more stressful events than do school-age boys (Goodyer, Kolvin, & Gatzanis, 1986), it is possible that girls experience more situations that fit the learned helplessness paradigm than do boys. Certainly, the data on sexual abuse suggest such a possibility. As I have discussed in some detail in Chapter 2, the degree of social support received—in particular, the degree of intimacy—is more closely associated with well-being among women than among men. Thus, the emotional dependence characteristic of borderline individuals may at times be simply an extreme variation of an interpersonal style common to many women. It is also possible that the dependent style characteristic of borderline individuals would not be viewed as pathological in other cultures.

Apparent Competence

"Apparent competence" refers to the tendency of borderline individuals to appear competent and able to cope with everyday life at some times, and at other times to behave (unexpectedly, to the observer) as if the observed competencies did not exist. For example, an individual may act appropriately assertive in work settings where she feels confident and in control, but may be unable to produce assertive responses in intimate relationships where she feels less in control. Impulse control while in the therapist's office may not generalize to settings outside his or her office. A patient who appears to be in a neutral or even positive mood when she leaves a therapy session may call the therapist hours later and report extreme distress as a result of the session. Several weeks or months of successful coping with life's problems may be followed by a crisis and behavioral retreat to ineffective coping and extreme emotion dysregulation. An ability to regulate affect expression in some social situations may seem completely absent in other situations. In many instances, borderline individuals exhibit very good interpersonal skills and are often good at assisting others in dealing with their own problems in living; yet they cannot apply these same skills to their own lives.

The idea for the apparent-competence pattern first came to me in working with one of my patients, whom I will call Susan. Susan was a systems analyst for a large corporation. She came to therapy well dressed, had an attractive demeanor, was humorous, and reported good performance reviews at work. Over a number of months, she repeatedly asked me for advice on how to handle interpersonal problems with her boss. She appeared very interpersonally competent, however, and I was convinced that she had the requisite skills. So I kept trying to analyze the factors inhibiting her use of skills I presumed she already had. She continued to insist that she simply couldn't think of how to approach her boss on particular matters. Although I still believed that she really had the requisite skills, I suggested one day, in exasperation and frustration, that we role-play how to handle a particular situation. I played her and she played her boss. After the role play, she expressed amazement at how I had handled the situation. She remarked that she had simply never thought of that way of approaching the problem. She readily agreed to approach her boss and use the new approach I had modeled. The next week she reported success. Certainly, this interaction did not prove that Susan did not have the requisite capabilities before our role play. Perhaps the role play conveyed information about the social rules for behavior with bosses; perhaps I simply gave her "permission" to use skills she already had. But I could not discount the possibility that I had insisted Susan had skills that she, in fact, did not have in the situation where she needed them.

A number of factors seem to be responsible for the apparent competence of the borderline individual. First, the individual's competence is extremely variable and conditional. As Millon (1981) has suggested, the borderline person is "stably unstable." The observer, however, expects competencies that are expressed under one set of conditions to generalize and be expressed under similar (to the observer) conditions. However, in the borderline individual, such competencies often do not generalize. Data on situation-specific learning suggest that generalization of behaviors across different situational contexts is not to be expected in many cases (see Mischel, 1968, 1984, for reviews); what makes the borderline patient unique is the influence of mood-dependent learning combined with situation-specific learning. In particular, behavioral capabilities that the individual has in one mood state she frequently does not have in another. If, furthermore, the individual has little control of emotional states (which is to be expected of persons with deficient emotional regulation), then for all practical purposes she has little control over her behavioral capabilities.

A second factor influencing apparent competence has to do with the borderline individual's failure to communicate her vulnerability clearly to the other significant people in her life, including the therapist. At times the borderline individual automatically inhibits nonverbal expression of negative emotional experiences even when such expression is appropriate and expected. Thus, she may be experiencing inner turmoil and psychic pain while at the same time communicating apparent calmness and control. Her manner often appears competent and communicates to others that she is feeling fine and in control. The competent appearance is sometimes enhanced by the borderline individual's adopting and expressing the beliefs of her environment— namely, that she is competent across related situations and over time. In one mood state or context, the individual has difficulty predicting herself in different states or situations. This smiling, competent facade is easily mistaken by others for an accurate reflection of transsituational reality under all or most conditions. When in another emotional state or situation the individual communicates helplessness, the observer often interprets such behavior as simply feigning helplessness to get attention or to frustrate others.

This inhibition of negative emotional expression probably stems from the social learning effects of being raised in an invalidating environment. As Chapter 2 has described, invalidating environments reward the inhibition of negative affect expression. Emphasis is put on achievement, personal control, and smiling in the face of adversity.[2] To make matters even more difficult, most borderline patients in my experience are unaware that they are not communicating their vulnerability. One of two things may be happening here. First, an individual sometimes communicates verbally that she is in distress, but her nonverbal cues do not support such a message. Or the patient may discuss a personally vulnerable topic and experience intensely negative affect, but may not communicate (verbally or nonverbally) the experience of that affect. In either instance, however, the patient typically believes that she has communicated clearly. In the first case, she believes that a simple description of how she feels, independent of nonverbal expressiveness, is sufficient. She may not be aware that the nonverbal message is discordant. In the second case, the patient believes that the context itself is sufficient communication. Yet when others fail to pick up the message, the individual is usually quite distressed. This failure is understandable, however, since most individuals faced with discrepant verbal and nonverbal affect cues will trust the nonverbal over the verbal cues.

I have had patients who calmly and in an ordinary tone say to me, almost offhandedly, that they are so depressed they are thinking of killing themselves. Or a patient may talk about a recent rejection, stating that she feels frantic at the loss, in a voice as casual as if she were discussing the weather. One of my patients, who was single and heavier than norms for women her age, would inevitably get extremely despondent when talking about either her weight or her marital status; however, except for the topic, I would never have known. Indeed, the patient presented such a cogent argument for a feminist perspective that I might have reasonably believed that she had mastered her cultural conditioning on the topics. Discussions of sexual abuse often have the same effect.

A third factor influencing apparent competence has to do with the borderline individual's reaction to interpersonal relationships. The typical patient I work with appears to have access to emotional and behavioral competence under two conditions: Either she is in the actual presence of a supportive, nurturing individual, or she perceives herself to be in a secure, supportive, and stable relationship with a significant other person even when the other person is not physically present. This is perhaps why the borderline individual often appears so competent when with her therapist; usually, the therapist is a supportive, nurturing individual. Rarely, however is the therapeutic relationship itself perceived as secure and stable. Thus, when the therapist is not present, the influence is reduced. Although this may be due to a failure in evocative memory, as Adler (1985) suggests, it also may have to do with the generally less secure nature of a therapeutic relationship. Indeed, therapy relationships are defined by the fact that they end. For many borderline patients, they end prematurely and abruptly. The beneficial effects of relationships, of course, are not unique to borderline patients; we all do better when we have stable, supportive social support networks (see Sarason, Sarason, & Shearin, 1986, for a review). The difference is the magnitude of the discrepancy between borderline patients' capabilities in and out of supportive relationships.

It is not clear why relationships have such an effect on these individuals. A number of factors may be important. It is not difficult to imagine how social learning can account for this phenomenon. If a child is reinforced for being competent and happy when around people and is sent to be alone when acting otherwise, it seems reasonable that the child may learn competence and happiness when with people. For an individual who is deficient in self-regulation and therefore relies on regulation from the environment, being alone may become fraught with danger. The anxiety that results from not having access to a helping relationship may disrupt the person's affect sufficiently to start the negative affect cycle that eventually interferes with competent behavior. In addition, the well-known phenomenon of performance facilitation in the presence of other individuals (Zajonc, 1965) may simply be more potent with borderline patients.

The appearance of competence can fool others, including the therapist, into believing that the borderline individual is more competent than she actually is. The discrepancy between appearance and actuality simply perpetuates the invalidating environment. The absence of expected competence is attributed to lack of motivation, "not trying," playing games, manipulations, or other factors discrepant with the individual's phenomenal experience. Thus, a major consequence of this borderline syndrome is that it supports the therapist and others in "blaming the victim" and blinds them to the patient's need for assistance in learning new behavioral patterns.

The Dialectical Dilemma for the Patient

The borderline individual is faced with an apparently irreconcilable dilemma. On the one hand, she has tremendous difficulties with self-regulation of affect and subsequent behavioral competence. She frequently but somewhat unpredictably needs a great deal of assistance, often feels helpless and hopeless, and is afraid of being left alone to fend for herself in a world where she has failed over and over again. Without the ability to predict and control her own well-being, she depends on her social environment to regulate her affect and behavior. On the other hand, she experiences intense shame at behaving dependently in a society that cannot tolerate dependency, and has learned to inhibit expressions of negative affect and helplessness whenever the affect is within controllable limits. Indeed, when in a positive mood, she may be exceptionally competent across a variety of situations. However, in the positive mood state she has difficulty predicting her own behavioral capabilities in a different mood, and thus communicates to others an ability to cope beyond her capabilities. Thus, the borderline individual, even though at times desperate for help, has great difficulty asking for help appropriately or communicating her needs.

The inability to integrate or synthesize the notions of helplessness and competence, of noncontrol and control, and of needing and not needing help can lead to further emotional distress and dysfunctional behaviors. Believing that she is competent to "succeed," the person may experience intense guilt about her presumed lack of motivation when she falls short of objectives. At other times, she experiences extreme anger at others for their lack of understanding and unrealistic expectations. Both the intense guilt and the intense anger can lead to dysfunctional behaviors, including suicide and parasuicide, aimed at reducing the painful emotional states. For the apparently competent person, suicidal behavior is sometimes the only means of communicating to others that she really can't cope and needs help; that is, suicidal behavior is a cry for help. The behavior may also function as a means to get others to alter their unrealistic expectations—to "prove" to the world that she really cannot do what is expected.

The Dialectical Dilemma for the Therapist

The dimension of active passivity versus apparent competence presents a dialectical challenge for the therapist as well. A therapist who sees only the competence of the apparently competent person not only may be too demanding in terms of performance expectations, but may also be unresponsive to low-level communications of distress and difficulty. An invalidating environment ensues. The tendency to attribute lack of progress to "resistance" rather than inability is especially dangerous. Not only is such a stance, adopted uncritically, invalidating; it also prevents the therapist from offering needed skills training. The all-too-usual experience of a patient's leaving a session apparently in a neutral or even positive emotional state, but calling shortly, thereafter to threaten suicide, may be a consequence of this pattern.

In contrast, it can be an equal problem if a therapist does not recognize a patient's true capacities, thus falling into the active-passivity pattern with her. It can be especially easy for the therapist to mistake escalating emotionality and demands for true deficiencies. Panic at times masquerades as inability. Naturally, it can be especially difficult to avoid this trap when the patient is insisting that if therapeutic expectations are not lowered and more assistance given, suicide will be the consequence. It takes a courageous (and, I might add, self-confident) therapist to avoid caving in and appeasing the patient under these circumstances. Behavioral principles of response shaping are especially relevant in these situations. For example, as I discuss further in Chapter 8, in the early stages of treatment the therapist may need to "mind-read" the patient's emotions more often from skimpy information and anticipate problems much more than during later stages, after the patient has improved her communications skills. The key, of course, is accurately judging where on the shaping gradient the patient is at a particular moment.

Breaking through the active passivity and generating coparticipation is a continuing task. The mistake the therapist must avoid is that of continuing the oversimplification of the patient's difficulties and assuming too soon that the patient can cope with problems alone. Such an assumption is understandable, given the apparent-competence pattern. However, such a mistake simply increases the passivity of the patient; otherwise, the patient risks going out on a limb and being left alone to climb down. In general, the easier the therapist makes progress sound, the more passive the individual is likely to be. But stressing the inherent difficulty of change, while at the same time requiring active progress nonetheless, can facilitate active work. The role of the therapist is to balance the patient's capabilities and deficiencies, once again flexibly alternating between supportive-acceptance and confrontational/change approaches to treatment. Exhortations to change must be integrated with infinite patience.

Unrelenting Crises versus Inhibited Grieving

Unrelenting Crises

Many borderline and suicidal individuals are in a state of perpetual, unrelenting crisis. Although suicide, parasuicide, and most other dysfunctional behaviors are conceptualized in DBT as maladaptive attempts at solving problems in living, a more accurate statement is that these behaviors are responses to a state of chronic, overwhelming crisis. This state is debilitating to the borderline individual not because of the magnitude of any one stressful event, but because of both the individual's high reactivity and the chronic nature of the stressful events. For example, simultaneous loss of job, spouse, and children and a concomitant serious illness would—theoretically, at least—be easier to cope with than the same set of events experienced on a sequential basis. Berent (1981) suggests that repetitive stressful events, coupled with an inability to recover fully from any one stressful event, result in "weakening of the spirit" and subsequent suicidal or other "emergency" behaviors. In a sense, the patient can never return to an emotional baseline before the next blow hits. From Selye's (1956) point of view, the individual is constantly approaching the "exhaustion" stage of stress adaptation.

This inability to return to baseline may be a result of several factors. Typically, a borderline individual both creates and is controlled by an aversive environment. Temperamental factors exacerbate the individual's initial emotional response and rate of return to baseline after each stressor. Both the magnitude and number of subsequent stressors are then increased by the individual's responses to the initial stressor. An inability to tolerate or reduce short-term stress without emitting dysfunctional escape behaviors creates still more stressors. Inadequate interpersonal skills both result in interpersonal stress and preclude solving many of life's problems. An equally inadequate social support network (the invalidating environment) may contribute to the inability to control negative environmental events; it also further weakens the person's chances to develop needed capabilities.

For example, a woman may be controlled by an abusive husband and several young, dependent children. It may be unrealistic, either financially or morally, to suggest that she leave her family. Poor skills and a deficient social support network may exacerbate her inability to control negative environmental events, in addition to preventing her from developing any new skills or strengths. Another woman may be in a job environment that offers few rewards and many punishments; it may be economically impossible, however, for her to leave the job in the foreseeable future. Long working hours may interfere with any chance she might have to learn the skills that would make a better job possible. The resulting chronic, unrelenting stress, combined with an initial low tolerance for stressful events and an inability to avoid them, leads almost inevitably to the experience of further events as overwhelming.

This experience of being overwhelmed is often the key to understanding borderline patients' repetitive tendency (sometimes almost determination) to commit parasuicidal acts, threaten suicide, or engage in other impulsive, dysfunctional behaviors. And, as Berent (1981) suggests, the cumulative weakening of the spirit can lead to actual completed suicide. Seemingly incomprehensible overreactions to apparently minor events, criticisms, and losses become understandable when viewed against the backdrop of the patients' helplessness in the face of the chronic crises they experience, The active-passivity pattern, described above, suggests that these individuals are usually unable to reduce the stress unaided. Both patterns—unrelenting crises and active passivity—predict the frequent, excessive demands that these patients make on therapists. However, the apparent-competence pattern leads to a certain unwillingness on the part of others to assist the patients. When this unwillingness extends even to their therapists, situations can escalate still more rapidly into unendurable crises.

Unremitting crises generally interfere with treatment planning. Critical problems change faster than either a patient or a therapist can deal with effectively. In my experience, the crisis-oriented nature of the borderline individual's life makes it particularly difficult—indeed, almost impossible—to follow a predetermined behavioral treatment plan. This is especially so if the plan involves teaching skills that are not intimately and obviously related to the current crisis and that do not promise immediate relief. Focused skills training with the borderline patient is a bit like trying to teach an individual how to build a house that will not fall down in a tornado, just as a tornado hits. The patient knows that the appropriate place to be during a tornado is in the basement, crouching under a sturdy table; it is understandable if she insists on waiting out an emotional "tornado" in the "basement."

I spent many years trying to get myself to apply consistently to chronically parasuicidal and borderline patients the behavioral therapies I knew to be effective with other patient populations. Generally, these treatment strategies required a consistent focus on some sort of skills training, exposure, cognitive restructuring, or self-management training. But I simply could not get myself or the patients to stick to my well-thought-out and articulated treatment plans for more than a week or two. In the face of new and multiple crises, I was constantly reanalyzing the problems, redeveloping the treatment plans, or simply taking time out from the current treatment to attend to the crises. New problems always seemed more important than old problems. Most of the time, I attributed my inability to get the therapy to work to my own inexperience as a behavior therapist or some other therapeutic weakness on my part. After a number of years, however, I decided that even if the problems were my lack of ability, there were probably many other therapists as unskilled as I. This insight was instrumental in my developing DBT. The solution to this dilemma in DBT has been to develop psychoeducational therapy modules to teach specific behavioral, cognitive, and emotional skills. Although the task of individual psychotherapy is to help the patient integrate the skills into daily life, the rudiments of the skills are taught outside of the context of ordinary individual therapy. My colleagues and I have found that it is far easier for a therapist to resist being pulled into individual crises in a group setting. In addition, it seems easier for patients to understand and tolerate a seeming absence of attention to their individual crises when they can attribute this to demands of the group setting rather than to lack of concern for their current helplessness; the sense of personal invalidation is reduced. A group is not essential, however. Any setting where the context is different from that of standard individual therapy—where the message conveyed is "Now we are doing skills training, not crisis intervention"—may work as well.

A further therapeutic problem with unrelenting crises is that it is often easy for both a patient and a therapist to get lost in the thicket of the crises. Once the patient is emotionally out of control, her crises can escalate and become so complex that neither patient nor therapist can maintain a focus on the original precipitating event or problem. Part of the problem at times is the patient's tendency to ruminate about traumatic events. The rumination not only perpetuates the crises, but can generate new crises whose relationship to the original crises is often overlooked. Such a patient is a bit like an overtired child on a family outing. Once overtired, the child may become upset at every minor frustration and disagreement, crying and having tantrums at the slightest provocation. If the parents focus on trying to resolve every individual crisis, little progress will be made. It is far better to attend to the original problem—lack of sleep and rest. Similarly, the therapist with a borderline patients must be attentive to the original event creating emotional vulnerability in a particular sequence or chain; otherwise, the therapist may soon be so distracted by the patient's accumulating distress that he or she becomes confused and disorganized in approaching the problem.

One patient of mine, whom I will call Lorie, was particularly sensitive to criticism and disapproval. She had been brought up in a home with an abusive father who could not control his temper. When the children did anything he disapproved of, violent outbursts sometimes followed, frequently accompanied by beatings. By the time Lorie was 35, a typical scenario would be as follows: She would make a decision and put into effect a plan she later feared her supervisor at work might not like. After much ruminating about the decision and her supervisor's likely negative reaction, she would retreat from the plan, deciding that her original decision was wrong. She would then fret over her apparent stupidity or problematic cognitive style. She might then have a discussion with other colleagues and decide that a joint work project, unrelated to the area of concern with her supervisor, was hopeless because of her cognitive impairment. After work she would buy liquor, go home to her room, and get drunk, rationalizing that she already had brain damage anyway. She would thereby disappoint her husband, who was near the end of his rope over her drinking. The next morning, with a hangover and unavoidable guilt about turning to alcohol again, she might overreact to a question from her husband about a college tuition bill for her daughter, and a heated argument with her husband over finances would ensue. She would then come to a session that day with me and begin with a calm request to discuss whether she should look for another job or sell her house, because she had decided that her family needed a higher income to put her children through college. All of my attempts at problem solving in regard to this particular crisis (not enough college money) would, understandably, be met by further escalation of emotion.

Inhibited Grieving

Balancing the tendency to perpetual crisis is the corresponding tendency to avoid or inhibit the experience and expression of extreme, painful emotional reactions. "Inhibited grieving" refers to a pattern of repetitive, significant trauma and loss, together with an inability to fully experience and personally integrate or resolve these events. A crisis of any type always involves some form of loss. The loss can be concrete (e.g., loss of a person through death, loss of money or job, or loss of a relationship through breakup or divorce). The loss can be primarily psychological (e.g., loss of predictability and control because of sudden, unexpected environmental changes, or loss of hope of ever having nurturing parents when a person once again recognizes their limitations). Or the loss can be perceptual (e.g., perceived loss of interpersonal acceptance when another's remark is interpreted as critical). The accumulation of such losses can have two effects. First, significant early or unexpected loss may result in sensitization to later loss (Brasted & Callahan, 1984; Osterweis, Solomon, & Green, 1984; Callahan, Brasted, & Granados, 1983; Parkes, 1964). Second, a pattern of many losses leads to "bereavement overload," to use a term coined by Kastenbaum (1969). It is as if the process of grieving itself is inhibited. As my description of this pattern indicates, inhibited grieving overlaps considerably with posttraumatic stress disorder.

Both BPD and parasuicidal behavior are associated with a history of one or more major losses (incest, physical or other sexual abuse, death of a parent or sibling, parental neglect) at an early age. A number of empirical literature reviews (Gunderson & Zanarini, 1989) have concluded that borderline patients experience more childhood loss of a parent through divorce or death, higher rates of early childhood separation from primary caretakers, and more physical abuse and neglect than do other types of psychiatric patients. As I have discussed in describing the invalidating environment (Chapter 2) most striking is the strong relationship of BPD with histories of childhood sexual abuse. These data on childhood trauma have led at least one investigator to suggest that BPD is a specialized case of posttraumatic stress disorder (Ross, 1989).

Normal Grieving

The empirical research on normal grieving is meager and generally focuses on the sequelae of deaths of loved ones. However, normal grief has a number of identifiable stages: (1) avoidance, including disbelief, numbness, or shock; (2) developing awareness of the loss, leading to acute mourning, which may include yearning and searching for the thing lost, various painful physical sensations and emotional responses, preoccupation with images and thoughts of the lost object, behavioral and cognitive disorganization, and despair; and (3) resolution, reorganization, and acceptance (see Rando, 1984, for a review of various formulations of the grief process). Grief is an exceptionally painful process consisting of a variety of characteristic emotional, physical, cognitive, and behavioral responses. Although not all responses typify each grieving individual, the following characteristics are sufficiently common to be considered part of "normal grief" when they do occur: hollowness of stomach, tightness of throat or chest, difficulty in swallowing, breathlessness, muscle weakness, lack of energy, dryness of mouth, dizziness, fainting spells, nightmares, insomnia, blurred vision, skin rashes, sweating, appetite disturbance, indigestion, vomiting, palpitations, menstrual disturbance, headache, general aching, depersonalization, hallucinations, and intense negative emotions (Worden, 1982; Maddison & Viola, 1968; Rees, 1975). It is important to note here that grief and the process of grieving include the full array of negative emotions—sadness, guilt and self-reproach, anxiety and fear, loneliness, and anger.

All social animals, including humans, mourn loss to one degree or another—a phenomenon with probable survival value for the species (Averill, 1968). Although there is a substantial clinical lore about the necessity of mourning, working through, and resolving loss, there is very little research to back up most claims about the process. Wortman and Silver (1989) suggest that there are at least three common patterns of adaptation to loss. Some individuals go through the expected pattern as described above. A sizeable minority enter into the mourning phase and continue in a state of high distress for much longer than would be expected. Finally, others do not show intense distress following loss, either immediately after the loss or at subsequent intervals. That, is some individuals appear to adaptively circumvent the grieving process.

Problems with Grieving in Borderline Patients

Borderline patients are not among those able to circumvent the process of grieving. Furthermore, they seem unable either to tolerate or to move through the acute mourning phase. Instead of progressing through the grief process to resolution and acceptance, they continually resort to one or more avoidance responses. Thus, the inhibition of grieving among borderline individuals serves to exacerbate the effect of stressful events and continues a vicious cycle.

Inhibited grieving is understandable among borderline patients. People can only stay with a very painful process or experience if they are confident that it will end some day, some time—that they can "work through it," so to speak. It is not uncommon to hear borderline patients say they feel that if they ever do cry, they will never stop. Indeed, that is their common experience—the experience of not being able to control or modulate their own emotional experiences. They become, in effect, grief-phobic. In the face of such helplessness and lack of control, inhibition and avoidance of cues associated with grieving are not only understandable, but perhaps wise at times. Inhibition, however, has its costs.

The common theme in pathological grieving is successful avoidance of cues related to the loss (Callahan & Burnette, 1989). The ability to avoid all cues associated with repeated losses, however is limited. Therefore, borderline individuals are constantly re-exposed to the experience of loss, start the mourning process, automatically inhibit the process by avoiding or distracting themselves from the relevant cues, re-enter the process, and so on in a circular pattern that does not end. Exposure to the cues associated with their losses and grief is never sustained long enough for desensitization to be achieved. Gauthier and Marshall (1977) have suggested that such brief exposure to intensive stimuli may create a situation analogous to the "Napalkov phenomenon." Napalkov (1963) found that following a single pairing of a conditioned stimulus and an aversive unconditioned stimulus, repeated brief presentations of the conditioned stimulus alone at full intensity produced a marked increase in a conditioned blood pressure response. Eysenck (1967, 1968) has elaborated this into a theory of the cognitive incubation of fear in humans. As Gauthier and Marshall (1977) point out, intrusive thoughts about one's loss or trauma, followed by attempts to suppress such thoughts, match the conditions described by Eysenck as ideal for the incubation of distressed responses.

Volkan (1983) describes an interesting phenomenon, "established pathological mourning," which is similar to the pattern I am describing. In established pathological mourning, the individual wishes to complete mourning, but at the same time persistently attempts to undo the reality of the loss. I have seen this pattern repeatedly in patients whose previous therapists precipitously terminated therapy with them. One of my patients was put in a hospital following a suicide attempt. Her therapist visited her in the hospital and informed her that therapy was over and there would be no further contact between them. Thereafter, this therapist consistently refused any contact with the patient, did not respond to any attempts at communication, and refused even to talk with me or send me a report, suggesting that such contact would only reopen hope on the part of the patient. The first 2 years of therapy with me consisted of the patient's continually trying to re-establish contact with her previous therapist, often by trying to persuade me to set up a joint meeting; expressing anger at me whenever I acted in ways inconsistent with the way her previous therapist had worked; continually entering into the grieving process with components of somatic, emotional, cognitive, and behavioral grief responses, including suicidal behaviors; and eventually short-circuiting the mourning response by returning to efforts to re-establish contact.

Although we know that long-term inhibition of grief is detrimental, it is not particularly clear why the expression of emotions associated with loss and trauma is beneficial. It may be that exposure to cues associated with emotional pain leads to extinction or habituation, whereas constant avoidance and insufficient exposure interfere with these processes. There is some evidence that talking or writing about traumatic or stressful events, especially when the disclosure includes the emotions aroused by the event, leads to reduced ruminating about the event, improved physical health, and increased feelings of well-being (see Pennebaker, 1988, for a review of this work).

The task of the therapist with a borderline patient is helping the patient to encounter the losses and traumatic events in her life and to experience and express grief reactions. The principal way of achieving this is to discuss the situations during therapy sessions. This is easier said than done, since often the patient actively resists such suggestions. Some patients insist on discussing previous traumas, particularly childhood abuse, before they are able to reverse the associated emotional inhibition. Even when the therapist is successful at beginning discussion of a trauma or loss, the patient will often simply shut down in the middle and be silent or only minimally communicative. For example, I have rarely had a patient who will continue talking about a topic if she feels that she is going to cry; the threat of tears generally stops our interaction until the patient regains control. One of my patients, whom I will call Jane, could almost never discuss emotionally charged topics for more than a minute or two. Almost immediately, her jaw and facial muscles would tighten, she would look away or curl up in a fetal position, and all interactions would cease. With previous therapists, who themselves fell silent when Jane did, she sometimes went for whole sessions without saying a word. Over time, I learned that during such episodes her mind usually either went blank or was flooded with racing thoughts; she felt as if she were choking, couldn't get her breath, and believed she might be dying.

Once confrontation and urging the patient to talk do not work, the therapist may be tempted to assume that since the experience is frustrating for him or her, the patient must *want* to be frustrating. The patient's behavior is then interpreted as an attack on the therapist or the therapy, as I have described earlier in this chapter in the discussion of anger and BPD. (The videotape of a therapy session with Jane, as noted in that discussion, is one of those that causes some professionals in the audience to assume that the frequent silences during the session are active attempts to attack me.) Often, my interpretation of such behavior as inhibited grief has been interpreted as naiveté on my part. Sometimes it seems to me that therapists think their own frustration and anger are infallible guides to the motives of the patient. The danger in such an approach is that it clearly invalidates the experience of the patient; thus, it perpetuates the invalidating environment that the patient has been exposed to all her life. Furthermore, it fails to offer the patient the help she needs.

In my experience, a more fruitful approach has been to focus on specific and concrete behaviors in which the patient can engage to reverse the emotional inhibition. The idea is to take the patient's expressive difficulty seriously and offer the help she needs. For example, with Jane, I progressed from specific instructions to remove mirrored sunglasses or unwrap her arms from around her knees to sessions where, when observing her jaw tightening, I reminded her to relax her face muscles and drop her jaw slightly. One can take this point of view to an extreme, however, and refuse to assess for hostile motivation and anger when it exists. The key point is that factors influencing behavior must be subject to assessment, not assumptions. The inhibited-grieving pattern offers an alternative to analyses of patients' sometimes contrary behaviors as manifestations of hostility directed at the therapist.

The Dialectical Dilemma for the Patient

The borderline patient is actually presented with two dilemmas on the dimension of unrelenting crises versus inhibited grieving. First, it is difficult if not impossible for her to inhibit grief reactions on demand and avoid exposure to loss and trauma cues when at the same time she is in a state of perpetual crisis. Second, although inhibition of affective responses associated with grief may be effective for short-term resolution of pain, it is not very effective in bringing about social support for the patient's crises, nor does it lead to tranquillity in the long run. Indeed, the escape behaviors typical of inhibited grieving are often impulsive behaviors such as drinking, driving fast, spending money, engaging in unprotected sex, and leaving situations. These behaviors are instrumental in creating new crises. Thus, the borderline individual tends to vacillate back and forth between the two extremes: At one moment, she is vulnerable to the crises; at the next, she inhibits all affective experiences associated with the crises. The key problem is that as the experience at each extreme intensifies, it becomes increasingly hard for the patient not to jump to the other extreme.

The Dialectical Dilemma for the Therapist

The dialectical dilemma for the therapist is to balance his or her response to the oscillating nature of the patient's distress—sometimes expressed as acute crises and overwhelming affect, and at other times presenting as complete inhibition of affective responding. An intense reaction by the therapist at either extreme may be all that is needed to push the patient to the other extreme. The task of the therapist is, first to help the patient understand her reaction patterns, and, second, to offer realistic hope that the patient can indeed survive the process of grieving. Such realistic hope requires the therapist to teach grieving skills, including the coping strategies needed for successful acceptance and reorganization of life in the present without that which is lost.

Concurrently, the therapist must also validate and support the patient's emotional experience and difficulties in the unrelenting crises of her life. Offering understanding without concrete help in ameliorating crises, of course, may be even more distressing than offering nothing at all. Yet the concrete help that the therapist has to offer requires the patient to confront rather than avoid the crises she is experiencing. The synthesis toward which the therapist works in the patient is the ability both to grieve deeply and to end grieving; the ultimate goal is for the patient to build and rebuild her life in the light of the current realities.

Concluding Comments

In this chapter, as well as the previous two, I have described the theoretical foundations of DBT. It is easy for many to believe that theory is not very relevant to practice. Practical help, especially ideas of what to do and when to do it, is what many therapists want and need. The rest of this book is an attempt to provide you with just such help—to take the theory and make it practical. However, no therapy manual or book can anticipate all of the situations you will run into. Thus, you will need to know the theory well enough to be able to create a new therapy with each patient. The purpose of theory is to give you a short-hand way to think about the patient—a way to understand her experience and to relate to it, even though you may not have experienced similar problems yourself. It is also intended to provide a conceptualization of the patient's difficulties that will give you hope when you are feeling hopeless, and to provide an avenue for new treatment ideas when you are desperate for something different to try.

Notes

1. Otto Kernberg is one of the most influential theorists proposing excess anger as crucial in the development of BPD. When I proposed this gender-linked hypothesis to account for our differences on this point, he pointed out that many of his teachers have been women.

2. At other times, expressive inhibition may function as an emotional control strategy. An alternate explanation for the "apparent nonemotionality" of some borderline patients may be that reduced nonverbal emotional expressiveness in general, or at certain levels of arousal, or for certain emotions, is a result of constitutional (i.e., biological) factors. If this is the case, it might be an important factor in eliciting invalidation from the environment at an early age.

Treatment Overview
and Goals

4

Overview of Treatment: Targets, Strategies, and Assumptions in a Nutshell

Crucial Steps in Treatment

In a nutshell, DBT is very simple. The therapist creates a context of validating rather than blaming the patient, and within that context the therapist blocks or extinguishes bad behaviors, drags good behaviors out of the patient, and figures out a way to make the good behaviors so reinforcing that the patient continues the good ones and stops the bad ones.[1]

At the onset, "bad" and "good" behaviors are defined and listed in order of importance. Commitment (even if only half-hearted) to work on the DBT behavioral targets is a requisite characteristic of the DBT patient. The requisite characteristics of the therapist are compassion, persistence, patience, a belief in the efficacy of the therapy that will outlast the patient's belief in its inefficacy, and a certain willingness to play "chicken" and take risks. Accomplishing these tasks requires a number of steps, which are discussed below.

Setting the Stage: Getting the Patient's Attention

Agreeing on Goals and Orienting the Patient to Treatment

Agreement on goals of treatment and general treatment procedures is the crucial first step before therapy even begins. At this point, the therapist has to get the patient's attention and interest. DBT is very specific on the order and importance of various treatment targets, as Chapter 5 discusses in detail. Suicidal, parasuicidal, and life-threatening behaviors are first. Behaviors that threaten the process of the therapy are second. Problems that make it impossible ever to develop a reasonable quality of life are third in importance.

Throughout treatment, the patient is learning coping skills to use instead of habitual, dysfunctional responses; fourth most important is the stabilization of these behavioral skills. Once progress has been made on these goals, work on resolving posttraumatic stress rises to the top in importance, followed by helping the patient achieve broad-based self-validation and self-respect.

Patients who do not agree to work on decreasing suicidal and parasuicidal behaviors and interpersonal styles that interfere with therapy, as well as on increasing behavioral skills, are not accepted into treatment. (Agreements to work on other DBT targets are developed as therapy progresses.) Prospective patients are then oriented to other aspects of the treatment, including the ways in which treatment is carried out and any ground rules. Patients who do not agree to the minimum ground rules (described later in this chapter) are not accepted. In settings where patients cannot legally or ethically be rejected from treatment, some sort of special "program within a program" is needed so that patients can be rejected. Patients' agreements to the terms of DBT are always brought up when they later try to violate the rules or get the rules changed. Therapists' agreements can also legitimately be brought up by the patients.

Establishing a Relationship

The therapist must work to establish a strong, positive interpersonal relationship with the patient right from the beginning. This is essential because the relationship with the therapist is frequently the only reinforcer that works for a borderline individual in managing and changing behavior. With a highly suicidal patient, the relationship with the therapist is at times what keeps her alive when all else fails. Finally, similar to many schools of psychotherapy, DBT works on the premise that the experience of being genuinely accepted and cared for and about is of value in its own right, apart from any changes that the patient makes as a result of therapy (Linehan, 1989). Not much in DBT can be done before this relationship is developed.

As soon as the relationship is established, the therapist begins to communicate to the patient that the rules have changed. Whereas the patient might have believed previously that if she got better she would lose the therapist, she is now told that if she does not improve she will lose the therapist much more quickly: "Continuing an ineffective therapy is unethical." DBT has been called "blackmail therapy" by some, since the therapist is willing to put the quality of the relationship on the line in a trade for improved behavior on the part of the patient. If the therapist cannot achieve the interpersonal power necessary to influence change, then the therapy should be expanded to include those who do have such power with the patient. For example, with adolescents, family therapy may be essential.

Staying Dialectical

The central dialectical tension in DBT is that between change and acceptance.

The paradoxical notion here is that therapeutic change can only occur in the context of acceptance of what is; however, "acceptance of what is" is itself change. DBT therefore requires that the therapist balance change and acceptance in each interaction with the patient. DBT treatment strategies can be organized in terms of their tendencies to fall primarily at the change end versus the acceptance end of the dialectical polarity. The secondary tension is between the exercises of control and freeing. The therapist exerts control of the therapy (and at times the patient) to enhance the patient's ultimate freedom and self-control. Staying dialectical also requires that the therapist model and reinforce dialectical response styles. Behavioral extremes (whether emotional, cognitive, or overt responses) are confronted, and new, more balanced responses are taught.

Applying Core Strategies: Validation and Problem Solving

The core of the treatment is the application of problem-solving strategies balanced by validation strategies. This is the "teeter-totter" on which the therapy rests. From the patient's perspective, maladaptive behaviors are often the solutions to problems she wants solved or taken away. From the DBT therapist's perspective, however, maladaptive behaviors are themselves the problems to be solved.

Validation

There are two types of validation. In the first type, the therapist finds the wisdom, correctness, or value in the individual's emotional, cognitive, and overt behavioral responses. The important focus here is the search for those behavioral responses, parts of responses, and patterns that are valid in the context of current, associated events. A key function of emotional suffering and maladaptive behaviors for borderline patients is self-validation. Thus, therapeutic changes cannot be made unless another source of self-validation is developed. A treatment focused only on changing the patient invalidates the patient. The second type of validation has to do with the therapist's observing and believing in the patient's inherent ability to get out of the misery that is her life and build a life worth living. In DBT, the therapist finds and plays to the patient's strengths, not to her fragility. The therapist both believes and believes *in* the patient.

Problem Solving

The core change strategies are those that fall under the rubric of problem solving. This set of strategies includes a (1) performing a behavioral analysis of the targeted behavior problem; (2) performing a solution analysis, in which alternate behavioral solutions are developed; (3) orienting the patient to the proposed treatment solution; (4) eliciting a commitment from the patient to engage in the recommended treatment procedures; and (5) appling the treatment.

A behavioral analysis consists of a moment-to-moment chain analysis to determine events that elicit or prompt maladaptive behavior, as well as a functional analysis to determine probable reinforcing contingencies for maladaptive behaviors. The process and outcome of the behavioral analysis lead into the solution analysis: The therapist and (optimally) the patient generate alternate behavioral responses and develop a treatment plan oriented to changing targeted behavior problems. Four questions are addressed:

1. Does the individual have the capability to engage in more adaptive responses and to construct a life worth living? If not, what behavioral skills are needed? The answers to this question leads to the focus on skills training procedures. Five sets of skills are emphasized: "core" mindfulness skills, distress tolerance, emotion regulation, interpersonal effectiveness, and self-management. (Chapter 5 discusses these in more detail.)

2. What are the reinforcement contingencies? Is the problem a result of reinforcing outcomes for maladaptive behaviors, or of punishing or neutral outcomes for adaptive behaviors? If either is the case, contingency management procedures are developed. The goal here is to arrange for positive behaviors to be reinforced, for negative behaviors to be punished or extinguished, and for the patient to learn the new rules.

3. If adaptive problem-solving behaviors exist, is their application inhibited by excessive fear or guilt? Is the patient emotion-phobic? If so, an exposure-based treatment is instituted.

4. If adaptive problem-solving behaviors exist, is their application inhibited or interfered with by faulty beliefs and assumptions? If so, a cognitive modification program must be instituted.

In most cases, the behavioral analysis will show that there are skill deficits, problematic reinforcement contingencies, inhibitions resulting from fear and guilt, and faulty beliefs and assumptions. Thus, a treatment program integrating skill training, contingency management, exposure strategies, and cognitive modification is likely to be required. The behavioral target of each strategy, however, is dependent on the behavioral analysis.

Balancing Interpersonal Communication Styles

DBT combines and balances two interpersonal communication styles: "irreverent" and "reciprocal" communication. Irreverent communication is designed to get the patient to "jump the track," so to speak. The therapist's reactions are not obviously responsive to the patient's communications, are sometimes experienced as "off the wall," and involve the therapist's framing the issue under consideration in a context different from the patient's. The main idea here is to push the patient "off balance" so that rebalancing can occur. The reciprocal communication style, in contrast, is warm, empathetic, and directly responsive to the patient. It includes therapeutic self-disclosure designed to provide modeling of mastery and coping with problems, as well as of normative responses to everyday situations.

Combining Consultation-to-the-Patient Strategies with Interventions in the Environment

In DBT, there is a strong bias toward teaching the patient to be her own case manager (the "consultation-to-the-patient" approach). The basic notion here is that rather than intervening for the patient to solve problems or coordinate treatment with other professionals, the DBT therapist coaches the patient in how to resolve the problems herself. The approach flows directly out of the therapist's believing in the patient. Problems and inappropriate behavior on the part of other mental health professionals, even when they are members of the DBT treatment team, are viewed as opportunities for learning. The consultation-to-the-patient strategies are the dominant DBT case management strategies. Interventions in the environment to make changes, solve problems, or coordinate professional treatment on behalf of the patient are used instead of the consultation strategies and balance them when (1) the outcome is important and (2) the patient clearly does not have the capability to produce the outcome.

Treating the Therapist

Staying in a DBT frame can be extraordinarily difficult for the therapist with a borderline patient. An important part of DBT is the treatment of the therapist by the supervision, case consultation, or treatment team. The role of the DBT case consultation group is to hold the therapist inside the treatment. The assumption is that treatment of borderline patients in solo practice, outside a team framework, is perilous at best. Thus, the treatment of the therapist is integral to the therapy.

Modes of Treatment

I use the term "mode" to refer to the various treatment components that together make up DBT, as well as the manner of their delivery. In principle, DBT can be applied in any treatment mode. In our research program validating the effectiveness of DBT as an outpatient treatment, however, treatment was delivered in four primary modes offered concurrently: individual psychotherapy, group skills training, telephone consultation, and case consultation for therapists. In addition, most patients received one or more ancillary treatment modes. In different settings (e.g., solo private practice or inpatient treatment), these modes may need to be condensed or supplemented.

Individual Outpatient Psychotherapy

In "standard" DBT (i.e., the original version of DBT), each patient has an individual psychotherapist who is also the primary therapist for that patient on the treatment team. All other modes of therapy revolve around the individual therapy. The individual therapist is responsible for helping the patient inhibit maladaptive, borderline behaviors and replace them with adaptive, skillful responses. The individual therapist pays close attention to motivational issues, including personal and environmental factors that inhibit effective behaviors and that elicit and reinforce maladaptive behaviors.

Individual outpatient therapy sessions are usually held once a week. At the beginning of therapy and during crisis periods, sessions may be held twice a week; this is usually done only on a time-limited basis, although for some patients twice a week may be preferable. Sessions generally last from 50–60 to 90–110 minutes. The longer sessions (i.e., "double sessions") are held with patients who have difficulty opening up and then closing up emotionally in the shorter sessions. Session length can vary over the treatment period, depending on the specific therapy tasks to be accomplished. For example, sessions may ordinarily last 60 minutes, but when exposure to abuse-related stimuli is planned, sessions may be scheduled for 90–120 minutes. Or one double session and one single session (or one half-session for "check-in") per week may be scheduled for a period of time. The therapist can shorten or lengthen a session on the spot to reinforce therapeutic "working" or to punish avoidance. When lengthening a session is impossible because of scheduling conflicts, a phone consultation may be planned for that same evening, or a session may be scheduled for the next day. Alternatively, patients who often need somewhat longer sessions may be scheduled at the end of the day. The key idea here is that session length should be matched to the tasks at hand, not the mood of either the patient or the therapist. Creative problem solving on the part of the therapist is sometimes called for.

Within clinic and research settings, assignment to therapists can pose special difficulties with borderline patients. Many borderline individuals have already had one or more "failed" therapeutic encounters and may have strong beliefs about what kind of person they want for a therapist. Therapists may have equally strong views about what kinds of patients they want to treat or feel comfortable with. Many women who have been sexually abused prefer to have a female therapist. In our clinic, my colleagues and I give information during the intake interview about the available therapists, and patients are asked for any preferences. A specific individual therapist is assigned following the treatment team's review of each individual's intake interview, history, and presenting complaints. Although I support the idea of patients' and therapists' interviewing each other to make an informed decision about working together, in our clinic such a procedure is not feasible. Instead, the first several sessions are structured as a way for each patient and therapist to decide whether they can indeed work together. A patient can switch therapists if she wishes to, if another one is available, and if that other therapist is willing to work with her. She may not participate in any other part of the treatment program, however, if she drops out of individual therapy without switching to another individual therapist (either inside or outside our clinic).

Skills Training

All patients must be in structured skills training during the first year of therapy. In my experience, skills training with borderline patients is exceptionally difficult within the context of individual therapy oriented to reducing the motivation for suicidal or other borderline behaviors. The need for crisis intervention and attention to other issues generally precludes skills training. Nor can sufficient attention to motivational issues be easily given in a treatment with the rigorous control of therapy agenda usually needed for skills training. The solution to this problem in standard DBT has been to split the therapy into two components; these are either conducted by different therapists or applied in different modes by the same therapist. In our program, patients cannot be in skills training without concurrent individual psychotherapy. The individual psychotherapy is necessary to help the patient integrate her new skills into daily life. The average borderline individual cannot replace dysfunctional, borderline coping styles with skilled behavioral coping without intensive individual coaching.

DBT skills training is conducted in a psychoeducational format. In our program, it is generally conducted in open groups that meet weekly for 2 to 2½ hours, but other group formats are possible. Some clinics have divided the group into two 1-hour sessions weekly (one session for homework review, one for presenting new material). In large clinics, there may be one large group meeting per week for new skill material, with numerous smaller weekly groups for homework review. In small clinics or private practice, groups may be small and meet for shorter periods.

Although my colleagues and I usually have six to eight members per group, a group needs only two patients. A patient who cannot be in a group for one reason or another, however, can be given skills training individually. In my experience, it is easier if a second therapist does the individual skills training; otherwise, there is a tendency (which I, at least, have difficulty resisting) to fall into the individual, non-skills-training psychotherapy mode. If, instead, the individual therapist folds the skills training into the ongoing psychotherapy, separate sessions tightly structured for skills training should be considered.

A point-by-point skills training program is described in the companion manual to the present volume.

Supportive Process Group Therapy

After completing skills training, patients in my program can join optional supportive process group therapy if they wish. These groups are ongoing and open; generally, patients make renewable, time-limited commitments to the group. To be in standard DBT supportive process groups, patients must have ongoing individual therapy or case management. The exceptions here are the most advanced groups, where group therapy may emerge as a long-term primary therapy for some borderline patients. The conduct of these groups is described more fully in the companion manual.

Although I have not collected any empirical data on this question, it is conceivable that the individual DBT described above could be duplicated within a group therapy context. In these cases, group DBT might supplement or replace the individual DBT component.

Telephone Consultation

Phone consultation with the individual outpatient therapist between psychotherapy sessions is an important part of DBT. There are several reasons for this. First, many suicidal and borderline individuals have enormous difficulty asking for help effectively. Some are inhibited from asking for help directly by fear, shame, or beliefs that they are undeserving or their needs are invalid; they may instead engage in parasuicidal behavior or other crisis behaviors as a "cry for help." Other patients have no difficulty asking for help, but do so in a demanding or abusive manner, act in a way that makes potential benefactors feel manipulated, or use other ineffective strategies. Telephone consultations are designed to provide practice in changing these dysfunctional patterns. Second, patients often need help in generalizing DBT behavioral skills to their everyday lives. Suicidal patients frequently need more therapeutic contact than can be provided in one individual session (and especially in one group skills training session) per week, especially during crises, when they may be unable to cope unassisted with problems in living. With a phone call, a patient can obtain the coaching needed for successful skill generalization to take place. Third, following conflict or misunderstandings, phone consultation offers an avenue for patients to repair their sense of an intimate therapeutic relationship without having to wait until the next session.

In day treatment programs, inpatient units, and residential programs, interactions with mental health technicians, nurses or other staff members can substitute for some of the phone consultations. In outpatient practice with an on-call system, other therapists can at times handle phone consultations within a DBT structure. This is particularly true for the first two goals of phone consultation (learning to ask for and receive help appropriately, and skill generalization).

Case Consultation Meetings for Therapists

There is no question about it: Treating borderline patients is enormously stressful for a therapist. Many therapists quickly burn out. Others (somewhat blindly, I suspect) fall into iatrogenic behaviors. As subsequent sections of this chapter indicate, one assumption of DBT is that therapists often engage in the problematic behaviors of which patients accuse them. They may do so for good reasons. Borderline patients can put enormous pressure on their therapists to ameliorate their pain immediately; therapists may thus feel pressured into making major (and at times precipitous) changes in the treatment, even when the treatment might have proved effective if held to. At other times, therapists react to such pressure by rigidly refusing to make any changes. When neither approach works and misery is not relieved, the therapists can easily respond by "blaming the victims." The stress of treating highly suicidal patients can lead to a cyclical pattern of appeasement followed by punitive reactions followed by reconciliation, and so on.

Problems that arise in a therapist's delivery of treatment are handled in DBT case consultation meetings. These meetings are attended by all therapists (individual and group) currently utilizing DBT with borderline patients. Similar to the requirement that patients participate in skills training, DBT therapists are required to be in a consultation or supervision relationship; either with one other person or (my own preference) with a group. During the first year of therapy, both the group and the individual therapists should attend the same meetings. In agency, day treatment, or inpatient settings applying DBT, all members of a patient's treatment team should attend the same meeting. Consultation meetings are held weekly.

Ancillary Treatments

Borderline patients may at times need more than the weekly individual, skills training, and telephone sessions. For example, some may need pharmacotherapy, day treatment, vocational counseling, or acute hospitalization, to name just a few. Many will also want to join nonprofessional groups such as Alcoholics Anonymous. There is nothing in DBT that proscribes the patient from obtaining additional professional or nonprofessional treatments.

If the additional treatment is offered by a therapist who regularly attends DBT consultation meetings and who applies DBT principles, then the DBT treatment is simply expanded to include these additional components. Although I have not written DBT protocols for these additional components, protocols based on DBT principles could (and should) be developed. For example, DBT is currently being adapted for day treatment and for both acute and long-term inpatient programs (see Barley et al., in press). More commonly, the additional treatment components will be delivered by non-DBT therapists using principles derived from other theoretical traditions. Or, even when additional treatment is applied by a DBT therapist, the therapist will not be able to consult regularly with the treatment team. In these cases the additional therapy is viewed as ancillary to the primary DBT treatment. There are specific protocols for the ancillary use of pharmacotherapy and acute psychiatric hospitalizations; these are described in Chapter 15. Guidelines for how the DBT therapist interacts with ancillary health professionals are discussed in Chapter 13.

Assumptions About Borderline Patients and Therapy

The most important thing to remember about assumptions is that they are just that—assumptions, not facts. Nonetheless, assuming and acting on the propositions discussed below can be useful in treating borderline patients. They constitute the context for treatment planning.

1. Patients Are Doing the Best They Can

The first philosophical position in DBT is that all people are, at any given point in time, doing the best they can. In my experience, borderline patients are usually working desperately hard at changing themselves. Often, however, there is little visible success, nor are the patients' efforts at behavioral control particularly obvious much of the time. Because their behavior is frequently exasperating, inexplicable, and unmanageable, it is tempting to decide that the patients are not trying. At times, when asked about problematic behavior, the patients themselves will respond that they just weren't trying. Such patients have learned the social explanation for their behavioral failures. The tendency of many therapists to tell these patients to try harder, or imply that they indeed are not trying hard enough, can be one of the patient's most invalidating experiences in psychotherapy. (This is not to say that in a well-thought-out strategic approach, a therapist might not use a phrase such as this to influence a patient.)

2. Patients Want to Improve

The second assumption is a corollary to the first, and is similar to the assumption therapists and crisis workers make with suicidal patients: If they are calling for help, they must want to live. Why else would they call? Borderline patients are so used to hearing that their behavioral failures and difficulties with therapeutic interventions stem from motivational deficits that they begin to believe it themselves. Assuming that patients want to improve, of course, does not preclude analysis of all of the factors interfering with motivation to improve. Fear- or shame-based inhibition, behavioral deficits, faulty beliefs about outcomes, and factors that reinforce behavioral regressions over improvement are all important. The assumption by therapists that failures to improve sufficiently or quickly are based on failure of intent, however, is at best faulty logic and at worst one more factor that interferes with motivation.

3. Patients Need to Do Better, Try Harder, and Be More Motivated to Change

The third assumption may appear to contradict the first two, but I do not think so. The fact that borderline patients are doing the best they can and want to do even better does not mean that their efforts and motivation are sufficient to the task; often they are not. The task of a therapist, therefore, is to analyze factors that inhibit or interfere with a patient's efforts and motivation to improve, and then to use problem solving strategies to help the patient increase her efforts and purify (so to speak) her motivation.

4. Patients May Not Have Caused All of Their Own Problems, but They Have to Solve Them Anyway

The fourth assumption simply verbalizes the belief in DBT that a borderline patient has to change her own behavioral responses and alter her environment for her life to change. Improvement will not result from the patient's simply coming to a therapist and gaining insight, taking a medication, receiving consistent nurturing, finding the perfect relationship, or resigning herself to the grace of God. Most importantly, the therapist cannot save the patient. Although it may be true that the patient cannot change on her own and that she needs help, the lion's share of the work nonetheless will be done by the patient. Would that it were not so! Surely if we could save patients, we would save them. It is essential that the DBT therapist make this assumption very clear to the patient, especially during crises.

5. The Lives of Suicidal, Borderline Individuals Are Unbearable as They Are Currently Being Lived

The fifth assumption is that borderline patients' frequently voiced dissatisfactions with their lives are valid. They are indeed in a living hell. If patients' complaints and descriptions of their own lives are taken at all seriously, this assumption is self-evident. Given this fact, the only solution is to change their lives.

6. Patients Must Learn New Behaviors in All Relevant Contexts

Borderline individuals are mood-dependent, and thus they must make important changes in their styles of coping under extreme emotions, not just when they are in a state of emotional equilibrium. With some exceptions, DBT does not generally favor hospitalization even during crises, since hospitalization takes individuals out of the environment where they need to learn new skills. Nor does DBT particularly favor taking care of patients when stress is extreme or seems unbearable. Times of stress are the times to learn new ways of coping.

Not taking care *of* a patient does not mean that a DBT therapist does not take care *for* the patient. The task of the therapist during crises is to stick to the patient like glue, whispering encouragement and helpful suggestions in her ear all the while. Such an approach, in which the therapist is biased toward producing self-care from the patient during crises rather than taking care of the patient, can result in a number of risky encounters for the therapist. Acceptance of the possibility that the patient may commit suicide is an essential requisite for conducting DBT. The other alternative, however—in which the patient stays alive, but within a life filled with intolerable emotional pain—is not viewed as tenable.

7. Patients Cannot Fail in Therapy

The seventh assumption is that when patients drop out of therapy, fail to progress, or actually get worse while in DBT, the therapy, the therapist, or both have failed. If the therapy has been applied according to protocol, and the patients still do not improve, then the failure is attributable to the therapy itself. This contrasts with the assumption of many therapists that when patients drop out or fail to improve, it can be attributed to a deficit in their motivation. Even if this assumption is true, the job of therapy is to enhance motivation sufficiently for the patients to progress.

8. Therapists Treating Borderline Patients Need Support

As noted throughout this book, borderline patients are one of the most difficult populations to treat with psychotherapy. Over and over, therapists seem to make mistakes that interfere with the patients' progress. Some of the problem stems from the patients' intense cries for immediate escape from suffering. Often therapists are capable of soothing the pain, but giving such relief frequently interferes with providing help for the longterm. Therapists get caught between these demands for immediate relief and for long-term cure. Many other factors make it difficult for therapists to remain therapeutic with borderline patients. A cosupervision group, a treatment team, a consultant, or a supervisor is important for keeping therapists on track.

Therapist Characteristics and Skills

"Therapist characteristics," in this context, are the attitudes and pervasive interpersonal positions that the therapist takes in relationship to the patient. Briefly, the therapist must balance the patient's capabilities and deficiencies, flexibly synthesizing acceptance and nurturing strategies with change-demanding strategies in a clear and centered manner. Exhortations to change must be integrated with infinite patience. Since the dialectical emphasis in DBT is large, a therapist must be comfortable with the ambiguity and paradox inherent in DBT strategies. Therapists who need black-and-white conceptualizations, goals, or methods are likely to experience DBT as dissonant when confronted with the dialectic inherent in actions to control patients' destructive behaviors while also promoting growth and self-reliance.

Requisite therapist characteristics are illustrated in Figure 4.1. Although they are presented in terms of bipolar attributes, the correct DBT stance is

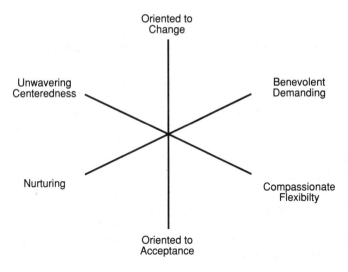

FIGURE 4.1. Therapist characteristics in DBT.

a synthesis or balance between the poles of each dimension; thus, the therapist stands at the center of each dimension. The synthesis of acceptance and change represents the central dialectical balance that the therapist must achieve in DBT. The other two dialectical dimensions—unwavering centeredness versus compassionate flexibility, and benevolent demanding versus nurturing—are reflections of this central dimension.

Stance of Acceptance versus Change

The first dimension is something I have been discussing throughout this book: the balance of an orientation toward acceptance with an orientation toward change. By "acceptance" here, I mean something quite radical—namely acceptance of both the patient and the therapist, of both the therapeutic relationship and the therapeutic process, exactly as all of these are in the moment. This is not an acceptance in order to bring about change; otherwise, it would be a change strategy. Rather, it is the therapist's willingness to find the inherent wisdom and "goodness" of the current moment and the participants in it, and to enter fully into the experience without judgment, blame, or manipulation. As noted previously, however, reality is change, and the nature of any relationship is that of reciprocal influence. In particular, a therapeutic relationship is one that originates in the necessity of change and the patient's wish to obtain professional help in the process of changing. An orientation toward change requires that the therapist take responsibility for directing the therapeutic influence, or change, to the advantage of the patient. Such a stance is active and self-conscious; it involves systematically applying principles of behavior change.

From the perspective of acceptance versus change, DBT represents a balance between behavioral approaches, which are primarily technologies of change, and humanistic and client-centered approaches, which can be thought of as technologies of acceptance. In DBT, the therapist not only models a change—acceptance synthesis but also encourages such a life stance to the patient, advocating change and amelioration of undesired aspects of herself and situations, as well as tolerance and acceptance of these same characteristics. Teaching mindfulness and distress tolerance skills is balanced by teaching skills in emotional control and interpersonal effectiveness in conflict situations.

Crucial to the balance of acceptance and change is the therapist's ability to express warmth and control simultaneously in therapy settings. Much of the control in changing patient behavior is achieved through the use of the relationship; without a significant level of concurrent warmth and acceptance, the therapist will probably be experienced as hostile and demanding rather than as caring and helpful.

Stance of Unwavering Centeredness versus Compassionate Flexibility

"Unwavering centeredness" is the quality of believing in oneself, in the therapy, and in the patient. It is calmness in the middle of chaos, much like the center of a hurricane. It requires a certain clarity of mind with respect to what the patient needs in the long run, as well as an ability to tolerate the intensity and pain experienced by the patient without flinching in the short run. Centeredness in DBT does not mean maintaining arbitrary boundaries as it does in some other therapies. Nor does it require more than the usual consistency (except in the commitment to the patient's welfare). Neither arbitrary boundaries nor consistency is particularly valued in DBT.

"Compassionate flexibility" refers to the contrasting ability of the therapist to take in relevant information about the status of the patient and to modify his or her position accordingly. It is the ability to let go freely of a position that was formerly clung to tenaciously. If centeredness is keeping one's feet on the ground, flexibility is moving your shoulders to the side to let the patient by. Flexibility is that quality of the therapist that is light, responsive, and creative. Dialectically, it is the ability to change the boundaries of the problem, finding and including what has been previously excluded.

Given the odds of making mistakes in conducting DBT, an overall willingness to admit and repair mistakes made in the course of the therapeutic relationship is essential. To put it another way, in such a complex and difficult therapeutic endeavor, mistakes are inevitable; what the therapist does afterwards is a better index of good therapy. Whether the mistake is smiling at the wrong moment and being perceived as mocking rather than warm, getting into power struggles, or becoming impatient with the patient's slow progress and then rejecting her by not returning telephone calls and behaving coldly, the effective therapist must be able to acknowledge such actions as errors. Higher-functioning patients may be able to experience both trust in their therapists and painful affect arising from some therapist actions, and thus may not require as much repair work. Borderline patients are not likely to be in this category, however, and their therapists may become identified with other abusive individuals in their lives. Without therapist validation of a patient's experience and flexible attempts at problem solving in the situation, the therapeutic relationship becomes for the patient one more mistaken trust, one more failed relationship that must be either fled or hopelessly endured. Furthermore, a therapist must be able to tolerate both frustration at the patient's rejection of seemingly appropriate interventions and progress that may appear glacial. Flexibility in strategies and timing is the key to any progress.

The balance between unwavering centeredness and compassionate flexibility means that the therapist must be capable of observing limits and conditions, often in the face of massive and often quite desperate attempts on the part of the patient to control the therapist's response, while at the same time flexibly changing, adapting, and "giving in" as the situation requires. The therapist must both be alert to his or her own rigidity (a natural reaction to the stress of the therapeutic situation) and falling into the trap of giving in to every wish, demand, or current need of the patient.

In working with a suicidal borderline patient, the balance between these two extremes becomes most salient when the therapist has placed a dysfunctional interpersonal behavior pattern of the patient on an extinction schedule. The ability to stay centered and maintain the schedule is imperative, lest the therapist inadvertently put the patient on an intermittent reinforcement schedule, in which case the dysfunctional behavior will become highly resistant to therapeutic change. This is a simple fact of operant learning schedules. But with a suicidal patient in particular, a therapist can be overly rigid in applying an extinction program and fail to respond adequately to the patient's legitimate needs. As one of my patients pointed out, it is normal in all societies to give people more care and attention when they are sick. Yet not everyone stays sick to get care and attention.

Stance of Nurturing versus Benevolent Demanding

In DBT, there is a high degree of nurturing of the patient. The qualities of "nurturing" in this context include teaching, coaching, assisting, strengthening, and aiding the patient, all from a stance of cherishing the patient's abilities to learn and change. A willingness and certain ease in taking care for and nurturing the patient are needed. Compassion and sensitivity are essential with patients who are as sensitive while simultaneously as constricted and limited in emotional expression as most borderline individuals. Without these qualities, a therapist is always two steps behind the patient's often subtle reactions to the therapist's statements, remarks of other group members, and internal or environmental cues. Although a major effort is devoted in DBT to teaching patients how to identify and verbalize emotions, therapists who cannot come very close to mind reading in the earlier stages of treatment are likely to believe that borderline clients deliberately sabotage therapy with capricious behavior, or that patients who are really experiencing fear and helplessness are hostile and attacking.

A therapist must balance giving a patient the real help she needs with not giving unneeded help. "Benevolent demanding" is the therapist's recognition of the patient's existing capacities, reinforcement of adaptive behavior and self-control, and refusal to take care of the patient when she can care for herself. Generally, adept use of contingencies (i.e., demanding change as a prerequisite for outcomes the patient desires) is crucial. A certain ability to be tough when the situation warrants it is a requisite therapist characteristic. The dialectical position here is to push the patient forward with one hand while supporting her with the other hand. Thus, nurturing is in the service of strengthening the capabilities of the patient. As I have noted above in discussing assumptions about the patient and the treatment, the balance is that between taking care *of* and taking care *for* the patient. It is using both the carrot and the stick to promote change.

Agreements of Patients and Therapists

Patient Agreements

DBT requires a number of patient agreements. Generally, these are required for formal acceptance into the treatment and are the conditions of treatment. They should be discussed and clarified during the first several sessions, and at least oral agreement should be obtained. A written contract can be used at the discretion of the therapist.

One-Year Therapy Agreement

Uses of a Renewable Time-Limited Approach. Following the first one or several sessions, the patient and therapist should agree explicitly on whether they will work together and for how long. It should not be automatically assumed that the patient wants to work with the therapist. Under ordinary circumstances, the patient and therapist make a 1-year agreement, renewable annually. At the end of each year of treatment, progress is evaluated, and the question of whether to continue working together is discussed. Therapists will differ on what is required for continuation. Some therapists are willing to work with patients on a long-term basis and will renew the agreement each year unless there is some problem or the patients have met their goals. Other therapists are much more oriented to time-limited therapy and will want to set up therapeutic relationships with a clear intent at the beginning to refer the patients elsewhere at the end of the year, if treatment is still necessary.

DBT conducted on an inpatient unit may be very time-limited.

Some borderline patients cannot tolerate a nonrenewable time-limited approach. They cannot open up emotionally or verbally when they know that the therapy is going to end at an arbitrary point. These patients should not be forced into nonrenewable time-limited therapy. Obviously, with nonrenewable time-limited approaches, the goals of therapy may be narrower than for long-term therapy. For example, I have taken several patients into time-limited DBT who have histories of many psychiatric hospitalizations; have burned out and been rejected by several previous therapists; are currently dysfunctional and chronically parasuicidal; and cannot find another therapist to work with them. Some have been on the no-admit lists of more than one area hospital. In these instances, I have made it very clear to the patients that I will work with them for 1 year and then help them find another therapist. My goal is to help them stop their parasuicidal behavior and learn how to function effectively in therapy, so that they can benefit from and keep their next therapist. I think of this as a sort of pretreatment for the long-term work that is needed.

Circumstances of Unilateral Termination. During the first several sessions, the therapist should make the circumstances that will lead to unilateral therapy termination very clear. DBT has only one formal termination rule: Patients who miss 4 weeks of scheduled therapy in a row, either required skills training or individual therapy, are out of the program. They cannot return to therapy until the end of the current contracted period, and then return is a matter of negotiation. There are no circumstances under which this rule is broken. There are no good reasons in DBT for missing 4 weeks of scheduled therapy. This rule was originally adopted for research reasons; we needed to have an operational definition of therapy termination. However, I have found that it is an excellent clinical rule. It very clearly defines what constitutes missed sessions (up to three in a row) and what constitutes dropping out (four missed individual or required skills training sessions in a row). Thus, patients who miss one, two, or three sessions in a row know that they will be welcomed back, and they know unequivocally that if they miss a fourth they will not be allowed to return. In this manner, the "drift-out-of-therapy" phenomenon is reduced.

Many borderline patients want their therapists to make an unconditional commitment to continue therapy indefinitely or until the end of the time-limited period (depending on the original agreement), no matter what. Such a patient will say that she cannot trust the therapist, self-disclose, or the like, because she is afraid that the therapist will end the relationship. She may worry constantly about this possibility. It is very tempting to reassure such a patient that no matter what she does or says in therapy, she will not be terminated before she is ready. DBT does not advocate this stance. Instead, the position taken is somewhat like that in a marriage. Although the therapist commits himself or herself to working with the patient, to sticking with difficult processes, and to trying to resolve any therapeutic problems that arise, the therapy commitment is not unconditional. If the therapist finds it impossible to help the patient further, if the patient pushes the therapist beyond his or her limits, or if an unexpected mitigating condition (such as moving out of town) arises, therapy termination will be considered. As I tell my patients, even a mother's love is not unconditional. The agreement that the therapist does make, however, is to do his or her best to protect the patient from unilateral termination. When the patient's behavior is precipitating termination, this means that the therapist will (1) alert the patient to impending danger of termination in enough time for the patient to make necessary changes in her own behavior, and (2) assist her in making the changes. (As the next two chapters indicate more clearly, behaviors that threaten to terminate therapy prematurely are the second most important treatment target.) Similarly, although the patient can terminate treatment at any time, it is expected that she will terminate by coming to a session and discussing the proposed termination with her individual therapist.

Attendance Agreement

The next agreement is that the patient will attend all scheduled therapy sessions. Individual skills training and therapy sessions will be rescheduled if both the therapist and the patient can do so conveniently. If a missed group session is videotaped, the patient can view the missed session before the next one. The therapist should communicate clearly to the patient that it is not acceptable for her to miss sessions because she finds them too aversive, is not in the mood for therapy, wishes to avoid a particular topic, or feels hopeless.

Suicidal Behaviors Agreement

If suicidal behaviors (including parasuicide without intent to die) are a problem for the patient, she should be advised that reducing such behaviors is a primary treatment goal. The basic agreement needed is that, all other things being equal, the patient will work toward solving problems in ways that do not include intentional self-harm, attempts to die, or suicide. It should be emphasized that if this is not one of her goals, then DBT may not be the appropriate program for her. The therapist must be especially attentive to the patient's ambivalence with regard to suicidal behaviors. Thus, although an explicit verbal commitment to reducing such behaviors is the goal, less explicit commitments can be accepted. At times, a patient may agree to attend therapy with the understanding that reducing suicidal behaviors is the goal of the therapy, but she may not be able to make an explicit statement that she will not commit suicide. Structuring this agreement is discussed in more detail in Chapter 14.

Therapy-Interfering Behaviors Agreement

The next agreement is simply to work on any problems that interfere with the progress of therapy. Making this agreement explicit highlights the nature of therapy as an interpersonal, collaborative relationship at the very beginning.

Skills Training Agreement

If one major aim of the therapy is to help the patient substitute skilled responses for previous dysfunctional responses, then it seems clear that she has to learn the needed behavioral skills somewhere. During the first year of DBT, all patients must take part in the DBT skills training program (or, if impossible, another equivalent program).

Research and Payment Agreement

If DBT is carried out in a research context, the patient must be informed of and agree to participate in the research condition. Patient fees should be made clear, and a method of payment should be agreed on.

Therapist Agreements

It is very important that the therapist state clearly what the patient can expect from him or her. Therapist agreements in our program are as follows.

"Every Reasonable Effort" Agreement

The maximum that patients can expect from therapists is that they will make every reasonable effort to conduct the therapy as competently as possible. Patients can expect therapists to make their best effort to be helpful, to help them gain insight and learn new skills, and to teach them some of the behavioral tools they need to deal more effectively with their current living situations. Therapists should make it clear that they cannot save the patients, cannot solve the patients' problems and cannot keep the patients from engaging in suicidal behavior. This point flows directly out of the assumption about patients, discussed earlier, that they have to solve their own life problems.

It is often useful for a therapist to go over common misconceptions about therapy. A major misconception is often that the therapist can somehow make everything better. The therapist's inability to take away the intense pain, or sometimes even to lessen it somewhat, is often interpreted as uncaring or unwillingness to help. It is important that the therapist not imply that when the patient "grows up" or is "less narcissistic" she will see that this is not true. Instead, the task of the DBT therapist is actively to counter such beliefs and assumptions. I find it useful to emphasize that although I can help a patient develop and practice new behaviors that may be helpful in reshaping her life, I cannot in the final analysis reshape her life for her. The metaphor of the therapist as guide can be helpful here. I can show someone the way, but I cannot walk the trail for her. The caring is in staying with the patient on the path. Statements to this effect are often needed periodically throughout the treatment process.

Ethics Agreement

Ethical conduct can be a very salient issue in treating borderline patients. In my clinic, many of our patients have had previous therapists who engaged in extremely questionable, and at times clearly unethical, behaviors. Sexual involvement and dual relationships that clearly cross the boundaries of effective therapy are cases in point. Thus, an explicit agreement to obey standard ethical guidelines and professional codes is particularly important.

Personal Contact Agreement

Like the patient (see above), the therapist agrees to come to every scheduled session, to cancel sessions in advance when needed, and to reschedule whenever possible. The length of sessions should be discussed, and the patient's preferences and prior therapy experience should be ascertained. The intent is to provide sessions of reasonable length that are not cut short for arbitrary reasons. In addition to providing reasonable backup coverage when the therapist is out of town or unavailable, the therapist also agrees to provide reasonable phone contact. How much contact is reasonable is determined both by the DBT telephone strategies (see Chapter 15) and by the observing-limits approach (see Chapter 10).

Respect-for-Patient Agreement

It seems obvious, but is helpful to discuss anyway, that the therapist must be willing to respect the integrity and rights of the patient. Although respecting the patient is essential to effective therapy, the agreement here goes beyond considerations of helping the patient make needed behavioral changes.

Confidentiality Agreement

The therapist agrees that all information revealed in therapy will be held in strict confidence. Generally, only the members of the treatment team and the research staff (if a research project is in progress) are allowed access to therapy videotapes or audiotapes, session notes, and assessment materials. (It should go without saying, of course, that appropriate release-of-information forms are signed.) Even within the DBT team and supervision meetings, the therapist agrees to keep sensitive, potentially embarrassing, and very private information confidential unless there is a compelling need to do otherwise. Records of sessions are kept secure. It should also be stressed, however, that the therapist is not bound to confidentiality when the patient is threatening suicide or in other circumstances where therapists are required by law to report things patients say to them. When doing so is necessary to maintain the patient's safety or that of others, such threats may be communicated to other people—either those in the patient's home environment or members of the legal or mental health professional community.

Consultation Agreement

Therapists agree to obtain therapy consultation when needed. In standard DBT, all therapists agree to attend regularly scheduled case consultation meetings, either with a supervisor, peer supervision group, or other members of the patient's treatment team. The basic idea, here, is that the patient can count on the therapist to get help when needed rather than, for example, continue indefinitely with ineffective treatment or blame the patient for problems in the therapy.

Therapist Consultation Agreements

Much as the therapist and patient do, therapists in cosupervision or a case consultation group agree to interact with one another in certain ways. The agreements have to do with following the general DBT guidelines within the context of the supervision or case consultation meetings. That is, therapists agree to treat each other at least as well as they treat their patients. In addition, the agreements are intended to facilitate staying within a DBT frame with patients.

Dialectical Agreement

The DBT case consultation group agrees to accept, at least pragmatically, a dialectical philosophy. There is no absolute truth; therefore, when polarities arise, the task is to search for the synthesis rather than for the truth. The dialectical agreement does not proscribe strong opinions, nor does it suggest that polarities are undesirable. Rather, it simply points to the direction therapists agree to take when passionately held polar positions threaten to split the consultation team.

Consultation-to-the-Patient Agreement

The spirit of treatment planning in DBT is that therapists do not serve as intermediaries for patients with other professionals, including other members of the treatment team. The DBT case consultation group agrees that the task of the individual therapists is to consult with their own patients on how to interact with other therapists, not to tell other therapists how to interact with the patients. Thus, when a therapist behaves fallibly (within reason), the task of the other therapists on the team is to help their patients cope with this therapist's behavior, not necessarily to reform the therapist. This does not mean that the team members do not conduct treatment planning together for their patients, exchange information about the patients (including their problems with other members of the treatment team), and discuss problems in treatment. This agreement is discussed more fully in Chapter 13.

Consistency Agreement

Failures in carrying out treatment plans are opportunities for patients to learn to deal with the real world. The job of the therapy team is not to provide a stress-free, perfect environment for the patients. Thus, the consultation group, including all members of the treatment team, agrees that consistency of therapists with one another is not necessarily expected; each therapist does not have to teach the same thing, nor do all have to agree on what are proper rules for therapy. Each therapist can make his or her own rules about conditions of therapy with himself or herself. Although it can make for smooth sailing when all members of an institution, agency, or clinic communicate the unit's rules accurately and clearly, mix-ups are viewed as inevitable and isomorphic with the world we all live in; they are seen as a chance for patients (as well as therapists) to practice almost all of the skills taught in DBT.

Observing-Limits Agreement

The case consultation group agrees that all therapists are to observe their own personal and professional limits. Furthermore, consultation group members agree not to infer that narrow limits reflect therapists' fears of intimacy, self-centeredness, problems with dominance and control, or generally withholding nature, or that broad limits reflect a need to nurture, problems with boundaries, or projective identification. Patients can learn to figure out the limits.

Phenomenological Empathy Agreement

The therapists agree, all other things being equal, to search for nonpejorative or phenomenologically empathic interpretations of patients' behavior. The agreement is based on the fundamental assumption (described earlier) that the patients are trying their best and want to improve, rather than to sabotage the therapy or "play games" with their therapist. When a therapist is unable to come up with such an interpretation, other consultation group members agree to assist in doing so, meanwhile also validating the "blame the victim" mentality of the therapist. Thus, consultation group members agree to hold one another nonjudgmentally in the DBT frame. They agree not to label therapists who always adopt the empathic interpretation as naive, unsophisticated, or overly identified with their patients; they also agree not to label therapists who always adopt the hostile, pejorative, "blame the victim" interpretation as aggressive, dominating, or vindictive.

Fallibility Agreement

In DBT, there is an explicit agreement that all therapists are fallible. Put in the vernacular, this means that, relatively speaking, "therapists are all jerks." Thus, there is little need to be defensive, since it is agreed ahead of time that therapists have probably done whatever problematic things they are accused of. The task of the consultation group members is to apply DBT to one another, in order to help each therapist stay within the DBT protocols. As with patients, however, problem solving with therapists must be balanced with validation of inherent wisdom of the therapists' stance. Because, in principle, all therapists are fallible, it is agreed that they will inevitably violate all of the agreements discussed here. When this is done, they will rely on one another to point out the polarity and will move to search for the synthesis.

Concluding Comments

The assumptions about therapy and borderline patients, as well as the patient, therapist, and consultation group agreements, form the ground work context on which DBT is built and provide a basis for therapeutic decision making throughout the treatment. The experienced therapist has no doubt noticed that DBT overlaps extensively with many other therapeutic schools, including those identified as behavioral and cognitive–behavioral as well as those that are not. Although there may be little if anything actually new in DBT, the threads of therapeutic advice (and I hope, wisdom) dispensed across many therapy manuals and treatises on the care of BPD are at times woven together slightly differently in DBT. The next two chapters, and the third section of the book, are devoted to outlining the specific therapist actions and decision rules that define DBT. In Chapters 5 and 6, I describe in much greater detail the behavioral patterns targeted in DBT. Telling therapists which patient behaviors to focus on is an important part of any treatment manual; for some, it forms the bulk of the therapy description. In Part III, I describe the specific treatment strategies and procedures used in contacts with patients. The application of treatment strategies in any approach is still more of an art than a science, but I try to elucidate as far as possible the rules that should guide this application in DBT.

Note

1. I have to thank Lorna Benjamin for this succinct summary of DBT.

5

Behavioral Targets in Treatment: Behaviors to Increase and Decrease

In standard cognitive–behavioral therapy, treatment goals are usually described in terms of behavioral targets— that is, behaviors to increase and behaviors to decrease. I have used the same convention here. In DBT, each target is a class of behaviors relating to a certain theme or area of functioning. The specific behaviors targeted within each behavioral class are individualized for each patient; target selection depends on initial and continuing behavioral assessment. This point cannot be overemphasized.

The Overall Goal: Increasing Dialectical Behavior Patterns

The overriding and pervasive target of DBT is to increase dialectical behavior patterns among borderline patients. Put simply, this means both enhancing dialectical patterns of thought and cognitive functioning, and also helping patients to change their typically extreme behaviors into more balanced, integrative responses to the moment.

Dialectical Thinking

Dialectical thinking is the "middle path" between universalistic thinking and relativistic thinking. Universalistic thinking assumes that there are fixed, universal truths and a universal order to things. Truth is absolute; in disagreements, one person is right and one person is wrong. Relativistic thinking assumes that there is no universal truth and that the order of things depends entirely on who is doing the ordering. Truth is relative; in disagreements, it is pointless to search for truth, since truth is in the eye of the beholder. By contrast, dialectical thinking assumes that truth and order evolve and develop over time. In disagreements, truth is sought through efforts to discover what is left out of the ways both participants are ordering events. Truth is created by a new ordering that embraces and includes what was previously excluded by both (Basseches, 1984, p. 11).

Thus, dialectical thinking is more akin to constructive thinking, where the emphasis is on observing fundamental changes that occur through people's interaction with their environments. The cognitive therapy approach of Michael Mahoney (1991), which he describes as a "developmental constructive" approach to therapy, is a good example of constructive thinking. It contrasts with a nondialectical pattern of thinking, such as structuralism, which emphasizes finding patterns that stay the same over time and circumstances.

As I have discussed in Chapter 2, dialectical thinking requires the abilities to transcend polarities and, instead, to see reality as complex and multifaceted; to entertain contradictory thoughts and points of view, and to unite and integrate them; to be comfortable within flux and inconsistency; and to recognize that any all-encompassing point of view contains its own contradictions. When one is stuck in considering a problem, a dialectical approach would be to consider what has been left out or how one has artificially narrowed the boundaries or simplified the problem. Borderline individuals, by contrast, think in extremes and hold rigidly to points of view. Life is black or white, viewed in dichotomous units. They often have difficulty receiving new information; they search instead for absolute truths and concrete facts that never change. The overall goal of DBT is not to get patients to view reality as a series of grays, but rather to help them see both black and white, and to achieve a synthesis of the two that does not negate the reality of either.

For those who are not dialectical thinkers, or even for those who are but have never thought about it, it can be difficult to grasp exactly what is being discussed here. Here is an example: Imagine a patient who grew up in a family with a very strong world view. As an adult, she rejects much of the world view important to her family and instead embraces a different view. Her family disapproves vehemently. She believes that either she is right and her family is wrong, or her family is right and she is wrong. Whoever is wrong should abandon that viewpoint in favor of the other point of view.

From a formalistic positon, the therapeutic task is to help the patient honestly examine which position is closest to the truth and understand factors that interfere with the acceptance of the truth. Either the patient is engaged in dysfunctional thinking and should change her thinking style, or she is viewing things accurately and needs assistence in validating and believing herself.

Relativistic thinking would imagine that neither world view is right or wrong. Therapy in this case might focus on helping the patient decide which world view is more useful to her. The focus might be on problems the patient has in taking responsibility for her own point of view and her dysfunctional need for others to decide for her or for others to agree with her.

In contrast, a dialectical therapist would assist the patient identify the influences over time on her world view and examine how her own actions, in turn, have influenced the world views of her family members and others she interacts with. Therapy here might focus on discovering whether anything is interfering with further development and change. Therapy might also focus on ways the family's world view has changed, as well as factors inhibiting further change. The therapist might lead the patient to explore how each world view adds to and follows from the other, suggesting that a different world view can be appreciated without invalidating one's own viewpoint.

Here is another example. Suppose a patient tells her therapist that she is having many urges to commit suicide. After prolonged efforts at problem solving in this situation without any success, the therapist suggests that the patient admit herself to the local hospital until the danger has passed. The patient decides against hospitalization and refuses. The therapist proceeds to have her committed involuntarily to an in-patient hospital. At one point the patient may analyze the situation from a formal position. She may see her own needs and values as more important and of a higher order than the therapist's. After all, her safety is her own business. The job of therapists is not to push their values down patients' throats, locking them up when they disagree. She may decide to withhold information or to lie about her suicidal feelings in the future—to "play the game," so to speak—and to give up getting help on solving problems that make her feel suicidal.

At other times, the patient's thinking may be more relative and less absolute. On the one hand, she thinks it is reasonable that she should be able to talk to her therapist about suicidal urges without threat of commitment. If she cannot refuse hospitalization, what is the point of the assertiveness training her therapist has given her? On the other hand, her therapist cares about her and wants her to stay alive, even if he or she has to use force to keep her alive. Both points of view make equal sense, but the conflict is unresolvable, so the patient is simply confused.

If the patient can assume a dialectical stance, she can come to see the problem as a clash between the therapist's goal of creating conditions that enhance her autonomy and the therapist's obligation to protect her from harm. The task of enhancing the patient's autonomy may lead to practices that are not optimal for protecting her from harm (teaching the patient assertion skills and encouraging trust in her own decision making). Conversely, the task of protecting the patient from harm may lead to practices that do not enhance her autonomy (committing the patient against her stated wishes). If the patient can come to accept and appreciate this state of affairs, she may decide to try working with the therapist on ways to deal with problems that make her feel suicidal, while at the same time working out ways to make her therapist feel secure about her safety. She will have to make some compromises between autonomy and safety, just as her therapist does. However, she is resolved not to lose sight of her own therapeutic goals. She may decide to work very hard in therapy, in order to move toward transforming the system so that these two values do not conflict.[1]

Dialectical Thinking and Cognitive Therapy

The pervasive focus on nondialectical thinking in DBT is very similar to the focus on dysfunctional thinking in cognitive therapy. For example, cognitive errors targeted in cognitive therapy are also examples of nondialectical patterns of thought. As in cognitive therapy, a task of the therapist in DBT is to help the patient identify her extreme and absolute thought patterns, and then to assist her in testing the validity of her conclusions and beliefs. Problematic thinking patterns targeted in both DBT and cognitive therapy are as follows:

1. Arbitrary inferences or conclusions based on insufficient or contradictory evidence.
2. Overgeneralizations.
3. Magnification and exaggeration of the meaning or significance of events.
4. Inappropriate attribution of all blame and responsibility for negative events to oneself.
5. Inappropriate attribution of all blame and responsibility for negative events to others.
6. Name calling, or the application of negative trait labels that add no new information beyond the observed behavior used to generate the labels.
7. Catastrophizing, or the presumption of disastrous results if certain events do not either continue or develop.
8. Hopeless expectancies, or pessimistic predictions based on selective attention to negative events in the past or present, rather than on verifiable data.

Some (but not all) forms of cognitive therapy emphasize an empirical form of reasoning, which holds that truth is what fits the facts, what works in actuality, what permits prediction in the material world, and what can be pointed to operationally. Thus, the main focus is on the truth or falsity of propositions, beliefs, and generalizations. If propositions were always "true and primary," the empirical approach would be sufficient, and there would be no need for the dialectical approach. However, the spirit of dialectics is never to accept a final truth, an immobile and indisputable fact. Although DBT favors the dialectical method of reasoning, it does not hold that such reasoning is sufficient in itself. Empirical logic is not viewed as "wrong," especially in problem solving, but it is treated as only one way to think. From this perspective, the synthesis of the two forms of reasoning is most useful for arriving at understanding.

Dialectical Behavior Patterns: Balanced Lifestyle

The easiest way to think about dialectical behavior patterns is to consider the idea of balance. Borderline individuals rarely lead balanced lifestyles. Not only their thinking, but their typical emotional responses and actions, are apt to be dichotomous and extreme. The borderline behavioral patterns— emotional vulnerability versus self-invalidation, unrelenting crises versus inhibited grieving, and active passivity versus apparent competence (see Chapter 3)—are examples here. A focus on dialectical behavior patterns emphasizes moving the patient toward more balanced and integrative responses to life situations. From a Buddhist perspective, this is walking the "middle path." In particular, the following dialectical tensions must be resolved:

1. Skill enhancement versus self-acceptance.
2. Problem solving versus problem acceptance.
3. Affect regulation versus affect tolerance.
4. Self-efficacy versus help seeking.
5. Independence versus dependence.
6. Transparency versus privacy.
7. Trust versus suspicion.
8. Emotional control versus emotional tolerance.
9. Controlling/changing versus observing.
10. Attending/watching versus participating.
11. Needing from others versus giving to others.
12. Self-focusing versus other-focusing.
13. Contemplation/meditation versus action.

Primary Behavioral Targets

Decreasing Suicidal Behaviors

As Mintz (1968) has pointed out, no psychotherapy is effective with a dead patient. Thus, when the life of a patient is under immediate threat, the focus of any therapy must shift to efforts to keep the patient alive. In most psychotherapy situations, the threat to life is posed by suicidal behavior, but other behaviors may also qualify (e.g., continued fasting in an anorexic patient, neglect of a potentially fatal illness, putting oneself in danger of a victim-precipitated homicide). As I have noted in Chapter 1, suicidal behaviors, including completed suicide and parasuicidal acts committed with intent to die, are particularly prevalent among borderline patients. In contrast to many other patient populations, however, and as Chapater 1 likewise notes, borderline patients also have a high incidence of parasuicidal behaviors not accompanied by any intent to die. At least among some patients, parasuicidal behaviors are unlikely to prove fatal, and thus do not represent an immediate threat to the patients' lives. Nonetheless, parasuicidal acts of any type are high-priority targets in DBT; the reasons for their importance are discussed below. Five subcategories of suicide-related behaviors are targeted in DBT: (1) suicide crisis behaviors, (2) parasuicidal acts, (3) suicidal ideation and communications, (4) suicide-related expectancies and beliefs, and (5) suicide-related affect.

Suicide Crisis Behaviors

Suicide crisis behaviors are behaviors that convince the therapist or others that the patient is at high risk for imminent suicide. In most instances, these behaviors consist of some combination of credible suicide threats or other communications of upcoming suicide; suicide planning and preparations; obtaining and keeping available lethal means (e.g., hoarding drugs or buying a gun); and high suicide intent. At times, indirect communications of suicide intent may also be suicide crisis behaviors. Whether or not the therapist believes that subsequent suicide is probable, these behaviors are never ignored

The desire to be dead among borderline individuals is often reasonable, in that it is based on lives that are currently unbearable. A basic tenet of DBT is that the problem is rarely one of distorting positive situations into negative situations. Instead, the problem is usually that a patient simply has too many life crises, environmental stressors, problematic interpersonal relationships, difficult employment situations, and/or physical problems to enjoy life or find meaning in it. In addition, the patient's habitual dysfunctional behavior patterns both create their own stress and interfere with any chance of improving the quality of life. In sum, borderline individuals usually have good reasons for wanting to be dead.

However, DBT therapists, even when confronted by lives of incalculable pain, are always on the side of life over death by suicide. The rationale for this stance against suicide is as follows. The agenda of many borderline patients seems at times to be to convince their therapists that life is indeed not worth living; such arguments may have many different functions. A patient may assume that if the therapist agrees, he or she will intervene directly (magically, from my point of view) and change the quality of the patient's life. Or the patient may be trying to work up courage to commit suicide. Or the patient may be using the process of arguing with the therapist to elicit reasons for hope and reassurance. Whatever the reason, I have at times been convinced by patients that they are right. Not only did I believe that their lives were unlivable, but I myself saw no way out for them. I felt hopeless myself.

My feelings of hopelessness about a particular patient, however, are no better as a guide to reading the future than are the patient's. That is, I have often felt hopeless about a patient who has subsequently improved the quality of her life dramatically. I do not believe that this is a particular deficit on my part; feelings of hopelessness, at least in regard to borderline patients, are not uncommon among therapists. But, the therapist's own current life events, the state of the therapeutic relationship, and transitory moods of both therapist and patient influence these feelings of hopelessness certainly as much as factors actually predictive of future progress do.

Although a therapist may believe that a life of any quality is worth living, the lives of many borderline individuals come perilously near the edge. Whether their intense suffering is a result of their own behavior or of uncontrollable environmental events is irrelevant; suffering is suffering. Indeed, one can make the case that keeping a patient alive within an untenable life is no admirable feat. This position has led me to assert that DBT is not a suicide prevention program, but a life improvement program. The desire to commit suicide, however, has at its base a belief that life cannot or will not improve. Although that may be the case in some instances, it is not true in all instances. Death, however, rules out hope in all instances. We do not have any data indicating that people who are dead lead better lives.

I believe that individuals at times make informed and rational decisions to commit suicide. I do not believe that this phenomenon is limited to those not in psychiatric or psychological treatment. Nor do I believe that borderline patients are incapable of making an informed decision about whether to commit suicide or not. However, these beliefs in individual liberty do not mean that I must agree with any person that suicide is a good or even an acceptable choice.

In the face of persistent attempts on the part of some borderline patients to convince their therapists that suicide is a good idea, as well as their occasional success in such attempts, a therapist has to have a predetermined, nonnegotiable position on suicide. It cannot be a debatable option, lest the patient lose. I have chosen to be on the side of life. Although I value those whose therapeutic task is to help patients choose whether to live or die, opening up such a possibility when treating borderline patients insures, it seems to me, that sometimes therapists will encourage suicide for individuals who, if they live, will not regret living. Knowing that some who live may regret that choice, therapists who take the stance of life must also, it seems to me, accept the responsibility of helping these individuals in every way possible to create lives that are worth living. There is an old saying that the person who saves a life is then responsible for that life.

Parasuicidal Acts

Like suicide crisis behaviors, parasuicidal acts (see Chapter 1 for a full definition and discussion) are never ignored in DBT. Reducing parasuicidal acts is a high-priority target in DBT for a number of reasons. First, parasuicide is the best predictor of subsequent suicide. Among borderline patients, the rate of completed suicide among individuals who engage in parasuicide is twice the rate among those who do not (Stone, 1987b). Second, parasuicide damages the body, often irrevocably. Cutting and burning, for example, cannot be undone; scars are permanent. Parasuicide not only damages the body, but holds out the possibility of accidental death. Third, actions based on the intent to harm one self are simply incompatible with every other goal of any therapy, including DBT. The effectiveness of all voluntary psychotherapy is based, at least to some extent, on developing an intent to help rather than harm one self. Thus, treatment of parasuicidal behavior goes to the heart of the therapeutic task. Fourth, it is quite difficult for a therapist to credibly communicate caring for a patient if the therapist does not react to the patient's harming herself. Responding to parasuicide by insisting that it must stop, and devoting the full resources of therapy to that end, are quintessential communications of compassion and care. The refusal to condone parasuicidal acts under any circumstances is, of course, a strategic therapeutic move, and it can be extraordinarily difficult for the therapist to maintain such a stance.

Suicidal Ideation and Communications

Another priority in DBT is to decrease the frequency and intensity of suicidal ideation and communications. Targeted responses include thinking about suicide and parasuicide, experiencing urges to commit suicide or inflict self-harm, having suicide-related images and fantasies, making suicide plans, threatening suicide, and talking about suicide. Borderline individuals often spend a considerable amount of time thinking about suicide. In these cases, suicidal ideation is a habitual response that may be unconnected to any desire to die at the moment. The possibility of suicide reassures them that if things get too bad, there is always a way out. (I am reminded here of the giving of cyanide capsules to spies during wars. If they are caught, they can always avoid torture by committing suicide.) Other borderline individuals habitually threaten suicide at almost any provocation, but immediately withdraw or dismiss their threats. Still other borderline individuals at times agonize over whether to commit suicide or not; usually, such agonizing is accompanied by what seems like intolerable pain. Suicidal threats are always targeted directly. In contrast, suicide ideation is targeted directly only when it is new or unexpected, is intense or aversive, is associated with parasuicide or suicide crises behaviors, or interferes with skillful problem solving.

Suicide-Related Expectancies and Beliefs

DBT likewise targets patients' expectations about the value of suicidal behavior as a problem-solving alternative. Unfortunately, many of these expectations may be quite accurate. If a patient wants to seek revenge, make others sorry for what they did or did not do, escape an intolerable life situation, or even save others pain, suffering, and money, suicide may be the answer.

Parasuicide can also have beneficial effects. As I described in Chapter 2, a sense of relief after cutting or burning is extremely common even when the behavior is carried out in private. Getting sleep, a consequence of overdosing and other methods that cause unconsciousness, often has a substantial beneficial effect on mood. Parasuicide of any sort, especially if it causes a great commotion, can be a very effective means of distraction from persistent negative affect and problematic situations. Finally, both suicide crisis behaviors and parasuicide are quite often effective ways for the patient to make others take her seriously, to obtain help and attention, to escape from situations, to resume or terminate relationships, or to achieve desired but otherwise unavailable hospitalizations.

Thus, the expectations that are perhaps most in need of attention are not those about the realistic short-term consequences of suicidal behavior. Rather, expectations regarding long-range negative outcomes for suicidal behavior need to be addressed, as do expectations about alternative problem-solving behaviors that may in the long run prove more effective. Suicide-related expectations and beliefs are generally attended to directly only if they are instrumental to parasuicide, or suicide crisis behaviors or if they interfere with more skillful behaviors.

Suicide-Related Affect

As noted above, both parasuicidal acts and thinking about suicide are associated with relief of intensely negative emotional states among some borderline and suicidal individuals. These individuals may report feelings of relaxation, calmness, and emotional "release" from feelings of panic, intense anxiety, overwhelming anger, and unbearable shame after they engage in parasuicide or make plans to commit suicide. Such a connection may be due the result of instrumental learning, classical conditioning, or some immediate neurochemical effect of self-injury. At times, positive affective experiences, including sexual arousal, may accompany parasuicidal acts. An important goal of DBT is to change the individual's emotional response both to parasuicide and to thoughts, images, and fantasies of suicide and parasuicide. Like suicide-related expectations, suicide-related affect is generally attended to directly only if it is functionally related to parasuicide or suicide crisis behaviors or if it interferes with skillful behaviors.

Postscript: Suicidal Behaviors as Maladaptive Problem Solving

As is perhaps obvious from the foregoing, DBT views all suicidal behaviors as maladaptive problem-solving behaviors. As I have noted previously, whereas the therapist typically views suicidal behaviors as a problem, the patient often (but not always) views them as a solution. Thus, a first task of therapy is to work actively toward resolution of this fundamental difference in viewpoints. A dialectical synthesis is the direction to head in. Once even a fragile synthesis is achieved (or reachieved), therapy is oriented to two fundamental targets: (1) helping the patient build a life worth living and (2) replacing maladaptive attempts at problem solving with adaptive, skillful problem-solving behaviors. Borderline patients often want to hold off on changing their problem-solving style until the factors that compromise the livability of their lives are reduced or removed. The emphasis in DBT is usually just the opposite: "First we will stop the suicidal behaviors, and then we will figure out how to improve your life." As Chapter 9 indicates, such a dichotomy is in fact arbitrary, since the problem-solving strategies that form the heart of DBT change interventions work incrementally on both reducing troublesome behaviors and changing the personal and situational circumstances that precipitate them.

Decreasing Therapy-Interfering Behaviors

The second target of DBT is the reduction of both patient and therapist behaviors that interfere with effective therapy, and, conversely, the increase of behaviors that enhance the continuation and effectiveness of therapy. The necessity of targeting this class of behaviors seems obvious. Patients who are not in therapy or who, though nominally in therapy, do not engage in or receive therapeutic activities, cannot benefit. Although the choice of whether to work together in the first place is a decision only a patient and therapist can make, whether they continue in a therapeutic relationship is a function of much more than simple decisional or choice behavior. Indeed, borderline patients frequently have great difficulty translating decisions and choices into congruent behaviors. Cognitive control over overt behavior is not one of their strengths. For therapists, many external factors, such as agency priorities, training needs, or financial considerations, may make following through on the decision to treat particular patients impossible. Furthermore, how a therapist chooses a patient is determined by a number of factors, including reinforcement history, behavioral capabilities, behavioral inhibitions, and current contingencies operating in the therapeutic environment. The aim of DBT is to create contingencies, enhance capabilities, and reduce inhibitions so that the probability of a patient's and therapist's continuing in therapy together is enhanced.

DBT requires active participation on the part of both the patient and the therapist. During both individual and group sessions, the patient must collaborate with the therapist in addressing therapeutic goals. Between sessions, the patient must carry out homework assignments; in addition, the patient is expected to keep a number of agreements having to do with living arrangements and suicidal behavior. Thus, a patient may exhibit many types of behaviors that can lead to problems in treatment. Similarly, a therapist who does not deliver effective therapy or who engages in behaviors that interfere with the patient's collaboration or continuation is rarely very helpful. The patient behaviors I am referring to here are similar to those included in the concept of "resistance" by psychodynamic and psychoanalytic therapists. The therapist behaviors I am referring to fall under the analytic rubric of "countertransference," at least when countertransference is evaluated in negative terms. They also fall under the rubric of "relationship factors" in more general discussions of psychotherapy.

"Butterfly" versus "Attached" Patients

Both borderline and parasuicidal patients are notorious for dropping out of therapy prematurely (Gunderson, 1984; Richman & Charles, 1976; Weissman et al., 1973). In my experience, however, borderline patients usually fall into one of two types: "butterfly" patients and "attached" patients. Butterfly patients have great difficulty attaching to therapy; they fly in and out of their therapists' hands, so to speak. Attendance at sessions is episodic, agreements are often broken, and therapy or a therapeutic relationship does not appear to be a high priority. Therapy with such patients rarely focuses on the relationship with the therapist, unless the therapist initiates such a discussion. Generally, the patient is involved in one or more primary relationships with someone else, either parents, a spouse, or a partner. Phone calls to the therapist usually concern the patient's personal crises rather than problems with the therapist. Most of her interpersonal energy goes into the alternate relationship(s) rather than into the therapeutic relationship. Whenever an alternate relationship is secure, the patient may miss or terminate therapy. Usually, she has not a had long history of prior psychotherapy. An important therapy-interfering behavior is the noninvolvement with the therapist.

On the other end of the spectrum is the attached patient. Such an individual usually forms an almost immediate, intense relationship with the therapist. She almost never misses a session, and if she does she often asks (or demands) to reschedule it. The patient asks for and may need longer than usual sessions, more frequent sessions, and more phone calls to the therapist between sessions. From the start, difficulties within the therapeutic relationship form an important focus of therapy. Often, the therapist is the patient's primary support person, and the therapeutic relationship is her primary interpersonal relationship. Attached patients rarely drop out of therapy, have great difficulties when their therapists go on vacation, and are afraid of termination from the beginning. Many of these individuals have had long histories of psychotherapy relationships, which have reinforced their attachment behaviors. With these patients, an important area of therapy-interfering behaviors is their inability to tolerate imperfect therapists who are often unable to meet their needs.

Traditional Cognitive and Behavior Therapy Approaches

In reading some cognitive and behavioral treatment manuals and research, one often has the impression that getting a patient to collaborate and actually engage in the therapy is so easy that it does not bear discussion. With some patient populations, this is indeed the case. The attention being given to patients' interfering behavior, however, is rapidly increasing. For example, Chamberlain et al. (1984) have developed a rating scale for patients' resistant behaviors. A number of articles and books have been written on patient compliance (Shelton & Levy, 1981; Meichenbaum & Turk, 1987). Cognitive–behavioral therapists regularly attend to the necessity of developing a collaborative relationship in therapy (Beck, Rush, Shaw, & Emery, 1979).

In contrast, cognitive and behavior therapists have paid little attention to therapists' behaviors (other than technique) that interfere with or enhance therapy. Generally, the behavioral position has been twofold on this question: First, the effect of therapist interpersonal factors on treatment outcome is an empirical question that cannot be answered without recourse to data; second, this empirical question must be addressed idiographically for each successive patient–therapist pair (Turkat & Brantley, 1981). Therapist behaviors that are effective for one patient–therapist pair may be completely ineffective for another pair. This twofold perspective is a direct outgrowth of the emphasis in cognitive and behavior therapy on applying empirical procedures to the remediation of clinical problems.

Therapy-enhancing behaviors discussed most frequently in the behavioral literature include those therapist qualities usually associated with client-centered therapy (e.g., warmth, accurate empathy, and genuineness) and those derived from social-psychological studies of interpersonal influence (e.g., therapist prestige, status, expertise and attractiveness). The precise role that these various qualities play in effective behavior therapy remains controversial. Some behaviorists stress the lack of consistent empirical data on the effects of many therapist variables traditionally thought to be important for therapeutic outcome, especially warmth and empathy (Morris & Magrath, 1983; Turkat & Brantley, 1981). Other behaviorists argue for their importance (Goldfried & Davison, 1976; Levis, 1980; Wilson, 1984). Even those who clearly view specific therapist interpersonal behaviors as important, however, argue for an idiographic implementation to fit each particular patient (Arnkoff, 1983; Wilson, 1984). Beck et al. (1979) perhaps express this behavioral view best when they advise that the individual therapist must proceed by observing the effects of his or her actions on the patient. DBT accepts such a point of view.

Therapy-Interfering Behaviors of the Patient

Three categories of behavior are included under the rubric of therapy-interfering behaviors of the patient. The first category consists of any behaviors that interfere with the patient's receiving the therapy offered. A second category, seen in group and inpatient therapy settings, consists of behaviors that interfere with other patients' benefiting from the therapy. The third category consists of patient behaviors that burn out the therapist; included are behaviors that push the therapist's personal limits or decrease the therapist's willingness to continue therapy.

Behaviors That Interfere with Receiving Therapy. The notion here is that a therapy applied but not received will fail. The idea is similar to the necessity of therapeutic blood levels for psychotropic medications. For DBT to be received, the patient must attend sessions, collaborate with the therapist, and comply with treatment recommendations.

1. *Nonattentive behaviors.* Behaviors that interfere with attending to therapy interfere with treatment effectiveness. Obviously, if a patient does not come to sessions or drops out prematurely, she will not benefit from therapy. Less obviously, if a patient comes to therapy physically but does not attend psychologically, it is difficult to understand how she will benefit from the experience. Attention-interfering behaviors that we have seen in our clinic are as follows: dropping out of therapy; threatening to drop out of therapy; missing sessions; canceling sessions for nontherapeutic reasons; experiencing continuous disruptive crises; getting admitted to hospitals excessively, and thus missing sessions; acting suicidal on inpatient units, and thus frightening the staff so that the patient cannot leave or receive a pass to come to individual or group therapy sessions; acting excessively suicidal or threatening suicide in the presence of people with legal power to commit the patient to a hospital (involuntary patients usually cannot obtain passes to attend outpatient therapy sessions); taking mind-altering substances before coming to sessions (unless required to by prescription); walking out of sessions before they end; fainting, having panic attacks, or having seizures during sessions; dissociating or daydreaming during sessions; and not getting sufficient sleep before sessions and coming too tired to stay awake. If these behaviors occur between one session and the next, or within the session, they are noted, and discussed, and relevant problem-solving strategies are applied.

2. *Non-collaborative behaviors.* Behavior therapists have historically emphasized the role played by a collaborative and collegial relationship between patient and therapist in therapeutic effectiveness, especially when treatments involve the patient's active participation within treatment sessions. Because direct modification of adults' environments is difficult or impossible, most behavioral treatment programs aimed at adults consist of some variation of self-management and skills training. Thus, therapists must teach adult patients how to modify their own environments so that functional behaviors and outcomes are enhanced. In such programs, patients' active collaboration is obviously essential.

Alternatively, in treatments emphasizing the reinforcing functions of the therapist and focusing primarily on in-session patient behaviors, collaboration may itself be a goal of treatment, rather than an essential patient behavior for achieving the goal. Such is the case with "functional analytic psychotherapy," a radical behavioral treatment based on Skinnerian principles, developed by Robert Kohlenberg and Mavis Tsai (1991). Collaborative behaviors are viewed in DBT both as essential to treatment and as a goal of treatment. Noncollaborative behaviors are considered instances of therapy-interfering behaviors. Examples include the following: inability or refusal to work in therapy; lying; not talking at all in therapy; withdrawing emotionally during sessions; arguing incessantly with anything and everything the therapist says; distracting and digressing from high-priority targets during sessions; and responding to most or all questions with "I don't know" or "I can't remember."

3. *Noncompliant behaviors.* An active sense of participation by the patient in therapy is consistently related to positive outcome (Greenberg, 1983). Behavior therapy in general, and DBT in particular, require very direct involvement of the patient in the treatment process. During sessions the patient may be required to engage in covert imaginal activities (e.g., relaxation training or systematic desensitization) or to practice new behaviors (e.g., role playing in social skills training), and also receives various homework assignments between sessions. Patients are expected to expose themselves to situations they fear and to produce responses they find very difficult. Courage, self-management skills, and a history in which both compliance behaviors and active problem-solving attempts have been reinforced are requisites to such behaviors. Not surprisingly, borderline individuals often lack these attributes. Noncompliant behaviors include not filling out or not bringing in diary cards; filling them out incompletely or incorrectly; not keeping agreements made with the therapist; refusing to complete or only partially completing behavioral homework assignments; refusing to comply with treatment recommendations, such as exposure strategies; and refusing to agree to treatment goals essential to DBT (e.g., refusing to work on reducing suicidal behaviors).

Behaviors That Interfere with Other Patients. In group and inpatient settings, interactions among patients can be crucial to the success or failure of therapy. In my experience, the behaviors that are most likely to make other patients unable to profit from therapy are openly hostile, critical, and judgmental remarks directed to them. Although it may be desirable for the other patients to learn to tolerate such remarks, this goal seems impossible for some borderline patients to reach when they feel open to attack at any moment. Borderline patients are very sensitive to any type of negative feedback, even if only implied. They will often experience appropriately given feedback as an attack. A patient's inability to accept reasonably given negative feedback from other patients may itself be a therapy-interfering behavior, but ill-timed expressions of negative feelings toward another patient or insistent attempts at solving a relationship problem with another patient are usually also therapy-interfering for the recipient.

Since one of the interpersonal targets in DBT is to help patients become more comfortable with conflict, however, conflict avoidance is not always (or even usually) viewed as actually desirable in DBT. Although almost any behavior that creates conflict may interfere with therapy for other patients, in my experience only openly hostile attacks on other patients threaten to destroy the possibility of therapy.

Behaviors That Burn Out Therapists. Borderline individuals want help from people in their environment, but often they either are unskilled at asking for and receiving help or burn out potential caregivers. Learning how to ask for and receive help appropriately, as well as how to care for the help giver, is an important life skill. A focus on enhancing help-requesting and help-receiving behaviors among borderline individuals, as well as the generalization of these behaviors to everyday life, enhances the quality of both therapy and everyday life. Of course, reducing behaviors that burn out therapists is also essential if a therapeutic relationship is to be maintained. Generally, research in this area suggests that burnout, once it occurs, can lead to a host of therapeutic mistakes (Cherniss, 1980; Carrol & White, 1981). It can be difficult to recover from. Thus, it seems important to prevent burnout rather than wait for it to occur and then try to remediate it. This same reasoning underlies the DBT strategy of observing limits, part of the contingency strategies discussed in Chapter 10; I discuss this point in much greater detail there.

Following from the above, the DBT individual therapist states clearly at the beginning that an important goal of DBT is to teach the patient to act in such a manner that the therapist not only can give the help that the patient needs, but also wants to do so. Generally, the therapist points out quickly that there is no such thing as unconditional positive regard or unconditional love. Even the most devoted person can be dissuaded from giving further help to a friend or relative; the same holds true for a therapist. Given the right behaviors, any patient can cause a therapist to reject her. This point is made very clear in the DBT therapy orientation, as Chapter 4 notes. The idea here is to cut off at the beginning any beliefs that the help the patient receives from the therapist is unrelated to her own interpersonal behaviors with the therapist. In my experience, most borderline patients welcome such an orientation on the part of their therapists. Many have been rejected from therapy at least once. The idea that therapy will assist them in preventing this from happening again is welcome news.

In my experience, therapists often have trouble identifying behaviors contributing to burnout that qualify as therapy-interfering behaviors. Most have no difficulty identifying patients' behaviors that interfere with attending therapy, collaborating with the therapists, and complying with treatment recommendations. However, patients' behaviors that push therapists' personal limits or decrease their motivation to work with the patient's are often not identified. In these instances, many therapists tend to believe one of two things: Either the behaviors are part of the patients' "psychopathology," or the therapists' reactions are somehow marks of their own inadequacy. When these behaviors are seen as part of "borderline pathology," they are often not targeted directly. Many therapists seem to believe that if patients can be "cured" of their "borderlineness," these behaviors will automatically cease. Alternatively, when a therapist's reactions are viewed as problems of the therapist, the patient's behaviors are often ignored in favor of focusing (usually in supervision or case conference meetings) on the inadequacies of the therapist.

1. *Pushing the therapist's personal limits.* Every therapist has personal limits both on what he or she is willing to do for a patient and on which patient behaviors are tolerable. Patient behaviors that exceed what the therapist is willing to tolerate, therefore, are therapy-interfering behaviors. Which behaviors constitute pushing personal limits vary over therapists, over time, and over patients. Within the therapy of one patient, limits vary with changes in the therapeutic relationship and with individual factors in the therapist's own life situation. Which behaviors are targeted at a given time depend both on the state of the therapist's limits at that time and on the capabilities of the patient.

The most important limit-pushing behavior of any borderline patient is refusing to engage in or accept therapeutic strategies that the therapist believes are essential to progress or effective therapy. Thus, if a patient refuses to comply with a therapeutic strategy that the therapist believes is essential to effective therapy, and other reasonably acceptable strategies are not available, then that refusal is a limit-pushing behavior and therefore may become the focus of therapy until it is resolved. The patient, the therapist, or both need to change. Other behaviors that can push the limits of a DBT therapist include phoning the therapist too much; going to the therapist's house or initiating interactions with the therapist's family members; demanding solutions to problems that the therapist cannot solve; demanding more session time or more sessions than the therapist can deliver; interacting with the therapist in an overly personal or familiar way, including sexually provocative or seductive behavior; infringing on the therapist's personal space; and threatening harm to the therapist or his or her family members. Almost any patient behavior can at times push some therapists' limits. Although at times limits must be stretched, there are no *a priori* personal limits that must be observed in DBT. Thus, limit-pushing behaviors can only be defined by each therapist in relation to each individual patient. Patients in a program where they interact with multiple therapists, therefore, must learn to observe multiple sets of limits.

Pushing a therapist's limits is often interpreted by nonbehavioral therapists as an absence of patient boundaries. Patient behaviors that make a therapist feel as if his or her personal boundaries are being intruded and infringed upon, and at times taken over, are assumed to be a result of the patient's having no personal boundaries of her own. The term "boundaries" is used as if it has a nonarbitrary meaning, independent of the effect of the patient's behaviors on the therapist. A therapist often sets such boundaries as if there is a "correct" placement for them. In my view, however, boundary setting is a social function; thus, there are no context-free, correct boundaries. The relevant task that a borderline patient often cannot or will not engage in is that of observing and respecting other people's interpersonal boundaries. Such failures may be determined by any number of factors other than the patient's sense of her own boundaries.

Focusing on the patient's own boundaries (instead of the infringement of the therapist's), however, has two unfortunate outcomes from a DBT point of view. First, it deflects the therapist from attention to the patient's problematic behavior. To change a construct, such as boundaries, requires at least that the therapist be able to specify the behaviors that operationally define the construct; this is rarely done. Second, since lack of boundaries is assumed to determine the problematic behaviors, there is little or no incentive to conduct a behavioral analysis to probe for other influences. Thus, important factors determining the behavior may be missed, making change that much more difficult.

2. *Behaviors that push organizational limits.* Although we do not ordinarily think of organizations, including treatment units, as having "personal limits," it is useful to consider limits from this perspective in DBT. Thus, inpatient unit rules (e.g., no loud radios), elements of day treatment contracts (e.g., no guns), or outpatient clinic rules (e.g., waiting for therapists in the designated waiting area) are instances of organizational limits. They are "personal" because each treatment unit has its own set of limits, often developed to satisfy many individuals (hospital and unit administrators, legal personnel, unit directors, etc.). For example, in my program, patients cross a limit when they do anything that might get my treatment unit kicked out of the larger clinic that gives us space. The only requirement in DBT is that the limits of organizations offering therapy should mimic as closely as possible organizational limits in everyday settings. Thus, limits requiring deferential or submissive behaviors, or proscribing interpersonal behaviors that would be tolerated in ordinary work, school, or home settings, are probably iatrogenic. In DBT, behaviors that cross organizational limits are treated in the same fashion as those that cross a therapist's limits. In both cases, the therapist must make it clear that the limits reflect the personality of the individual or the organization.

As in the case of a therapist's personal limits, a most important type of organizational limit has to do with the treatment unit's bottom-line requirements for conducting effective treatment. This type of limit comes the closest to an arbitrary limit, since it is constructed with a class of patients in mind (e.g., borderline patients), without considering the needs of any particular patient. For example, in the first year of standard DBT, all patients are required to be in both individual psychotherapy and some sort of structured skills training. On many inpatient units, all patients are required to take part in a specified number of unit activities or therapy groups. In a research treatment setting, all patients may be required to participate in periodic assessments. The key here is for the unit to be very careful in developing these limits, keeping only those that everyone is sure are necessary for the treatment program to work.

3. *Behaviors that decrease the therapist's motivation.* A prerequisite to continuation of therapy is motivation to continue on the part of both therapist and patient. Motivation, in turn, is dependent on reinforcement history in a particular situation or context. In the best of cases, the patient's progress toward treatment goals is the primary reinforcer for the therapist; when

progress is slow, other behaviors of the patient can assume greater importance. The unwillingness of many therapists to work with borderline patients
is directly tied to the relative absence of reinforcing behaviors from these patients and to the presence of many behaviors that the therapists experience
as aversive. Failure to attend to therapy, noncollaborative behaviors, noncompliance, and pushing the therapist's limits all qualify here. Other behaviors
I have experienced include a hostile attitude; impatience and statements that
the therapist should do better or is not a good therapist, especially when these
are sarcastic or caustic; criticisms of the therapist's person or personality; criticisms of the therapist's values, place of work, or family; lack of gratitude or
appreciation of the therapist's efforts; inability or unwillingness to see or admit progress that does occur; and comparisons of the therapist to others who
are viewed as better therapists. Particularly stressful patient behaviors are
threats to sue the therapist, reporting the therapist to the licensing board, or
otherwise engaging in a public rebuke of the therapist. One patient in our
clinic brought and sent her therapist an overwhelming number of letters, es-
says, poems, drawings, and gifts. The therapist once took home an essay to
read and somehow misplaced it. The patient at a later date asked for it back,
and when informed that the therapist had misplaced it at home, she took
the therapist to small-claims court to request damages of several hundred dol-
lars. Needless to say, the therapist was not highly motivated to continue therapy with the patient even after she located the missing essay.

4. *Behaviors that reduce milieu or group members' motivation.* In group,
milieu, and family therapy, the typical expectation is that patients or family
members will assist one another. In this sense, each patient and family member can also be considered a therapist. Any individual behaviors that decrease
the motivation of other group, milieu, or family members to continue offering help and stay interested in the patient's welfare are therapy-interfering behaviors.

Therapy-Enhancing Behaviors of the Patient

During the initial orientation to DBT, and sometimes frequently thereafter,
I make it clear to patients that one of their tasks is to interact with me in
such a way that I want to continue working with them. (I have a similar
reciprocal obligation to them.) This idea is often a new one to our patients.
Of course, during interactions with a patient, a therapist has an obligation
to act in helpful ways no matter what the patient is doing. If this is not possible, then the interactions should be terminated. To prevent such an
outcome—for example, losing phone calls or therapy altogether—the patient
is taught the specific behaviors that will enhance the likelihood of interaction's continuing.

As noted above, the chief therapy-enhancing behavior is simply making
progress toward behavioral goals. Behaviors important to therapists, besides
the converse of the therapy-interfering behaviors described above, are specif-

ic to each therapist and vary with context. Those that have been important to me and therapists I work with consist of asking for help in avoiding suicide or parasuicide (rather than threatening suicide or parasuicide if help is not given); trying out behavioral suggestions given by the therapist (rather than saying that they will not work); asking whether this is a convenient time to talk when calling the therapist, and taking no for an answer when necessary; accepting with good grace a phone call shorter than desired; keeping agreements made to the therapist; calling to cancel appointments (rather than simply not showing up); and showing a sense of humor, or at least appreciation of the therapist's sense of humor. The key point I want to make is that therapy-enhancing behaviors must often be taught, not expected.

Therapy-Interfering Behaviors of the Therapist

Therapy-interfering behaviors on the part of the therapist include any that are iatrogenic, as well as any that unnecessarily cause the patient distress or make progress difficult. The basic idea here is that the therapist should, first, do no harm. Second, all other things being equal, the therapist should implement the most benign therapy possible. Third, the therapist should be nondefensive about mistakes and flexibly open to repairing and changing response patterns when necessary.

A broad array of factors may increase therapist-interfering behaviors. Those that have consistently influenced me and others in my clinic include the following: personal factors, such as life stress at home or at work, not enough sleep, or illness; too many time demands other than those created by the patient; compartmentalizing clinical work into a small part of the week, so that clinical demands at other times are experienced as intrusive (a particular problem for those in the academic world); insecurity about one's skills as a therapist, especially in comparison to other therapists on the team; comparisons of the patient's seeming lack of progress to the progress everyone else's patients seem to be making; anger, hostility, and frustration directed at the patient; "blaming the victim" attitudes, especially if one cannot remember another way to think about the patient's behavior; a sense of being pushed up against the wall by the patient, or of losing control of the therapy situation; fear of being sued; anxiety and/or panic that the patient will commit suicide; and unrealistic beliefs about what is possible in the moment, with corresponding unreasonable expectations of the patient.

One of the most common, and most debilitating, factors leading to therapeutic mistakes is a therapist's inability to tolerate a patient's communications of suffering in the present. Attempts to ameliorate patient suffering often lead to reinforcements of dysfunctional behaviors, which, rather than reducing suffering, actually increase it in the long run; this point has been discussed in more detail in Chapter 4. Therapists' therapy-interfering behaviors, however, can be generally classified into two categories: (1) those that concern balance within the therapy delivery, and (2) those that concern respect for the patient.

Behaviors Creating Therapeutic Imbalance. Typically, behaviors that imbalance the therapy are consistent behaviors located at one extreme or the other (e.g., acceptance vs. change or stability vs. flexibility) of a continuum of therapist behaviors.

1. *Imbalance of change versus acceptance.* From a DBT perspective, the worst offenders of this sort are behavior patterns that create and maintain a lack of balance between change and acceptance treatment strategies. A therapist who is overly focused on change may so invalidate the patient's sense of herself and her view of reality that years may be spent in subsequent therapies undoing the damage. A patient who rebels in such an environment may be blamed as excessively defensive, and her objections may go unheeded. In contrast, a therapist who accepts the patient unconditionally, but does not teach her new, more competent behavior patterns, does the patient little good. Indeed, such an approach rarely accepts the patient's own view of what she needs for change to occur. It is a rare borderline patient who is not eager for behavioral coaching, especially in situations she finds difficult or impossible to handle.

2. *Imbalance of flexibility versus stability.* A second group of therapy-interfering behaviors consists of those indicating an inability to balance flexibility in modifying treatment approaches with stability of therapeutic focus. Such a problem most often occurs with the therapist who, without a theoretical perspective to guide therapy, switches strategies endlessly in an effort to achieve some behavioral progress. Essentially, the problem is one of patience. Almost any therapeutic strategy with a borderline patient takes a fair amount of time to succeed. Equally problematic is a therapist's modification of therapy according to non-theory-linked criteria. Examples include skipping skills training in favor of "heart-to-heart" discussions when the therapist is bored or not "in the mood" for the effort imposed by skills training; locking a patient in a hospital out of anger or to appease family members, rather than as a theory-linked response to the patient's suicide crisis behavior; or appeasing the patient because the therapist is too tired or does not have time to cope with conflict. Needless to say, trying to convince the patient that these therapeutic behaviors are for the patient's own good simply compounds the problem. At the other pole, rigidly maintaining therapeutic strategies that produce no progress or extreme distress for the patient, especially if other potentially therapeutic strategies are available, is also therapy-interfering. Unfortunately, all humans become more rigid under stress—a condition that often accompanies treating the borderline patient. In my experience, under the stress of treating difficult patients, therapists often vacillate between being too rigid and stubborn and being too flexible. Keeping a balance between stability and flexibility depends on ongoing therapeutic assessment and application of the interventions described in great detail in Chapters 8–11.

3. *Imbalance of nurturing versus demanding change.* A third type of imbalance is that between nurturing and doing for the patient on one hand,

and withholding help on the other, assuming that the patient will help herself when she is sufficiently motivated. In the first case, the patient is seen as excessively fragile, incompetent, and too vulnerable to help herself. The therapist may infantilize the patient, treat her as unable to make decisions, and do things for and help her in ways that the therapist would not consider for other patients. Out of context, examples of this may include regularly meeting the patient in a coffee shop for sessions because the patient is viewed as too afraid to come to the office; taking her places (or ignoring missed sessions) because she is unable to drive and is believed too fragile to learn to ride public transportation; changing difficult topics; believing that the patient is too intimidated to speak for herself and allowing her to be silent while answering for her in a family meeting; and taking charge of her money and paying bills for her. In contrast, a therapist at times may refuse to accept that a patient needs more support and nurturing than she is receiving—a stance that insures failure. At times the patient may actually exaggerate her needs and incompetence to make the therapist take her seriously, thus continuing the cycle of failure. Difficulties in keeping a balance between intervening for and taking care of a patient versus consulting with and teaching her how to care for herself are discussed extensively in Chapter 13.

4. *Imbalance of reciprocal versus irreverent communication.* Therapists also err when they lose their balance between reciprocal and irreverent communication (see Chapters 4 and 12). On the one hand, borderline patients seem to encourage vulnerability and personal sharing on the part of their therapists. Two factors operate here. First, borderline patients can be quite persuasive in their arguments that the therapeutic relationship is artificially unegalitarian and one-sided. "Why should I be the one taking all the risks?" they may ask. Second, borderline individuals are often extremely capable caregivers; thus, all too often, therapists make the mistake of becoming overly vulnerable within the therapy. It is not unusual for therapists to develop the habit of sharing their own personal trials and tribulations with borderline patients, regardless of their relevance to the patients' therapy. Sexual involvement with a patient is the most exaggerated example here. At the other extreme, therapists can overemphasize the distance between themselves and their patients. Non-DBT therapists justify this by referring to "boundary issues" or the "therapeutic frame." DBT therapists can resort to irreverent communication strategies. Irreverent communication, therapeutic frames, and boundary issues, however, can all be distorted to condone cruel jokes at patients' expense; hostile criticism; unwarranted attacks on patients' beliefs, emotional responses, decisions, and behavior; and inflexible emotional and physical distancing from patients.

Behaviors Showing Lack of Respect for the Patient. Behaviors that communicate lack of respect to a patient sometimes communicate accurately. At other times they are inadvertent, resulting more from thoughtlessness than from genuine lack of respect. Typical disrespectful behaviors of therapists are

TABLE 5.1. Examples of a Therapist's Disrespectful Behaviors

1. Misses or forgets appointments
2. Cancels appointments without rescheduling
3. Arbitrarily changes his or her policies with the patient (e.g., changes phone policy, fees, appointment times)
4. Does not return messages or phone calls, or delays calling back
5. Loses papers/files/notes
6. Does not read the notes/papers patient gives him or her
7. Is late for appointments
8. Appears or dresses unprofessionally
9. Has poor physical hygiene
10. Has a messy or unclean office space
11. Smokes during appointments
12. Eats/chews gum during appointments
13. Does not close the door during therapy sessions
14. Allows interruptions such as phone calls or messages
15. Is inattentive during sessions or phone calls, or engages in other activities
16. Forgets important information (name, relevant history/information)
17. Repeats self, often forgets what he or she said
18. Appears visibly tired or fatigued
19. Dozes off when with the patient
20. Avoids eye contact
21. Talks about other patients
22. Talks about how he or she would rather be doing something else
23. Watches the clock when with the patient
24. Ends sessions prematurely
25. Refers to patient in a sexist, paternalistic, or maternalistic manner
26. Treats patient as inferior to the therapist

Note. From *Developing a Scale to Measure Individuals' Stress-Proneness to Behaviors of Human Service Professionals* by M. Miller, 1990, unpublished manuscript, University of Washington. Reprinted by permission of the author.

listed in Table 5.1; this list was put together from a number of resources by Marian Miller (1990). Many of the behaviors listed here are indicative of therapist burnout, either in general or with a particular patient. Although an occasional instance of behavior communicating lack of respect is perhaps not very detrimental to therapy, an accumulation over time can interfere seriously with the therapeutic endeavor. Even more crucial than avoiding disrespectful behaviors, however, is the therapist's response when such behaviors are pointed out by the patient. The task of repairing disruptions and tears in the fabric of the relationship can be one of the most therapeutic processes the patient experiences. Certainly the necessity to repair relationships is typical in the patient's life; the repair in this case, however, can prove extraordinarily healing.

Decreasing Behaviors That Interfere with Quality of Life

As I have indicated in Chapter 4 and again in this chapter, DBT assumes that borderline patients have good reasons for being suicidal and unhappy.

The solution, from my point of view, is for the patients to change the quality of their lives. Behaviors that might be categorized as interfering with the quality of life are listed in Table 5.2. The list is not exhaustive, and other problems may surface with a particular patient. To be included in this category, a patient's behavior must be seriously problematic—enough so that if not changed, it surely will interfere with any chance of a reasonable quality of life. A good way to determine whether the behavior pattern is serious enough to qualify here is to consider the pattern both in terms of DSM-IV diagnostic criteria (in particular, Axes I and V) and in terms of the effects of the behavior on the patient's ability to progress further in therapy. Behavioral patterns that are not serious enough to meet diagnostic criteria, cause serious impairment, or interfere with the further conduct of therapy do not qualify under this heading. Instead, less serious or less harmful patterns should be treated in the second and third stages of DBT.

Usually, the determination of which behavior patterns meet this criteria will be made by therapist and patient jointly. However, in many instances,

---

TABLE 5.2. Behaviors That Interfere with Quality of Life

1. Substance abuse (examples: alcohol drinking; abuse of illicit or prescription drugs)

2. High-risk or unprotected sexual behavior (examples: unsafe sex practices; abusing others sexually; excessively promiscuous sex; sex with inappropriate persons)

3. Extreme financial difficulties (examples: overwhelming unpaid bills; difficulties in budgeting; excessive spending or gambling; inability to manage public assistance agencies)

4. Criminal behaviors that if not changed may lead to jail (examples: shoplifting; setting fires)

5. Serious dysfunctional interpersonal behaviors (examples: choosing or staying with physically, sexually, and/or emotionally abusive partners; excessive contact with abusive relatives; ending relationships prematurely; making other people feel so uncomfortable that few friends are possible; incapacitating shyness or fear of social disapproval)

6. Employment- or school-related dysfunctional behaviors (examples: quitting jobs or school prematurely; inability to look for or find a job; fear of going to school or getting needed vocational training; difficulties in doing job or school-related work; inappropriate career choices; getting fired or failing in school excessively)

7. Illness-related dysfunctional behaviors (examples: inability to get proper medical care; not taking necessary medications; overtaking medication; fear of physicians; refusal to treat illness)

8. Housing-related dysfunctional behaviors (examples: living in shelters, in cars, or in overcrowded housing; living with abusive or incompatible people; not finding stable housing; engaging in behaviors that cause evictions or rejections from housing possibilities)

9. Mental-health-related dysfunctional behaviors (examples: going into psychiatric hospitals; pharmacotherapist hopping; not finding needed ancillary treatments)

10. Mental-disorder-related dysfunctional patterns (examples: behavioral patterns that meet criteria for other severe or debilitating Axis I or Axis II mental disorders)

the recognition that a particular behavior pattern is problematic is the first step on the path to change. In such instances, the therapist must be very careful to keep the focus on behaviors that indeed are functionally related to quality-of-life issues for the particular patient. Opinions and personalized judgments can often interfere here (instances of therapy-interfering behaviors by the therapist).

Case conferences and supervisory sessions can be invaluable for helping a therapist sort through his or her own values, differences between these and the patient's values, and the influence of the therapist's values on therapeutic priorities. Such sorting through is especially important when a therapist and patient come from differing cultural backgrounds. Whether or not a therapist can work within the context of the patient's values, however, depends on the therapist's own personal limits. For example, I once had a patient who set fires in postal pickup boxes. She did not view this as a high-priority problem. When we were negotiating for a second year of therapy, I told her that I could not work with her unless one goal of therapy was to stop this behavior. I did not want to tolerate my images of the patient's getting arrested or other people's not getting important letters.

One basic premise of DBT is that a structured lifestyle is functionally related to therapeutic gains across all target areas. In an early version of DBT, I required patients to have structured activities that took them out of their homes at least part of each week, preferably daily. Such activities could consist of employment, volunteer jobs, school, or other obligations. The reason for this requirement was that my colleagues and I found it difficult (if not impossible) to have an effect on borderline patients' mood-dependent behaviors if the patients stayed home all day. Generally, staying home was related to increasing depressive affect, escalating fear and agoraphobia-like behaviors, behavioral passivity, and increased suicidal behaviors. I changed this requirement to a recommendation in subsequent versions of the treatment; the reason this had to do with the DBT policy on termination of treatment. Generally, the approach is to avoid unilateral termination of therapy, if at all possible. Termination is not only the most powerful but also the last contingency available to the therapist, and we found that it had to be used too often when structured activities were *required*. The current policy is to make dysfunctional behaviors as uncomfortable as possible within the treatment. Conditions that can lead to termination of DBT are discussed further in Chapter 10.

Increasing Behavioral Skills

Skills training in DBT is designed to remediate behavioral skill deficits typical of individuals meeting criteria for BPD. As Chapter 1 has suggested (see especially Table 1.5), the nine criteria for BPD designated in DSM-IV can be collapsed reasonably well into five categories: self dysfunction (inadequate sense of self, sense of emptiness); behavioral dysregulation (impulsive, self-damaging, and/or suicidal behaviors); emotional dysregulation (emotional

TABLE 5.3. Goals of Skills Training in DBT

General Goal

To learn and refine skills in changing behavioral, emotional, and thinking patterns associated with problems in living that are causing misery and distress.

Specific Goals

Behaviors to decrease	Behaviors to increase
Interpersonal dysregulation	Interpersonal skills
Emotional dysregulation	Emotion regulation skills
Behavioral and cognitive dysregulation	Distress tolerance skills
Self dysregulation	Core mindfulness skills: observing, describing, participating, taking a non-judgmental stance, focusing on one thing in the moment, being effective)

lability, problems with anger); interpersonal dysregulation (chaotic relationships, fears of abandonment); and cognitive dysregulation (depersonalization, dissociation, delusion). The behavioral skills taught in DBT target these problem areas. The relationship of DBT skills training to the broad categories of BPD criteria is outlined in Table 5.3. Emotion regulation skills, interpersonal effectiveness skills, distress tolerance skills, and DBT "core" mindfulness skills are taught in a structured format. Self-management skills, which are needed for learning all other skills, are taught as needed throughout the treatment.

Core Mindfulness Skills

Mindfulness skills are central to DBT; they are so important that they are referred to as "core" skills. They are the first skills taught and are listed on the diary cards that patients fill out every week. The skills are psychological and behavioral versions of meditation skills usually taught in Eastern spiritual practices. I have drawn most heavily from the practice of Zen, but the skills are compatible with most Western contemplative and Eastern meditation practices. There are three "what" skills (observing, describing, participating) and three "how" skills (taking a nonjudgmental stance, focusing on one thing in the moment, being effective). These skills are outlined and described in great detail in the companion manual to this volume; a brief summary is given below.

Core "Whats." The mindfulness "what" skills include learning to observe, to describe, and to participate. The goal is to develop a lifestyle of participating with awareness; it is assumed that participation without awareness is a key characteristic of impulsive and mood-dependent behaviors. Generally, actively observing and describing one's own behavioral responses are only necessary when new behavior is being learned, there is some sort of problem, or a change is necessary. For example, beginning piano players pay close attention to the location of their hands and fingers, and may either count beats out loud or name the keys and chords they are playing. As skill improves, however, such observing and describing cease. But if a habitual mistake is made after a piece is learned, the player may have to revert to observing and describing until a new pattern has been learned.

The first "what" skill is observing—that is, attending to events, emotions, and other behavioral responses, even if these are distressing ones. What the patient learns here is simply to allow herself to experience with awareness, in the moment, whatever is happening, rather than leaving a situation or trying to terminate an emotion, (behaviors discussed below as among those that must be decreased). Generally, the ability to attend to events requires a corresponding ability to step back from the event; observing an event is separate or different from the event itself. (Observing walking and walking are two different responses, for example.) This focus on "experiencing the moment" is based on both eastern psychological approaches and Western notions of nonreinforced exposure as a method of extinguishing automatic avoidance and fear responses.

The second "what" skill is that of describing events and personal responses in words. The ability to apply verbal labels to behavioral and environmental events is essential for both communication and self-control. Learning to describe requires that the individual learn not to take her emotions and thoughts literally—that is, as literal reflections of environmental events. For example, feeling afraid does not necessarily mean that a situation is threatening to one's life or welfare. However, borderline individuals often confuse emotional responses with precipitating events. Physical components of fear (e.g., "I feel my stomach muscles tightening and my throat constricting") may be confused with perceptions of the environment ("I am starting an exam in school") to produce a thought ("I am going to fail the exam"). Thoughts also are often taken literally; that is, thoughts ("I feel unloved") are confused with facts ("I am unloved"). Indeed, one of the principal aims of cognitive therapy is to test the association of thoughts with their corresponding environmental events. The individual who cannot identify thoughts as thoughts, outside events as events, and so on, will have great difficulty in most treatment approaches. Interestingly, almost every therapeutic approach stresses the importance of helping the patient observe and describe events. Free association in psychoanalysis; keeping behavioral diaries in behavior therapy; recording thoughts, assumptions, and beliefs in cognitive therapy; and reflective responding in client-centered therapy are all instances of the patient's or the therapist's observing and describing behavioral responses and ongoing events in the patient's life.

The third core "what" skill is the ability to participate without self-consciousness. "Participating" in this sense is entering completely into the activities of the current moment, without separating oneself from ongoing events and interactions. The quality of action is spontaneous; the interaction between the individual and the environment is smooth and based in part, but not by any means entirely, on habit. Participating can, of course, be mindless. We have all had the experience of driving a complicated route home as we concentrated on something else, arriving home without any awareness whatsoever of how we got there. But it can also be mindful. A good example of mindful participating is that of the skillful athlete who responds flexibly but smoothly to the demands of the task with alertness and awareness, but not with self-consciousness. Mindlessness is participating without attention to the task; mindfulness is participating with attention.

Core "Hows." The next three mindfulness skills have to do with *how* one observes, describes, and participates; they include taking a nonjudgmental stance, focusing on one thing in the moment, and being effective (doing what works). As taught in DBT, taking a nonjudgmental stance means just that—judging something as neither good nor bad. It does not mean going from a negative judgment to a positive judgment. Although borderline individuals tend to judge both themselves and others in either excessively positive terms (idealization) or excessively negative terms (devaluation), the position here is not that they should be more balanced in their judgments, but rather that judging should in most instances be dropped altogether. This is a very subtle point but a very important one. The notion is that, for instance, a person who can be "worthwhile" can always become "worthless." Instead, DBT stresses a focus on the consequences of behaviors and events. For example, behaviors may lead to painful consequences for oneself or for others, or the outcome of events may be destructive. A nonjudgmental approach observes these consequences, and may suggest changing the behaviors or events, but does not necessarily add a label of "bad" to them. Everything simply is as it is. Or, as Albert Ellis is reputed to have said when asked how a rational–emotive therapist would handle the prospect of an imminent plane crash, "If you die, you die."

Mindfulness in its totality has to do with the quality of awareness that a person brings to activities. The second "how" goal is to learn to focus the mind and awareness on the current moment's activity, rather than splitting attention among several activities or between a current activity and thoughts about something else. Achieving such a focus requires control of attention, a capability that most borderline patients lack. Often borderline patients are distracted by thoughts and images of the past, worries about the future, ruminative thoughts about troubles, or current negative moods. Rather than focusing their entire attention on current worries (which would be an instance of mindful worrying) and perhaps resolving some aspect of a current worry, they often worry while at the same time trying to do something else. This problem is readily observable in their difficulties in attending to the DBT skills training program. The patients must be taught how to focus their attention on one task or activity at a time, engaging in it with alertness, awareness, and wakefulness.

The third "how" goal, being effective, is directed at reducing the patients' tendency at times to be more concerned with what is "right" than with doing what is actually needed or called for in a particular situation. Being effective is the opposite of "cutting off your nose to spite your face." As our patients often say, it is "playing the game" or "doing what works." From an Eastern meditation perspective, focusing on effectiveness is "using skillful means." The inability to let go of "being right" in favor of achieving goals is, of course, related to borderline patients' experiences with invalidating environments. A central issue for many patients is whether they can indeed trust their own perceptions, judgments, and decisions — that is, whether they can expect their own actions to be correct or "right." However, taken to an extreme, an emphasis on principle over outcome can often result in borderline patients' being disappointed or alienating others. In the end, we all have to "give in" some of the time. Borderline patients at times find it much easier to give up being right for being effective when it is viewed as a skillful response rather than as a "giving in."

Distress Tolerance Skills

DBT emphasizes learning to bear pain skillfully. The ability to tolerate and accept distress is an essential mental health goal for at least two reasons. First, pain and distress are part of life; they cannot be entirely avoided or removed. The inability to accept this immutable fact leads itself to increased pain and suffering. Second, distress tolerance, at least over the short run, is part and parcel of any attempt to change oneself; otherwise, impulsive actions will interfere with efforts to establish desired changes.

Distress tolerance skills constitute a natural progression from mindfulness skills. They have to do with the ability to accept, in a nonjudgmental fashion, both oneself and one's current situation. Essentially, distress tolerance is the ability to perceive one's environment without putting demands on it to be different; to experience one's current emotional state without attempting to change it; and to observe one's own thoughts and action patterns without attempting to stop or control them. Although the stance advocated here is a nonjudgmental one, this should not be taken to mean that it is one of approval. It is especially important that this distinction be made clear to the patient: Acceptance of reality is not equivalent to approval of reality. Or, as a cognitive restructuring therapist might put it, "The fact that something is not a catastrophe does not mean it is not a pain in the ass."

The distress tolerance behaviors targeted in DBT are concerned with tolerating and surviving crises and with accepting life as it is in the moment. Four sets of crisis survival strategies are taught: distracting (with activities, doing things that contribute, comparing oneself to people less well off, opposite emotions, pushing away painful situations, other thoughts, and intense other sensations), self-soothing (via vision, hearing, smell, taste, and touch), improving the moment (with imagery, meaning, prayer, relaxation, focusing on one thing in the moment, taking vacations, and self-encouragement), and thinking of pros and cons. Acceptance skills include radical acceptance (i.e., *complete* acceptance from deep within), turning the mind toward acceptance (i.e., choosing to accept reality as it is), and willingness versus willfulness. The idea of "willingness" is Gerald May's (1982); he describes it as follows.

> Willingness implies a surrendering of one's self-separateness, an entering into, an immersion in the deepest processes of life itself. It is a realization that one already is a part of some ultimate cosmic process and it is a commitment to participation in that process. In contrast, willfulness is the setting of oneself apart from the fundamental essence of life in an attempt to master, direct, control, or otherwise manipulate existence. More simply, willingness is saying yes to the mystery of being alive in each moment. Willfulness is saying no, or perhaps more commonly, "yes, but. . ." (p. 6)

Although borderline patients and their therapists alike readily accept crisis survival skills as important, the DBT focus on acceptance and willingness is often viewed as inherently flawed. This viewpoint is based on the notion that acceptance and willingness imply approval. This is not what May (1982) means; indeed, he points out that willingness demands opposition to destructive forces, but goes on to note that it seems almost inevitable that this opposition often turns into willfulness:

> But willingness and willfulness do not apply to specific things or situations. They reflect instead the underlying attitude one has toward the wonder of life itself. Willingness notices this wonder and bows in some kind of reverence to it. Willfulness forgets it, ignores it, or at its worst, actively tries to destroy it. Thus willingness can sometimes seem very active and assertive, even aggressive. And willfulness can appear in the guise of passivity. Political revolution is a good example. (p. 6)

Emotion Regulation Skills

Borderline individuals are affectively intense and labile. As noted in Chapter 1, many studies have suggested that borderline and parasuicidal individuals are characterized by anger, intense frustration, depression, and anxiety; as noted in Chapter 2, DBT postulates that difficulties in regulating painful emotions are central to the behavioral difficulties of the borderline individual. From the patient's perspective, painful feelings are most often the "problem to be solved." Suicidal behaviors and other dysfunctional behaviors, including substance abuse, are often behavioral solutions to intolerably painful emotions.

Such affective intensity and lability suggest that borderline patients might benefit from help in learning to regulate their affective levels. In my experience, most borderline individuals try to regulate affect by simply giving themselves instructions not to feel whatever it is that they feel. This tendency is a direct result of the emotional invalidating environment, which mandates that people should smile when they are unhappy, be nice and not rock the boat when they are angry, and confess and feel forgiven when they are feeling guilty.

Affect regulation skills can be extremely difficult to teach, because borderline individuals have often been overdosed with instructions that if they would just "change their attitude" they could change their feelings. In a sense, many borderline individuals come from environments where everyone else exhibits almost perfect cognitive control of their emotions. Moreover, these very same individuals have exhibited intolerance and strong disapproval of the patients' inability to exhibit similar control. Often borderline patients will resist any attempt to control their emotions; such control would imply that other people are right and they are wrong for feeling the way they do. Thus, affect regulation can be taught only in a context of emotional self-validation.

Like distress tolerance, affect regulation requires the application of mindfulness skills—in this case, the nonjudgmental observation and description of one's current emotional responses. The theoretical idea is that much of the borderline individual's emotional distress is a result of secondary responses (e.g., intense shame, anxiety, or rage) to primary emotions. Often the primary emotions are adaptive and appropriate to the context. The reduction of this secondary distress requires exposure to the primary emotions in a nonjudgmental atmosphere. In this context, mindfulness to one's own emotional responses can be thought of as an exposure technique. There are a number of specific DBT emotion regulation skills, described below.

Identifying and Labeling Affect. The first step in regulating emotions is learning to identify and label ongoing, current emotions. Emotions, however, are complex behavioral responses. Their identification often involves the ability not only to observe one's own responses, but also to describe accurately the context in which the emotions occur. Thus, learning to identify an emotional response is aided enormously if one can observe and describe (1) the event prompting the emotion; (2) the interpretations of the event that prompt the emotion; (3) the phenemonological experience, including physical sensation, of the emotion; (4) the expressive behaviors associated with the emotion; and (5) the aftereffects of the emotion on one's own functioning.

Identifying Obstacles to Changing Emotions. Emotional behavior is functional to the individual. Changing emotional behaviors can be difficult when they are followed by reinforcing consequences; thus, identifying the functions and reinforcers for particular emotional behaviors can be useful. Generally, emotions function to communicate to others and to motivate a person's own behavior. Emotional behaviors can also have two other important functions. The first, related to the communication function, is to influence and control other people's behaviors; the second is to validate the person's own perceptions and interpretations of events. Although the latter function is not fully logical (e.g., if one person hates another, this does not necessarily mean that the other is worthy of being hated), it can nonetheless be important for borderline patients. Identifying these functions of emotions, especially negative emotions, is an important step toward change.

Reducing Vulnerability to "Emotion Mind." All people are more susceptible to emotional reactivity when they are under physical or environmental stress. Accordingly, patients are assisted in achieving balanced nutrition and eating habits, getting sufficient but not too much sleep (including treating insomnia if needed), getting adequate exercise, treating physical illnesses, staying off nonprescribed mood-altering drugs, and increasing mastery by engaging in activities that build a sense of self-efficacy and competence. The focus on mastery is very similar to activity scheduling in cognitive therapy for depression (Beck et al., 1979). Although these targets seem straight forward, making headway on them with borderline patients can be exhausting for both patients and therapists. With respect to insomnia, many of our borderline patients fight a never-ending battle in which pharmacotherapy often seems of little help. Poverty can interfere with both balanced nutrition and medical care. Work on any of these targets requires an active stance by the patients and persistence until positive effects begin to accumulate. The typical problem-solving passivity of many borderline patients can be a substantial difficulty here.

Increasing Positive Emotional Events. Once again, DBT assumes that most people, including borderline individuals, feel bad for good reasons. Although people's perceptions tend to be distorted when they are highly emotional, that does not mean that the emotions themselves are the result of distorted perceptions. Thus, an important way to control emotions is to control the events that set off emotions. Increasing the number of positive events in one's life is one approach to increasing positive emotions. In the short term, this involves increasing daily positive experiences. In the long term, it means making life changes so that positive events will occur more often. In addition to increasing positive events, it is also useful to work on being mindful of positive experiences when they occur, as well as unmindful of worries that the positive experience will end.

Increasing Mindfulness to Current Emotion. Mindfulness to current emotions means experiencing emotions without judging them or trying to inhibit them, block them, or distract from them. The basic idea here is that exposure to painful or distressing emotions, without association to negative consequences, will extinguish their ability to stimulate secondary negative emotions. The natural consequences of a patient's judging negative emotions as "bad" are feelings of guilt, anger, and/or anxiety whenever she feels "bad." The addition of these feelings to an already negative situation simply makes the distress more intense and tolerance more difficult. Frequently, the patient could tolerate a distressing situation or painful affect if only she could refrain from feeling guilty or anxious about feeling bad in the first place.

Taking Opposite Action. As discussed in Chapter 2, behavioral-expressive responses are important parts of all emotions. Thus, one strategy to change or regulate an emotion is to change its behavioral-expressive component by acting in a way that opposes or is inconsistent with the emotion. The therapist should focus on the patient's overt actions (e.g., doing something nice for someone she is angry at, approaching what she is afraid of) as well as her postural and facial expressiveness. But, with respect to the latter, the therapist must make it clear that the idea is not to block expression of an emotion; rather, it is to express a different emotion. There is a very big difference between an constricted facial expression that blocks the expression of anger and a relaxed facial expression that expresses liking. This technique is discussed extensively in Chapter 11.

Applying Distress Tolerance Techniques. Tolerating negative emotions without impulsive actions that make matters worse is, of course, one way to modulate the intensity and duration of negative emotions. Any or all of the distress tolerance techniques may be helpful here.

Interpersonal Effectiveness Skills

The particular behavioral patterns needed for social effectiveness depend almost entirely on one's goals in a particular situational context. The first section of the interpersonal skills module addresses this problem. As noted in connection with the apparent-competence syndrome in Chapter 3, borderline individuals quite often have many conversational skills in their repertoire. Social effectiveness, however, requires two complementary behavioral-expressive skills: (1) skills in producing automatic responses to situations encountered habitually; and (2) skills in producing novel responses or a combination of responses when the situation calls for them.

The interpersonal response patterns taught in DBT are very similar to those taught in assertiveness and interpersonal problem-solving classes. They include effective strategies for asking for what one needs, saying no, and coping with interpersonal conflict. "Effectiveness" here means obtaining the changes one wants, keeping the relationship, and keeping one's self-respect. Although the skills included in this progoram are quite specific (see the skills training manual for further details), I suspect that any well-developed interpersonal training program could be substituted for the DBT package.

Again, borderline and suicidal individuals frequently possess good interpersonal skills in a general sense. The problems arise in the application of these skills to the situations that the patients encounter. They may be able to describe effective behavioral sequences when discussing another person encountering a problematic situation, but may be completely incapable of generating or carrying out a similar behavioral sequence when analyzing their own situation. Usually, the problem is that both belief patterns and uncontrollable affective responses are inhibiting the application of social skills.

A behavioral mistake that borderline individuals often make is premature termination of relationships. This probably results from difficulties in all of the target areas. Problems in affect tolerance make it difficult to tolerate the fears, anxieties, or frustrations that are typical in conflictual situations. Problems in affect regulation lead to inability to decrease chronic anger or frustration; inadequate self-regulation and interpersonal problem-solving skills make it difficult to turn potential relationship conflicts into positive encounters. Borderline individuals frequently vacillate between avoidance of conflict and intense confrontation. Unfortunately, the choice of avoidance versus confrontation is based on the patients' affective state rather than on the needs of the current situation. In DBT in general, therapists challenge patients' negative expectancies regarding their environment, their relationships, and themselves. The therapists should assist the patients in learning to apply specific interpersonal problem-solving, social, and assertiveness skills to modify aversive environments and develop effective relationships.

Self-Management Skills

Self-management skills are needed to learn, maintain, and generalize new behaviors and to inhibit or extinguish undesirable behaviors and behavioral changes. Self-management skills include behavioral categories such as self-control and goal-directed behavior. In its widest sense, the term "self-management" refers to any attempt to control, manage, or otherwise change one's own behavior, thoughts, or emotional responses to events. In this sense, the DBT skills of mindfulness, distress tolerance, affect regulation, and interpersonal problem solving can be thought of as specific types of self-management skills. The term is used here, however, to refer to the generic set of behavior capabilities that an individual needs in order to acquire further skills. To the extent that the borderline individual is deficient in self-management skills, her ability to acquire the other skills targeted in DBT is seriously compromised. The self-management skills that should be targeted are discussed below.

Knowledge of Principles of Behavior Change and Maintenance. Borderline individuals are often seriously lacking in knowledge of fundamental principles of changing and maintaining behavior. A patient's belief that people change complex behavior patterns in a heroic show of willpower sets the stage for an accelerating cycle of failure and self-condemnation. The failure to master a goal becomes one more proof that trait explanations of failure (laziness, lack of motivation, no "guts") are really true. The therapist must undermine this notion of how people change. Frequently, analogies to the learning of common everyday skills (e.g., learning to write, ride a bicylce, etc.) serve to illustrate that willpower does not in itself produce success; it merely allows a person to persist in the face of the failure that is typically part of learning new behaviors.

Borderline individuals need to learn principles of reinforcement, punishment, shaping, environment–behavior relationships, extinction, and so forth. Thus, principles of learning and behavioral control in general, as well as knowledge about how these principles apply in each individual's case, are important targets in teaching self-management skills. Learning these targeted concepts often involves a substantial change in a patient's belief structure, especially of her beliefs about those factors controlling her own behavior.

Realistic Goal Setting. Borderline patients also need to learn how to formulate positive goals in place of negative goals, to assess both positive and negative goals realistically, and to examine their life patterns from the point of view of values clarification. Borderline patients typically believe that nothing short of perfection is an acceptable outcome. Behavior change goals are often sweeping in context and clearly exceed the skills the patients may possess. Encouraging patients to "think small" and "accumulate small positives" can be helpful here.

Environmental/Behavioral Analysis Skills. Therapists will need to teach patients such skills as self-monitoring and environmental monitoring, setting up and evaluating baselines, and evaluating empirical data to determine relationships between antecedent and consequent events and their own responses. These skills are very similar to the hypothesis-testing skills taught in cognitive therapy (Beck et al., 1979).

Contingency Management Skills. Borderline individuals frequently have great difficulty in formulating and carrying out contingency management plans. In my experience, most have enormous difficulty with the concept of self-reward. Usually, the problem is that their thought patterns center around deserving versus not deserving rewards or punishments. Since the entire notion of deserving versus not deserving is based on judgments, work on contingency management has to be interwoven with teaching mindfulness skills. A patient will often admit to believing that administering self-punishment or deprivation is the only effective way to change her inadequate behavior. The therapist should specifically point out the numerous negative effects of this strategy (e.g., "If you do overeat again, what additional problems are you creating by then starving yourself as punishment?") and attempt to generate nonaversive behavior management contingencies. In my experience, the therapist has to be both knowledgeable about the rules of learning and persuasive about the problematic effects of misapplying contingencies.

Environmental Control Techniques. A invalidating environment's belief that an individual can overcome any set of environmental stimuli is based on the assumption that individuals can function independently of their environments. Given this set of beliefs, it is understandable that borderline patients are not particularly skilled at utilizing their environments as a means of controlling their own behavior. As I have discussed in Chapter 3, however, borderline individuals are likely to be more responsive to transitory environmental cues than are others. Thus, the ability to manage their environmental surroundings effectively can be particularly crucial. Techniques such as stimulus narrowing (e.g., reducing the number of distracting events in the immediately surrounding environment) and stimulus avoidance (avoiding events that precipitate problematic behaviors) should be targeted in particular, to counteract a patient's tendencies to believe that "willpower" alone is sufficient.

Relapse Prevention Plans. Like the alcoholic individuals described so well by Alan Marlatt (see Marlatt & Gordon, 1985), borderline individuals frequently respond to any relapse or small failure as an indication that they are total failures and may as well give up. For example, they will develop a self-management plan and then unrealistically expect perfection in adhering to the plan. The target here is attitudinal change. It is important to teach the patients to plan realistically for relapse, as well as to develop strategies for accepting relapse nonevaluatively and for mitigating the negative effects of relapse.

Ability to Tolerate Limited Progress.   Because borderline individuals have little tolerance for feeling bad, they have difficulties carrying out behavior change action plans that require a "wait-and-see" approach. Rather, they will often engage in the "quick-fix syndrome," which involves setting unreasonably short time limits for relatively complex changes. To put it another way, progress is expected to occur overnight, otherwise, the plan has failed. Once again, emphasizing the gradual nature of behavior change and the need to tolerate some negative affect in the interim should be a major focus of therapists' efforts.

What About Other Behavioral Skills Training Programs?

You may be wondering whether you need to stick to DBT-specific behavioral skills training or whether you can use other skills training programs instead. Different programs may be available in your area or to your patients, or you may be more familiar with another program. Mindfulness skills can be learned in meditation programs based on principles similar to mindfulness, or from a meditation teacher. There are dozens of self-help books and classes on personal self-management and on interpersonal skills and effectiveness, including assertiveness classes. A number of specific programs are designed to help individuals with emotion regulation—most notably, structured cognitive and cognitive–behavioral programs for depression, anxiety and/or panic, and anger control—and more such programs are being developed every day. Distress tolerance is perhaps the one area of DBT skills training that is not covered in numerous other publications and programs.

There is no *a priori* reason why one skills training program cannot be substituted for another. A number of considerations besides practicalities, however, must be taken into account. First, you must thoroughly know the skills each patient is learning. Your task will be to help the patient learn them and apply them, often in situations of great stress. You cannot teach what you do not know. In my clinical program, therapists often learn the DBT skills by studying the DBT skills training manual that accompanied this book and trying out the homework assignment themselves. It is something of a "learn as you go" program, often with both therapists and patients learning the skills together (at least at first). Although the skills I discuss in DBT are organized in a somewhat idiosyncratic manner and are described in terminology you may not use, they are actually reasonably basic skills that most people have at least some familiarity with.

Second, if you send your patient somewhere else for skills training, it is important that you use the same skills terminology as that used in skills training; otherwise, the patient may feel confused and overwhelmed. You need to have access to the training materials used by the skills trainer. Third, you need to be sure that the skills you teach are relevant to BPD and to the specific problems of each patient. Fourth, it is important to interrelate the skills taught in each module and to develop a method of tracking the use of skills over time, especially when you are not actively teaching a specific set of skills at the moment. In a sense, what I am recommending is that if you do not use the DBT skills training manual as is, you consider either writing one of your own or modifying the manual to suit your own purposes.

Decreasing Behaviors Related to Posttraumatic Stress

When a borderline patient has serious, unresolved, and untreated traumatic life events, reduction of related stress response patterns is a primary DBT target. As Chapter 2 has indicated, a majority of patients in DBT can be expected to report at least one instance of sexual abuse in childhood. A number of these patients, as well as others with no history of sexual abuse, will report physical and emotional trauma and neglect during childhood, which in some cases may have been especially violent, intrusive, pervasive, and/or chronic. The therapist must be very careful, however, not to assume that all borderline patients have histories of severe sexual or physical abuse, or even of traumatic neglect; some do not. This does not mean, however, that they may not have experienced trauma. Some have experienced loss of important persons through death, divorce, or relocation; others have suffered traumatic threats of loss; still others have experienced parental alcoholic rages, unexpected or persistent traumatic rejections, or chaotic life circumstances. At a minimum, if the biosocial theory proposed in Chapter 2 is correct, all borderline patients will have experienced pervasive invalidating environments.

The work done in this target area is similar to that done in "uncovering" work or to the focus on childhood precursors to dysfunctional behaviors in psychodynamic therapies. The difference is that no *a priori* assumptions are made about which particular event(s) or what developmental phase of an individual's life is functionally related to current traumatic stress.

Information about the facts of previous sexual, physical, or emotional trauma and/or physical or emotional neglect should be obtained on a continuing and as-needed basis as therapy progresses. Some patients will give this information readily; others will only disclose information about abuse gradually or after some time in therapy. The therapist should read all records of previous treatment for clues about abuse history. At times, however, the facts of all or some abuse history may not have been disclosed during previous therapies. Because of the trauma associated with even therapeutic exposure to abuse-related cues, eliciting of details and events associated with early trauma generally does not take place until suicidal, therapy-interfering, and serious quality-of-life interfering behaviors have been substantially reduced and behavioral skills are in place. This issue is discussed in more depth in the next chapter.

Characteristic sequelae of childhood sexual abuse have been described by Briere (1989) and are listed in Table 5.4. A number of these sequelae are the behavioral problems targeted directly in DBT, while others overlap with characteristics of posttraumatic stress disorder. As noted earlier, some authors have suggested that BPD itself should be reconceptualized as posttraumatic stress associated with childhood abuse. Although DBT does not take this position, certainly many of the behavioral problems of borderline patients may be directly related to previous abusive experiences.

Accepting the Fact of Trauma and/or Abuse

Coming to terms with and accepting the facts of the trauma that took place is both the first and the last target in treating the sequelae of traumatic experiences. Individuals who have been severely traumatized often have little memory of the experience. The first target, therefore, is for the patient to verbalize the traumatic incidents sufficiently to begin work. When one or more events (or fragments of events) are remembered, the next task is for the individual to believe that the events she remembered (or some approximation of the events) actually took place. This can be a very difficult part of therapy, since trauma victims often fear that they have simply imagined or made up the traumatic events or abuse.

It is also difficult because retrospectively one never has direct access to events that took place in the past. Thus, an important task for the patient (and sometimes for the therapist also) is to learn to trust herself even when the actual facts of her life may be uncertain. The goal for many patients is to synthesize both *knowing* that something happened, on the one hand, and *not knowing* exactly what happened, on the other. Comfort with ambiguity

TABLE 5.4. Characteristic Sequelae of Childhood Sexual Abuse

1. Intrusive memories of flashbacks to and nightmares of the abuse.
2. Abuse-related dissociation, derealization, depersonalization, out-of-body experiences, and cognitive disengagement or "spacing out."
3. General posttraumatic stress symptoms, such as sleep problems, concentration problems, impaired memory, and restimulation of early abuse memories and emotions by immediate events and interactions.
4. Guilt, shame, negative self-evaluation, and self-invalidation related to the abuse.
5. Helplessness and hopelessness.
6. Distrust of others.
7. Anxiety attacks, phobias, hypervigilance, and somatization.
8. Sexual problems
9. Long-standing depression.
10. Disturbed interpersonal relatedness, including idealization and disappointment, overdramatic behavioral style, compulsive sexuality, adversariality, and manipulation.
11. "Acting out" and "acting in," including parasuicidal acts and substance abuse.
12. Withdrawal.
13. Other-directedness.
14. Chronic perception of danger.
15. Self-hatred.
16. Negative specialness—that is, an almost magical sense of power.
17. Impaired reality testing.
18. A heightened ability to avoid, deny, and repress.

Note. From *Therapy for Adults Molested as Children* by J. Briere, 1989, New York: Springer. Copyright 1989 by Springer Publishing Company. Reprinted by permission.

and uncertainty, discussed at the beginning of the chapter, becomes part of the goal. As the story unfolds, the task of grieving and radically accepting the reality of one's life becomes at once both crucial and extremely difficult for many to negotiate. It is within this context that radical acceptance, taught as a core mindfulness skill, must be learned and practiced. The inability to grieve, discussed in Chapter 3, is one of the main impediments to successful passage through this phase. Judith Herman (1992) has called this the remembrance and mourning phase of treating traumatic people and describes most eloquently both the immense difficulty and the courage needed.

Reducing Stigmatization, Self-Invalidation, Self-Blame

The second goal is to reduce the stigmatization, self-invalidation, and self-blame associated with trauma. Victims of abuse typically believe that they are somehow reprehensibly different from others; otherwise, the abuse would not have occurred. They often believe that they caused the abuse, or that because they did not stop it (and at times might have found it pleasurable,

TABLE 5.5. Denial and Intrusive Stress Response Phases

Denial phase

Perception and attention
   Daze
   Selective inattention
   Inability to appreciate significance of stimuli
   Sleep disturbance (for example, too little or too much)

Consciousness of ideas and feelings related to the event
   Amnesia (complete or partial)
   Nonexperience of themes that are consequences of the event

Conceptual attributes
   Disavowal of meanings of current stimuli in some way associated with the event
   Loss of a realistic sense of appropriate connection with the ongoing world
   Constriction of range of thought
   Inflexibility of purpose
   Major use of fantasies to counteract real conditions

Emotional attributes
   Numbness

Somatic attributes
   Tension–inhibition responses of the autonomic nervous system, with sensations such
      as bowel symptoms, fatigue, headache, and muscle pain

Activity patterns
   Frantic overactivity
   Withdrawal
Failure to decide how to respond to consequences of the event

Perception and attention
   Hypervigilance, startle reaction
   Sleep and dream disturbance

Intrusive phase

Consciousness of ideas and feelings related to the event
   Intrusive–repetitive thoughts, emotions, and behaviors (illusions, pseudohallucina-
      tions, nightmares, unbidden images, and ruminations)
   Feelings of being pressured, confused, or disorganized when thinking about themes
      related to the event

Conceptual attributes
   Overgeneralization of stimuli so that they seem related to the event
   Preoccupation with themes related to the event, with inability to concentrate on
      other topics

Emotional attributes
   Emotional "attacks" or "pangs" of affect related to the event

Somatic attributes
   Sensations or symptoms of flight or fight readiness (or of exhaustion from chronic
      arousal), including tremor, diarrhea, and sweating (adrenergic, noradrenergic, or
      histaminic arousals with sensations such as pounding heart, nausea, lump in
      throat, and week legs)

Activity patterns
   Compulsive repetitions of actions associated with the event or of searching for lost
      persons or situations

Note. From "Stress-Response Syndromes: A Review of Posttraumatic and Adjustment Disord-ers" by M. J. Horowitz, 1986, *Hospital and Community Psychiatry, 37,* 241–249. Copyright 1986 by American Psychiatric Association. Reprinted by permission.

in the case of sexual abuse), they are "bad" or "sick" or both. Even when they do not feel responsible for the occurrence of traumatic events, victims often believe that they are responsible for, and feel ashamed of, their reactions to the trauma. At times they minimize the severity of the trauma.

Reducing Denial and Intrusive Stress Responses

When an individual is confronted with severe trauma, responses occur in two phases, which often repeat themselves in a cyclical fashion: a "denial" phase and an "intrusive" phase. Responses occurring in these two phases have been outlined by Horowitz (1986) and are listed in Table 5.5. Even when the facts of the trauma have been accepted, the individual may continue to disavow the implications of the traumatic event and to exhibit the other denial-phase responses listed in the table. In individual or group sessions, when cues associated with the trauma are brought up, the individual may become mute and stare blankly into space. The denial phase is quite similar to the borderline syndrome I have described as "inhibited grieving" (see Chapter 3).

The intrusive phase is similar to what I have described in Chapter 3 as the emotional vulnerability syndrome. During the intrusive phase, a wide range of stimuli originally unrelated to the trauma may become associated with trauma cues and responses. Over time, if this phase lasts long enough, these responses and associations tend to extinguish. However, when the denial phase follows quickly, the extinction does not occur, and a cycle in which one phase rapidly follows the other can continue over many years. Such is the case with the borderline patient.

Synthesizing the "Abuse Dichotomy"

The "abuse dichotomy" is a phrase coined by Briere (1989) to refer to the tendency of victims of childhood abuse to conceptualize responsibility for their abuse in black-and-white terms: Either their abusers are all bad for abusing them, or they are all bad because they were abused. Often their views of who is all bad vacillate from moment to moment. This is a case of nondialectical thinking, or "splitting" in psychoanalytic terms. Resolution of this dialectical tension is the target here. The therapist must be careful, however, not to imply that the only synthesis possible for a patient is forgiveness of the abuser. Although acceptance of the facts of abuse is essential, and some understanding of the abusive behavior as a consequence of events surrounding the abuser may be important, forgiveness itself may not always be possible. In addition, the therapist must be equally careful not to paint the abuser in entirely negative terms, especially when the abuser was a caregiver or parent. For most individuals, it is important to salvage at least some positive relationship with parental figures. Pushing a patient to stop loving a parent denies the valuable parts of the relationship, and thus results in a loss to the patient. Many victims of abuse cannot tolerate that further loss. Instead, the goal must be to achieve a synthesis in which a patient does not have to lose her own integrity to retain a relationship with the abuser.

Increasing Respect for Self

"Respect for self" encompasses the ability to value, believe, validate, trust, and cherish oneself, including one's own thoughts, emotions, and behavior patterns. The idea here is not that anyone's emotional, cognitive, and behavioral responses are entirely adaptive or beneficial. Indeed, the ability to evaluate one's own behavior nondefensively is an important characteristic of adaptive functioning and an outcome of enhanced self-respect, and the ability to trust one's own self-evaluations is crucial to growth. The borderline patient, however, is usually unable to evaluate her own responses and hold on to her self-evaluations independently of the opinions of important others, including the therapist. She is unable to respect her own self-evaluative capabilities. Thus, she is buffeted by changes in opinions and the presence or absence of important others—opinions and events that are usually out of her control. Much of this difficulty is a result of excessive fear of social disapproval. Borderline individuals often operate as if their well-being is totally dependent on the approval of all persons important to them. One goal of the therapist, therefore, is to increase appropriate self-evaluation and tolerance of social disapproval, and to extinguish behaviors contradictory to these goals.

Many borderline patients react to themselves with extreme loathing, bordering on self-hate. All but a few feel enormous shame in general, and shame about their own abuse history, the troubles they have caused, and their present emotional reactivity in particular. Cherishing oneself is the opposite of these emotional reactions. Thus, the therapist must target the self-hate, the self-blame, and the sense of shame. Although work on this target is a lifelong process, substantial progress should be made before therapy ends.

One thing the therapist must be especially careful to do before therapy ends is to reinforce patient self-respect that is independent of the therapist. That is, the therapist must ultimately pull back and relentlessly reinforce within the therapeutic relationship self-validation, self-care, self-soothing, and problem solving without reference to the therapist. I hasten to add, however, that this stance does not suggest that patients should learn to be independent of all people. Interpersonal dependence, asking for and accepting nurturing, soothing, and active assistance from others are crucial for most people's well-being. Indeed, the ability to be related to and to depend on others without invalidating one self is an important target of DBT.

Secondary Behavioral Targets

A number of response patterns may be functionally related to the primary target problems of borderline patients. These patterns are secondary DBT targets. The importance of any secondary target for the individual patient in DBT, however, is entirely dependent on its relationship to achieving the primary target goals. In the individual case, it is crucial that the presence of each secondary pattern and the functional relationship of the pattern to primary targets be assessed, rather than assumed. If changing a particular secondary pattern is not instrumental in achieving primary goals, the response pattern is not targeted. Thus, the secondary target list is a set of hypotheses to be tested.

The secondary target list proposed in DBT is based on the poles of the dialectical dilemmas I have described in Chapter 3. The targets are as follows: (1) increasing emotion modulation and decreasing emotional reactivity; (2) increasing self-validation and reducing self-invalidation; (3) increasing realistic decision making and judgment, and reducing crisis-generating behaviors; (4) increasing emotional experiencing and decreasing inhibited grieving; (5) increasing active problem solving and decreasing active-passivity behaviors; and (6) increasing accurate expression of emotions and competencies and decreasing mood dependency of behavior.

Increasing Emotion Modulation; Decreasing Emotional Reactivity

The first secondary target is to increase the emotion modulation and reduce the lightning-quick emotional reactivity of the borderline individual. The specific behavioral skills that are most helpful in this regard are mindfulness (especially nonjudgmental observation of events precipitating emotional responses), the distress tolerance attitudes of acceptance and willingness, and emotion regulation practices included under the rubric of reducing vulnerability.

Increasing modulation and reducing reactivity should be clearly distinguished from emotional nonreactivity. The idea is not to get rid of emotions; indeed, DBT assumes that former borderline individuals will continue to be the emotionally intense, colorful, and dramatic people of the world. Nor is the focus on the irrationality of a patient's responses. Rather, the focus is on the extremity of the responses. The idea is to reduce intolerable rage to tolerable anger, incapacitating panic to prudent fear, immobilizing grief to reflective sadness, and humiliating shame to transitory guilt. In other words, the assumption is not that extreme emotions are based on irrational beliefs about a rational world; rather, they are seen as overshooting the mark.

Increasing Self-Validation; Decreasing Self-Invalidation

Self-acceptance and self-soothing are specific skills included in the distress tolerance skill package. Since patients pick and choose their distress tolerance strategies, it is common for patients to ignore these two. However, self-invalidation and self-hate are often related to suicidal behaviors, failures in self-management programs, and increases in emotional vulnerability. When such is the case, these behaviors should be targeted directly by the individual therapist. Increasing self-validation and reducing self-hate are important components of self-respect, and thus become primary targets in the later stages of therapy.

Increasing Realistic Decision Making and Judgment; Decreasing Crisis-Generating Behaviors

DBT does not assume that borderline individuals precipitate all of their own crises. But it also does not assume the opposite—that patients have nothing to do with generating crises. The two patient characteristics most related to crises are mood dependency and the resulting mood-related behavioral choices (to be discussed below), and difficulty in predicting realistic outcomes for various behavioral choices—that is, poor judgment. To a certain extent mood dependency further exacerbates poor judgment, since an individual often cannot predict how her reactions will change from one mood to another, and thus cannot predict her own behavior. The invalidating environment teaches the individual to look to others for behavioral solutions, instead of shaping individual problem-solving and decision-making skills. In a chaotic family, there is little modeling and teaching of realistic decision making. A patient from such a family needs to learn to predict realistic outcomes (both short-term and long-term) of behavioral choices. Many of the self-management skills needed in DBT are related to issues of making realistic judgments about oneself.

Increasing Emotional Experiencing; Decreasing Inhibited Grieving

The ability to experience emotions as they occur, especially negatiave emotions, is crucial to their reduction. The rationale for this has been discussed extensively in Chapter 3 and is not repeated here. Thus, an important target of treatment for many patients is increasing their ability to experience rather than inhibit negative emotions. In extreme cases, where patients are almost totally incapable of experiencing negative affect for more than a moment, this target may take on the status of a primary target.

Increasing Active Problem Solving; Decreasing Active-Passivity Behaviors

Borderline patients have a tendency to react to problems passively—a tendency that not only interferes with achieving some life goals, but also can be extremely frustrating for the therapist. As discussed in Chapter 3, borderline "active passivity" is perhaps the result of a biologically mediated passive self-regulation style combined with learned helplessness. An important target of DBT is to disrupt this interaction style and increase the use of active problem solving. All of the DBT behavioral skills both rely on and feed back into active problem-solving behaviors.

Attempting to increase borderline patients' ability and motivation to generate problem solutions, try them out, and evaluate their effectiveness is the point at which therapy can become derailed. The problem is quite similar, of course, to problems that arise for the patients outside of therapy. A mistake that many therapists make is trying to make apples into oranges. That is, therapists often try to make patients who prefer a passive self-regulation style into people who prefer an active self-regulation style. I suspect that this approach is doomed to failure a good percentage of the time. The focus in DBT is on helping patients become good passive self-regulators. The notion here is that an individual who prefers a passive self-regulation style (i.e., allowing persons or events in the environment to regulate her behavior) can learn to control her own behavior by skillfully controlling the structure of the environment. Signing contracts, setting up deadlines, making lists and written schedules, and arranging to be around people are all examples of passive self-regulation.

Increasing Accurate Communication of Emotions and Competencies; Decreasing Mood Dependency of Behavior

Borderline individuals often miscommunicate their current emotional state, as noted in Chapter 3. Although at times they communicate exaggerated emotional responses, at other times they inhibit expressions of negative emotions. Such a pattern is predictable for anyone brought up in an invalidating environment. Borderline individuals, however, are often unaware that they are not expressing emotions accurately; instead, they frequently believe that other persons are aware of how they feel but are "withholding" in their responses to the patients' distress. Thus, it is crucial that the individuals learn how to express emotions accurately (both nonverbally and verbally), as well as to assess whether their emotional expression has been understood.

Similarly, borderline individuals also have problems with communicating to others when they are having difficulty or are not competent to handle a particular situation. Part of the problem here is that patients often are not good judges of their own competencies; frequently, they believe they are unable to cope with a situation when they are simply afraid. At other times, however, patients communicate competency when in fact they are not able to cope. The net result is that people tend to see them as the boy who cried "wolf" too many times, and falsely believe that the patients are comfortable in a situation when they themselves feel that they are "falling apart." All people, including borderline patients, must be able to communicate needs for assistance or help in such a way that others will heed the message. Much of interpersonal effectiveness skills training addresses just this topic.

The rule that action must be in accord with mood is a dysfunctional opposite extreme that is also typical of borderline individuals. Separating current mood from current behavior is essential if primary target goals are to be reached in DBT. The emphasis in DBT on distress tolerance and acceptance of life as it is, without necessarily changing it, is based on precisely this point. Although I am discussing mood dependency of behavior last, it is by no means least important. In many ways, all of DBT focuses on this target, since the link between negative mood and congruent maladaptive behavior is extinguished (and sometimes punished) consistently throughout therapy.

Concluding Comments

DBT target priorities are a defining characteristic of the therapy. Knowing or being able to list the targets in order of priority, however, is only the first step. The crucial second skill, which can only be learned by practice, is the ability to monitor the great influx of a patient's behavior as it rushes by and to organize it into the relevant categories. Once you can pigeonhole what the patient is doing on a continuing basis, then you can survey the array of behaviors, look at your priorities, and decide what to focus on at the moment. It is a bit like learning to read a complex piece of music. First, you must be able to identify the notes. Once you can read the notes, you have to be able to play the music. That is the topic of the next chapter.

Note

1. These examples are transformations of examples offered by Basseches (1984).

6

Structuring Treatment Around Target Behaviors: Who Treats What and When

The unrelenting crises and behavioral complexity of a borderline patient often overwhelm both the patient and the therapist. At times, so many environmental problems and maladaptive behaviors are occurring simultaneously that the therapist has difficulty deciding how to focus therapy time. The fact that the patient often makes intense efforts to focus sessions on her current life crises does not help in this situation. Mood dependency can make it difficult for a borderline individual to address any problem not related to her current emotional experience; the intensity of her communications of emotional pain can make it equally difficult for the therapist to focus on anything else. DBT targets priorities, which are guidelines for how to structure therapy time, are designed to help out here. When a therapist is feeling overwhelmed by the clinical situation, DBT target priorities indicate what to focus on.

The spirit of DBT is that treatment targets, as well as the priorities accorded to them, must be clear and specific. Targets as well as priorities are different in each mode (e.g., individual therapy, group therapy, telephone consultation) of DBT. Thus, it is essential that each individual providing treatment for the borderline patient be clear and specific about which targets that individual is responsible for. Even if a therapist is the only therapist for a particular patient, it is important to have a clear idea of priorities in each interaction; priorities in a psychotherapy session, for example, may be very different from priorities during a phone conversation.

In this chapter, I describe how treatment targets are organized in standard DBT. The most important point is that although specific priorities can change (and probably must change in some settings), the requirement for clarity and specificity should not be dropped. If the target order, the division of target priorities across treatment modes, or the responsibility for achieving target goals is changed, the therapist must be clear and specific about what is being changed and how.

The General Theme: Targeting Dialectical Behaviors

The goal of increasing dialectical behavior patterns among borderline patients is the theme that guides DBT's approach to all other target behaviors. This target differs from the others in three ways. First, it is a target of all modes of treatment. The attention accorded to other behavioral targets varies by treatment mode; in contrast, all modes of DBT attend to dialectical behavior patterns. All therapists try both to model and to reinforce a dialectical style of thinking and approaching problems and to challenge nondialectical thinking or approaches to problems, as Chapter 5 has described.

Second, in contrast to other therapy targets, increasing dialectical behavior patterns as a specific therapy target is rarely discussed with the patient. That is, the patient does not make an explicit commitment to work at becoming more dialectical. The main reason for this is that I have believed that the concept of dialectics is overly abstract, and feared that explanation and instruction might get in the way instead of facilitating learning. In addition, I have thought that the very absence of dialectical thinking patterns would prevent commitment to work toward adopting such a style of thought. For example, the individual who believes that there is a universal order to reality, and thus that absolute truth is knowable, is not likely to agree to let go of this approach to knowing and ordering the universe. My reluctance to teach dialectical patterns explicitly, however, may be an overly timid approach. Several cognitive therapists (e.g., Bech et al., 1990) focus treatment directly on changing cognitive style, with good results. At a minimum, one might emphasize balanced thinking and action (as opposed to dichotomous thinking and extreme action) in teaching the sets of skills discussed in Chapter 5.

A third difference between targeting dialectical behavior patterns and targeting other behaviors is that, because it forms an aspect of each of the other goals to be achieved, dialectical behavior is not on the hierarchical list of targets to be discussed next.

The Hierarchy of Primary Targets

The remaining seven primary behavioral targets outlined in Chapter 5 can be assigned to a hierarchy in order of importance. The hierarchy for the treatment as a whole is shown in Table 6.1; it reflects the order in which these targets have been discussed in Chapter 5. This is also the order of priority for targets in outpatient individual therapy. The hierarchies for other modes of therapy differ slightly, as I discuss later in this chapter. Although the list

TABLE 6.1. The Hierarchy of Primary Targets in DBT

Pretreatment targets:
  Orientation to treatment and agreement on goals

First-stage targets:
  1. Decreasing suicidal behaviors
  2. Decresing therapy-interfering behaviors
  3. Decreasing quality-of-life-interfering behaviors
  4. Increasinng behavioral skills
     A. Core mindfulness skills
     B. Interpersonal effectiveness
     C. Emotion regulation
     D. Distress tolerance
     E. Self-management

Second-stage targets:
  5. Decreasing posttraumatic stress

Third-stage targets:
  6. Increasing respect for self
  7. Achieving individual goals

was developed specifically for parasuicidal borderline patients, a moment's reflection suggests that the list, at least through the first phase of therapy could be applied to any severely dysfunctional patient population.

Treatment Targets and Session Agenda

Although the importance of each target does not change over therapy, the relevance of a target does change. Relevance is determined by the patient's current day-to-day behavior, as well by as her behavior during the therapy interaction. Problems not evident in the patient's current behavior are not currently relevant. Relevance and importance determine what the therapist should pay the most attention to when interacting with the patient. The basic idea here is that the therapist applies the DBT strategies and techniques (discussed in Chapters 7–15) to the highest-priority treatment target relevant at the moment. If a particular target goal has already been reached, or if problems in the target area have never arisen for the patient, are not evident in the patient's current behavior, or have already been addressed in the current session, then targets next on the list become the principal focus of the treatment.

Treatment Targets and Modes of Therapy

Responsibility for achieving specific target goals is spread across the various modes of DBT (individual psychotherapy behavioral skills training, supportive process groups, phone calls). The priority assigned to each treatment target, the amount of attention each target receives, and the nature of that attention vary, depending on the mode of therapy. Thus, as noted above, each mode of therapy has its own unique hierarchical ordering of treatment goals.

The individual therapist pays attention to one order of targets, the skills training therapists another, and the process group therapists another; in telephone interactions, yet another order of targets guides the conversation. In some settings, the milieu and unit or clinic director may be part of the DBT team. If so, then the milieu and unit director have their own lists of target priorities as well. If other modes are added to the treatment, prioritized target lists must be drawn up for each mode. In principle, the division of responsibility for targets can be divided up in any number of ways to reflect various treatment settings and modes of therapy. These possibilities are discussed more fully later in this chapter.

The key point to be made here is that all DBT therapists in a particular setting must understand clearly what their own hierarchies of targets are with each patient and how those hierarchies fit into the overall hierarchy of DBT behavioral targets. Generally, the targets and their order are tied to each specific mode of treatment. Thus, if therapists are carrying out more than one mode of treatment (e.g., if the individual therapist is also the process group therapist, or if the individual therapist or skills trainer also takes phone calls), then they must be able to remember the order of targets specific to each mode, and must be able to switch smoothly from one hierarchy to another as they switch from one mode to another.

The Primary Therapist and Responsibility for Meeting Targets

In each treatment unit, one therapist is designated the primary therapist for a particular patient. In our outpatient unit, as in individual clinical practice, the therapist is the patient's individual psychotherapist. The primary therapist is responsible for treatment planning, working with the patient on progress toward all targets, and helping the patient integrate (or occasionally decide to discard) what is being learned in other modes of therapy. In my experience, if the primary therapist does not help the patient to integrate and strengthen what is being learned elsewhere, such learning is often seriously weakened. All therapists in a common setting may take part in treatment planning, have input into which specific behaviors should receive attention in each category of targets, and together decide a division of target responsibilities among treatment modes and therapists. However, the primary therapist has the task of helping the patient remember and take into account the "big picture," so to speak. As I emphasize in discussing the consultation-to-the-patient strategies in Chapter 13, the primary therapist consults with the patient on how to interact effectively with all other members of the treatment unit and professional community. (Conversely, other therapists consult with the patient on how to interact with her primary therapist.)

Progress Toward Targets Over Time

In my experience, progress toward treatment targets can be grouped into phases. Although the stages of therapy are presented here in chronological order for heuristic purposes, therapy usually develops in a circular fashion. Thus, although orienting the patient to therapy and focusing on therapy expectations ordinarily occur during the first several sessions, these issues are likely to be important throughout therapy. The first stage of therapy includes behavioral analysis and treatment of suicidal behaviors, therapy-interfering behaviors, behavioral patterns that seriously interfere with the quality of life, and skill deficiencies. For some patients, however, problems in these areas may be continuing concerns throughout therapy. The second stage of treatment, oriented to reducing posttraumatic stess, at times requires attention right from the beginning of therapy; moreover, such stress is unlikely to be fully remediated even by the end of therapy. The final stage targets goals of self-respect, generalization, integration, and termination. These issues, however, are dealt with from the very beginning of treatment and arise sporadically throughout the entire treatment.

Pretreatment Stage: Orientation and Commitment

A continuing concern in conducting treatment with borderline and parasuicidal patients is the possibility that a significant percentage will terminate therapy prematurely. The use of pretreatment orientation sessions has been empirically linked to a reduced dropout rate in several treatment studies (Parloff, Waskow, & Wolfe, 1978). Thus, the first several sessions of individual therapy focus on preparations for therapy. The goals of this stage are twofold. First, the patient and therapist must arrive at a mutual, informed decision to work together on helping the patient make changes she wants to make in herself and in her life. Second, the therapist attempts to modify any dysfunctional beliefs or expectations of the patient regarding therapy that are likely to influence the process of therapy and/or the decision to terminate therapy prematurely.

With respect to the first goal, the patient must find out as much as possible about the therapist's interpersonal style, professional competence, treatment goals, and intentions regarding the conduct of therapy. The therapist has to assist the patient in making an informed decision about committing to therapy, and must also obtain sufficient information about the patient to decide whether he or she can work with the patient. Diagnostic and assessment interviewing, plus history taking, should occur at this point. With respect to the patient's therapy-oriented beliefs and expectations, the therapist describes the treatment program and the rate and magnitude of change that can be expected to occur within it; determines and discusses the patient's beliefs about psychotherapists and psychotherapy in general; and attempts to "reframe" psychotherapy as a learning process. Details on how to conduct these orientation sessions are provided in Chapters 9 and 14.

Stage 1: Attaining Basic Capacities

As noted above, the first phase of therapy centers on suicidal behaviors, therapy-interfering behaviors, major quality-of-life-interfering behaviors, and deficits in behavioral skills. With severely dysfunctional, highly suicidal patients, it may take a year of more to get control of the first two targets. Progress on quality-of-life-interfering behaviors depend to some extent on what the actual interfering behaviors are. For addictive behaviors, simply getting a commitment from the patient to work on these behaviors can take a long time. I once had a patient with a serious drinking problem who took over 2 years to commit to work on reducing her excessive alcohol consumption; even then it took a conviction for driving while intoxicated, a court-ordered 2-year treatment program, and my putting her on a "vacation" from therapy to persuade her to make the commitment. (The strategy of "vacation from therapy" is discussed in Chapter 10.)

Generally, by the end of the first year of therapy, patients should also have at least a working knowledge of and competence in the major behavioral skills taught in DBT. Although application of these skills to various target problem areas is a continuing focus of therapy, the large amount of time devoted to acquisition of skills during the first stage is usually not required in subsequent phases of therapy, except in cases when the primary therapist does not sufficiently help the patient integrate the skills she is learning. Again, my experience is that if the primary therapist does not value the skills and help the patient integrate them into her daily life, the patient will often forget what she has learned.

Stage 2: Reducing Posttraumatic Stress

The second phase of therapy, begun only when previous target behaviors are under control, involves working directly on posttraumatic stress. The status of posttraumatic stress as a second-stage target may be questioned by some. Those who believe that BPD is a special case of posttraumatic stress disorder may suggest that resolving early trauma, especially sexual abuse, should be the first priority of treatment; once that is resolved, all other problems will become manageable. Although I have some sympathy for this point of view, I believe that the resulting havoc in the patient's life and the suicide risk are such that the treatment of posttraumatic stress has to be very carefully timed.

My experience with patients whose therapists began therapy with an "uncovering" approach, where the initial focus of therapy sessions was on discussing childhood trauma (including sexual, physical, and/or emotional trauma or neglect), was that many of these patients simply could not handle the re-exposure to the traumatic events. Instead, they often became extremely suicidal, engaged in near-lethal parasuicidal acts or compulsively mutilated themselves, and/or had to be admitted and readmitted to inpatient psychiatric units. Thus, DBT does not focus on traumatic stress until a patient has the necessary capabilities and supports (both within therapy and in her environment outside therapy) to resolve the trauma successfully. Satisfactory progress through the first-stage targets readies the patient for subsequent work on previous tramatic experiences. In psychodynamic terms, the patient must have the necessary ego strength to do the therapy.

This does not mean, of course, that previous trauma is ignored during the first stage of therapy if the patient brings it up. How it is responded to, however, depends on its relationship to other target behaviors. If the aftereffect of trauma (memories, flashbacks, self-blame, emotional responses to trauma-associated cues, etc.) are functionally related to subsequent suicidal behaviors, for example, then they are attended to just as any other precipitant of suicidal behavior would be. That is, their association to subsequent suicidal behavior becomes the focus of treatment. In any case, painful sequelae of trama are treated as problems to be solved (i.e., quality-of-life-interfering behaviors) when they arise in therapy. As part of treatment, the therapist ordinarily would also target the development of distress tolerance skills and mindfulness skills (see Chapter 5), both of which are required in dealing with posttraumatic stress. The therapist takes a very here-and-now approach to managing dysfunctional behavioral and emotional patterns. Although the connection between current behavior and previous traumatic events, including those from childhood, may be explored and noted, the focus of the treatment is distinctly on analyzing the relationship among current thoughts, feelings, and behaviors and on accepting and changing current patterns. What the therapist does *not* do during the first stage of therapy is refocus the major activities of therapy on addressing the prior trauma. Again, the rule here is that such trauma is not brought into therapy before the patient can cope with the consequences of exposure to it.

Because of its middle position in the three stages, the reduction of posttraumatic stress reactions is often started, stopped, and restarted. For many patients, such a resolution will be a lifelong task with many beginnings and leavings. Some patients may enter therapy ready for Stage 2 of therapy: They are not actively engaged in suicidal behaviors, are able to work in therapy, and have adequate stability and resources. Conversely, some patients who appear ready to work on Stage 2 goals may not be ready. Their apparent competence may fool both therapist and patient. At times, a therapist will not even suspect that a patient meets criteria for BPD until attempts to resolve earlier traumas precipitate extreme reactions typical of Stage 1. This is especially likely when the therapist has not conducted a comprehensive clinical assessment at the beginning of therapy. As I have mentioned previously, borderline individuals sometimes function quite well when in supportive and nurturing relationships with little or no interpersonal stress. Although a patient may often be "crying on the inside," the therapist may not see the patient's distress until she is exposed once again to the trauma-associated cues.

Stage 2 of DBT, however, requires exposure to the trauma-related cues. (See Chapter 11 for a thorough discussion of exposure techniques.) There is simply no other way to work on the stress responses to such cues. For some patients, the rate of exposure may need to be extremely gradual; for others, Stage 2 may go quite rapidly. The length of time and the pacing of therapy in Stage 2 will depend on the severity of the previous trauma and the patient's behavioral and social resources to cope with the therapy process. At times, therapist and patient may find it useful to take a break from therapy for a while. For example, one of my patients took several years to get through Stage 1 of therapy. When she was finally ready to focus on the severe sexual abuse she had received from ages 9 to 13 years, I was planning an 8-week trip out of the country for 8 months later. The patient's fear that she would be in the middle of a crisis period when I left was so great that it inhibited her ability to work hard on Stage 2 goals. We agreed to have monthly check-in meetings until I left and to wait until I returned from my trip to begin Stage 2 therapy. The patient stayed in her ongoing supportive process group therapy. Another patient left therapy after completing most of Stage 1. During the vacation time, she entered and completed a 1-year substance abuse program. She then returned to therapy with me to work on resolving traumatic relationships within her family of origin.

It is extremely important that the therapist not mistake adequate coping with posttraumatic stress responses (a successful completion of Stage 1 of therapy) for a satisfactory conclusion of therapy. Although the stability is now there for constructing a life worth living, the posttraumatic stress patterns themselves (see Chapter 5 for a detailed review) are nonetheless a source of considerable emotional pain and suffering. Although some individuals may be able to tolerate for long periods of life with much pain and suffering, others will finally go back to Stage 1 behaviors as a way to ameliorate the pain or to get further help. Thus, the gains of Stage 1 of therapy may be lost if Stage 2 is not negotiated successfully.

Stage 3: Increasing Self-Respect and Achieving Individual Goals

Overlapping with the first two phases, and forming the final phase of therapy, is work on developing the ability to trust the self; to validate one's own opinions, emotions, and actions; and, in general, to respect oneself independently of the therapist. Work on the patient's individual goals also occurs largely during this stage. It is of utmost importance that the skills the patient learns in therapy be generalized to nontherapeutic situations. The ordinary course of events in therapy with a borderline patient is that the patient will initially have great difficulty in trusting the therapist, in asking the therapist for help, and in arriving at an optimum balance between independence and dependence. Quite often during the first months of therapy, the patient will have trouble trusting the therapist, will not call the therapist even when it would be appropriate to do so, and will vacillate between extreme dependence on the therapist to solve her problems and an independent attitude of "I don't need anything or anybody." Exploration of these patterns will often indicate that the same interpersonal patterns are also occurring with others in the patient's environment. Thus the ability to trust, to ask for help appropriately, and both to depend on and to be independent from another person will often be the focus of treatment. As the patient begins to develop trust in the therapist, she will generally begin to be more honest with the therapist about her need for help. During the initial stages of therapy, strong emphasis is put on reinforcing the patient for asking the therapist for help when the patient is having trouble coping with a particular situation. However, if this request for help is not transferred to other people in the patient's environment, and if the patient is not taught to render assistance to herself or self-soothe the termination of therapy will be extremely traumatic. The transition from reliance on the therapist to reliance on self and others must begin almost immediately. Once again, there is a dialectical emphasis on being able to rely on other people while learning to be self-reliant. Thus, the goal is to be able to rely on oneself while remaining firmly within reciprocal interpersonal networks.

Enhancing self-respect also requires the reduction of self-hate and shame. In my experience, residual patterns of shame about oneself and one's past usually surface during Stage 3 of therapy. In particular, the individual may need to work out how she will construe her own history and how she will present it to others. Especially if there is visible scarring, the patient must decide how to respond to queries about her past. At times, the re-emergence of intense shame or fears of terminating therapy may be such as to precipitate a return of Stage 1 behaviors or Stage 2 stress reactions. Usually, these relapses are brief. It is particularly important that the therapist not further shame the patient or overly pathologize the return of maladaptive behavior patterns. The situation is much like that of a smoker who stopped smoking 5 years ago and is re-exposed to a cue strongly associated with smoking. If there have not been sufficient learning experiences with that cue, the ex-smoker may experience an unexpected, intense urge to smoke. In DBT, one would suggest that a bit of new learning may be needed, rather than that the individual has regressed.

As between Stages 1 and 2, patients may sometimes take a break from therapy before or during Stage 3. At times, patients may enter other therapies or work with other therapists during the intervals. There is no reason not to encourage this in DBT.

Setting Priorities within Target Classes in Outpatient Individual Therapy

As noted above, the individual psychotherapist in outpatient DBT is the primary therapist, and thus is responsible for organizing treatment to achieve all primary treatment goals. The selection of behaviors to focus on within target classes, however, can at times be a challenge for the primary therapist. The hierarchies of behaviors within classes are outlined in Table 6.2 and are discussed below.

TABLE 6.2. Hierarchies of Target Behaviors within Target Classes in Outpatient Individual Therapy

Suicidal behaviors:
1. Suicide crisis behaviors
2. Parasuicidal acts
3. Intrusive suicidal urges, images, and communications
4. Suicidal ideation, expectations, emotional responses[a]

Therapy-interfering behaviors:
1. Patient or therapist interfering behaviors likely to destroy therapy
2. Immediately interfering behaviors of patient or therapist
3. Patient or therapist interfering behaviors functionally related to suicidal behaviors
4. Patient therapy-interfering behaviors similar to problem behaviors outside of therapy
5. Lack of progress in therapy

Quality-of-life-interfering behaviors:
1. Behaviors causing immediate crises
2. Easy-to-change (over difficult-to-change) behaviors
3. Behaviors functionally related to higher-order targets and to patient's life goals.

Increasing behavioral skills
1. Skills currently being taught in skills training
2. Skills functionally related to higher-order targets
3. Skills not learned yet

[a]Background suicide ideation is not targeted directly. It is seen as a by-product of quality-of-life-interfering behaviors.

Decreasing Suicidal Behaviors

The first task of the individual therapist is to assess, keep track of, and focus treatment on the reduction of suicidal behaviors (see Chapter 5 for a full discussion). The particular DBT response to suicide crisis behaviors, however, depends on the assessed likelihood of suicide; the function of the behavior; the therapist's assessment of the patient's capabilities to change to more adaptive problem solving; and, most importantly, which behaviors the therapist is willing to reinforce. Although suicide crisis behaviors are never ignored, this does not mean that the proper DBT response is always to "save" the patient.

When parasuicidal acts occur, they are *always* discussed in the next individual psychotherapy session. The conduct of a detailed behavioral analysis and subsequent solution analysis after every instance of parasuicide is a crucial aspect of DBT (see Chapter 9 for a description of these strategies). The only thing that would take precedence is suicide crisis behavior occurring during the session. From my experience in consulting with therapists treating suicidal and/or borderline patients, this refusal to allow parasuicidal behavior to occur unattended differentiates DBT from many other approaches to treating borderline patients.

Intrusive or very intense suicide thoughts, images, and communications are addressed directly in individual therapy sessions subsequent to their occurrence. However, unlike suicide crisis behaviors and parasuicidal acts, habitual or what I think of as "background" suicide ideation is not always addressed directly when it occurs. To do so would rule out attention to any other behavior for many borderline patients. For the most part, the assumption in DBT is that ongoing suicide ideation is an outcome of low-quality lives; thus, the treatment consists of focused attention to enhancing the quality of life (see below).

Decreasing Therapy-Interfering Behaviors

The second task in individual treatment is to deal with any behaviors that interfere with the therapy process. These behaviors are considered second in importance only to high-risk suicidal behaviors, including parasuicidal acts. Violations of terms for continuing therapy (e.g., missing 4 consecutive weeks of scheduled therapy) or other problems that threaten continuation for either the patient or the therapist take highest priority, of course. Next in importance are the following, in this order:

1. Patient or therapist behaviors that interfere with the immediate process of treatment (e.g., the patient's not coming to therapy sessions, remaining mute in sessions, or engaging in behaviors that are so aversive to the therapist that, if they do not stop, they will result in the therapist's terminating therapy; the therapist's making unreasonable or overly rigid demands that the patient cannot meet).

2. Patient or therapist behaviors that are functionally related to suicide crisis behaviors or parasuicidal acts (e.g., the therapist's pushing too hard, too fast, or insensitively in topic areas that overwhelm the patient and often precipitate a suicidal crisis; the patient's retraction of the agreement to work on reducing suicidal behaviors; the patient's fears of calling or confiding in the therapist before rather than after parasuicidal behaviors; the patient's threatening suicide in such a manner that it is too scary for the therapist not to overreact, and/or the therapist's overreaction that further reinforce suicidal behaviors.

3. Patient behaviors that mirror problem behaviors outside the therapist's office (hostile, demanding remarks to the therapist similar to interactions with close family members; avoidance of difficult topics and problems similar to avoidance of problem solving outside of therapy).

These problem behaviors, whether brought up by the patient or observed by the therapist, are addressed directly whenever they occur. They are not ignored. If a patient is engaging in multiple therapy interfering behaviors, the therapist may want to select one or two for comment and ignore the others until progress is made on the ones selected. One of the most common, but nonetheless harmful, mistakes that therapists make with borderline patients is to tolerate the patients' therapy-interfering behaviors until it is too late. What often happens is that a patient engages in behaviors that frustrate both the therapist and the therapy; the therapist says nothing about it directly; and then suddenly the therapist hits his or her wall of tolerance, is burned out, and terminates the therapy unilaterally. Usually, this is done in a way that makes it look as though the patient is at fault or the therapist had no choice. The patient is shocked, and begs for a chance to repair the relationship, but is not taken back. With some of our patients, this has happened repeatedly; no wonder that by the time they get to us they have little trust!

The lack of progress as a therapy-interfering behavior should also be mentioned here. Clearly, if a patient is not progressing in therapy, this must be a primary target of therapeutic interactions. If progress still does not occur, therapy should be terminated at the end of the contracted period. That lack of progress will lead to therapy termination is often a new contingency for the patient. Indeed, a borderline patient's central fear is at times that if she *does* make progress, therapy will be terminated. Clarifying this switch in contingencies is an important topic of initial therapy orientation.

The central questions here in treating the borderline patient are these: How long should therapy continue without discernible progress toward goals; how much behavioral regression should be expected, especially when the patient is put on an extinction program; and how should progress be measured? Answers to these questions will be intimately tied to the therapist's theories of treatment, of behavioral functioning in general, and of BPD in particular. Borderline patients, relative to many other patients, often make very slow progress. For example, one study found that significant improvement in adjustment might require over 10 years to achieve (McGlashen, 1983), despite the fact that almost half of the patients were in therapy at the time of the follow-up assessment. At 5 years after the index diagnosis, borderline patients typically remain dysfunctional across many areas (Pope et al., 1983). The therapist must balance tolerance for slow progress in therapy with an openness to the possibility that the therapy he or she is offering is simply ineffective.

Unfortunately, a patient often tolerates ineffective and at times iatrogenic behaviors by the therapist for too long. We have had several patients who stayed in ineffective therapies and showed gradual but remarkable behavioral deterioration over time. Some stayed with therapists for over 10 to 12 years, and were still frequently engaging in parasuicidal acts and going in and out of hospitals monthly when they came into our program. Others tolerated therapists who engaged in inappropriate sexual behaviors; used the patients as surrogate therapists for themselves; refused to respect the patients' knowledge of themselves or to modify the treatment in any way to fit the patients better; or interacted defensively and "blamed the victims," further undermining the patients' sense of competence and worth. These behaviors, if they should occur, are a primary focus of DBT treatment. As one might expect, the treatment of the therapist by the DBT consultation supervisory group is often crucial here.

Decreasing Quality-of-Life-Interfering Behaviors

The third set of targets for treatment consists of maladaptive behaviors that are serious enough to jeopardize any chance the patient has for a life of reasonable quality. It is not unusual for patients to have more than one quality-of-life-interfering behavior; several patients in my clinic have such problems in five or six areas. Guidelines for choosing which of these behaviors to work on in a given therapy session are as follows. First, behaviors that are immediate take priority. That is, if the patient has no money for food or housing now, focusing on financial issues takes precedence over working on substance abuse (unless, perhaps, the patient has spent the entire week in detoxification). Second, easy problems should be solved before hard problems. This strategy is intended mainly to increase the likelihood of reinforcement of active problem solving for the patient. The idea is that if the patient acquires some experience in solving problems, she will be more likely to work actively on solving larger problems.

Third, behaviors functionally related to higher-priority targets and to the patient's life goals take precedence. Loosely speaking, the order of importance in working on these types of interfering behaviors (from high to low priority) is to address those functionally related to (1) suicide crisis behaviors and parasuicidal acts; (2) therapy-interfering behaviors; (3) suicide ideation and a sense of "misery"; (4) maintenance of treatment gains; and (5) other life goals of the patient. For example, if alcohol abuse is a reliable precursor of parasuicide, working on substance abuse should take precedence over inability to complete a semester of school, which may be functionally related only to suicide ideation. If living on the streets is causally related to missing therapy sessions, finding housing should take precedence over getting a job, which may be functionally related only to maintenance of treatment gains. And so on. Once again, principles of shaping determine pacing.

Increasing Behavioral Skills

Teaching behavioral skills (mindfulness, emotional regulation, interpersonal effectiveness, distress tolerance) is on the one hand intertwined with success in achieving the first three targets, and on the other hand constitutes a fourth independent treatment target in its own right. If the patient and therapist are to succeed in reducing the patient's suicidal, therapy-interfering, and quality-of-life-interfering behaviors, those behaviors have to be replaced with something. That "something," in DBT, consists of the behavioral skills described briefly in Chapter 5 and in detail in the companion manual to this volume. The therapist must either pull skillful behaviors from the patient that she already possesses to some degree or teach her new ones. In either case, a substantial amount of energy must be focused on strethening and generalization of behavioral skills, so that the patient can use those skills in contexts that previously elicited maladaptive, unskillful responses.

Borderline patients' unrelenting crises and mood dependency, as well as intense negative reactions to focusing sessions on teaching skills, can make it very difficult to structure the teaching of new behavioral skills into individual psychotherapy. These problems cannot be entirely avoided; one way or the other, the teaching must be accomplished. In my clinic, all new patients in individual psychotherapy also take part in 1 year of group skills training. In this situation, the individual therapist during the first year focuses primarily on application of skills the patient is learning rather than on acquisition of new skills *per se*. The aim in individual therapy is to integrate these skills into the patient's daily life and to increase the frequency of their use.

This absence of a skill acquisition focus in individual therapy in our program is not a hard and fast rule. If a patient needs a skill that has not yet been covered in the skills training part of the therapy, then the individual therapist teaches the skill "ahead of time," so to speak. Also, if the patient misses several skills training sessions, and remedial teaching is not conducted by the skill trainers (as is often the case), the individual therapist may choose to teach the missed skills in individual therapy. Doing so will depend on the therapist's and patient's opinions about the functional value of the skills in relationship to other target problems.

In some situations, independent skills training may not be possible or even preferable. A patient's insurance may not pay for it; a group skills training program may not be running at the moment; available skills training programs may be inappropriate for the patient; or the therapist may be isolated within a setting where independent skills training is not valued or supported. With well-functioning borderline patients (i.e., those entering therapy already well past Stage 1), or those eager to learn new skills and able to focus attention on doing so, there may be little need for separate skills training. When this is the case, the individual therapist can fold skills training into the individual psychotherapy.

Once substantial progress has been made in achieving the first three targets, the therapist should assess whether the patient has sufficient behavioral skills to cope with the second stage of therapy, in which residual posttraumatic stress responses are treated. The key thing to remember is that the treatment for posttraumatic stress is almost always traumatic in itself, as noted earlier. Therapy should not proceed until the therapist is reasonably sure that the patient has at least the rudimentary skills necessary to cope with that trauma. Thus, if the teaching of new behavoral skills has been incidental to other aspects of individual therapy thus far, the therapist at this point may need to program a period of intensive focus on skill acquisition and strengthening before proceeding. In a sense, the therapist is filling in the "learning holes" before taking the next step.

The therapist also must be alert to the re-emergence of first-stage problems (suicidal, therapy-interfering, and quality-of-life-interfering behaviors) in subsequent stages of therapy. When this happens, the focus on later-stage issues is momentarily suspended and the higher-order targets are readdressed. Treatment of posttraumatic stress will usually fade into the last phase of therapy, where the primary target is remediating any residual problems with self-respect.

Reducing Posttraumatic Stress

The primary work on posttraumatic stress reduction is done in individual therapy, although joining ancillary groups for victims of sexual or physical abuse or the like is encouraged for some. During the second stage of treatment, DBT moves to a focus on previous sexual, physical, and emotional abuse, and neglect. This phase is also the time to focus on any other early childhood experiences, such as losses, "misfits," or other traumas that are related to current stress responses. Thus, the second phase of individual therapy generally begins the "uncovering," cognitive and emotional processing, and resolution of pathogenic childhood events. Individual treatment will usually involve a heavy emphasis on exposure and cognitive modification strategies, focused on changing patients' emotional responses to trauma-related stimuli and cognitive reinterpretations of both the trauma and the patient's subsequent responses to the trauma.

The four goals within this target area (accepting the facts of trauma; reducing stigmatization, self-invalidation, and self-blame; reducing denial and intrusive stress response patterns; and reducing dichotomous thinking about the traumatic situation) have been discussed in Chapter 5. In the ordinary case, these goals are worked on concurrently, with session focus dictated by problems that arise during the course of exposure to traumatic cues.

Increasing Self-Respect and Achieving Individual Goals

During the final stage of individual therapy, self-respect is targeted. Since the greatest threats to self-respect for the borderline individual often originate in the social environment, treatment at this stage focuses primarily on self-respect behaviors as they occur (or fail to occur) in the interpersonal relationship between the patient and the therapist. Attention to such behaviors requires a very close focus by the therapist on moment-to-moment interactions between therapist and patient, as well as on the verbal, emotional, and overt behavioral responses of the patient. Generalization of newly acquired behavior patterns to the everyday world is targeted simultaneously. The treatment at this point closely resembles psychodynamic as well as client-centered therapy, although the interpretations of behavior offered may differ substantially between them. An even closer fit may be found between DBT at Stage 3 and functional analytic psychotherapy (Kohlenberg & Tsai, 1991)

Stage 3 is also the time for working on any other residual life problems the patient may want assistance with. At this point, goals are arrived at much as they are in any therapy. Preferences of the patient and skills of the therapist are most important. For example, I have had patients work on making more friends, resolving problems at work, making career or later-in-life choices, and learning to cope with chronic physical pain. The work on self-respect may thus be woven within the fabric of working on other issues.

Using Target Priorities to Organize Sessions

How an individual therapy session is used is determined by the patient's behaviors during the particular week preceding a session and/or during the session itself. Two types of behaviors are relevant. The first consists of the patient's negative or problem behaviors—for example, committing parasuicidal acts, telephoning the therapist too much, spending the rent money on clothes, having flashbacks of childhood sexual abuse, or invalidating her own point of view during the session. The second consists of positive behaviors that indicate the patient's progress on a targeted behavior—for example, resisting strong urges to engage in parasuicide, coming to a session on time after being late many times previously, overcoming fears and applying for a job, using behavioral skills to confront a family member, or holding on to an opinion in the face of disapproval. Treatment time is oriented to current behaviors; the structure of the session is somewhat circular, in that target focal points revolve over time.

The priority for attention during a given therapy interaction is determined by the hierarchical list (see Table 6.1). If either parasuicidal behaviors or substantial progress on such behaviors occurs during a particular week, attention to it takes precedence over attention to therapy-interfering behavior. In turn, a focus on therapy-interfering behaviors (both problems and progress) takes precedence over working on quality-of-life-interfering behaviors, and so on. Although more than one target behavior can often be worked on in a given therapy session, if time is short or a problem is complex a higher-priority target always takes precedence, even if it means slighting some other problem the patient or therapist wants to address in a session. Thus, the treatment targets and their order of precedence determine to a large extent what is talked about in therapy sessions. The amount of time spent on a particular target, which can range from a simple highlighting comment by the therapist to an entire session devoted to a thorough analysis, depends on the valence of the behavior (positive or negative) and whether or not talking about the behavior is reinforcing. Naturally, the idea is to reinforce positive behaviors and to withhold reinforcement following negative behaviors.

With respect to each target, the key task in problem solving is to elicit (at times, repeatedly) the patient's commitment to work on the target behavior. Every treatment strategy in DBT works better with cooperation from the patient. Thus, if the therapist is working on a behavioral target without the patient's active commitment to work on the same target, little progress is likely. In my experience, obtaining at least the initial commitment is rarely difficult for suicidal behaviors. The long-term negative effects of parasuicide and suicide are generally obvious to patients, and commitment to a goal of reducing such behavior is difficult to resist credibly. In any case, my colleagues and I simply do not accept patients in treatment if they do not agree that a goal of therapy is to reduce suicidal behaviors. (To date, only one has been rejected for this reason.) Thus, retraction of the commitment to work toward this goal at a later point would be considered a therapy-interfering behavior; as such, it would be second in importance only to the risk of imminent suicide.

The necessity for being in therapy, if therapy is to work, is also self-evident. And a logical case can usually be made that for therapy to continue, any therapy-interfering behaviors that arise have to be dealt with. The rationale given to the patient here is that if such behaviors are allowed to continue, the patient, the therapist, or both will build up resentment or burn out, and commitment to maintaining the therapeutic relationship will decrease. Since the therapeutic work is the glue that binds the relationship together, any behaviors that interfere with that work interfere with the relationship. Borderline patients have often been unilaterally terminated from one or more therapy regimens. Thus, a goal of developing and maintaining a working relationship with their therapist(s) is usually an attractive idea, at least at the beginning of therapy.

Work on a target problem will involve a number of coordinated treatment strategies, which are described in detail in the remainder of this book. At a minimum, the emergence of either the problem behavior or detectable progress is commented on by the therapist. Since determinants of problems and progress vary over time and situational context, each time the target problem behavior or substantial progress emerges, a behavioral analysis is usually conducted. For a negative behavior, the therapist analyzes, often in excruciating detail from the patient's point of view, what led up to the problematic response. For a positive behavior, the therapist analyzes exactly how the problem behavior was avoided. At the beginning of therapy, the conduct of such analyses may take up whole sessions, and little else will be accomplished. However, as therapy progresses the time needed to conduct these analyses shortens, and the therapist can then move to solution analyses, which are analyses of how the patient could have prevented (or did prevent) the problem behavior. Such analyses may then lead to employment of any number of other treatment strategies to remediate problems functionally related to the targeted problem behavior. I describe how to work on a target behavior in much more detail when I discuss individual treatment strategies. One entire strategy—the targeting strategy, which is a substrategy under the structural strategies—pertains to the allotment of treatment time and attention to various targets (see Chapter 14).

Patient and Therapist Resistance to Discussing Target Behaviors

The importance in DBT of focusing time and attention directly on target behaviors according to the hierarchical list cannot be overemphasized. It is a defining characteristic of DBT. From my experience in teaching and supervising DBT, however, this aspect of treatment is one of the most difficult parts for many therapists. Usually, neither a patient nor a therapist wants to focus therapy on high-priority targets, for very good reasons. Discussion of high-priority topics often leads to immediate aversive outcomes for patient and therapist alike. The therapist who is working alone, without support, is very likely to drift into a pattern of alternately appeasing and attacking the patient in regard to the issue of addressing these topics. When this pattern continues, therapy is likely to become so aversive that one or both parties terminate the relationship. Keeping the individual therapist focused on high-priority behaviors in a validating, problem-solving approach is the task of the DBT consultation team.

Patient Resistance

Patients usually do not want to discuss their own dysfunctional behaviors in a problem-solving way. For example, I have never met a patient who likes to talk about previous parasuicidal acts during individual therapy sessions. A patient may want to discuss the problem that "caused" the behavior, or to have heart-to-heart discussions about her feelings about the behavior or the events surrounding the behavior. Rarely, however, does the patient want to discuss in moment-to-moment, second-by-second detail the behavioral and environmental events leading up to and following a parasuicidal act, and then to generate a list of behaviors she could substitute for such an act the next time. Some patients not only do not want to talk about suicidal behaviors; they also do not want to talk about anything associated with it. Often, these are emotion-phobic patients who are afraid that talking about the problems will expose them to overwhelming negative affect.

Borderline patients may resist these discussions for any number of other reasons. Once parasuicidal behavior has occurred, patients often "move on" to new problems, so to speak. Focusing a discussion on past behavior does not address the current problems they may want to discuss in a therapy session. At times, borderline patients feel too ashamed of their parasuicidal behavior to bear discussing it. Or the matter-of-fact, analytical approach to the behavior in DBT may make patients feel that their emotional suffering is being invalidated. The idea that other behaviors are possible may be interpreted as blame and criticism, leading to feelings of extreme anxiety, panic, or anger at the therapist. However, the point to be remembered here is that a discussion is required every time parasuicidal behavior occurs between sessions. Noncompliance with this treatment requirement is a therapy-interfering behavior (at least when the therapay is DBT), and thus should be the next issue discussed in the therapy session.

Borderline patients do not usually want to discuss therapy-interfering behaviors either, at least not when their behaviors are the ones interfering. Reasons for this reluctance are often similar to the reasons given above for avoiding discussions of parasuicide. Whether or not quality-of-life-interfering behaviors are desirable topics for discussion from a patient's point of view depends heavily on whether the patient agrees that the behavioral pattern is problematic; if not, she can be expected to resist such discussions. At such points, it is important that the therapist be open to the possibility that he or she has misassessed the actual effects of the behavior on the patient's life. If the behavior does not seriously interfere with the patient's chances of constructing a high-quality life, then the behavior should not be high on the target list. Although there is room for true disagreement between patient and therapist, often the best direction for the therapist to take in such a situation is to find the synthesis between both points of view.

Patients also may not want to discus positive behaviors. Sometimes they have more pressing problems to discuss; in these instances, to reinforce the postive behavior, the patients' preference should probably take precedence. At other times, patients may fear that if success is noticed, more will be expected. Or patients may be uncomfortable with praise because they feel they do not deserve it. To many, progress threatens loss of therapy and of the therapeutic relationship. Each of these latter instances is viewed as a therapy-interfering behavior, and thus should be second in priority only to analyzing parasuicidal behaviors or suicide crisis behaviors that have occurred since the last session. As discussed in Chapter 10, controlling the focus of therapy discussions is a powerfful contingency management strategy.

Therapist Resistance

Some therapists find controlling the focus of sessions difficult in any case. This is especially true when therapists have been trained in nondirective types of therapy. Some patients can make such control difficult for any therapist. These patients may withdraw and refuse to talk further in a session, continually respond to questions with "I don't know" or "It doesn't matter," threaten suicide, become extremely agitated or otherwise emotional, or react in any number of other ways that therapists find punishing. (All of these responses are instances of therapy-interfering behaviors, of course.)

Some therapists do not want to hear about dysfunctional behaviors of their patients. Such reports might threaten their sense of competence or control as therapists, or remind them of behavioral problems of their own or of people close to them. One therapist I supervised told me that she didn't like to hear about "weird" behaviors from anyone. Other therapists are afraid they will make patients more suicidal if they force them to talk about things they are reluctant to discuss, especially suicidal behavior. Still others feel that the patients are in enough misery; why make it worse by forcing the topic of discussion? These reactions by therapists are viewed in DBT as therapy-interfering behaviors: They may make patients feel better in the short term, but long-term change requires that patients' high-priority problem behaviors be dealt with directly.

Interestingly, many therapists are also reluctant to discuss patients' therapy-interfering behaviors directly with the patients. In my supervision experience, many therapists put off discussing such behaviors with patients until they are burned out and it is too late. The problems are brought up in supervision, but not easily with the patients. Generally, these therapists seem to believe that "nontherapeutic" responses to patients (e.g., feelings of anger, burnout, reluctance to continue treatment) are indications of their own inadequacies. By contrast, DBT approaches such responses as indications that there are problems in the therapeutic relationship—that is, therapy-interfering behaviors are going on. With very few exceptions, such problems are discussed with patients in a direct, problem-solving manner. More is said on this topic in Chapters 9 and 15. Like patients, therapists often do not want to discuss or work on their own therapy-intefering behaviors, either. Indeed, some therapists are quite adept at turning patients' complaints about their own behavior into discussions of the patients' excessive demands, oversensitivity, or the like.

Individual Therapy Targets and Diary Cards

How does a therapist come to know about parasuicidal and other targeted behaviors that occur during the week between sessions? Certainly, the therapist can ask. This is a simple thing to do when negative high-priority behaviors are occurring often or positive behaviors are occurring infrequently. For example, if a person enters therapy cutting herself daily, and wants help in stopping the cutting, it is easy for the therapist to ask about self-mutilation at the beginning of each session. However, in my experience, it gets increasingly difficult for the therapist to ask about such behavior after it has not occurred for a number of weeks or months. Likewise, if drug or alcohol use is not a problem at the moment, the therapist may feel uncomfortable or silly asking about it each and every week. If increased use of behavioral skills is a focus, but the patient is diligently applying such skills week after week, it may be difficult to ask for a progress report every single week. But, in my experience, problems with drugs and alcohol are very unlikely to be reported spontaneously. Parasuicide may or may not be reported, depending on whether the function of the act is communication to the therapist. And once the patient forgets to work at applying behavioral skills, she is unlikely to report this to the therapist as a problem.

The easiest solution to these difficulties is to have the patient fill out a diary card each and every week, in order to obtain information on a daily basis about relevant behaviors. The front of a DBT diary card is shown in Figure 6.1. As can be seen, information is obtained about type and amount of alcohol ingested each day; types and amounts of prescription, over-the-counter, and illicit drugs taken; and degree of suicide ideation, degree of misery, degree of urges to commit parasuicidal acts, and occurrence of such acts. A rating for amount of behavioral skills practice is also obtained each day. The card can be used for a variety of purposes, but one major purpose is

Dialectical Behavior Therapy
DIARY CARD

Name: _____   Date started: _____

Date	Alcohol		Over-the-Counter Medications		Prescription Medications		Street/ Illicit Drugs		Suicidal Ideation (0-5)	Misery (0-5)	Self-Harm					Used Skills (0-7)*
	#	Specify	#	Specify	#	Specify	#	Specify			Urges (0-5)	Action Yes/No					
Mon																	
Tue																	
Wed																	
Thu																	
Fri																	
Sat																	
Sun																	

*
0 = Not thought about or used
1 = Thought about, not used, didn't want to
2 = Thought about, not used, wanted to

3 = Tried, but couldn't use them
4 = Tried, could do them but they didn't help
5 = Tried, could use them, helped

6 = Didn't try, used them, they didn't help
7 = Didn't try, used them, helped

FIGURE 6.1. The front of a DBT diary card. The blank columns at right enable the patient to record behaviors in addition to those listed; these are decided upon with the therapist.

to elicit information about targeted behaviors that have occurred during the previous week. If the card indicates that a parasuicidal act has occurred, it is noted and discussed. If very high suicide ideation is indicated, it is assessed to determine whether the patient is at high risk for suicide. If a pattern of excessive alcohol or drug use appears, it is discussed (as a quality-of-life-interfering behavior). Failure to take prescribed drugs may be a therapy-interfering behavior. If the card is not brought in or is inadequately filled out, this constitutes a therapy-interfering behavior and, of course, is discussed as such. Finally, there are blank columns for recording any other behaviors that the patient and therapist may decide upon. Generally, at least at the beginning of therapy, these columns are used to record other quality-of-life-interfering behaviors. For example, I have had patients record hours per day at work, hours per day fantasizing, bulimic episodes, amount of exercise, number of urges to avoid situations that are resisted, and number of dissociative experiences.

Patients fill out diary cards during at least the first two stages of therapy. As problems with parasuicide and substance abuse are resolved, patients generally resist continuing to fill out the cards. However, since there is a high likelihood that these behaviors will return during work on posttraumatic stress, diary cards should not be stopped until the third phase. At that point, continuation is a matter of negotiation between patient and therapist. This is not to say that a fair amount of negotiation does not take place during the end of the first phase and throughout the second phase of therapy. As patients learn more assertion skills, they can be expected to use these skills in therapy more frequently. Diary cards afford an almost perfect vehicle for this practice. I have one patient who, on general principle, refuses to fill out diary cards when I am out of town. She reasons that if I am on vacation, she should also be allowed to go on vacation. This seems reasonable to me.

Skills Training: Hierarchy of Targets

By definition, skills training has as its primary focus the acquisition and strengthening of behavioral skills. Skills training in DBT has four distinct modules covering mindfulness, distress tolerance, interpersonal effectiveness in con-

---

TABLE 6.3. The Hierarchy of Primary Targets in DBT Skills Training

1. Stopping behaviors likely to destroy therapy
2. Skill acquisition, strengthening, and generalization
   A. Core mindfulness skills
   B. Interpersonal effectiveness
   C. Emotion regulation
   D. Distress tolerance
3. Decreasing therapy-interfering behaviors

TABLE 6.4. The Hierarchy of Primary Targets in DBT Supportive Process Groups

1. Decreasing therapy-interfering behaviors
2. Strengthening interpersonal skills
3. Increasing behaviors instrumental to a positive quality of life; decreasing behaviors interfering with a positive quality of life:
   A. Emotional reactivity
   B. Self-invalidation
   C. Crisis-generating behaviors
   D. Grief inhibition
   E. Active-passivity behaviors
   F. Mood dependency of behavior

flict situations, and emotion regulation. The order of targets for skills training is given in Table 6.3. The targets and their ordering are reviewed in detail in the companion manual to this volume; thus, I do not discuss them here. The important point, however, is that the target hierarchy in skills training is not the same as that in individual psychotherapy.

Supportive Process Groups: Hierarchy of Targets

In contrast to skills training, where very little direct attention is given to in-session process issues, supportive process group therapy in DBT utilizes the behaviors that occur during group meetings—that is, the group process—as the vehicle for change. Thus, the principal targets are in-session behaviors that exemplify in some way the problems each patient is having outside of group meetings. This comparability is crucial if the therapy is to be effective. Teaching patients to behave as good group members when those same behaviors are not functional in their everyday lives does them a disservice. Because the agenda in process groups is far less strictly controlled by the group therapists than in any other mode of DBT, the hierarchy of targets is less rigidly adhered to. However, through orienting patients to treatment and through in-session comments and questions, therapists can have some influence on the therapeutic focus as well as on which behaviors are reinforced.

The hierarchy of process group targets is outlined in Table 6.4. The most important target class is that of therapy-interfering behaviors (e.g., not coming to sessions, coming late, missing for unimportant reasons, not keeping agreements, violating group rules, withdrawing, attacking others, etc.). In individual DBT and skills training groups, therapists take primary responsibility for addressing these issues. In the process group, by contrast, therapy-interfering behaviors of group members or of the group therapists offer an opportunity for patients to work on the second most important target—strengthening use of interpersonal skills, especially in the resolution of conflict situations. The third target class includes any other behavioral patterns exhibited in group interactions that, outside of the group, would interfere

TABLE 6.5. The Hierarchy of Primary Targets for Telephone Calls

Calls to the individual therapist:
 1. Decreasing suicide crisis behaviors
 2. Increasing generalization of behavioral skills
 3. Decreasing the sense of conflict, alienation, distance from therapist
Calls to the skills trainer or other therapists:
 1. Decreasing behaviors likely to destroy therapy

with (behaviors to decrease) or enhance (behaviors to increase) the quality of life for a particular patient. Two points must be attended to. First, the focus in on behaviors that show up within the therapy session, not on outside events or behaviors. Second, the particular behaviors stressed and reinforced, punished, or extinguished are specific to each patient. That is, not every target is necessarily accorded the same importance for each patient.

Telephone Calls: Hierarchy of Targets

Targets for phone conversations with a patient depend on whether a call is made to the primary therapist or to a skills training or ancillary therapist. The hierarchy of targets is outlined in Table 6.5.

Calls to the Primary Therapist

Telephone calls between sessions to the primary therapist are encouraged in DBT. (A therapist who is immediately worried about getting too many calls, however, should remember that a patient's calling too often is considered therapy-interfering behavior.) To understand the hierarchy of targets for phone calls, the primary therapist needs to remember the three reasons why DBT favors phone calls. First, for the individual who has difficulty asking for help directly, and instead attempts suicide as a "cry for help" or otherwise suffers adverse consequences as a result of her difficulty, the very act of telephoning is practice in changing this dysfunctional behavior. It offers the therapist an avenue to intervene to stop suicidal behavior.

Second, a patient often needs help in generalizing DBT behavioral skills to her everyday life. A phone call can obtain the coaching needed for successful generalization. In DBT, the primary therapist is much like a high school basketball coach. Individual psychotherapy sessions are like the daily, after-school practice sessions where fundamentals are taught and attention is given to building the basic skills for the game. Phone calls, in contrast, are like the interaction of the coach with team members during an actual competitive game. The coach helps team members remember and apply what they have learned during the weekly practice sessions. In sports, it is inconceivable that a coach would refuse to go to games and help team members. No coach would suggest that this is not part of the job, that helping players during games is making them dependent, or that asking for advice during the game is a hostile attack on the coach.

Third, when interpersonal conflicts or crises arise in an intimate relationship, it does not seem reasonable that the person having difficulty has to wait an arbitrary amount of time, set by the other person, to resolve the crises. Phone calls in these instances offer an opportunity to increase the interpersonal bonding between patient and therapist, but they also offer an opportunity to equalize the power distribution in therapy. As other therapy perspectives would put it, such calls "empower" the patient.

These three reasons for phone calls dictate the targets for such calls. In order of importance, these are as follows: (1) decreasing suicide crisis behaviors; (2) increasing application of skills to everyday life; and (3) resolving interpersonal crises, alienation, or a sense of distance between patient and therapist. As in other interactions with a borderline patient, it can at times be extremely difficult for the therapist to keep a phone session on track. With respect to suicide crisis behaviors, the main focus is on assessing risk and using a problem-solving approach to identify alternative behaviors. Generally, such problem solving will lead into a discussion of how the patient can apply DBT behavioral skills to the current situation. Or, if the problem is the relationship with the therapist, a discussion of this may ensue. However, keeping the patient alive in a crisis generally takes precedence over other targets.

With respect to skill generalization, the modal comment of the DBT therapist on a phone call is "What skills could you use in this instance?" Thus, the therapist relentlessly keeps the focus on how the patient can use her skills to cope with the current problem until she has another session. At least at the beginning of treatment, getting the patient to utilize distress tolerance (including crisis survival) skills is the primary goal here. Analyzing the current crisis and generating solutions is a focus of therapy sessions but not of phone sessions; resolving the problem or crisis is definitely not the target of phone sessions. It is crucial that the therapist remember and attend to this point, since problem resolution is usually the patient's primary objective during the phone call.

A borderline patient often feels angry, alienated, or distant from her therapist; therapy sessions frequently set off these feelings. However, such a patient also often has delayed reactions to interactions with the therapist. Thus, emotions of anger, sadness, alienation, or other distress may not occur until some time after an interaction. Calling the therapist is appropriate in this situation. The target of these calls, from the DBT point of view, is a decrease in the patient's sense of alienation or distance from the therapist. The difficulty for the therapist is helping the patient with this issue while not reinforcing dysfunctional behaviors at the same time. I discuss this issue in much greater detail in Chapter 15. In the beginning of therapy, phone interactions not only may be frequent, but also may last a fair amount of time. The therapeutic strategies of observing limits, discussed in Chapter 10, can be especially critical here if the therapist is not to burn out. As therapy progresses and trust in the relationship increases, both the frequency and duration of calls should decrease.

Calls to Skills Trainers and Other Therapists

Although the skills trainer might seem to be the logical person to call for help in applying behavioral skills to everyday life, in DBT, where skills training is conducted in groups, the patient is instead directed to call the individual therapist for this purpose. Generally, the individual therapist will have a much better appreciation of the patient's current abilities and limitations, and thus will be in a better position to require and reinforce "just-noticeable improvement." In other settings, this limitation on phone calls and ancillary contact may not be necessary. For example, if an individual skills training model is used, it may make sense for the patient to be able to call the skills trainer for help in applying specific behavior skills outside of treatment sessions. If milieu treatment is used, as is typical in inpatient and day treatment settings, consultations for help in skill generalization might ordinarily be directed to milieu staff. In these instances, the second target is application of skills to everyday life.

In my program, the only purpose of a call from the skills trainer's point of view is to keep the patient in skills training—that is, to decrease any behavior that threatens the continuation of therapy. Obviously, keeping the patient alive is useful to achieving this target goal. A similar position is taken by other therapists in the DBT program, including the program director. The only appropriate focus is on those problems that threaten the patient's continuation in the program. All other problems are handled by the individual therapist.

If a patient calls the skills trainer or any other therapist, including the program or unit director, for help in a crisis or for help in applying skills to a situation, that therapist will refer her to her individual therapist and will help the patient with distress tolerance skills until her therapist is available. If the patient is in immediate danger of suicide, the therapist does what is needed to insure the patient's safety and then turns the problems over to the individual therapist. A more detailed discussion of these points is provided in the accompanying skills training manual.

Target Behaviors and Session Focus:
Who Is in Control?

When the patient does not want to discuss high-priority target behaviors, the therapist is faced with controlling the therapy focus against the patient's wishes. DBT requires that the therapist adhere resolutely to the target hierarchy for the particular type of session being conducted. Although at times such a focus can create a power struggle that derails attention to other pressing problems, this does not need to be the case. The therapist must remember and attend to a number of points. The most important one is that the therapist must believe in attending directly to high-priority behaviors. That is, the therapist must believe in the value of applying problem-solving approaches to such behaviors. Clearly, the patient usually does not believe in this approach, and frequently punishes persistence and reinforces moving on to other topics. If the therapist also does not believe in confronting the problem behaviors directly, it is very difficult to resist the patient's pressure to attend to other topics. The solution here is for the therapist to keep a resolute focus on long-term gain rather than short-term peace during the session (i.e., the therapist practices the crisis survival strategies taught to the patient in the distress tolerance module of skills training).

Although high-priority behaviors do not have to be the very first topics discussed during a session, they nonetheless cannot be ignored. If the therapist agrees to discuss something other than these behaviors, he or she may unwittingly be reinforcing avoidance behaviors; by insisting on discussing the high-priority behaviors, the therapist is extinguishing avoidance behaviors. At times a patient will respond to the therapist's insistence by withdrawing, refusing to speak, attacking the therapist or therapy, or other behaviors that can be loosely described as "throwing a behavioral tantrum." If these behaviors work—that is, if the therapist is dissuaded from discussing the high-priority behaviors by these patient responses—the therapist is then rewarding the patient's often dysfunctional style of resistant behaviors. It is much like trying to help a person lost in a snowstorm who has hypothermia and wants to lie down and sleep. A good friend will do what is necessary to keep the hypothermia victim moving. (This metaphor can be useful in gaining cooperation from the reluctant patient.)

As I discuss in more detail in Chapter 10, the key here is the combination of unwavering nonappeasement with equally unwavering soothing. Soothing, in this instance, may consist of orienting the patient to the importance of discussing the high-priority behaviors, reminding the patient of her commitment to work on the behaviors, compromising on both timing and amount of time spent on unwanted topics, and validating her difficulties with such an approach. Unwavering nonappeasement means continuing with the behavioral and solution analyses, taking each response of the patient at face value, and staying on track, but all the while responding with warmth and attention. In my experience, once a patient learns the rules and knows that without exception the therapist will not avoid high-priority behaviors in therapy, one of two things happens: Either the patient makes enough progress on the behaviors that they do not have to be discussed, or she cooperates with the therapeutic guidelines.

Modification of Target Hierarchies in Other Settings

There is no *a priori* reason why the particular targets or divisions of targets described above must be invariant. The hierarchies described here have worked well in an outpatient treatment setting; however, in other treatment settings, modification in the divisions of targets and orderings of importance may be indicated. Any program that develops treatment plans with specified behavioral targets is compatible with a DBT approach. In many settings, however, treatment targets will necessarily be much more limited than in the full DBT program, although reduction of suicide risk and reduction of therapy-destructive behaviors have to be primary targets in any setting.

Responsibility for Decreasing Suicidal Behaviors

In my view, the primary therapist should always give first priority to the reduction of suicidal behaviors, including parasuicide. That is, this target cannot be downplayed or ignored by the primary therapist. On an acute unit, the person whose chief responsibility it is to help the patient decrease suicidal behaviors may be the individual contact person, or any other person who is reasonably familiar with the patient. Because of the short-term nature of an acute unit, the designated person may be whoever fills a particular role rather than a specific individual. For example, the primary contact person may change every day, or may stay the same each day but change with each shift. If the individual's outpatient therapist is also her attending therapist on the inpatient unit, that therapist is the ideal person. In day treatment, the designated person may be the case manager. The point here is that if suicidal behavior occurs or is threatened while the person is receiving treatment in the setting, DBT treatment strategies focus directly on the behavior need to be implemented by someone. Such behavior should not be ignored.

In my clinic, the individual psychotherapist is the only person who directly targets reducing suicidal behaviors. All other treatment team members do the minimum necessary to keep the patient alive. In addition, they may utilize suicidal or parasuicidal crises as opportunities to help the patient with skill implementation (e.g., stress tolerance instead of parasuicidal activity until she can see her individual contact person). Otherwise, all members of the treatment team send the patient to the individual psychotherapist for extensive work on suicidal behavior, including crisis management.

Others using DBT have developed different systems. For example, all milieu therapists (nurses, mental health technicians, etc.) may respond to suicidal or parasuicidal behavior with immediate application of problem-solving strategies. If patient–staff community meetings are a part of treatment, the entire unit may target parasuicide episodes. Reviewing the behavioral and solution analyses (see Chapter 9) of any parasuicidal activities that week, for example, may be part of the weekly agenda. In process group sessions following parasuicidal behavior, the entire group may assist in such analyses. Even if the targets are kept entirely as I have described above for outpatient DBT, who is responsible for which targets will vary by treatment location and setting. In principle, there is nothing in DBT that prohibits these changes if each segment of the treatment team has a clear and specific understanding of its targets, its limits, and its rules. The most relevant principle here, as I discuss in Chapters 10 and 15, is to apply change strategies that do not simultaneously reinforce the behaviors therapy is intended to reduce.

Responsibility for Other Targets

Depending on the setting and the length of treatment available, treatment targets may be a blend of general targets for all patients in the setting (e.g., increasing skills taught in groups everyone participates in) and individualized targets developed for each patient. For example, each patient may have her own set of targeted quality-of-life-interfering behaviors. In my experience, an important quality-of-life-interfering behavior that can be usefully targeted on acute inpatient units is active passivity with respect to finding affordable housing or coping with other crises situations. Because suicidal behaviors can recur as a result of initial attempts to treat posttraumatic stress due to sexual abuse, especially when the treatment strategy involves exposure to stress cues, an inpatient unit is often an ideal environment for at least much of the early work on this target. A structured substance abuse setting will, of course, have decreasing substance abuse as a primary target. Many settings other than outpatient therapy also target some variation of the behavioral skills taught in DBT. It is not unusual, for example, to have life skills classes and groups for teaching assertion, cognitive skills for reducing depression, anger management, and the like.

Specifying Targets for Other Modes of Treatment

As I have said, DBT modes in my clinic include individual psychotherapy, group skills training, supportive process group therapy, telephone calls, and therapist case consultations. In some settings, however, other modes of treatment may be very important. For example, on inpatient and day treatment units there is a milieu mode of treatment. Patient–staff community meetings constitute another mode. Vocational counseling, "wellness" or exercise classes, high school classes, and others may be important modes of treatment in some settings. In community mental health settings, case management, crisis outreach, and emergency room management are often important modes. The essential idea here is that regardless of the mode of treatment being provided, it is imperative to list clearly and in order the targets of each mode. This does not mean that there cannot be overlap between modes. For example, both crises outreach and emergency room management may target reducing immediate suicide crises behaviors and, secondarily, skills generalization.

In one long-term inpatient hospital unit, directed by Charles Swenson at Cornell Medical Center/New York Hospital at White Plains, DBT skills training groups are a regular part of the therapy. In addition, a unit skills consultant has been designated (a new mode of treatment). This consultant has daily office hours, and patients can go to him or her with questions and problems regarding the application of their new skills in everyday life in the hospital. Thus, generalization of behavioral skills is the primary target for the consultant, rather than a target for the individual psychotherapist. Such an approach may be particularly useful when individual psychotherapists do not themselves provide DBT.

DBT is nonetheless increasingly being applied in milieu settings. The success of the application in such a setting is closely linked to the unit's ability to think clearly about the milieu's behavioral targets and to organize DBT treatment strategies to address these targets. The hierarchical list of targets for milieu interactions might be as follows: (1) preventing parasuicide and suicide; (2) decreasing behaviors that interfere with unit functioning and cohesiveness; (3) increasing generalization of DBT behavioral skills to on-unit interactions; and (4) decreasing quality-of-life-interfering behaviors and increasing quality-of-life-enhancing behaviors as these behaviors occur on the unit.

The limits of an inpatient unit with respect to suicidal and therapy-interfering behaviors may be quite different from those of an individual psychotherapist. Outright control of their behavior may be more important, if only because society expects behavior to be controlled in such a setting. Thus, milieu staff members may develop rules and contingencies for behavior that differ from those set by the individual psychotherapists. These rules may reflect the milieu staff's need to target the welfare of the entire unit, as well as that of each individual patient. It is more than likely that a more precise and context-specific set of therapy-interfering behaviors will be needed to assist staff members in pinpointing when these behaviors (by either staff or patients) are occurring. In a long-term inpatient setting, the milieu may have primary responsibility for increasing skill generalization. In such a setting, a patient may more appropriately call on the milieu staff than on her individual psychotherapist. As in supportive process group therapy, the value of this approach depends heavily on a similarity between behaviors that work on the unit and behaviors that work in the outside world. Teaching a patient to be a good patient is not in itself a very useful target for the borderline individual. Indeed, in my experience, many borderline individuals have this role down very well.

In milieu and other institutional settings, there will be at least one organizational leader and sometimes many more. In such settings, the treatment targets of these individuals need to be specified. Usually, they will be responsible for patients' and therapists' observation of unit or organizational limits. They also are generally responsible for the therapists' behaviors; thus, they target delivery of DBT by the therapists.

Turf Conflicts with Respect to Target Responsibilities

As I have discussed in Chapter 4, the mode of DBT for the therapist is the weekly case consultation/supervision meeting. In my experience, if this is well attended and if the entire treatment team accepts the spirit of DBT and its dialectical framework, little conflict about target responsibilities emerges. The key to this cooperation is clarity about which treatment targets are specific to which modes of treatment, as well as clarity about the hierarchy of targets in each mode of treatment. For example, in standard DBT as delivered in my clinic, skills trainers must understand clearly that decreasing parasuicidal and high-risk suicidal behaviors is not their top-priority target; rather, it is that of the primary therapist. Thus, when such behavior is threatened, a skills trainer calls or refers the patient to her primary therapist, instead of working out a no-harm contract on the spot or sending the patient to the hospital. A second component of cooperation, as I discuss in Chapter 13, is the philosophy of DBT that team members do not have to agree, say the same things to patients, or be particularly consistent with patients. Thus, if two team members focus on teaching interpersonal skills and teach opposite behaviors, it is the responsibility of the patient (with help from the primary therapist, if needed) to sort out what to learn and what to discard. A third aspect of keeping the team on track is mutual respect among team members. Dialectical and problem-solving strategies are applied when conflicts arise. However, defensiveness and judgmental attitudes can quickly derail such efforts.

In contrast, patients' use of ancillary treatment is rife with possibilities for conflict. A psychologist consulted for behavioral work on a specified problem — for example, desensitization of fear of flying — may expand treatment to target general fears and problems with passivity and avoidance. A pharmacotherapist may decide that another mode of treatment is required for depression or suicidal ideation (e.g., hospitalization), without referring the patient back to her primary therapist. A member of the inpatient hospital staff may develop an entirely different treatment plan and send the patient to a new outpatient therapist. Although DBT seeks to control the treatment priorities of the DBT team, it has no necessary agenda for directly influencing treatment priorities of ancillary therapists. The consultation-to-the-patient approach, which puts the burden of influence on the patient, is used here. I discuss this much more extensively in Chapter 13.

Concluding Comments

Structuring therapy in DBT requires two things: a clear understanding of what stage of therapy a patient is in, and a clear understanding of the specific targets with this specific patient and of how those targets relate to the total treatment picture. Even when you are a patient's only therapist, you must understand your goals and make them clear during each interaction with the patient. Once you have achieved this clarity, you have to get yourself to follow the treatment guidelines. It is this aspect of the treatment that has proved to be the most difficult for many therapists. It is probably impossible to follow the treatment guidelines in this chapter unless you believe firmly in them. Once you believe in them, you have to take a protective stance toward the patient and be unwilling to allow continued pain and dysfunction. As one of my students said about doing DBT, you have to be "warmly ruthless" in your determination to help the patient change. It also helps (if you are empirically minded) to remember the empirical data on the efficacy of the treatment.

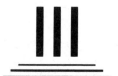

Basic Treatment Strategies

7

Dialectical Treatment Strategies

DBT treatment strategies are coordinated activities, tactics, and procedures that the therapist employs to achieve the treatment goals described in Chapters 5 and 6. Strategies also describe the role and focus of the therapist and may refer to coordinated responses that the therapist should give to a particular problem presented by the patient. The term "strategies" in DBT means the same thing as terms such as "procedures," "protocol," and "techniques" in other treatment approaches. I prefer the term "strategies" because it implies both a plan of action and finesse in carrying out the plan. Although each set of strategies has a number of components, not all of these are required in every instance. It is more important to apply the intent of a group of strategies than to adhere rigidly to the exact guidelines as presented here. In this section of the book, I define and outline the major strategies in DBT.

Basic treatment strategies in DBT are depicted in Figure 7.1. They are grouped into four major categories: (1) dialectical strategies, (2) core strategies, (3) stylistic strategies, and (4) case management strategies. (Specific integrative strategies, which involve various combinations of strategies from these four categories, are discussed in the last two chapters of this book.) Dialectical strategies are pervasive and inform the entire treatment. The core strategies consist of problem-solving and validation strategies; as the label "core strategies" implies, they are at the heart of the treatment, together with dialectical strategies. Stylistic strategies specify interpersonal and communication styles compatible with the therapy. Case management strategies have to do with how the therapist interacts with and responds to the social network in which the patient is enmeshed. With specific patients, some strategies will be used more often than others, and it is possible that one or more of the strategies will be needed only rarely. Not all strategies may be necessary or appropriate for any given session, and the pertinent combination may change over time.

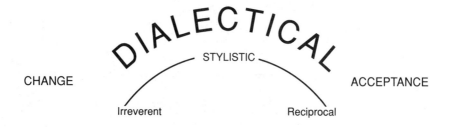

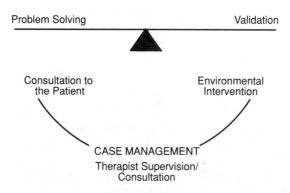

FIGURE 7.1. Treatment strategies in DBT.

The strategies described in this and the following chapters no doubt have many things in common with aspects of the other varieties of psychotherapy currently in use. To the extent that those who develop therapy models learn how to do therapy from their patients—that is, what works and what does not—there should be many overlaps among the various approaches to working with similar types of patients and problems. Although the formulation of how and why a particular treatment approach works with borderline patients may differ across theoretical orientations, the therapeutic behaviors that are actually effective as probably much less variable. In writing the original draft of this volume, I read every other treatment manual I could find, both behavioral and nonbehavioral. I also read books that tell new therapists how they are supposed to behave in therapy. My intent was to see how others described the behaviors specific to their treatment. Whenever I found a treatment component or strategy that was the same as or similar to one used in DBT, I tried to use similar language to describe it. Thus, in a sense, much of this manual has been "stolen" from preceding manuals. When I give workshops on DBT, a very common response from therapists, regardless of their theoretical orientation, is that I am telling them what they already do with borderline patients. Thus, I suspect that many therapists will find much of their own therapeutic behavior described in these chapters.

Defining Dialectical Strategies

Dialectical strategies permeate all aspects of treatment in DBT. These strategies grow out of a dialectical philosophical position (discussed more fully in Chapter 2) that views reality as a wholistic process in a state of constant development and change. Dialectical strategies stress the creative tensions generated by contradictory emotions and oppositional thought patterns, values, and behavioral strategies, both within the person and in the person–environment system. As I have noted repeatedly throughout this book, the primary therapy dialectic is that of change in the context of acceptance of reality as it is. The therapist facilitates change by responding strategically to optimize the dialectical tensions arising within therapeutic interactions, and by highlighting each side of the dialectical oppositions arising in therapy interactions as well as in everyday life. The object is to foster successive reconciliation and resolution at increasingly functional and viable levels. Rigid adherence to either pole of a dialectic by therapist or patient contributes to stagnation, increases tension, and inhibits reconciliation and synthesis.[1]

The dialectical focus of the therapist involves two levels of therapeutic behavior. Although they may occur simultaneously, they are very different in their point of view and in their application. First, the therapist is alert to the dialectical tensions and balance occurring within the treatment relationship itself. From this perspective, the focus is on the therapeutic interaction and on movement within that relationship. The therapist pays attention to the dialectics of the relationship by combining acceptance and change strategies and by moving back and forth within the current dialectic during each interaction in such a way as to maintain a collaborative working relationship with the patient.

Second, the therapist teaches and models dialectical behavior patterns. From this perspective, the focus is on the patient, independent of her interactions with the therapist. The strategies in ths case include directly teaching the patient; questioning her in order to open up new avenues of behavior; offering alternative ways of thinking and behaving; and, most importantly, modeling dialectical behavior. The message communicated to the patient is that truth is neither absolute nor relative, but rather evolves and is constructed over time. Thus, it is not possible at one point in time to grasp the totality of the truth in any state of affairs. Either extreme of a dialectic, by definition, is not the place to be. No rigid position is possible, and process and change are inevitable. Teaching dialectical patterns of thinking is essentially an application of cognitive restructuring procedures (see Chapter 11), with a specific focus on replacing nondialectical with dialectical thinking and underlying assumptions. Both attention to the dialectics of the therapeutic relationship and teaching dialectical behavior patterns are essential in every interaction with the patient; they also inform the treatment supervision and case consultation meetings.

BALANCING TREATMENT STRATEGIES:
DIALECTICS OF THE THERAPEUTIC RELATIONSHIP[2]

The primary dialectical strategy is the balanced use of specific strategies and therapeutic positions by the therapist during interactions with the patient. Constant attention to combining acceptance with change, flexibility with stability, nurturing with challenging, and a focus on capabilities with a focus on limitations and deficits is the essence of this strategy. The goal is to bring out the opposites, both in therapy and the patient's life, and to provide conditions for syntheses. The key idea guiding the therapist's behavior is that for any point, an opposite or complementary position can be held.

Thus, change may be facilitated by emphasizing acceptance, and acceptance by emphasizing change. The emphasis upon opposites sometimes takes place over time—that is, over the whole of an interaction, rather than simultaneously or in each part of an interaction. The wisdom of this approach with borderline individuals was noted much earlier by Sherman (1961), who commented that "whichever side the therapist aligns himself with, the patient will usually feel impelled to leave" (p. 55). Conversely, a rigid adherence to either pole of a dialectic leads to increased tension between therapist and patient, and usually to increased polarization rather than to synthesis and growth. Thus, synthesis and growth require attention to balance. The therapist must search for what is left out of both the therapist's and patient's current behaviors and ways of ordering reality, and then must assist the patient (while being open himself or herself) to create new orderings that embrace and include what was previously excluded.

Maintaining a dialectical stance in the therapeutic interaction has a number of essential characteristics. First, speed is often of the essence. The idea is to keep the patient sufficiently off balance that she cannot find a secure foothold to maintain her previous behavioral, emotional, and cognitive rigidity. Quick and light footwork is important here. Second, the therapist must be awake, observing and sensing each movement of the patient. The idea is to "go with the flow," responding with just enough movement each time the patient moves. The therapist has to be as alert as if he or she and the patient really were balanced at opposite ends of a teeter-totter perched on a high wire over the Grand Canyon. Third, a dialectical approach requires that the therapist move with certainty, strength, and total commitment. When a position is taken, it must be taken whole-heartedly. Half-hearted, tentative movements with borderline patients will have half-hearted tentative effects. Sheldon Kopp (1971) made a similar point when he described gifted and charismatic psychotherapists as follows:

> the central quality. . . is that such a man [sic] trusts himself. It is not so much that he is responding in ways which are beyond other men [sic] (or lesser therapists). Rather it seems that he is past worrying about how he is doing. No longer expecting to be unafraid or certain or perfect, he gives himself over to being just as he is at the moment. (p. 7)

Dialectics in the context of the relationship can be compared to ball-room dancing. The therapist must respond to and with the patient just where she is. The idea is to move the patient slightly off balance but with a hand firmly guiding her, so that eventually she can allow herself to relax and let the music move her. However, the patient is frequently like a dancer twirling out of control. The therapist has to move in quickly with a counterforce to stop the patient from moving off the dance floor. "Dancing" with the patient often requires the therapist to move quickly from strategy to strategy, alternating acceptance with change, control with letting go, confrontation with support, the carrot with the stick, a hard edge with softness, and so on in rapid succession.

The return to the teeter-totter image, the object is for the therapist and patient to move to the middle together so that both can move up a notch to a higher platform and teeter-totter. Although the natural tendency when one or the other moves back on the teeter-totter is to balance it by moving back oneself, if both continue to move backwards, both will fall off and the therapy will be derailed or destroyed. A typical dialectical tension in the treatment of a borderline patient is between the patient's "I can't stand it" or "I can't do it" and the therapist's "Yes, you can." Thus, as the patient moves back slightly, the task of the therapist is to move slightly to the middle, hoping that the patient will then also move toward the middle: "I can see that it is terribly difficult. Perhaps you can't do it alone, but I will help you. I believe in you."

Such a strategy with a suicidal patient is risky, and from this risk comes the notion that DBT is like a game of "chicken" played by therapist and patient. For example, a patient at my clinic hated group skills training and wanted to quit, but did not want to have to leave her individual therapist as well. Her individual therapist, however, said that she was not willing to break the original therapy agreement. The patient left the session and called her therapist, saying she was at the bus station and was going to take a bus to a distant spot, get off, and kill herself. If her therapist went to the bus station to get the patient, or immediately changed the rules of therapy, it would have been the same as jumping to the patient's side of the teeter-totter. If the therapist had called the patient a "manipulator" and refused to talk to her, it would have been the same as moving back on the teeter-totter to maintain balance. The problem with that strategy, however, was that the patient might move back again herself. Instead, the therapist moved slightly toward the middle by expressing faith in the patient, validating her suffering, and encouraging her to find it in herself to get off the bus (if she indeed got on it), come back, and work with the therapist to solve the problem. The therapist would be waiting and hoping that the patient would come back.

In the example just presented, jumping over the patient to the other end of the teeter-totter would have been an instance of a paradoxical move. Used skillfully, such moves will induce the patient to jump quickly to the other side to maintain the balance. The therapist may say something like this: "I can see that life is just unbearable for you. You really can't take care of yourself any more. Perhaps therapy is too difficult at this point in your life. Do you think I should just take over for you for the time being? Perhaps I should send the police or an aid car to get you. Maybe this is the wrong program for you? Should we explore taking a break?" Or, more irreverently, "Perhaps staying in bed for 6 months is a good idea."

All DBT strategies are arranged to highlight their dialectical character. As shown in Figure 7.1, strategies can be categorized as primarily emphasizing change or acceptance. Many treatment impasses result from the therapist's failing to balance treatment strategies on one side (change or acceptance) with their polar counterparts. The categorization is artificial, since in many ways every strategy comprises both acceptance and change. Indeed, the best strategies are those that clearly combine the two, as I found in dealing with one patient who was referred to me. At the time of her referral, her options were to get into treatment with me or to be committed involuntarily to a state hospital (yet again). The patient repeatedly engaged in parasuicidal behavior and had burned out almost all mental health resources in the Seattle area. Her behavior seemed out of control. Her inpatient physicians were trying to get her involuntarily committed; the nurses were trying to get her into a program with me. At our first appointment, I told her that she was the perfect kind of person for our program and I would accept her into therapy (an acceptance strategy), but only if she agreed to work on changing her suicidal behavior (a change strategy). She was free to choose therapy with me or not (letting go), but I was also free to choose whether to work with her or not (control). The aspects of change and acceptance are discussed in more detail later.

TEACHING DIALECTICAL BEHAVIOR PATTERNS

Throughout therapy, an emphasis is put on dialectical reasoning, both on the part of the therapist and as a style of thinking taught to patients. Dialectical reasoning requires the individual to assume an active role, to let go of logical reasoning and intellectual analysis as the only route to truth, and to embrace experiential knowledge. Meanings are generated and new relationships are found by opposing any term or proposition with its opposite or an alternative. The primary message to be communicated to the patient is that concerning every subject, opposite statements are possible. The dialectical therapist helps the patient achieve syntheses of oppositions, rather than focusing on verifying either side of an oppositional argument. The therapist helps the patient move from "either–or" to "both–and." Thus, many statements should be closely followed by their inherent opposites with the therapist modeling for the patient the ambiguity and inconsistency that reside therein. The key here is not to invalidate the first idea or polarity by asserting the second. The position is "Yes, but also. . ." rather than "Yes, but no, I was mistaken."

A similar position is adopted with respect to action and emotional responses. Two ideas are important here. The first is that the possibilities for personal and social change do not emerge from some point outside of or transcendent to the system, but lie within the existing contradictions of each specific social context (Sipe, 1986). The person and the environment both challenge and limit each other reciprocally. Change, both in the person and in her social context, involves refinements and transformations of current capacities in light of these challenges and limits (Mahoney, 1991).

The second idea is that extremes and rigid behavior patterns are signals that a dialectic has not been achieved. Thus, a middle path, similar to that advocated in Buddhism, is advocated and modeled: "The important thing in following the path to Enlightenment is to avoid being caught and entangled in any extreme, that is, always to follow the Middle Way" (Kyokai, 1966). This point holds for therapist and patient alike. Thus, the therapist should not hold to flexibility in a rigid fashion or avoid extremes at all costs. As Robert Aitken, a Zen master, has said, we must even "be detached from our non-attachment" (Aitken, 1987 p. 40).

Dialectics, from the point of view of behavior, can be most clearly seen in the treatment targets advocated in DBT. The DBT behavioral skills are good examples here. Emotion regulation is balanced with mindfulness, where the emphasis is on observing, describing, and participating, instead of regulating emotional or any other experience. Even in the teaching of emotional control, both distraction and control of attention on the one hand, and experiencing with attention and letting go of control on the other, are advocated. Interpersonal effectiveness focuses on changing problematic situations; by contrast, distress tolerance emphasizes accepting problematic situations.

SPECIFIC DIALECTICAL STRATEGIES

Specific techniques that target the therapist–patient relationship and dialectical behavior patterns are described below and summarized in the bottom half of Table 7.1. Although I believe that each of these strategies can be described in strictly behavioral terms, I have not attempted to translate from dialectical discourse to behavioral terms in every instance. It would, it seems, violate the spirit of the dialectics I am trying to convey.

I. ENTERING THE PARADOX

Allen Frances (1988) once said that one of the first and most important tasks in psychotherapy with borderline patients is to get their attention. "Entering the paradox" is a powerful way to do just that. It works, in part, because paradox contains within itself surprise; like humor, it presents the unexpected. When confronted with a paradox, one has to sit up and take notice. Entering the paradox is a strategy much like *koan* practice for the Zen student. *Koans* are dilemmas or enigmatic stories that Zen students are given to solve, even though there seem to be no logical answers; they force students to

TABLE 7.1. Dialectical Strategies Checklist

____ T BALANCES TREATMENT STRATEGIES within session.
    ____ T alternates between acceptance and change strategies in such a way that a collaborative working relationship is maintained in the session.
    ____ T balaces nurturing the patient with demanding that the patient help herself.
    ____ T balances persistence and stability with flexibility.
    ____ T balances focus on capabilities with focus on limitations and deficits.
    ____ T moves with speed, keeping P slightly off balance.
    ____ T is awake, responsive to P's movements.
    ____ T takes positions whole-heartedly.

____ T MODELS dialectical thinking and behaviors.
    ____ T looks for what is not included in P's and own points of view.
    ____ T gives developmental descriptions of change.
    ____ T questions permanence and intransigence of boundary conditions of the problem.
    ____ T makes synthesizing statements, including aspects of both ends of the continuum.
    ____ T makes statements highlighting the importance of interrelationships in determining identity.
    ____ T advocates a middle path,

____ T highlights PARADOXICAL contradictions of the following:
    ____ P's own behavior.
    ____ The therapeutic process.
    ____ Reality in general.

____ T speaks in METAPHORS and tells parables and stories.

____ T plays the DEVIL'S ADVOCATE.

____ T EXTENDS the seriousness or implications of P's communication.

____ T helps P activate "WISE MIND."

____ T makes LEMONADE out of lemons.

____ T allows NATURAL CHANGES in therapy.

____ T ASSESSES DIALECTICALLY, examining both the individual and the broader social context, for an understanding of P.

Note. In this checklist and those in the chapters to follow, T refers to the therapist and P to the patient.

go beyond intellectual understanding to direct experiential knowledge. Knowing how sugar tastes by reading about its taste qualities in a book is very different from knowing how sugar tastes by directly experiencing sugar on one's tongue. The solution to a *koan* is not logical or intellectual. It is an experience.

In this therapeutic strategy, the therapist highlights for the patient the paradoxical contradictions of the patient's own behavior, of the therapeutic process, and of reality in general. The patient's attempts at rational explanations of a paradox meet silence, another question from the therapist, or a story or slightly different paradox that may throw some (but not too much) light on the enigma to be solved. Suler (1989) suggests that a *koan* "becomes a desperate struggle around personal issues, including the personal conflicts that led the student to Zen. It is a struggle for one's very life" (p. 223). So, too, a therapeutic paradox well constructed and highlighted becomes for the borderline patient a struggle for life. Innumerable paradoxical dilemmas that take on life-and-death qualities typically arise in therapy with a borderline patient. For example, the therapist may say, "If I didn't care for you, I would try to save you." The patient says, "How can you say you care for me if you won't save me when I am so desperate?" The ultimate synthesis here is "You are already saved." However, interim insights have to do with the fact that, in reality, the therapist can not save the patient. Trying to do so, therefore, would divert therapy into pseudo-help rather than the real help that the patient needs. Also, even if the therapist could save the patient in the current moment, it takes infinitely more care and patience for the therapist to help the patient save herself than for the therapist to rescue the patient.

Another example has to do with the typical borderline patient's perennial dilemma of deciding who is right and who is wrong whenever a disagreement or confrontation arises. The idea that the answer is both (or neither) is difficult for the patient to grasp. Often, the therapeutic relationship is the first one the patient has ever been in where, during a confrontation, the other person asserts that "I'm OK and you're OK." In particular—and this is a crucial point—the therapist in DBT often validates the patient's point, but simultaneously does not "give in" or change his or her behavior. For example, in the strategy of observing limits (see Chapter 10), the therapist validates the patient's need ("Yes, it would be better for you if I were not going out of town this weekend") while meanwhile continuing with plans to go out of town. The patient is portrayed as the "good guy" ("You really do need what you say you do"), but so is therapist ("And I'm still OK for not giving it to you and going out of town").

The essence of the strategy of entering the paradox, however, is the therapist's refusal to step in with logic or intellectual explanation to pull the patient out of the struggle. As Suler (1989) goes on to state, "The cracking open of the double-binding self-contradiction and the insightful reframing of one's crisis can only occur if, in the words of Zen, one 'lets go of the hold'. . . letting things happen of their own accord" (p. 223). Some paradoxes inherent in psychotherapy and in the life of a borderline patient may take years to resolve.

By entering the paradox, the therapist continually stresses to the patient that things can both be true and not true, that an answer can be both yes and no. The therapist is not drawn into the patient's wish to assert one side of an oppositional argument as absolutely true, to the exclusion of the truth of the oppositional point of view. Neither does the therapist unconditionally assert the other side of the argument. The therapist continues to maintain that both sides can be true and that an answer to any question can be both yes and no. As noted earlier, "both–and" is offered as an alternative to "either–or." The therapist need not be overly concerned about clearing up the patient's confusion about this; the confusion will clear up as the patient becomes more comfortable with the dialectical approach. To return to the teeter-totter metaphor, when the patient sits on the very end of one side of the teeter-totter, the therapist both sits at the other end to provide balance and simultaneously focuses attention on the oneness of the teeter-totter.

A central paradox of DBT and all therapies is that all behavior is "good," yet the patient is in therapy to change "bad" behavior. DBT stresses validation of a patient's responses, but only to counter the invalidation she has been exposed to. Validation is a strategic necessity. As long as the patient (or the therapist) is mired in invalidation or in validation, she cannot see that the dichotomy itself is an artificial one. Behavior is neither valid nor invalid, neither good nor bad. Once the balance is achieved, both therapist and patient must move to a position of neither validation nor invalidation. Responses simply are. They arise as a consequence of causes and conditions that are both past and immediate, and that are both internal and external to the person. In turn, responses have consequences, which may either be desired or not.

The paradox of change versus acceptance runs throughout therapy. Entering the paradox, the therapist highlights and amplifies the seeming incongruity that even the inability to accept must be accepted. (As we say to patients, "Don't judge judging.") A patient is exhorted to accept herself just as she is in the moment. But, of course, if she does that, she will have changed substantially; indeed, the very admonition to learn to accept conveys a nonacceptance of the status quo. The patient is told that she is perfect just as she is, neither good nor bad, and completely understandable, yet she must change her behavior patterns. In this way, the therapist heightens the naturally arising dialectical tensions facing the patient, so that she has no way out other than to move away from the extremes. Patrick Hawk, a master of Zen and Christian contemplation, suggests that "*Koans* are themes to be clarified in engagement with one's teacher. . . .This act of making clear is called realization" (personal communication, 1992). In DBT, as in Zen, clarification and realization are arrived at via the engagement of the student/patient with the teacher/therapist. In particular, the therapist must enter the multiple paradoxes the patient encounters in trying to solve the dialectical dilemmas of extreme vulnerability versus invalidating the vulnerability; unrelenting crises versus blocking and inhibiting the experience of the emotional components of the crises; and a passive inability to resolve problems and painful emotional states versus apparent independence, invulnerability, and competence.

A number of dialectical tensions arise naturally in the course of the psychotherapy relationship. The patient is free to choose her own behavior, but she can not stay in therapy if she does not choose to reduce suicidal behaviors. The patient is taught to achieve greater self-efficacy by becoming better at asking for and receiving help from others. The patient has a right to kill herself, but if she ever convinces the therapist that suicide is imminent, she may be locked up. The therapist is paid to care for the patient, but the patient's doubts about the genuineness of the therapist's caring are usually interpreted as instances of the patient's problems showing up in the therapeutic relationship. And if the patient stops paying, the therapy stops. The therapist is both detached and intimate, modeling autonomy and independence, yet encouraging attachment and dependence on the part of the patient. The patient is not responsible for being the way she is, but she is responsible for what she becomes.

The patient is urged to get in control of excessive attempts to control. The therapist uses highly controlling techniques to increase the patient's freedom. Struggling with, confronting, and breaking through these paradoxes forces the patient to let go of rigid patterns of thought, emotion, and behavior so that more spontaneous and flexible patterns may emerge. Likewise, genuine entering of the paradox, within both the therapeutic relationship and the consultation group, forces the therapist to let go of rigid theoretical positions and inflexible therapy rules, regulations, and patterns of action.

2. THE USE OF METAPHOR

The use of metaphor and storytelling has been stressed by many psychotherapists, most notably by Milton Erickson, who was famous for his teaching stories (Rosen, 1982). Likewise, the use of metaphor, in the form of simple analogies, anecdotes, parables, myths, or stories, is extremely important in DBT. Metaphors are alternative means of teaching dialectical thinking and opening up possibilities of new behaviors. They encourage both patient and therapist to look for and create alternate meanings and points of reference for events under scrutiny. Ones from which multiple meanings can be drawn are usually the most effective in encouraging different views of reality.

As many other writers have discussed (Barker, 1985; Deikman, 1982; Kopp, 1971), the use of metaphor is a valuable strategy in psychotherapy for a number of reasons. Stories are usually more interesting and easier to remember than straight lecturing or instruction. Thus, a person whose attention wanders when she is presented with behavioral information or instruction, may find it much easier to attend to a story. Stories also allow an individual to use them in her own way, for her own purposes. Thus, the sense of being controlled by the therapist or teacher is lessened, and the patient may be more relaxed and open to a new way of thinking or behaving; she is thus less likely to stop listening immediately or to feel overwhelmed. She can take from the story what she can use, either immediately or at a later point. Finally, metaphors, when constructed properly, can be less threatening to the individual. Points can be made indirectly, in a way that softens their impact.

The use of stories can be especially helpful when the therapist is trying to communicate the harmful effects of the patient's behavior on others in a way that normalizes the responses of others while not directly criticizing the patient. They can also be useful in talking about the therapist's own responses (especially when the therapist's own motivation to continue working is flagging), or in telling the patient what she can expect from the therapist. Metaphors can also redefine, reframe, and suggest solutions to problems; help the patient recognize aspects of her own behavior in or reactions to situations; and give the patient hope (Barker, 1985). Generally, the idea is to take something the patient understands, such as two people climbing a mountain, and compare it by way of analogy to something the patient does not understand, such as the therapeutic process.

Over the years, my colleagues and I have developed a large number of metaphors to discuss suicidal and therapy-interfering behaviors, acceptance, willingness, therapy, and life in general. Therapy-interfering behaviors have been compared to a mountain climber's refusing to wear winter gear when climbing in the snow, hiding the climbing gear, or sitting on a rock looking at the scenery when a storm is threatening; to a mule's climbing out of the Grand Canyon and refusing to go forward or backward (not an analogy that gained me a lot of points with the patient!); and to one cook's throwing cups of salt instead of sugar into cherry pies while the other cook is out of the room. Passive behavior and emotional avoidance (and, by contrast what the patient has to do) have been compared to cringing in the corner of a room on fire when the only way out is through the flaming door (the person has to wrap herself in wet sheets and run through the door) and to clinging to an icy mountain ledge when the only way to safety is to keep going (the person has to move slowly across the ledge without looking down). Suicidal behaviors have been compared to a climber's jumping off the mountain, sometimes with the rope still tied to the guide (who then has to pull the climber up) and sometimes after cutting the rope; to demanding a divorce from an unwilling partner; and to addictive behaviors such as drinking and drugs. Learning distress tolerance is like learning to be a blanket spread on the ground on a fall day, letting leaves fall as they may without fighting them off. Learning acceptance is like a gardener's learning to love the dandelions that come into the garden year after year, no matter what the gardener does to get rid of them. Trying to be what others want the patient to be is like a tulip's trying to be a rose just because it happens to have been planted in a rose garden. Life led willingly is like playing a game of cards (the object is to play each hand as well as possible, not to control what cards are dealt), or like hitting baseballs or tennis balls thrown by a ball-throwing machine (the person can't stop or even slow down the balls coming, so she just swings as well as she can and then focuses on the next ball).

We have used more extended metaphors to describe therapy and the process of growth and change. Here is one: Therapy, for the patient, is like climbing out of hell on a red-hot aluminium ladder with no gloves or shoes. Continually jumping off or letting go is therapy-interfering behavior by the patient. Holding a blowtorch on the patient's feet to get her to climb faster is therapy-interfering behavior by the therapist. The problem here is that the bottom of hell is usually hotter even than the ladder, so that after a while the patient always gets up, gets back on the ladder, and has to climb again. Another extended metaphor for therapy is learning how to swim in all kinds of conditions. The patient is the swimmer; the therapist is the coach, sitting in a rowboat circling the patient, providing directions and encouragement.

The tension often is between the swimmer's wanting to get in the boat so the coach can row her to shore and the coach's wanting the swimmer to stay in the water. If the coach rows the swimmer to the shore, she will never learn to swim, but if the swimmer drowns in rough seas she won't learn to swim either. Clinging to the boat and refusing to swim, and swimming under water to scare the coach into jumping in after her, are instances of patient therapy-interfering behaviors. Refusing to hold out an oar when the swimmer keeps going under, and rowing the swimmer to shore every time a black cloud comes by, are examples of therapist therapy-interfering behaviors.

Patients often feel misunderstood whenever their therapists push them to make changes to improve their lives. "If you understood me, you wouldn't ask me to do something I can't do," or, put another way, "If you took my suffering seriously, you wouldn't ask me to do something that makes me feel worse than I already do," is a common message sent from borderline patient to therapist. This message and the problems it creates for the therapist are so common in the treatment of BPD that Lorna Benjamin (in press) has described BPD interpersonal patterns as playing out a scenario of "My misery is your command." In this situation, stories can be particularly useful to validate both the patient's emotional pain and sense of helplessness, and the therapist's attempt to get the patient moving. My favorite story is an elaboration of one I have described elsewhere in this book. A woman with no shoes is standing on a white-hot bed of burning coals. The bed is very deep and very wide. The woman is paralyzed with pain and calls out to her friend to run and get a pitcher of cooling water to pour on her feet. But there is not enough water to cool down all the coals. So the friend, very anxious for the woman to get out of her suffering as quickly as possible, yells "Run!" And if that does not work, the friend jumps into the coals and starts pushing the patient toward the cool grasses by the side. Does the friend understand the woman's pain? If she *really* understood it, would she have poured on the cool water instead?

A similar story and question can be fashioned around the metaphor of the room on fire, mentioned briefly above. The woman is so afraid of the fire that she wants to remain pressed into the corner of the back room. Does the friend who truly understands her pain stay back there with her, perishing with her in the fire? Or does the good friend grab her despite her protests and pull both to safety through the flaming door? In a slight variation, I asked the patient to imagine that she and I were alone on a raft in the middle of the ocean following a shipwreck several days earlier. Her arm was badly cut and she was in desperate pain. Over and over she was asking me for pain medicine, or for anything to take away the pain. I asked her to imagine further that the first aid kit was washed out to sea. If I didn't find and give her pain medicine, would that mean that I did not understand or take seriously her pain? What if I only had three more pain capsules and I said, "Let's ration them and take only one a day so we won't run out so quickly?" Or would the patient believe that I really had lots of pain capsules and just didn't want her to have any—perhaps because I thought she was a drug addict? Honest discussion of such story variations can often clarify difficult therapeutic impasses.

These analogies, or any other that the therapist thinks of, can be spun into shorter or longer stories as the situation calls for (and as I have demonstrated). In some cases, I have spent almost entire sessions wholly within a metaphorical story spun alternately by myself and the patient. Teaching stories and metaphors have been used in all spiritual traditions (Vedanta, Buddhism, Zen, Hasidic, Christian, and Sufi), as well as in philosophy, literature, and children's stories. (See Appendix for other sources.)

3. THE DEVIL'S ADVOCATE TECHNIQUE

In the "devil's advocate" strategy, developed by Marvin Goldfried (Goldfried, Linehan, & Smith, 1978), the therapist presents an extreme propositional statement, asks the patient whether she believes the statement, and then plays the role of devil's advocate to counter attempts by the patient to disprove the proposition. The therapist presents the thesis and elicits the antithesis from the patient; in the process of argument, they arrive at a synthesis. The extreme proposition presented by the therapist should relate to dysfunctional beliefs that the patient has expressed or to problematic propositional rules that the patient seems to be following. It is used best to counteract new, oppositional patterns. The technique is similar to the use of paradox, in which the therapist holds down the maladaptive end of the continuum and thereby forces the patient to the adaptive end.

The devil's advocate technique is always used in the first several sessions to elicit a strong commitment to change on the part of the patient. The therapist argues against change and commitment to therapy, because change is painful and difficult; ideally, this moves the patient to take the oppositional position in favor of change and commitment. This use of the strategy is discussed further in Chapter 9.

The argumentative approach often used in cognitive restructuring therapy is another example of the devil's advocate strategy. For example, the thesis may be an irrational belief of the type proposed by Ellis (1962), such as "Everyone has to love me, and if there is one person who doesn't, then I am a worthless person," or "If I offend anyone for any reason, it is a mortal catastrophe." The therapist argues in favor of the irrational belief, questioning why the patient does not agree. For example, the therapist may present the second proposition given above by suggesting that even if a total stranger is offended at some legitimate activity of the patient's (such as driving the speed limit on the highway), or if someone is offended because of a distortion, or if someone is offended by the patient's refusal to behave illegally or immorally (such as cheating), the patient should alter her behavior to conform to what is expected and approved of. Anything the patient proposes can be countered by exaggerating her usual position until the self-defeating nature of the belief becomes apparent.

A number of things are necessary to carry this technique off. First, the therapist must be alert to the patient's actual dysfunctional rules and generalized beliefs. Second, the therapist has to engage the patient with a straight face and with a rather naive-seeming expressive style. Third, a kind of offbeat but very logical response to each of the patient's argument is helpful. Fourth, the therapist's position has to be reasonable enough to seem "real," but extreme enough to allow counterargument by the patient. A position that simultaneously validates the patient's attachment to an idea and invalidates the wisdom of the idea is the ideal. A certain lightness and ability to modify an argument unobtrusively are also necessary. Finally, the therapist has to know when to stay deadly serious and when to "lighten up" and play the argument for tongue-in-cheek humor.

4. EXTENDING

"Extending" is the therapist's taking the patient more seriously than she takes herself. Whereas the patient may have been saying something for effect, or expressing an extreme emotion in order to induce reasonably minor changes in the environment, the therapist takes the communication literally. This strategy is the emotional equivalent of the devil's advocate strategy.

For example, the patient may make an extreme statement about the effects or consequences of some event or problem in her life ("If you don't schedule an extra session with me, I will kill myself"). The therapist first takes the patient's statement of the effects or consequences literally, and then responds to the seriousness of the consequences ("I will kill myself"), independently of their relationship to the event or problem identified by the patient (not scheduling an extra therapy session). The therapist may say, "We've got to do something immediately if you are so distressed that you might kill yourself. What about hospitalization? Maybe that is needed. How can we discuss such a mundane topic as session scheduling when your life is in danger? Surely, this threat to your life must be dealt with first. How are you planning to kill yourself?" The aspect of the communication that the therapist takes seriously is not the aspect that the patient wants taken seriously. The patient wants the *problem* taken seriously, and indeed is often extending its seriousness. The therapist takes the dire *consequences* seriously and extends them even further by refusing to stop focusing on them until they are resolved.

Used well, this strategy has the effect of making the patient see that she is exaggerating the consequences. When this happens ("OK, maybe I am exaggerating. I'm not feeling that suicidal"), it is crucial that the therapist then move to taking the problem very seriously. The patient must be reinforced for reducing the emotional consequences of the problem. Used poorly, the strategy can be a cover for a therapist's failing to take legitimate problems of the patient seriously. This technique is best used when the patient is not expecting the therapist to take her seriously, or when escalating a crisis or set of emotional consequences is maintained by its instrumental effect on the

environment. It can be particularly effective when the therapist feels manipulated. It has the advantage that it manages both the patient's behavior and,
at times, the therapist's affect and desire to attack, in one response. Done
successfully, it is very satisfying.

The term "extending" to describe this technique has been borrowed from
aikido, a Japanese art of self-defense. Extending is an aikido practitioner's
allowing the movements of a challenger to reach their natural completion,
and then extending the end point of the movement slightly further than it
would go naturally; this leaves the challenger off balance and vulnerable to
a shift in direction. Extending is always preceded by "blending," which in aikido means accepting or joining or moving with the challenger's energy flow
in the direction in which it is going (Saposnek, 1980). For example, the patient may say to the therapist, "If you don't act different, this therapy isn't
going to help me" [the challenge]. The therapist says, "If therapy isn't helping you [blending], we need to do something about that [going to the natural
conclusion of the response]. Do you think you should fire me? Perhaps we
should get you a new therapist? This is very serious [extending]." Each of
the characteristics noted above in regard to the devil's advocate technique (picking up overly extreme consequences, naiveté, an offbeat but very logical
response, a response reasonable enough to seem "real" but extreme enough
to allow the patient to see that she is being extreme, lightness, and unobtru-
sive modification of the therapist's position) is equally important here.

5. ACTIVATING "WISE MIND"

In DBT, patients are presented with the concept of three primary states of
mind: "reasonable mind," "emotion mind," and "wise mind." A person is in
"reasonable mind" when she is approaching knowledge intellectually, is thinking rationally and logically, attends to empirical facts, is planful in her behavior, focuses her attention, and is "cool" in her approach to problems. The
person is in "emotion mind" when thinking and behavior are controlled
primarily by her current emotional state. In "emotion mind," cognitions are
"hot"; reasonable, logical thinking is difficult; facts are amplified or distorted to be congruent with current affect; and the energy of behavior is likewise
congruent with the current emotional state.

"Wise mind" is the integration of "emotion mind" and "reasonable mind";
it also goes beyond them. "Wise mind" adds intuitive knowing to emotional
experiencing and logical analysis. There are many definitions of intuition.
Deikman (1982) suggests that it is knowing that is not mediated by reason
and goes beyond what is received via the senses. It has qualities of direct experience, immediate cognition, and the grasping of the meaning, significance,
or truth of an event without relying on intellectual analysis. Intuitive knowing is guided by "feelings of deepening coherence" (Polanyi, 1958). Although
experience and reason play a part, the quality of the intuitive experience is
unique. "Wise mind" depends upon a full cooperation of all ways of know-

ing: observation, logical analysis, kinetic and sensory experience, behavioral learning, and intuition (May, 1982).

Borderline patients have to learn how to access "wise mind." In effect, they have to let go of emotional processing and logical analyses, of set ideas and extreme reactions; they must become calm enough to allow wise knowing to proceed uncomplicated and unintruded upon by other, more volitional ("reasonable mind") or overdetermined ("emotion mind") modes of knowing. The first task for some patients (though certainly not all) is to convince them that they are indeed capable of this. A borderline patient may question the very idea that she has an ability to achieve wisdom of any sort. First, the therapist simply has to insist that all humans have "wise mind," much as all humans have hearts. The fact that a patient cannot see her heart doesn't mean she doesn't have one. Second, it is often helpful to give a number of examples of times when the patient may have experienced "wise mind." Many people experience it immediately following a crisis or enormous chaos in their lives. It is the calm that follows the storm. It is that experience of suddenly getting to the heart of a matter, seeing or knowing something directly and clearly. Sometimes it may be experienced as grasping the whole picture instead of only parts; at other times it may be the experience of "feeling" the right choice in a dilemma, when the feeling comes from deep within rather than from a current emotional state. Third, it can be useful to lead the person through exercises in which she may be able to experience that inner calmness that surrounds "wise mind." Generally, I have patients follow their breath (attend to their breath coming in and out), and after some time try to let their attentional focus settle into their physical center, at the bottom of their inhalation. That very centered point is "wise mind." Almost all patients are able to sense this point.

When asked to go into "wise mind" later, a patient is instructed to take this stance and then to respond from that center of calmness. It can be compared to going deep within a well in the ground. The water at the bottom of the well—and, indeed, the entire underground ocean—is "wise mind." But on the way down there are often trap doors that impede progress. Sometimes the doors are so cleverly built that the person actually believes that there is no water at the bottom of the well. A trap door may look like the bottom of the well. The task of the therapist is to help the patient figure out how to get each trap door open. Perhaps it is locked and she needs a key. Perhaps it is nailed shut and she needs a hammer, or it is glued shut and she needs a chisel. But, with persistence and diligence, the ocean of wisdom at the bottom can be reached.

Borderline patients may have difficulty distinguishing "wise mind" from "emotion mind." Both have a quality of "feeling" something to be the case; both rely on a type of knowing that is different from reasoning or analysis. To go back to our story, if there has been a hard rain, water can collect on top of a trap door in the well. If the trap door stays shut, the pool of water can be confused with the ocean at the bottom of the well. It can be easy for both therapist and patient to get confused. Rain water can look like ocean water. The intensity of emotions can generate experiences of certainty that mimic the stable, calm certainty of wisdom. There is no simple solution to this. If intense emotion is obvious, the suspicion that a conclusion is based on "emotion mind" instead of "wise mind" is probably correct. Generally, time is the best ally here.

A borderline patient often makes statements that represent her emotional or feeling state ("I feel fat or unlovable," "I don't want to live without him," "I'm afraid I'm going to fail") as if the feeling state provides information about the empirical reality ("I am fat or unlovable," "I can't live without him," "I'm going to fail"). When this occurs, it is effective at times simply to question the patient in this manner: "I'm not interested in how you feel. I'm not interested in what you believe or think. I am interested in what you know to be true (in your 'wise mind'). What do you know to be true? What is true?" The dialectical tension here is between what the patient feels to be true and what she thinks to be true; the synthesis is what she knows to be true. The refusal of the therapist to entertain "emotion mind" or "reasonable mind" is an example of a controlling strategy in the service of letting go.

The push toward "wise mind" by the therapist can be easily abused; especially when the therapist confuses "wise mind" with what the therapist believes to be the case: "If I agree with you, then you are functioning from 'wise mind.' " This can be particularly difficult when the therapist trusts the wisdom of his or her own knowledge or opinions. How can one person's "wise mind" conflict with another's? This is an interesting paradox. The value of therapeutic humility cannot be overstated. In DBT, one of the major functions of the consultation/supervision group is to provide a balance to the arrogance that can easily accompany such a powerful position as the therapist's.

6. MAKING LEMONADE OUT OF LEMONS

"Making lemonade out of lemons" requires that the therapist take something that seems apparently problematic and turn it into an asset. The idea is similar to the notion in psychodynamic therapy of utilizing the patient's resistances: The worse the patient acts in therapy, the better it is. If problems did not show up in the therapeutic encounter, how could the therapist be helpful? Problems in everyday life are opportunities to practice skills. Indeed, from the point of view of practicing skills, not having problems would be a disaster, since there would be nothing to practice on. Suffering, when accepted, enhances empathy, and those who have suffered can reach out and help others. A variation here is the notion that the patient's greatest weaknesses are ordinarily also her greatest strengths (e.g., her persistence in "resisting" change is just what will keep her going until changes are made).

The idea that lemons can be made into lemonade should not be confused with the invalidating refrain, repeatedly heard by borderline patients, that the lemons in their lives are actually already lemonade if only they could realize it. One of the dangers of this strategy is that a patient may feel that the therapist is not taking her problems seriously. The trick is not to over-simplify how hard it can be to find such positive characteristics; in fact, it can be like looking for a needle in a hay stack. Thus, the strategy cannot be used in a cavalier manner. Its effectiveness rests on a therapeutic relationship where the patient knows that the therapist has deep compassion for her suffering. In that context, however, the strategy can be used lightly and with humor. When I conduct skills training, for instance, patients soon realize that I may rejoice over even the worst crisis as an opportunity to practice or learn a skill. The incongruity of my response ("Oh, how wonderful!") to a patient's distress ("I got fired") forces the patient to stop and take in new information (i.e., this is a chance to practice interpersonal effectiveness, emotion regulation, or distress tolerance skills, depending on the current skill module). The skill of the therapist is in finding the silver lining without denying that the cloud is indeed black.

7. ALLOWING NATURAL CHANGE

Dialectics assumes that the nature of reality is process, development, and change. Thus, to introduce arbitrary stability and consistency into therapy would be nondialectical in character. In contrast to many other therapeutic approaches, DBT does not avoid introducing change and instability into therapy, nor is emphasis put on maintaining a consistent therapeutic environment. Arrangement of the physical setting may change from time to time; appointment times may vary; rules may be changed; and different therapists interacting with the patient may all say different things. The change, development, and inconsistency inherent in any environment are allowed to proceed naturally. The key words here are "allowed" and "naturally." Allowing change is not the same thing as introducing change for the sake of change; that would be arbitrary change. Natural changes are those that evolve from current conditions rather than those that are imposed from without.

Stability and consistency are more comfortable for borderline patients, and many have enormous difficulty with change. The notion here is that exposure to change, in a safe atmosphere, can be therapeutic. Avoidance of change within the therapeutic relationship offers little opportunity for the patient to develop comfort with change, ambiguity, unpredictability, and inconsistency. (Indeed, the opportunity to learn to cope effectively with change is the "lemonade" made from the "lemon" of experiencing the occasional inconsistency of the therapist's behavior.) An artificial stability and predictability within the therapeutic relationship also limit the generalizability of learning within that relationship to more natural relationships, where ambiguity and a certain amount of unpredictability often prevail.

Does this strategy mean that there is no consistency in DBT? No. But the consistencies that do exist are like the still water underneath the waves that come and go in the ocean. They are more real than apparent. Technically, the only consistency required is that behavioral progress be reinforced and the dysfunctional status quo as well as backsliding not be reinforced. Thus, the therapist must be consistently on the side of the patient, willing to bend the therapy to promote the welfare of the patient. Indeed, it is this consistency of care that makes the relationship safe enough for exposure to change to be beneficial.

8. DIALECTICAL ASSESSMENT

Much of what goes on in any psychotherapy can be thought of as "assessment." That is, the therapist and the patient try to figure out just exactly what is influencing what; what factors are causing the person to act, feel, and think as she does; what is going wrong or right in the patient's life and in therapy; and what is going on at this very moment. Where the therapist directs the patient to look for answers depends on the theoretical persuasion of the therapist. American psychology and psychiatry in general, and most theoretical approaches to BPD in particular, have a penchant for locating the source of disorder within the individual rather than within the social and physical context surrounding the person. Although psychological theories typically ascribe primary importance to early environmental events in the development of the problems of the borderline patient, most theories pay scant attention to the role of the current environment in eliciting and maintaining the individual's problems. Disordered biology, dysfunctional cognitive schemas, inadequate object relations, and skill deficits, however, all receive extensive attention. Borderline individuals are notable for their acceptance of the premise that their problems are the results of personal deficiencies or disorders. Indeed, many see themselves as fatally flawed, forever unable to change.

Remember, however, that a dialectical world view is a wholistic, systems view. Patterns of influence are reciprocal and developmental. Identity is relational. Dialectical assessment requires that the therapist, along with the patient, constantly look for what is missing from individual or personal explanations of current behaviors and events. The question always being asked is "What is being left out here?" The assessment does not stop at the immediate environment, or at the historical family or other past learning experiences (although these are not ignored); it also examines social, political, and economic influences on the patient's current behavior. Robert Sipe (1986, pp. 74–75), quoting Trent Schroyer (1972, pp. 30–31), describes a similar point:

> Dialectical awareness. . . [is that] which "restores missing parts to historical self-formulation, true actuality to false appearance" so that we can "see through socially unnecessary authority and control systems." In seeing our psychological and social world as it really is, we can see real possibilities for its transformation. . . . As missing parts are restored, new insights into the potential for psychosocial change emerge that previously could not be comprehended.

In work with women in particular, dialectical assessment directs attention to the role of culturally institutionalized sexism and sex-role expectations in individuals' problems. Indeed, the frequent double binds that sex-role, social class, religious, regional, and racial expectations place on individual behavior are viewed dialectically as important influences on individual behavior, including the behaviors that borderline individuals find problematic. The possibility that BPD is a joint person–environment disorder is entertained.

Borderline patients often say that they feel as if they don't "fit in"; they feel alienated or disconnected from the culture they are living in. Their behavior certainly suggests that they have great difficulty adapting or adjusting to the social world they must live in. The traditional solution to this is to figure out how such an individual can change herself to fit in better or to better accept her fate. The social context that the person finds herself in, however, is often presented as natural ("the way things are") and unchangeable. The notion that there might be a fatal flaw in the social fabric—in the human and social relationships of the society in which the person finds herself—is frequently not considered. The illusion is so pervasive that the individual has little choice but to believe that she is indeed inadequate or fatally flawed. Dialectical assessment requires an analysis of the larger social network and its interrelationship with the more narrow personal context. The shoe is put on the other foot, so to speak, and changes the person can make in the environment are explored. Dialectical assessment is aimed at introducing the idea that another culture—a culture into which the borderline individual can fit—is possible.

These very same points also apply to analyzing the influence of the structure of therapy on the well-being of the borderline patient. Over the years, rules and regulations about how psychotherapy should progress have been developed. It seems at times that these rules and regulations are also natural, the only way things can be. Such a position leads to a certain rigidity of therapeutic behaviors. The implication once again is that if a patient does not improve, there is something wrong with her rather than with the therapy. The patient is taught to fit the therapy; we do not ordinarily think of fitting the therapy to the patient. Dialectical assessment requires an openness to examining the oppressive or iatrogenic nature of some therapeutic rules and styles when working with borderline patients. Such an analysis will expand the possibilities of therapy, and perhaps allow a development of the therapeutic procedures and relationship for the maximum benefit of both patient and therapist.

Concluding Comments

The dialectical strategies proposed here can easily be confused with gimmicks or with playing of a game (albeit a quite sophisticated game). And without care, honesty, and commitment to what is actually said and done, this would be the case. A dialectical stance requires the therapist to hold both sides of every polarity, to believe that he or she does not have absolute truth, and to search in earnest for what is missing in both the therapist's and the patient's way of construing and responding to the world. In short, it takes some humility—just the opposite of the superior position one takes when using sleight of hand or gimmicks. Of course, this does not rule out playing games, in the true sense of having fun with the patient. But such games must be mutual and gentle to be effective.

Each strategy described in this chapter can be misused or falsely applied. An aspect of paradox is that the statements appear to make no sense, to be nonsense; however, not all nonsense is paradoxical. Metaphor and storytelling can be used to get out of answering a question directly, to divert attention, to fill time, or to show off. The story may be fascinating but may have no relationship to the problem at hand. The devil's advocate technique is best used when the therapist selects a position to argue that has merit and validates the patient's tenacious hold on the particular dysfunctional rule or belief. It is most badly used when the therapist humiliates the patient or makes her appear to be stupid or foolish. Extending can easily become hostile and sarcastic, especially when the therapist feels manipulated by the patient's threats or extreme responses. Activating "wise mind" has great potential to validate the patient's inherent wisdom; it can just as easily be used, however, to validate the therapist's sense of his or her own wisdom at the expense of the patient. Similarly, it is easy to forget that making lemonade requires a fair amount of sugar. When the therapist fails to recognize that the patient does not have ready access to sugar herself, the result can leave a sour taste and diminish the patient's faith and confidence in the therapist. Natural change strategies can be a cover for a therapist's arbitrary inconsistency, failure to keep a promise, failure to plan therapy, or moodiness. Finally, dialectical assessments, if not rigorously tested and evaluated, can create and justify their own illusions. Time-tested traditions and rules of therapeutic encounter can be violated thoughtlessly, sometimes with terrible consequences for the patient or for the therapist. The baby can indeed be thrown out with the bath water.

Notes

1. To a greater or lesser extent, all therapeutic approaches highlight the same dialectical principles as discussed here. Psychodynamic therapies, for example, attend to dynamic tensions and conflicts within the person. Behavioral approaches attend to the wholistic relationship between the person and his or her environment. Cognitive approaches focus extensively on observing and accepting reality as it is in the moment in a context of helping the patient change. Thus, in a very real sense, the emphasis on dialectics in DBT is "nothing new."

2. In this and the following chapters, subheads in capital letters call attention to particular treatment strategies.

8

Core Strategies:
Part I.
Validation

As noted at the beginning of Chapter 7, validation and problem-solving strategies form the core of DBT; all other strategies are built around them. Validation strategies are the most obvious and direct acceptance strategies in DBT. Validation communicates to the patient in a nonambiguous way that her behavior makes sense and is understandable in the current context. The therapist engages the patient in trying to understand her actions, emotions, and thoughts or implicit rules. Problem-solving strategies, by contrast, are the most obvious and direct change strategies in DBT. In problem solving the therapist engages the patient in analyzing her own behavior, committing to change, and taking active steps to change her behavior.

As discussed in Chapter 4, maladaptive behaviors are often the solutions to problems the patient wants solved or taken away. However, from the therapist's point of view, these same behaviors are the problems to be solved. To oversimplify matters somewhat, validation strategies highlight the wisdom of the patient's point of view, and problem-solving strategies highlight the therapist's. This statement is overly simple because sometimes the perspectives are switched: The patient views her own behavior as problematic and in need of change, whereas the therapist is focused on acceptance of the patient and her behavior just as it is. Both validation and problem-solving strategies are used in every interaction with the patient. Many treatment impasses result from an imbalance of one strategy over the other.

A borderline patient presents herself clinically as an individual in extreme emotional pain. She pleads, and at times demands, that the therapist do something to change this state of affairs—to make her feel better, stop doing destructive things, and live her life more satisfactorily. It is very tempting, given the high distress of the patient and the difficulties in changing the world around her, to focus the energy of therapy on changing the patient. Depending on the therapist's orientation, treatment might focus on how the patient's irrational thoughts, assumptions, or schemas contribute to dysfunctional negative emotions; how her inappropriate interpersonal behaviors or motives contribute to interpersonal problems; how her abnormal biology interferes with functional adaptation; how her emotional reactivity and intensity contribute to her overall problems; and so forth. Therapy typically consists of applying technologies of change, with the focus of change on the patient's behavior, personality, or biological patterns.

In many respects, this focus recapitulates the invalidating environment, in which the patient was the problem and the patient needed to change. When promoting change, a therapist may validate a patient's worst fears: The patient indeed cannot trust her own emotional reactions, cognitive interpretations, or behavioral responses. Mistrust and invalidation of one's own responses to events, whether self-generated or coming from others, however, are extremely aversive. Depending on circumstances, invalidation may elicit fear, anger, shame, or a combination of all three. Thus, the entire focus of change-based therapy can be aversive, since by necessity the focus contributes to and elicits self-invalidation. No wonder the patient often avoids or resists.

Unfortunately, a therapeutic approach based on unconditional acceptance and validation of the patient's behaviors proves equally problematic and, paradoxically, can also be invalidating. If the therapist urges the patient to accept and validate herself, it can appear that the therapist does not regard the patient's problems seriously. The desperation of the borderline individual is discounted in acceptance-based therapies, since little hope of change is offered. The patient's personal experience of her life as unacceptable and unendurable is thereby invalidated.

To resolve this impasse, DBT attends to the balance of acceptance-based with change-based treatment strategies. A primary focus of treatment is teaching the patient both to validate herself and to change. Most importantly, the therapy strives to help the patient understand that responses may prove both appropriate or valid and, at the same time, dysfunctional and in need of change (see Watts, 1990, for a similar point). This balance point, however, constantly changes; as a result, the therapist must be able to move and react flexibly and quickly in therapy. The recognition of the need for flexibility and for the synthesis or balance of complementary or opposite poles is the reason why dialectics is used as a foundation for the therapy.

Defining Validation

The essence of validation is this: The therapist communicates to the patient that her responses make sense and are understandable within her *current* life context or situation. The therapist actively accepts the patient and communicates this acceptance to the patient. The therapist takes the patient's responses seriously and does not discount or trivialize them. Validation strategies require the therapist to search for, recognize, and reflect to the patient the validity inherent in her responses to events. With unruly children, parents have to catch them while they're good in order to reinforce their behavior; similarly, the therapist has to uncover the validity within the patient's response, sometimes amplify it, and then reinforce it. In the early period of individual treatment, validation strategies may be the principal strategies used in therapy.

Sometimes it is easier to understand what validation means by understanding what it does not mean. Pointing out that a response was functional in the past, but is not now, is invalidating rather than validating. For example, a patient may say that the therapist is always angry at her. If the therapist immediately denies it, and then points to how the patient's experiences in other intimate relationships might have reasonably led her to expect the therapist to be angry, the therapist is invalidating the patient's comment. The therapist may be showing that the patient is not crazy, and that in the context of her previous experience her response would be valid, but not that her response is valid in the current context. Validating the patient's history is not the same as validating her current behavior.

Similarly, the therapist is invalidating the patient's response if her comment is interpreted as a projection of her own anger onto the therapist. Almost any *ad hominem* (or, in this case, *ad feminam*) response, such as this one, invalidates the content of the patient's viewpoint. Although such arguments may also have validity, they do not validate the patient's comment, nor are they likely to be experienced as validating. A validating response would be for the therapist to first search openly for any expressive behavior on his or her part that might communicate anger, and then thoughtfully discuss with the patient the emotion or attitude that these behaviors reflect. Finally, validating is not simply making patients feel good or building up their self-esteem. If a patient says that she is stupid, saying that she is smart invalidates her experience of being stupid.

There are three steps in validating. The first two are part of almost all therapy traditions; the third step, however, is essential to DBT. The steps are as follows.

1. *Active observing.* First, the therapist gathers information about what has happened to the patient or what is happening in the moment, and listens to and observes what the patient is thinking, feeling, and doing. The essence of this step is that the therapist is awake. The therapist lets go of theories, prejudices, and personal biases that get in the way of observing the actual emotions, thoughts, and behaviors of the patient. In agency and hospital settings, the therapist lets go of gossip about the patient and other professionals' opinions about the patient. The therapist listens to direct communications and observes public acts. In addition, the therapist listens with a "third ear"

to hear the unstated emotions, thoughts, values, and beliefs; the therapist also observes with a "third eye" to guess the unstated action of the patient. At the beginning of therapy, the therapist often needs the ability to "read the patient's mind"; it can be similar to taking a photo in the dark on infrared film. Via therapeutic shaping, the patient progresses over time to being able to take such "photos" for herself.

2. *Reflection.* Second, the therapist accurately reflects back to the patient the patient's own feelings, thoughts, assumptions, and behaviors. In this step, a nonjudgmental attitude is fundamental. The therapist communicates to the patient, in a way that the patient can hear, that the therapist is awake and listening. Accurate emotional empathy; understanding of (but not necessarily agreement with) beliefs, expectations, or assumptions; and recognition of behavioral patterns are required. Through back-and-forth discussion, the therapist helps the patient identify, describe, and label her own response patterns. Thus, the patient has a a chance to say that the therapist is wrong. The therapist frequently asks "Is that right?" In reflecting, the therapist often states what the patient observes but is afraid to say or admit. This simple act of reflection, especially when the therapist "says it first," can be a powerful act of validation: A borderline patient often observes herself accurately in the first place, but invalidates and discounts her own perceptions because of self-mistrust.

3. *Direct validation.* Third, the therapist looks for and reflects the wisdom or validity of the patient's response, and communicates that the response is understandable. The therapist finds the stimuli in the current environment that support the patient's behavior. Even though information regarding all the relevant causes may not be available, the patient's feelings, thoughts, and actions make perfect sense in the context of the person's current experience and life to date. Behavior is adaptive to the context in which it occurs, and the therapist must find the wisdom of that adaptation. The therapist is not blinded by the dysfunctional nature of a patient's response but, instead, attends to those aspects of the response that may be either reasonable or appropriate to the context. Thus, the therapist searches the patient's responses for their inherent accuracy, appropriateness, or reasonableness before considering their more dysfunctional characteristics. Even if only a small part of the response is valid, the therapist searches out that portion of the behavior and responds to it. It is this third step that takes the most searching by the therapist and that defines validation most clearly. By finding the validity in the patient's response, the therapist can honestly support the patient in validating herself.

The search for validity is dialectical, in that the therapist must find the grain of wisdom and authenticity in a patient's responses that on the whole may have been dysfunctional. At times, validating a patient's response is like finding for a nugget of gold in a cup of sand. The assumption of DBT is that there is a nugget of gold in every cup of sand; there is some inherent validity in every response. Attention to the nugget of gold does not preclude attention to the sand, however. Indeed, validation strategies are balanced by problem-solving strategies, which focus on finding and taking action on characteristics of the patient that must be changed.

There are four types of validation strategies. The first three, emotional, behavioral, and cognitive validation, are very similar to one another. They are distinguished in this chapter only to provide an opportunity to discuss some specific points that are often important in treating borderline patients. "Cheerleading" is different, in that the therapist is validating the inherent capabilities of the patient—ones that are not always obvious to the patient. Thus, emotional, cognitive, and behavioral validation are experienced by the patient as validating; cheerleading sometimes is not. Although each of these four strategies includes the three steps above, how the therapist puts these steps together can vary.

Why Validate?

Although the need for validation in treatment of borderline patients may be self-evident, especially to anyone who has read the previous seven chapters of this book, therapists often experience so much difficulty in maintaining a validating stance with borderline patients that the point cannot be repeated too often. To summarize the points I have made earlier, validation is needed first to balance change strategies. The amount of validation needed per unit of change focus will vary among patients and for a particular patient over time. Generally, the patient who is unassertive, is nonverbal, and tends to withdraw when confronted will need a higher validation-to-change ratio that the combative patient who, though equally vulnerable and sensitive, can "stay the course" when feeling attacked. For all patients, when stress in the environment (both within and outside of the therapy relationship) goes up, the validation–change quotient must also go up accordingly. Similarly, when particularly sensitive topics are being addressed, validation should be increased. Even within a particular session, the need for therapist validation can be expected to vary. Therapy with a borderline patient can be likened to pushing an individual ever closer to the edge of a sheer cliff. As the back of the person's heel rubs the edge, validation is used to pull the person back from the precipice toward the safe ground where the therapist is.

Second, validation is needed to teach the patient to validate herself. As I have discussed in Chapter 2, the borderline individual is often faced with two incompatible but very strong sources of information: her own intense response to events on the one hand, and others' discrepant, but often equally intense, responses on the other hand. Although DBT does not assume that borderline patients do not at times distort events, the first line of approach is always to discover the aspect of an event that is not being distorted. Distortion of events is often a consequence rather than a cause of emotional dysfunction. The experience of self-mistrust is intensely aversive when it is long-standing and pervasive. At a minimum, people have to trust their own decision on whom to believe—themselves or others. Exaggeration of events is often an attempt to obtain validation for an original, quite valid perspective on events. I often point out to patients that one of my goals in therapy is to help them learn to trust their own response.

The secrets to effective use of validation are knowing when to use it and when not to, and, once it is begun, when to cut it off. This can be a special problem when intense emotions are present or elicited. For some patients, if the therapist allowed it, therapy would be little more than emotional catharsis. The ability to shut off emotional expression and get to problem solving is important if progress is to be made. In particular, it is important that the therapist not use validation strategies immediately following dysfunctional behaviors that are maintained by their tendency to elicit validation from the environment. (The use of therapeutic contingencies to modify behavior is discussed at length in Chapter 10.) At times the best strategy is to ignore a patient's current distress and plunge into problem solving, dragging the patient along, so to speak, as best one can. Validation can be a brief comment or digression while working on other issues, or it can be the focus of an entire session. As with other DBT strategies, the use of these must be goal-oriented and purposeful. That is, they should be used when the immediate goal is to calm a patient who is too emotionally aroused to talk about anything else; to repair therapeutic errors; to develop the patient's skills in nonjudgmental self-observation and nonpejorative self-descriptions (i.e., to teach her self-validation); to learn about the patient's current experiences or experiences accompanying an event; or to provide a validating context for change.

EMOTIONAL VALIDATION STRATEGIES

Borderline patients vacillate between emotional inhibition and intense emotional reactivity. Some patients characteristically inhibit emotional expression during therapy interactions; other patients always seem to be in a state of emotional crisis; still others cycle back and forth. These phases have been described in detail in Chapters 3 and 5. Emotional validation poses different challenges, depending on which phase the patient is in. With the inhibited individual, emotional expression is like the small flame of a campfire on a rainy day. The therapist has to be very careful not to smother the emotion with overly facile observations, explanations, and interpretations. Teaching the patient to observe her own emotions, being able to read emotions from minimal information, and remaining open to the possibility of guessing wrong are all important. With the emotionally reactive patient, by contrast, the challenge is to validate the emotion without escalating it at the same time. Providing opportunities for emotional expression and reflecting emotions are important in this case.

Emotional validation strategies contrast with approaches that focus on the overreactivity of emotions or the distorted basis of their generation. Thus, they are more like the approach of Greenberg and Safran (1987), who make a distinction between primary or "authentic" emotions and secondary or "learned" emotions. The latter are reactions to primary cognitive appraisals and emotional responses; they are the end products of chains of feelings and thoughts. Dysfunctional and maladaptive emotions, according to Greenberg and Safran, are usually secondary emotions that block the experience and expression of primary emotions. These authors go on to suggest that "all primary affective emotion provides adaptive motivational information to the organism" (1987, p. 176). The important point here is the suggestion that dysfunctional and maladaptive responses to events are often connected or interwoven with "authentic" or valid responses to events. Finding and amplifying these primary responses constitute the essence of emotional validation. The honesty of the therapist in applying these strategies cannot be overstressed. If emotional validation strategies are used as change strategies — that is, if lip service is given to validation in order simply to calm the patient down for the "real work"— the therapist can expect the therapy to backfire. Such honesty, in turn, depends on the therapist's belief that there is substantial validity to be found, and that searching for it is therapeutically useful.

A borderline individual commonly cannot identify the emotions she is experiencing, usually because she is experiencing a variety of emotions simultaneously or in rapid succession. In some instances, the patient's secondary emotional response (e.g., fear, shame, or anger) to her primary emotion may be so intense or extreme as to disrupt or inhibit the primary emotion before the patient has a chance to experience, process, or articulate. At other times, the patient may experience a single emotion intensely and may report being upset, but cannot get past that depiction to a fuller description of the emotion. The patient may report that in daily encounters she becomes aware of her emotions only after the fact. An important focus of therapy is on helping the patient observe and describe her current emotional state in a nonjudgmental fashion, taking care to separate descriptions of the emotion from descriptions of the events that led to the emotion.

A borderline patient often withdraws from very intense emotions, showing few overt indications of emotional arousal. Very passive behavior is sometimes an indication that the patient is avoiding or inhibiting all emotional responses that would otherwise be elicited under the current conditions. At times, the escape or avoidance will be incomplete, and the individual will react with part of an emotional response while inhibiting other parts. For example, the patient may have a phenomenological experience of sadness or fear without the facial or postural expressive aspect of the emotion, or vice versa. Or the patient may have an action urge usually associated with an emotion (e.g., to scream, to run out of the session, or to hit the therapist) with no corresponding emotional experience or physiological changes. DBT does not assume that the patient is experiencing the emotion unconsciously, and thus just doesn't know it. The patient who wants to hit the therapist is not necessarily assumed to be angry at him or her. In fact, in this latter case the problem may be that the patient is *not* reacting with anger. That is, she is avoiding or inhibiting the flow of a response that would ordinarily occur.

For the patient who is inhibiting emotional experience and expression, the therapist must be careful to validate both the emotion that is being inhibited and the difficulties the patient is having in expressing it spontaneously. Understanding the inhibition will generally require skillful behavioral assessment (described in detail in Chapter 9). For example, the patient may automatically avoid emotional responses or inhibit emotional expression as a result of classical conditioning experiences. (See Chapter 3.) Secondary emotions, as noted above, typically cut off or interfere with the full experience and/or expression of the primary emotions. Finally, many patients have very strong moral beliefs about the appropriateness of various emotions.

For the patient who is in an emotional crisis or is expressing intense emotions, the therapist has to take great care not to use invalidation as a technique to dampen the emotion—an all-too-common strategy. In my experience, one of therapists' greatest fears is that if they recognize or validate borderline patients' emotional experiences, they are rewarding the emotional behavior and it will continue and even escalate. At other times, therapists, like their patients, feel that if they validate the patients they are invalidating themselves. The temptation is then to try punishment to reduce the emotion. This rarely works; even when it does, the patients usually revert to emotional inhibition, only to respond intensely the next time the same situation is encountered. Once a patient feels heard, listened to, and taken seriously, however, she will usually calm down. Indeed, if the therapist takes the patient's emotions more seriously than the patient is taking them (the dialectical strategy of extending), the patient may actually start to reassure the therapist. Specific emotional validation strategies are discussed below and summarized in Table 8.1.

I. PROVIDING OPPORTUNITIES FOR EMOTIONAL EXPRESSION

A patient in a state of overwhelming crisis often requires a substantial part of the session for emotional expression and processing. Efforts on the part of the therapist to control intense emotional expressions may be met with strong resistance, including statements that the therapist does not understand her. In these instances, the therapist should simply listen, identify, clarify, and directly validate the patient's feelings in a nonjudgmental manner. As noted above, the patient will gradually calm down and be ready for more focused problem solving. Open-ended questions about feelings at this point are probably not useful. Generally, they will simply prolong the emotional intensity, whereas reflective statements about either the patient's feelings or environmental state may help diffuse the intensity.

Opportunities for emotional expression are just as important for the inhibited patient. Here, however, the task is to provide enough structure to in-

TABLE 8.1. Emotional Validation Strategies Checklist

_____ T provides opportunities for EMOTIONAL EXPRESSION; T empathizes and accepts P's feelings.

     _____ T listens with a nonjudgmental and sympathetic attitude to emotional expression of P.

     _____ T surrounds attempts to modulate emotional expression or refocus topic of discussion with statements that provide structure while indicating sympathy for P's emotional pain and difficulty.

_____ T helps P OBSERVE AND LABEL feelings; T helps P slow down, step back, and attend to components of emotional responses.

     _____ T directs P to attend to her own phenomenological experiences of emotion.

     _____ T helps P describe and label bodily sensations associated with feelings.

     _____ T helps P describe and label thoughts, assumptions, and interpretations of situations associated with feelings.

     _____ T helps P describe desires and wishes associated with feelings.

     _____ T help P describe action tendencies and urges associated with feelings.

     _____ T helps P observe and describe facial and postural expressions that may be associated with feelings.

_____ T READS EMOTIONS; T expresses in nonjudgmental fashion emotional responses that P may be only partially expressing.

     _____ T times reading of emotions, tapering as P progresses in therapy.

     _____ T offers P multiple-choice suggestions about how she might be feeling.

_____ T COMMUNICATES that P's feelings are valid.

     _____ T communicates that P's emotional response (or part of P's response) is reasonable, is wise, or makes sense in the context of the situation ("but of course you would feel that way").

     _____ T points out that even when P is overreacting or is reacting to a possibly "distorted" view of the situation, P is nonetheless picking up something from her own behavior or environment (i.e., there is some stimulus setting off the emotion).

     _____ T teaches that all behaviors (including emotions) are caused.

     _____ T offers/elicits a developmental, learning-based explanation for emotional responses, countering P's judgmental theories.

Anti-DBT tactics

_____ T insists upon T's perception of P's feelings; T appears closed to possibility of P's feeling different than T supposes.

_____ T criticizes P's feelings.

_____ T stresses irrationality or distorted basis of feelings without ever acknowledging the "kernel of truth."

_____ T responds to painful emotions as something to get rid of.

     _____ T expresses only discomfort with P's painful emotions.

     _____ T reinforces dysfunctional emotional expressions by consistently stopping change procedures for lengthy validation whenever such expressions occur.

duce communication of emotions, while not imposing so much structure that the patient withdraws further. "Enough structure" generally involves asking questions about emotional reactions and leaving enough silence for the patient to respond. Patience and the ability to tolerate silence are requisite here. Needed also is the ability to judge when a silence has gone on too long. Long silences can induce further withdrawal. Instead, after a reasonable silence the therapist should engage in solitary verbal patter, punctuated with questions about what the patient is feeling and silences for response, until the patient begins to talk again.

2. TEACHING EMOTION OBSERVATION AND LABELING SKILLS

Skills in observing and labeling emotional experiences and states are an important target of the skills training module in emotion regulation. The therapist must know these skills and help the patient integrate them into daily life. The therapist may also need to teach these skills explicitly when there is no separate skills training component to the therapy or when that portion of the skills training occurs too long after the skills are needed. Some borderline patients are quite good at observing and describing emotions; others have minimal abilities, often existing in an emotional fog. They know they are feeling something, but they have little or no idea of what they are feeling or how to put it into words. With these patients it is often useful to teach them first how to observe and describe the components of emotions, without necessarily having to put labels on their feelings right away.

There are many theories of emotions, and just as many theories of the components of emotional responses. In DBT we teach patients how to observe and describe the prompting events (either internal or external); thoughts and interpretations associated with the event; sensory and physical responses associated with the emotional experience; desires and wishes associated with the experience (e.g., wanting the best for a person or wanting to be close to a loved one); and associated action tendencies (e.g., "I feel like hitting him," "My feet want to run"). Information about the emotion being experienced can also be obtained from overt reactions that may be expressions of the emotion, such as facial and body expressions, words used or things said, and actions. Finally, it can also be useful to examine the aftereffects of an emotion. For example, feeling secure and trusting when near someone is more indicative of love than of anger.

At times, information about prompting events is all that is needed to figure out an emotional response. If one person threatens to kill another, the other will most likely respond with fear; sadness usually follows the death of a loved one. Because of their idiosyncratic and cultural learning experiences, however, individuals may vary in their emotional responses to different situations. A further complicating factor is that most individuals, including borderline patients, have difficulty discriminating prompting events (e.g., "He spoke to me with a curt tone of voice," "My heart is racing") from their interpretations of the events (e.g., "He hates me," "I am having a panic attack and will humiliate myself"). The ability to separate actual events from inferences about the events is an important first step in cognitive therapy approaches and is also important in DBT.

Self-observation requires further that a patient step back and note the presence of physical sensations, feelings, emotion-laden, or "hot" thoughts, and action tendencies. At times, getting the patient to slow down and observe her own responses is the only way for the therapist to get enough information to respond helpfully to the patient. Although the DBT therapist is expected to "read the patient's emotions," at least in the initial stages of therapy (see below), information about how the patient is actually responding makes this much easier. Otherwise, identifying the patient's emotions can sometimes feel like a guessing game. Most people, including borderline patients, find it extremely difficult to observe emotional responses without being carried away by them. Indeed, emotion observation is also an emotion regulation technique. Thus, it can be useful to help the patient practice reflective self-observation during therapy sessions and in phone interactions.

Techniques for helping a patient learn to observe, describe, and label ongoing emotions include questioning and making comments about the prompting events; instructing the patient in how to step back and observe her ongoing cognitive, physiological, and nonverbal action responses; and focusing on normative responses of other people in similar situations. Filling out "Observing and Describing Emotions" homework sheets from the emotion regulation skills training module (see the companion manual to this volume) can also be quite useful. The advantage of these sheets is that the patient can use them between sessions to work on identifying emotions.

Sometimes a patient expereinces the very idea that one can reflectively observe an emotion as invalidating of the emotion. The patient's tendency to take the emotion literally, as information about the precipitating event rather than about her response to the precipitating event, is the difficulty here. The suggestion that one can or should observe the emotion implies that the "problem" is the emotion, not what set it off. To counter this, the therapist should surround the request to observe with communications that validate the emotion.

3. READING EMOTIONS

Reading emotions is the emotional equivalent of reading someone's mind. A therapist who is a good reader of emotions can figure out how the patient feels just by knowing what has happened to her; he or she can make the link between precipitating event and emotion without being given any information about the emotion itself. This is almost always experienced as validating of the patient's emotional experience. The message communicated is that the patient's emotional responses to events are normal, predictable and understandable; how else would the therapist know how the patient feels? In contrast, when the therapist cannot figure out how the patient feels unless the patient spells it out in detail, this is often experienced as invalidating, insensitive, or uncaring.

Many therapists are unwilling or unable to read patients' emotions, insisting instead that the patients state verbally how they are feeling or what they want. It is not unusual to hear therapists say to patients, "I can't read your mind," in a tone of voice clearly implying that expecting the therapists to know how the patients feel without being told is somehow pathological. Patients' demands that therapists do this are common complaints at case conferences. Yet a moment's reflection tells us that the ability to know how another feels without being told directly is an essential and expected social skill in ordinary interpersonal relationships. If a loved one dies, a person is fired, a house is burned in a fire, a large account is won or lost at work, or a child wins a coveted prize, most people would expect others to know how they feel and to act accordingly. In many conflicts between groups, the issue is just this — the complaint of one group that the other is insensitive and cannot understand the first group's emotions unless everything is spelled out in detail. Men don't understand women; Caucasians can't see life from the perspective of African-Americans; the rich misunderstand the poor; and so on. Demanding that others understand us better, or develop the ability to read our emotions, is not unique to borderline patients. In each case, the problem is that people of one cultural background have difficulty reading the emotions of those from another background. And this is the state of affairs between borderline patients and most therapists. They have very different life experiences, making it difficult for each to understand the other. Patients have not had the inculturation that makes a therapist; most therapists have not had experiences close to those of the borderline patient.

Among the more common and important emotional assertions made by borderline and suicidal patients are variants of the statement that they "don't care any more." Such comments are important because they afford the potential of invalidating emotions that are very central to the patients' opinion of themselves. A patient may say that she doesn't want to try any more, or that she doesn't care about something she previously cared very much about. When taken literally, these comments cut off further collaborative work between patient and therapist, at least with respect to the topic under consideration. At times, the patient's statement that she doesn't care reflects the therapist's secret belief ("If she cared, she would try harder, do better, etc."). Thus, there is a temptation to agree with the patient that she doesn't care or doesn't want to improve. At other times, the therapist experiences the patient's statement as manipulative ("Obviously she cares; she is just saying that to play games or get something from me"). The therapist responds with veiled hostility or coldness. Both responses can be experienced by the patient as invalidating of her true emotional state. Not caring any more is usually a frustration response and an attempt on the part of the patient to avoid the cycle of caring and subsequent disappointment. It is useful for the therapist to respond to this by stating to the patient that she would probably care if she let herself, and that the problem may be one of feeling helpless and hopeless rather than one of not caring. Simply recognizing the patient's sense of being out of control can be useful in helping the patient identify her avoidance strategy.

Reading emotions requires some familiarity by the therapist with the culture of the patient. Knowledge of the patient's current situation or the precipitating situation, together with observations of the patient's verbal and nonverbal behavior, can be useful in arriving at a description of the patient's emotional responses. The link between events and emotions is in part universal but in part learned. Thus, to the extent that the therapist's and patient's learning histories are similar, the therapist will be adept at emotion reading. In the absence of such similarity, clinical experience (especially with borderline patients) and books and movies about people like the patient can be helpful. A very important task of the case consultation group is to assist the therapist in this work.

Timing

Reading emotions is essential at the beginning of therapy with the borderline patient, but it should be tapered off as therapy progresses. As a strategy, it is both very powerful as a validating technique and at the same time is fraught with difficulty. The main problem is that when the therapist reads the patient's emotions, the patient does not have to learn how to read her own emotions. The therapist is doing the work, not the patient. Second, having the therapist read her emotions is usually very comforting to the patient. Thus, when the therapist starts to taper it off — to insist on the patient's improving her ability to read her own emotions — this can be experienced as punishing and uncaring. Third, when the therapist verbalizes the patient's emotions, it lets the patient avoid verbalizing them herself. Thus the exposure to talking about her emotions is further avoided, and the development of comfort in discussing emotions may be impeded. Finally, avoiding emotional expressiveness allows the patient to avoid emotional self-validation.

In the beginning of therapy, and sometimes well after therapy has begun, the therapist's refusal to read the patients' emotions often produces escalation of an emotion until it is finally expressed openly, but in an extreme and often maladaptive way. In other words, the emotion is only expressed when the experience of it is more intense than the counterbalancing experience of shame, fear, or self-invalidation. At this point, the patient may cut herself or attempt suicide, or may rigidly adhere to a point of view that supports an extreme emotional response. Before the patient has learned to inhibit such maladaptive behaviors, the therapist's withholding of emotion reading to force the patient to express her emotions is probably counterproductive. However, once these behaviors are under control and the patient can adequately tolerate distress, continuing to read emotions is itself counterproductive. In effect, the therapist's task becomes teaching the patient the skills of emotional experiencing and expression. This is especially true of the final stage of DBT, in which developing self-respect and learning self-validation are the primary targets. Principles of skills training (including shaping, discussed in Chapter 11) are relevant here.

Offering Multiple-Choice Emotion Questions

One danger in emotion reading is that the therapist will misread an emotion but the patient will agree anyway. She may do this because of simple confusion, fear of disagreeing with or disappointing the therapist, or a belief that her actual emotions are so bad that she can not admit them. An alternative strategy is to offer the patient a range of emotion labels to choose from—for instance, "Are you feeling angry, hurt, sad, or all three?" The advantage here is that such questions are not open-ended. Borderline patients often simply can not answer open ended questions about their current emotions. Multiple-choice emotion questions give the patients some choice but not too much.

4. COMMUNICATING THE VALIDITY OF EMOTIONS

The single best way to validate a patient's emotional experience is for the therapist to communicate directly that he or she finds the emotional response understandable. Two types of understanding can be communicated here. First, the patient can be informed that almost anyone (or at least many people) would respond to the emotion-generating situation in much the same way that she is responding. This is normative validation. Second, the patient can be helped to see that given her past learning experiences, her emotional reaction (even if others would react differently) is understandable within that context. In both instances, however, the emphasis is on identifying those aspects of the current situation that prompt the emotion.

It is important that the therapist validate not only the primary emotional experience, but also the secondary emotional response. For example, a patient often feels guilty, ashamed, angry at herself, or panicky if she experiences anger or humiliation, feels dependent on the therapist, begins to cry, grieves, or is afraid. These secondary responses are often the most debilitating for the patient. Patients who hold religious beliefs about the morality of various emotional responses should be helped to explore the validity of these beliefs. Although the therapist must be careful not to challenge such patients' moral standards, a patient's prohibitions against various emotions are often based on a faulty understanding of her own religious tradition.

Emotional validation is an essential first step in any attempt to help the patient moderate her responses. Thus, it is rarely useful to respond to what seems to be an unwarranted emotion by instructing the patient that she need not feel that way. The therapist may frequently be tempted to do this when the patient is responding emotionally to the therapist. For example, if a patient calls the therapist at home (according to the treatment plan) and then feels guilty or humiliated about doing so, it is a natural tendency for the therapist to tell the patient that she need not feel this way. This should be recognized as an invalidating statement. Although the therapist may want to communicate that calling the therapist is acceptable and understandable, it is also understandable that the patient feels guilty and humiliated.

Most often, invalidation of a patient's feelings will arise from the therapist's overanxious attempts to help the patient feel better immediately. Such tendencies should be resisted, because they counter an important message that the therapy is attempting to communicate—namely, that negative and painful emotions are not only understandable but tolerable. In addition, if the therapist responds to the patient's negative emotions by either ignoring them, telling the patient that she need not feel that way, or focusing too quickly on changing the emotions, the therapist runs the risk of behaving just as others in the patient's natural environment have done. The attempt to control emotions by willpower, or to "think happy" and to avoid negative thoughts, is a key characteristic of the invalidating environment. The therapist must be sure not to fall into this trap.

BEHAVIORAL VALIDATION STRATEGIES

Behavioral validation strategies are used in every session. They constitute the main response to the tendency of borderline patients to invalidate and punish their own behavior patterns. Behavioral validation can focus on behaviors a patient notes on her diary card, other behaviors during the week, or behaviors occurring during the therapy session or interaction with the therapist. The basic idea is to elicit a clear description of the behaviors in question and then to communicate their essential understandability. Behavioral validation is based on the notion that all behavior is caused by events occurring in time, and thus (in principle, at least) is understandable. The therapist's task is to search out the validity of the patient's response and to reflect that aspect of the behavior. Although these strategies are being discussed in terms of overt behaviors and actions, they can be applied equally well to helping patients accept their own emotional reactions, decisions, beliefs, and thoughts; they are discussed here for convenience's sake. The behavioral validation strategies are summarized in Table 8.2.

I. TEACHING BEHAVIOR OBSERVATION AND LABELING SKILLS

Describing behavior and its patterns is an essential part of any psychotherapy. Borderline patients can be remarkably unaware of both their own behavior patterns and the effects of their behavior on others. Often this is the case because other people have described their behavior to them in terms of pre-

TABLE 8.2. Behavioral Validation Strategies Checklist

____ T helps P OBSERVE AND DESCRIBE (points out or elicits P's recognition — e.g., by Socratic questioning) her own behavior.

    ____ T helps P differentiate behavior from inferred motives and judgmental labels.

____ T helps P IDENTIFY THE "SHOULD"; T observes and describes self-imposed behavioral demands, unrealistic standards for acceptable behavior.

    ____ T identifies P's ineffective strategies for behavior modification.

    ____ T observes and describes uses of guilt, self-berating, and other punishment strategies.

____ T COUNTERS THE "SHOULD"; T communicates that all behavior is understandable, in principle.

    ____ T communicates that any standard not realized is by definition unrealistic in the present moment.

    ____ T communicates that everything that happens "should" happen, given the context of the world (i.e., in principle, everything is understandable).

    ____ T is careful to distinguish understanding that the conditions necessary for something to happen have occurred (on the one hand) from approving of the event itself (on the other).

    ____ T makes use of stories, analogies, parables, examples, and instructions about principles of behavior to help P see that whatever happens, including her own behavior, is a natural product of reality as it is at present.

____ T ACCEPTS P's behavior, including the "shoulds" she places on herself.

    ____ T responds to P's behavior in nonjudgmental fashion.

    ____ T explores with P the validity of her "should in order to."

    ____ T looks for nugget of truth in P's behavior.

____ T validates P's DISAPPOINTMENT in her own behavior.

Anti-DBT tactics

____ T imposes his or her own behavioral preferences as absolute "shoulds."

____ T communicates that P should be (feel, act, think) differently than she does.

____ T communicates that others should be different.

---

sumed motives (e.g., "You are trying to control me") or the effects of the behavior on the observers (e.g., "You are manipulating me"), rather than in purely behavioral terms ("You are changing the topic"). Although these may be accurate descriptions of the observers' experience, they often are not accurate descriptions of the patients' experience; thus, the feedback is dismissed or argued against. Energy that could go into understanding their own actual behavior patterns and their effects, regardless of the motives or intended effects, is diverted into self-defense.

Both behavioral analysis and insight strategies, discussed in the next chapter, are important techniques for teaching a patient how to observe and describe her own behavior. The point I want to make here is that describing behavior, without adding inferred motives and judgments, can itself be a validating response. This is all the more so when the therapist helps the patient recognize self-invalidating and self-judgmental descriptions of her own behavior. For a borderline patient, "I was stupid" may be a more typical description of missing a bus than "I went to the bus stop too late to catch the bus."

2. IDENTIFYING THE "SHOULD"

Borderline and suicidal patients often express extreme anger, guilt, or disappointment in themselves because they have behaved in ways that they find unacceptable. Almost without exception, such feelings will be based on some belief system that they "should not" have acted in the manner they did, or that they "should" have acted differently. In other words, these patients place unrealistic demands upon themselves to behave differently than they do. A key step in behavioral validation is helping a patient identify this type of self-imposed demand. Although the patient may state openly that she shouldn't have done what she did, other statements communicate the same message only indirectly (e.g., "Why did I do that?", "How could I have done that?", "That was stupid!"). Learning to identify unspoken "shoulds" is an important skill.

The use of magical "shoulds" by a borderline individual is one of the most important factors interfering with behavioral shaping. Believing that she should be different already prohibits the patient from putting together a realistic plan to bring about desired changes. Indeed, in an invalidating family it is the imposition of unrealistic "shoulds" that substantially inhibit teaching the patient how to change her own behavior. Thus, imposing "shoulds" recapitulates the invalidation that the individual experienced in growing up. Highlighting this for the patient can be helpful in promoting change.

3. COUNTERING THE "SHOULD"

The first step in countering "shoulds" is to make a distinction between understanding how or why something happened and approving of the event. The main resistance to believing that an event should have happened, given the circumstances surrounding it, is the belief that if a behavior is understood it is also approved of. The therapist must emphasize that the act of refusing to accept a given reality means that one cannot act to overcome or change that reality. Simple examples can be given here. The therapist can point to a nearby wall and suggest that if an individual wants the wall to be chartreuse in color and refuses to accept the fact that the wall is currently not chartreuse, it is unlikely that the person will ever paint the wall chartreuse. A second point is being made here as well: Wishing that reality were different does not change it; believing that reality is what one wants it to be does not make it so. At times, a statement that something shouldn't be is also tantamount to denying its existence: "Since it isn't acceptable, it couldn't happen."

The counterstatement to this is "It is" or "It happened." The task is to get the patient to agree that neither wishing nor denying will change reality.

A useful step in countering "shoulds" is to present a mechanistic explanation of causality, indicating that every event has a cause. The therapist can go through a number of examples of unwanted, undesirable behaviors with step-by-step illustrations of the factors that brought the events about. The strategy is to show that thoughts ("I don't want it") and emotions (fear, anger) are not sufficient to keep an event from happening. The notion to be communicated is that everything that happens should happen, given the context of the world; in principle, everything is understandable.

Countering the "should" can require a substantial amount of time, and the therapist may need to have many stories and metaphors at hand to illustrate the point. For example, I usually tell a story about boxes rolling down a conveyor belt and out of a building. The boxes tumble out of the building everywhere. A person driving by would not believe that he or she could get the boxes to stop tumbling out of the building just by yelling at them to stop, or just by wanting desperately enough for them to stop. No, the person would assume that he or she would have to get out of the car and go into the building to figure out what is wrong. Knowing what is going on in the building will make it clear why the boxes are rolling out into the yard. People, together with their pasts, are often like buildings that no one can see into. Another example I use is to hold something in my hand and pretend that it is a glass of red wine, simultaneously pretending that the carpet is a brand-new white carpet. As I keep dropping the object on the floor, I keep asking whether the glass should not drop when let go. Why does it drop if I don't want it to? After this point is made, I move my hand under the object as it drops, catching it. The point is that for the glass not to drop on the carpet (once my hand opens), something has to be done to stop it.

It is very important to cover these principles in a rather abstract way near the beginning of therapy and to get the patient to agree on the abstract principles. If the skills training modules are being administered, these points are usually discussed while the patient is learning both mindfulness skills and distress tolerance. Getting a patient to accept the idea that a nonjudgmental stance is preferable to a judgmental stance almost always requires a thorough discussion of these ideas. Throughout the remainder of therapy, the therapist can refer back to these principles, noting that the patient has already agreed to them, and can point out their application in the individual case. As therapy progresses, the patient will begin catching herself and her "shoulds." This, of course, is to be encouraged and reinforced.

4. ACCEPTING THE "SHOULD"

Often one event must occur for a second event to occur. ("If A, then B"; "If not A, then not B"). It is common and appropriate to use the term "should" in a statement when one is referring to something that must happen in order for something else to happen. Thus, the following phrase is appropriate: "*A* should happen in order to produce *B*." It is very important that the therapist accept the patient's preferences about her own behavior. The patient may often prefer to behave in certain ways or may want various outcomes that demand prior behavior patterns. In these instances, the therapist must be alert to accepting the "shoulds," and communicate to the patient the validity of her preferences. Together, the therapist and patient can explore the validity of the "should in order to" sequence. At times, a patient will be making inaccurate predictions (e.g., "*A* is not needed in order for *B* to occur"). At other times, a patient's predictions are quite accurate. In this instance, the therapist is looking for the nugget of truth in the patient's behavior.

5. MOVING TO DISAPPOINTMENT

It is easy for the therapist to get caught up in invalidating the patient's "shoulds" without recognizing that it is important to avoid invalidating the patient's quite understandable disappointment in her own behavior. In the context of any brief discussion, it is important for the therapist to alternate between validating the events as understandable and validating the disappointment as equally understandable. Certain behaviors both should and should not occur. When this happens, an appropriate response is disappointment.

COGNITIVE VALIDATION STRATEGIES

Intense emotions can precipitate emotion-congruent thoughts, memories, and images; conversely, thoughts, memories, and images can have powerful influences on mood. Thus, once an intense emotional response starts, a vicious circle is often set up: The emotion sets off memories, images, and thoughts and influences perceptions and processing of information, which in turn feed back into the emotional response, keeping it going. In such instances, distortions can take on a life of their own and may color many, if not most, of the individual's interactions and responses to events. Not all mood-related thoughts, perceptions, expectancies, memories, and assumptions, however, are dysfunctional or distorted. This point is crucial in conducting DBT.

DBT does not assume that borderline individuals' problems stem primarily from dysfunctional cognitive styles, faulty interpretations and distortions of events, and maladaptive underlying assumptions or cognitive schemas. Because borderline patients sometimes distort, sometimes exaggerate, and sometimes remember selectively, it is common for the people around them (including therapists) to assume that their thinking and perceptions are always faulty, or at least that in disagreements the borderline individuals are more likely to be incorrect. Such assumptions are especially likely when full information about events precipitating an individual's emotional response is not available—that is, the stimuli setting off the individual's reaction are not public. Especially when the borderline individual is experiencing intense emotions, it is easy for another person to assume that the individual is distorting somehow. Things are not, or cannot be, as bad as she says. The trap here is that assumptions take the place of assessment; hypothesis and interpretations take the place of analysis of the facts. The other person's private interpretation is taken as a guide to public facts. Such a scenario replicates the invalidating environment.

The task of the therapist in cognitive validation is to recognize, verbalize, and understand the patient's expressed and unexpressed thoughts, beliefs, expectations, and underlying assumptions or rules, and to find and reflect the essential truth of all or part of these. The strategies for "catching thoughts," identifying assumptions and expectancies, and uncovering rules that are guiding the individual's behavior, especially when these rules are operating outside of awareness, differ little from the guidelines outlined by cognitive therapists such as Beck and his colleagues (Beck et al., 1979; Beck et al., 1990). The essential difference is that the task in DBT is validation rather than empirical refutation or logical challenge.

A borderline individual has usually been raised in a "crazy-making" family where her perceptions of reality were often invalidated. The struggle for the patient, then, is to learn to discriminate when her perceptions, thoughts, and beliefs are valid and when they are not—when she can trust herself and when she cannot. The task of the therapist is to assist in this process. An exclusive focus on the patient's invalid beliefs, assumptions, and cognitive styles is counterproductive, since it leaves the patient unsure of when (if ever) her perceptions and thoughts are adaptive, functional, and valid. Specific cognitive validation strategies are described below and summarized in Table 8.3.

1. ELICITING AND REFLECTING THOUGHTS AND ASSUMPTIONS

The first task in cognitive validation is to figure out exactly what the patient is thinking, what her assumptions and expectancies are, and what constructs she is using to organize her world. This is easier said than done, because borderline individuals often cannot articulate exactly what they are thinking. At times, thoughts rush through their minds too quickly for them to identify; at other times, their assumptions and expectancies are implicit rather than explicit. Passive expectancies, for example, are automatic, effortless, and difficult to verbalize, as opposed to active expectancies, which are conscious, occupy attention, and are easy to describe (Williams, 1993).

2. DISCRIMINATING FACTS FROM INTERPRETATIONS

It is easy to assume that a patient is distorting what she observes; it is much more difficult to ascertain just what a patient is observing. The task here is to make private events public. The therapist should carefully question the pa-

TABLE 8.3. Cognitive Validating Strategies Checklist

_____ T helps P OBSERVE AND DESCRIBE (points out or elicits P's recognition— e.g., by Socratic questioning) her own thought processes (automatic thoughts, underlying assumptions).

    _____ T identifies constructs P uses to organize her world.

    _____ T identifies meaning P attaches to events.

    _____ T identifies P's basic assumptions about herself and the world.

    _____ T helps P observe and describe "crazy-making" experiences.

    _____ T listens to and discusses P's point of view in nonjudgmental fashion.

_____ T helps P assess the facts and DIFFERENTIATE EVENTS FROM INTER-PRETATIONS of events.

_____ T searches for the "KERNEL OF TRUTH" in P's way of viewing events.

    _____ When appropriate, T uses T-P interactions to demonstrate to P that while her grasp of reality may not be complete, neither is it incomplete.

_____ T ACKNOWLEDGES "WISE MIND"; T communicates to P that intuitive knowledge can be as valid as empirically verifiable knowledge.

_____ T RESPECTS DIFFERING VALUES; T does not insist on validity of his or her own values over P's.

Anti-DBT tactics

_____ T pushes a particular set of values or philosophical position on reality and truth.

_____ T presents a rigid view of events.

_____ T is unable to see reality from the perspective of P.

---

tient about just what has happened and who did what to whom. As I have noted earlier, discriminating events from the interpretations of the events can be very difficult. Often the patient offers an interpretation of the observed behavior of another ("He wants to fire me") or an expectation derived from an observation ("He is going to fire me"). The therapist should ask, "What did he do to make you believe that?" The crucial element here is the initial assumption that the other person did something, and that the patient's interpretation is likely to be reasonable in some fashion. The goal in this case is to uncover the empirical basis of the patient's beliefs.

3. FINDING THE "KERNEL OF TRUTH"

The next task is to find and highlight the thoughts and assumptions of the patient that are valid or make sense within the context she is operating in. The idea is not that individuals (including borderline individuals) always "make sense," or that they do not at times exaggerate or minimize, think in extremes, devalue what is valuable and idealize what is ordinary, and make dysfunctional decisions. Indeed, in both popular and professional opinion, borderline individuals are notorious for just such distortions. But it is essential not to prejudge the opinions, thoughts, and decisions of a borderline patient. When a therapist disagrees with a patient, it is all too easy simply to assume that the therapist is right and the patient is wrong. In looking for the "kernel of truth," the therapist takes a leap of faith and assumes that with proper scrutiny, some amount of validity or reason or sense can be found. Although the patient's grasp of reality may not be complete, neither is it wholly incomplete. At times, the patient's thoughts on the matter may make substantial sense. Borderline patients have an uncanny ability sometimes to see that the "emperor has no clothes"—to observe or attend to stimuli in the environment that others do not observe. The task of the therapist is to separate the wheat from the chaff and to focus, in this moment, on the wheat.

4. ACKNOWLEDGING "WISE MIND"

As I have discussed in Chapter 7, DBT presents to patients the concept of "wise mind," in contrast to "emotion mind" and "reasonable mind." "Wise mind" is the integration of both, and also includes an emphasis on intuitive, experiential, and/or spiritual ways of knowing. Thus, one aspect of cognitive validation is the therapist's acknowledgment and support of this type of knowing on the part of the patient. The therapist takes the position that something can be valid even if the patient cannot prove it. The fact that someone else is more logical in an argument does not mean that the patient's points are not valid. Emotionality does not invalidate a position any more than logic can necessarily validate it. Each of these therapeutic positions counteracts aspects of the invalidating environment.

5. RESPECTING DIFFERING VALUES

At times a patient and therapist will have differing opinions and values. Respecting these differences, while not assuming superiority, is an essential component of cognitive validation. It is easy for a therapist to take a "one-up" view of his or her own opinions and values as more respectable than the patient's, and thereby to invalidate the patient's point of view. For example, one of my patients believed that I should be available to her by phone any time, night or day. She herself had a job in the mental health area and stated that she was available to the people she worked with, because she believed that it was the compassionate and right thing to do. I pointed out to her that the problem was that she was trying to get me to be like her (to have fewer limits on what I could give), and I was trying to get her to be more like me (to observe more limits). Although I did not change my position about my own behavior, I could appreciate the value of her point of view also.

CHEERLEADING STRATEGIES

In many ways, working with a borderline patient is like being the football coach of the lowest-rated high school team in the league during the final game of the season. The team is behind 92 to 0 in the fourth quarter; three people are left in the stands. It is cold, snowing, and muddy, and the other team is threatening another touchdown. A time out is called by the team captain. The team huddles and wants to quit. What does the coach do? The coach acknowledges that the situation is grim, but nonetheless stands firm, shouts encouragement, and inspires the team to keep going. In short, the coach cheerleads.

Borderline and suicidal patients are often discouraged, hopeless, and unable to see any nonsuicidal solution to their problems in living. Life and therapy are very difficult for them. Their self-concept, and frequently the opinions others have of them as well, are at a low ebb. During a session, such a patient may vacillate between hope and discouragement. The most minor confrontation may be enough to precipitate discouragement. Even when the patient is momentarily not discouraged, the therapist can be certain that between sessions the feeling is likely to return. Cheerleading strategies can be helpful both in counteracting current hopelessness and in anticipating and counteracting demoralizing episodes in the upcoming days. Cheerleading is one of the principal strategies for combating the active-passivity behavior of the borderline patient.

In cheerleading, the therapist is validating the inherent ability of the patient to overcome her difficulties and to build a life worth living. Although the form of that life may differ from what is hoped or even expected at any given point, the potential for overcoming obstacles and for creating value is what is attended to and observed. The trick of cheerleading is to get the person to perform up to her ability and to give her hope that her abilities can be expanded, while being realistic as to both what those abilities are and how much they can be expanded. A key therapist attitude is "I believe in you." At its very simplest, cheerleading is believing in the patient. For some patients, this will be their first experience of having someone believe in and have confidence in them. In cheerleading, the therapist is validating the inner capabilities and wisdom of the patient; at times, therefore, the cheerleading strategy will balance, contrast, and contradict the emotional, behavioral, and cognitive validating strategies.

Cheerleading strategies are used in just about every interaction (e.g., every session, every phone call). Frequency should be highest with the extremely dysfunctional patient. As the patient improves — and particularly during the last phase of therapy, which targets self-respect and self-validation — the amount of cheerleading should be tapered off. However, it is important to recognize that almost everyone needs a certain amount of cheerleading to get through life comfortably. This is particularly true when someone undertakes a difficult task, such as psychotherapy. Thus, although cheerleading should be reduced over the course of therapy, and certainly the focus of the cheerleading will change, it remains an important part of the therapeutic relationship throughout.

Cheerleading is sometimes experienced by the patient as invalidating. If the therapist understood how really awful it is, and how really incapable the patient is, the therapist wouldn't believe that the patient can change or accomplish anything or do what is being requested. In cheerleading, the therapist believes that the patient can save herself; the patient, in contrast, often believes that she needs to be saved. The task here is to balance an appreciation for the difficulties of making progress and realistic expectations with hope and confidence that the patient can indeed change. Cheerleading has to be laced with emotional validation and a large dose of realism. Without these elements, it can indeed be invalidating. Thus, the therapist must be vigilant in recognizing the difficulty of the patient's problem, even while never giving up on the idea that the problem can be overcome eventually. The therpaist cheers the patient toward goals that are realistic for her, and considers individual differences in capabilities. Some specific techniques are discussed below and summarized in Table 8.4.

I. ASSUMING THE BEST

One of the most demoralizing things that happens to borderline patients is that others attribute their lack of progress or ineffective behavior to an absence of motivation or to lack of effort. As discussed in Chapter 4, a fundamental assumption of DBT is that patients want to improve and are doing their best. Frequent comments to the patient that the therapist knows that she wants to improve, and that she is doing her best, are often helpful. These comments are most needed when the patient is expressing doubts about her desire to improve or reporting that she could have done better. Almost always, the patient's statement that she could have done better should be followed by a comment from the therapist that she did the best she could. Such a statement follows directly from the behavioral validation strategies described above.

Maintaining this belief—that the patient is doing the best she can—is both essential and extremely difficult. It often feels as if the patient is manipulating the therapist or is being obstinate. I find the following story useful for keeping myself and the therapists in my case consultation group in a cheerleading (rather than punishing) frame of mind:

Imagine that you have just been in a terrible earthquake. Huge buildings have crashed down. Fires are all around. Police, firefighters and construction workers are overtaxed, and no one is available to help you. The child you love most in the world is still alive, but trapped in a small space under a building. There is a tiny opening she could crawl through to escape if she could get to it, or, if she could move just 2 feet closer to the opening, you could grab her and pull her out. The opening is too small for you to crawl in and get her. Time is of the essence because a loudspeaker truck just went by telling everyone to clear the area; when the next aftershock comes, more of the building will fall down. You search for a stick or something to throw to her to grab hold of, with no success. The child is crying for help. She can't

TABLE 8.4. Cheerleading Strategies Checklist

____ T communicates a belief that P is DOING HER BEST.

____ T ENCOURAGES and actively expresses hope.
     ____ T expresses faith that P will make it.
     ____ T tells patient that she will be able to cope or handle a problem or situation.
     ____ T says, "You can."

____ T focuses on P's CAPABILITIES.
     ____ T redirects P's attention from problematic response patterns to areas of capability.
     ____ T surrounds confrontation with observations about P's strengths, criticisms with praise.
     ____ T expresses belief that P has what she needs to overcome her difficulties and construct a life worth living.
         ____ T refers to, acknowledges, and expresses belief in P's "wise self."

     ____ T expresses faith in T and P as a team.

     ____ T validates emotions, thoughts, behavior.

____ T MODULATES EXTERNAL CRITICISM.
     ____ T points out that the criticisms are often not accurate, and that even when accurate they do not mean the situation or P is hopeless.
     ____ T communicates a stance of being on P's side.

____ T PRAISES AND REASSURES P.

____ T is REALISTIC in expectations and deals directly with P's fears of T's insincerity.

____ T STAYS NEAR in a crisis.

Anti-DBT tactics

____ T overgeneralizes, overestimates P's capabilities.

____ T uses cheerleading to "get rid" of P.

____ T calls P a "manipulator," or accuses her of "playing games," "splitting," "not trying," or the like, either to her face or to other therapists during case consultations.

---

move because every one of her bones are broken! You can't reach her if she doesn't move. Would you decide that she is manipulating you or just being obstinate? Would you sit back and wait for her to move, reasoning that when she wants to get out she will? Probably not. What would you do? Cheerlead. Cry out, command, yell, cajole, sweet-talk, insist, plead, suggest, threaten, direct, distract—all of these, in proper context and with proper modulation of tone, are methods of cheerleading.

2. PROVIDING ENCOURAGEMENT

Providing encouragement simply means expressing the belief that the patient will eventually overcome her difficulties, will engage in requisite behaviors, will cope with a given situation, or the like. Essentially, it is a way of communicating hope that the patient can achieve what she wishes to achieve. Encouragement can be specific (e.g., "I know you can handle the upcoming job interview well") or general (e.g., "I know you will someday overcome your problems and make it in life"). It can express faith in the patient's abilities to cope or change in the short term (e.g., "I believe you can get through just this night without a drink") or in the long term (e.g., "I have confidence that someday you will overcome alcoholism"). However it is stated, it is absolutely essential for the therapist not to give up hope in the patient, as well as to express that hope and confidence directly to the patient.

One of the common mistakes both patients and therapists make is to underestimate the patients' available ability and strength. Some therapists, like their patients, oscillate between underestimating and overestimating. It is important, however, that encouragement be based on clear assessment of a patient's abilities and not on the mood of a therapist. Generally, it is good to encourage the patient to do just a little more than she may be able to do with ease. That is, the therapist encourages the patient to do hard things. Believing that the patient can do something does not mean believing that it will be easy. Often, the patient will believe that she is not capable of doing it. In such a case, the therapist must balance cheerleading against validating the patient's sense of herself and her own abilities. The therapist must be adept at fading from "I think you can do it now" to "I think you can learn to do it."

When the patient rejects encouragement, saying that the therapist does not understand, the therapist should consider whether he or she is are being too specific. In these instances, it can be helpful to fall back on the more general statement that the therapist simply believes in the patient, has confidence in her, or believes that somehow she will find a way. It can also be useful to discuss with the patient the dilemma that she creates if she always feels misunderstood if the therapist believes in her. What is the therapist to do? Stop believing in her?

3. FOCUSING ON THE PATIENT'S CAPABILITIES

It is very easy to focus too closely on helping the patient gain insight into her maladaptive thinking patterns, problematic emotions, and dysfunctional action patterns. It is essential that the focus on problems be followed by a focus on and encouragement of the patient's capabilities. It is most helpful here to pinpoint specific capabilities specifically.

Communicating That the Patient Has Everything She Needs to Succeed

As noted in Chapter 3, borderline patients often subscribe to the "fatal flaw" theory: They believe that somehow they do not now and never will have what they need to overcome their difficulties. A therapist should periodically communicate that a patient has everything she needs to overcome her difficulties. According to this perspective, the problem is a developmental one rather than a problem of critical and irremediable flaws. Thus, the strategy is to affirm the patient's inner strength, the presence of a "wise self," in a rather nonspecific way. Indeed, since the qualities alluded to are not directly observable, the therapist should not be trapped into trying to prove the validity of the affirmation. Statements such as "I simply know it to be true" or "I simply feel it" may be sufficient. Since a borderline patient often feels that she has to prove the validity of any thought or emotion she experiences, such statements on the part of the therapist can also help to model for the patient the acceptability of intuitive knowledge. When the patient argues with encouragement, the therapist can always fall back on this strategy.

Expressing a Belief in the Therapeutic Relationship

The therapist should periodically express a belief in the therapy team. This can be even more reassuring and encouraging to the patient than believing in the patient. If the patient believes in the therapist and the therapist believes in the patient, believing in the two as a team can be a good synthesis. Patients often doubt whether therapy can help them. Some, of course, constantly tell their therapists that; others keep their doubts to themselves. In either case, however, it is useful for a therapist to remark periodically that he or she has faith in the therapy and in the therapy team. Although the patient may often argue back, the power of this simple statement should not be underestimated.

Validating the Patient's Emotions, Behavior, and Thinking

The strategies for emotional, behavioral, and cognitive validation discussed above can be quite appropriate in the context of cheerleading.

4. CONTRADICTING/MODULATING EXTERNAL CRITICISM

When the therapist is cheerleading the patient, the patient will often refer to other people's stated lack of belief in her or criticisms of her as justification for her hopelessness and lack of self-belief. The therapist should point out that whether these criticisms are valid or not, they do not necessarily imply that the patient is hopeless. The therapist can (if honest) flatly disagree with the criticism. The therapist should not invalidate any negative feelings that the patient may be having in response to others' criticisms. Such emotional responses are understandable, and this understanding should be communicated.

5. PROVIDING PRAISE AND REASSURANCE

Praising the patient's behavior can be both reinforcing and encouraging. The therapist should make a determined effort to find and highlight evidence of improvement. An area that can always be praised is the patient's steadfastness in working on her problem, as evidenced by her remaining in therapy. As I discuss extensively in the next chapter, a borderline patient often experiences praise as threatening. Thus, for it to be an effective cheerleading technique, the therapist should surround it with reassurances. The content of the reassurance, of course, depends on the source of the threat. For example, if praise threatens termination of help or therapy, the therapist may say, "I know you still need help." If praise threatens too high expectations in the future, the therapist may say "I know how difficult it still is." And so on.

Some borderline patients seem to request reassurance endlessly. Therapists often feel that no matter how often they reassure such patients, their reassurances fall on deaf ears; they have no effect. When this occurs, it should be treated as a therapy interfering behavior and addressed directly. As I discuss further in Chapter 10, praise and reassurance should be gradually reduced as the patient learns to validate and soothe herself. This is, of course, especially important in Stage 3 (see Chapter 6) where self-respect is the primary target.

6. BEING REALISTIC, BUT DEALING DIRECTLY WITH FEARS OF INSINCERITY

A patient will sometimes respond to cheerleading with statements that she finds it hard to trust the therapist's sincerity. The first response to this should be to validate the lack of trust. The rules of therapy are so different from those of other relationships that the patient's uncertainty may well be understandable. At least, it may not be clear whether praise, encouragement, and cheerleading from a therapist have the same meaning as they do from someone else. After all, providing praise, encouragement and cheerleading is what the therapist is paid to do. Trust takes time to build; acknowledging that can be extremely validating for the patient.

Second, it is essential that the therapist be realistic in her or his cheerleading. To make this point in my case consultation group, I add the following to the story of the child in the earthquake (see above):

> Now, imagine the same earthquake situation. But add to it your knowledge that a huge boulder has fallen on the child. crushing her legs and hips, pinning her in the space where she is. Would you urge her to crawl, saying she can do it? No, you would soothe. You would console. You might search for more help, or you might stay near, no matter the danger to you. This is the balance that is needed with cheerleading.

Effective cheerleading is contingent on realistic goals. It is not helpful for the therapist to tell the patient that she can do anything in a situation when in fact her chance of even minimal success is limited. Although a therapist's faith in a patient's general ability to overcome difficulty may always be warranted, faith in her ability to achieve specific objectives should be tempered with a clear focus on reality.

7. STAYING NEAR

Cheerleaders and coaches do not leave a game early just because the team is doing well. Similarly, it is important that the therapist be available to offer coaching or other assistance if the patient runs into trouble. If the therapist tells a patient she can do something on her own, and then leaves her alone instead of standing in the wings, so to speak, it is understandable that the patient would suspect the therapist's motives in cheerleading. Since it is a habit of most busy people to "get rid" of others by telling them, "You don't need me," it is very important for the therapist to guard against inadvertently falling into this habit.

Concluding Comments

It is difficult to overestimate the importance of validation in DBT. Many problems in therapy are the result of insufficient validation and an excessive focus on change. The general rule to keep in mind is that every change strategy must be surrounded by validation. Often the excessive focus on change stems froms the therapist's anxiety about helping the patient; the therapist, like the patient, is having problems tolerating the distress. Validation has many roles in DBT. It soothes the patient through very difficult times in therapy. Done well, it enhances the therapeutic connection of patient and therapist. The patient feels understood and supported. The therapist strengthens his or her own empathetic attitude. Therapist validation teaches the patient to trust and validate herself. Finally, encourages the patient to keep going when she wants to throw in the towel.

9

Core Strategies:
Part II.
Problem Solving

Problem-solving strategies are the core DBT change strategies. In DBT, all dysfunctional behaviors, in and out of sessions, are viewed as problems to be solved—or, from another perspective, as faulty solutions to problems in living. Problem-solving strategies with borderline patients are designed to foster an active approach that can counteract the passive, helpless response commonly encountered among this population.

Levels of Problem Solving

First Level

At the first level, the entire DBT program can be seen as a general application of problem solving. The problem to be solved is a patient's overall life, and the solution is implementation of DBT. Problem-solving effectiveness here depends on whether DBT is the appropriate treatment for this particular patient. To date, the empirical data suggest that the treatment is appropriate for severely impaired borderline women; it may or may not be appropriate for other groups.

Second Level

DBT is a very flexible treatment and includes many treatment strategies and procedures. The second level of problem solving is figuring out which strategies and procedures should be applied to this specific patient, at this moment, for this problem. Most importantly, the therapist has to figure out which change strategies are most likely to be helpful. Problem-solving effectiveness here depends on whether the therapist correctly determines what is causing and maintaining the problem behaviors in need of change. Application of a specific change procedure is the problem solution at this level. The four main change procedures used in DBT (contingency management, skills training, cognitive modification, and exposure) are described in the next two chapters.

Third Level

At the third level, problem solving addresses specific problems that come up in the patient's day-to-day life. A DBT treatment session often begins with the patient's describing events that have occurred during the past week. This description may take place in the context of reviewing diary cards and responding to questions about suicide ideation or parasuicide during the previous week. During the initial stages of this discussion, the patient may describe situations involving emotions, thoughts, or actions that she felt unable to control. Or she may have reacted to her problems with suicidal or other dysfunctional behaviors. If the problem is ongoing, she may present a plan of action (suicidal or nonsuicidal) that she intends to pursue but that the therapist believes is either impulsive or likely to be dysfunctional.

Usually, the patient's problem is not as clearly articulated as the preceding statements might suggest. Sometimes the problem must be "dragged out" of the patient, so to speak, especially when the patient feels she has already solved the problem and wants to move on to a new problem. (This is especially likely, for example, when the patient has "solved" her problem via parasuicidal behavior.) At other times, the patient's problems will be presented in the context of emotional ventilation, involving anger, desperation, anxiety, or tearful depression. In either of these instances, the task of the therapist is to elicit a collaborative effort from the patient in developing and implementing new, more effective solutions to her current problems in life. Problem-solving effectiveness here depends on whether the therapist and patient can generate a solution to the specific problem the patient brings in, and whether the patient can or will carry out the solution.

Mood and Problem Solving

The effect of mood on problem solving is essential to understand in working with borderline patients. As I have noted repeatedly in this book, borderline patients are characterized by volatile mood swings. A baseline negative mood is most typical for chronically suicidal borderline patients, but all are sensitive to any mood-relevant therapeutic behaviors. Thus, a negative mood can at times be improved and a positive mood can be ruined by incidental or inadvertent therapist responses.

Problem solving, cognitive flexibility, and mood are inextricably linked. Flexibility is related to the ability to actively choose cognitive strategies that fit one's goals at a particular time, to adapt to one's environment, and to find creative yet relevant solutions to problems (Berg & Sternberg, 1985; Showers & Cantor, 1985; Simon, 1990). The ability to analyze problems (particularly aspects of one's own behavior and one's environment that are related to the problem) and to generate effective solutions, therefore, requires a certain amount of cognitive flexibility. A number of research studies suggest strongly that positive mood facilitates cognitive flexibility, and thus problem solving in general.

Positive mood enhances a person's ability to develop multiple, alternative interpretations of a situation and to see interconnections or similarities when required by a task, as well as to see important distinctions when that is required (Murray, Sujan, Hirt, & Sujan, 1990; Showers & Cantor, 1985). These abilities in turn are requisite to collaborating with the therapist in analyzing and interpreting behavioral patterns. Positive mood also enhances creativity, including generation of problem solutions (Isen, Daubman, & Nowicki, 1987; Isen, Johnson, Mertz, & Robins, 1985). When asked to generate solutions to problems, individuals in a positive mood, relative to others, may organize information differently, see relationships they would not ordinarily see, and use more creative and intuitive cognitive strategies (Fiedler, 1988). Evaluating the outcomes associated with particular solutions is also affected by mood. For example, subjective estimates of risk and the likelihood of positive versus negative outcomes are related to an individual's current positive or negative mood (see Williams, 1993, for a review of this literature).

These points are essential to keep in mind when applying problem solving with borderline patients. In particular, the therapist should expect that problem solving will often go more slowly and be more difficult than with many other patient populations. The need for sympathetic understanding and for interventions aimed at enhancing current positive mood during problem solving can be extremely important. The effectiveness of validation strategies may result in part from their mood-enhancing effects. Understanding these points and mentally rehearsing them while interacting with the patient may also be helpful in heading off inappropriate interpretations of the patient's passive problem solving or negative attitudes toward proposed solutions as simply not trying or not wanting to change.

A primary task of the therapist is to orient the patient to seeing maladaptive behavior as in fact a result of attempting to solve problems in living. With help, these problems can be solved in a more functional and adaptive fashion. The six groups of problem-focused strategies discussed in this chapter—behavioral analysis, insight strategies, didactic strategies, solution analysis, orienting strategies, and commitment strategies—may be repeated as new problems are brought up for discussion. In some cases, the sequence will be modified and/or several sections will need to be repeated (seemingly over and over) in dealing with a single problem issue. The application of problem-solving strategies to the more general case of selecting DBT as the treatment for a particular patient is discussed more extensively in Chapter 14.

Overview of Problem-Solving Strategies

Problem solving is a two-stage process: (1) understanding and accepting the problem at hand, and (2) attempting to generate, evaluate, and implement alternative solutions that might have been used or could be used in the future in similar problematic situations. The acceptance stage employs behavioral analysis, insight strategies, and didactic strategies; the second stage, that of targeting change, employs solution analysis, orienting strategies, and commitment strategies.

Although it may seem obvious, solving problems requires first accepting of the existence of a problem. As noted earlier, therapeutic change can only occur within the context of acceptance of what is. In the case of borderline patients, problem solving is enormously complicated by their frequent tendency to view themselves negatively and their inability to regulate the consequent emotional distress. On the one pole, they have difficulty correctly identifying problems in their environment, tending instead to view all problems as somehow self-generated. On the other pole, viewing all problems as self-generated is so painful that the patients often respond by inhibiting the process of self-reflection. Repeated attempts to address both the failures in dialectical thinking that have led to these positions and the accompanying negative emotions may be necessary before the patients can acknowledge the existence of the more painful problems. The validation strategies described in Chapter 8, and the irreverent communication strategies, described in Chapter 12, aid this process without reinforcing suicidal or other extreme behaviors.

Behavioral analysis requires a chain analysis of the events and situational factors leading up to and following the particular problematic response at hand. The analysis is conducted in great detail, with close attention to the reciprocal interaction between the environment and the patient's cognitive, emotional, and behavioral responses. Insight strategies, which are pulled apart from behavioral analysis arbitrarily for the purposes of the present discussion, include observing and labeling patterns of behavior and situational influence over time. The analysis of the problem proceeds in a nonjudgmental fashion, with attention to the patient's tendency both to experience panic and to engage in ruthless, vindictive evaluative judgments whenever behaviors or behavioral outcomes are less than expected or desired. Typically, the target of these judgments shifts, sometimes with lightning speed, from the self as generating the problem to other people or the environment as the sole source of the problem. Throughout, the therapist provides information to the patient in a didactic fashion about characteristics of behavior and people in general, and of borderline behavior in particular. This information both normalizes the patient's own behavior and serves as a source of hypotheses about what may be maintaining the patient's behavior, as well as what may help in the change process.

The second problem-solving stage begins with the generation and evaluation of alternative solutions that can be used in the future. Once a range of solutions has been generated, the therapist and patient review what is required to implement the change procedures. That is, the therapist orients the patient to the change process. Finally, the therapist and patient commit themselves to the implementation of the solutions generated. Putting commitment at the end of problem solving is done purely for illustrative purposes; in reality, it precedes, accompanies, and follows change procedures.

BEHAVIORAL ANALYSIS STRATEGIES

Behavioral analysis is one of the most important and most difficult sets of strategies in DBT. Many, if not most, therapeutic errors are assessment errors; that is, they are therapeutic responses based on a faulty understanding and assessment of the problem at hand. Behavioral analysis is the first step in problem solving. Treatment of any new patient, or of any new problem behavior with a current patient, requires an adequate behavioral analysis to guide the selection of an appropriate intervention. In addition, the emergence (or omission) of currently targeted problem behaviors between one session and the next, as well as failures in self-control programs (e.g., attempts to increase positive behaviors, and decrease negative behaviors) or problems arising within the therapy process itself, should be responded to first with a behavioral analysis.

The purpose of a behavioral analysis is to figure out what the problem is, what is causing it, what is interfering with the resolution of the problem, and what aids are available to help solve the problem. In some instances, some of this information is already known or can be surmised. Thus, the process of conducting a behavioral analysis may be brief, involving only a few questions, or quite lengthy, requiring one or more entire therapy sessions. The point in either case, however, is to check out in an empirical fashion what the therapist is either surmising from experience with the particular patient or hypothesizing from theory; in a way, it is a counterpoint to therapist bias. Thus, it should not be dispensed with or run through in a cavalier fashion. The only exceptions are cases when intervention, even without an assessment, is urgent; when other activities clearly take priority; or when the therapist is very sure of his or her assessment of the situation.

As noted earlier, behavioral analysis is presented separately from insight strategies in this chapter for purely instructional purposes. In reality, behavioral analysis will always include insight strategies; in turn, insight into a patient's problems and behavioral patterns depends on the judicious use of behavioral analysis. In most textbooks on behavioral assessment, the two sets of strategies are combined, with the whole being labeled "behavioral analysis" or "functional analysis." For our purposes, the two sets of strategies can be separated as follows. Behavioral analysis in DBT refers specifically to the in-depth analysis of one particular instance or set of instances of a problem or a targeted behavior. Thus it is a self-conscious and focused attempt on the part of the therapist (and, one hopes, the patient) to determine the factors leading up to, following, and "controlling" or influencing the behavior. Therapeutic insight is the feedback the therapist gives the patient about patterns of behavior that have emerged either within the relationship, during session-to-session discussion, or over the course of a number of separate behavioral analyses.

Three aspects of the behavioral analysis process are critical: (1) The analysis must be carried out collaboratively (this necessitates the concurrent use of other strategies, such as validation and contingency management); (2) it must provide sufficient detail to give an accurate and reasonably complete picture of the sequence of internal and external events associated with the problem behavior; and (3) conclusions must be accepted in a manner that will permit their abandonment if they are later disconfirmed. The ultimate goal is to teach the patient to perform a competent behavioral analysis on her own. Behavioral analysis includes a number of steps, which are discussed below and summarized in Table 9.1.

There are any number of ways to divide up the conduct of such as analysis. Not every aspect of the steps discussed below is always required, and the order is not invariant. But the therapist should, at a minimum, obtain all of the indicated information.

I. DEFINING THE PROBLEM BEHAVIOR

Choosing a Focus

The focus of problem definition is determined by a number of factors. At the first level (see "Levels of Problem Solving," above), when therapy is beginning or when its targets or goals are shifting, the target priority list (see Chapter 6, Table 6.1) is used as a guideline. Problems are explored in all seven of the specified areas: suicidal behaviors, therapy-interfering behaviors, behaviors that interfere with quality of life, behavioral skills deficits, posttraumatic stress responses, problems with self-respect, and difficulties in achieving individual goals. At the second level, when therapy is in progress, the focus of assessment is determined by the order of targets within the DBT hierarchy. Thus, during the first phase of therapy, any suicidal, therapy-interfering, or quality-of-life-interfering behaviors that have occurred since the last session are addressed explicitly (in that order of priority, although not necessarily that order in time). During the second phase of therapy, posttraumatic stress responses are probed and analyzed. During the final phase of therapy, failures in self-respect and in meeting individual goals are observed and responded to. At the third level, if no prioritized problem behaviors have occurred, the patient sets the agenda and focus.

TABLE 9.1. Behavioral Analysis Strategies Checklist

____ T helps P DEFINE THE PROBLEM BEHAVIOR.

    ____ T helps P formulate the problem in terms of behavior.

    ____ T helps P describe the problem behavior specifically, in these terms:
        ____ Frequency of behavior.
        ____ Duration of behavior.
        ____ Intensity of Behavior.
        ____ Topography of behavior.

    ____ T weaves validation throughout.

____ T conducts a CHAIN ANALYSIS.

    ____ T and P select one instance of problem to analyze.

    ____ T attends to small units of behavior (the links of the chain), with attention to defining the chain's beginning (antecedents), middle (the problem instance itself), and end (consequences) in terms of the following:
        ____ Emotions.
        ____ Bodily sensations.
        ____ Thoughts and images.
        ____ Overt behaviors.
        ____ Environmental factors.

    ____ T conducts brief chain analyses as necessary of in-session events.

    ____ T maintains P's (and own) cooperation.

    ____ T helps P develop methods to monitor her behavior between sessions.

____ T GENERATES HYPOTHESES with P about variables influencing or controlling the behaviors in question.

    ____ T uses the results of previous analyses to guide the current one.

    ____ T is guided by DBT theory.

Anti-DBT tactics

____ T colludes with P in avoiding behavioral analysis of targeted behaviors.

____ T unduly biases information gathering to prove T's own theory of P's behavior.

This process of arriving at a problem to be analyzed differs from the behavioral case formulation method of Turkat (1990) in that the highest-priority targets are not so much those "primary" problems that may be seen as giving rise to all other symptoms, but those problems that embody the gravest immediate threat to continued life, therapy, and minimal quality of life, in that order. From the DBT point of view, assessment of any problem will soon lead to the "primary" problem through the interrelationships between behavioral systems and across problems that emerge through repeated behavioral analyses. Arrival at these primary problems is dependent on conduct of very thorough chain analyses, as described later.

Formulating the Problem in Terms of Behavior

Although at times the problem to be solved is the environment's behavior, not the patient's, the therapeutic task is to formulate the problem in terms of some aspect of the patient's or therapist's feelings, thoughts, or actions. For example, with a patient in a severely abusive marriage the problem may be cast as the patient's not finding the situation acceptable. The eventual solution may then be to leave the partner or act in a way that causes the partner to either stop the abuse or be controlled by others. By defining the patient's behavior of not leaving the partner or not acting to change the partner's abusive interaction as the problem, I am not suggesting that the environment is not dysfunctional, maladaptive, and aversive. Nonetheless, a defining characteristic of all psychotherapy with adults, including DBT, is that the primary focus is on the patient's behavior in situations, not on the situations themselves.

As I have noted previously, a borderline patient often presents a solution to a problem (e.g., "I'm going to kill myself") without being able to identify the problem. The patient may present extremely painful emotions or discuss aversive environmental situations without being able to label such events as problem situations to be solved. At other times, the patient will describe a situation or event in such ambiguous and nonspecific terms that it is difficult to isolate the problem with any precision. In either case, the therapist should tell the patient that the first task is to identify the specific problem clearly and in terms of behavior. At times, the patient will be unwilling to engage in such a discussion; in these instances, the therapist should simply repeatedly formulate for the patient what the problem behavior appears to be. As noted in Chapter 8, however, it is critical for the therapist not to assume automatically that the problem is the patient's distortion of a situation rather than the aversiveness of a situation itself.

Describing the Problem Specifically

Problem definition should be specific, not general. Defining a problem as "feeling upset and blue every day" is general. Saying the problem is "feeling depressed every day" is more specific but still too general. The goal is to describe precisely and in detail exactly what the individual means by "depression" and by "every day." Thus, once the problem behavior pattern is identified in general, the therapist should obtain a precise description of the behavior in terms of its topography (i.e., exactly what the patient did), the frequency of its occurrence since the last session, and its intensity (i.e., strength or depth of the behavior).

Some examples of useful questions for eliciting specific descriptions are as follows: "What do you mean by that, exactly?" "How many times did that happen last week?" "How long [how many minutes] did that feeling stay with you?" "Did a thought run through your mind at that point? What was it?" "How intense was the feeling or desire on a 1–100 scale?" Although after a few behavior analyses the therapist and patient may not need such detailed questioning, the therapist must nonetheless be very careful not to assume that things are clear when they have not been made clear. The assumption of facts not in evidence seems to be one of the most common mistakes people make when learning how to do behavior analysis.

Specific therapeutic strategies for obtaining this information and arriving at a definition of the problem include the validation strategies of active observing, reflection, helping the patient observe and label emotions reading emotions, asking multiple-choice emotion questions, eliciting noninferential and nonjudgmental descriptions of behavior, eliciting and reflecting the patient's thoughts, and assessing the facts (see Chapter 8).

Validating the Patient's Distress

It is difficult to focus on solving a problem if one has not first accepted the validity of having the problem in the first place. As noted in Chapter 8, borderline and suicidal individuals quite often have difficulty experiencing and admitting to having painful emotions or needing help. Thus, validating strategies must be interwoven with all of the assessment strategies.

2. CONDUCTING A CHAIN ANALYSIS

Choosing a Specific Instance of Behavior to Analyze.

Once the problem behavior is identified, the next task is to develop an exhaustive, step-by-step description of the chain of events leading up to and following the behavior. At the first level, when therapy is beginning, the therapist will need to mix more general analyses of the overall pattern of problem behaviors, their antecedents, and their consequences with more detailed analyses of some specific instances. Chapter 14 describes how to do this.

At the second level, chain analyses will focus on any instances of DBT target behaviors that have occurred since the last session or that are ongoing in the current therapeutic interaction. The important point here is that although the therapist should get an overview each session of how often a particular problem behavior occurred, a chain analysis requires that one instance of the behavior be selected. This point cannot be overstressed. The essence of conducting a chain analysis is examining a particular instance of a specific dysfunctional behavior in excruciating detail. Much of the therapeutic work in DBT is the ceaseless analysis of specific instances of targeted behaviors, each time integrating new information with old information to evolve a definition of patterns and to explore possible new behavioral solutions to continuing problem events.

Why such an emphasis on detailed assessment of individual episodes? It is because the therapist does not rely on the patient's unaided ability to remember, analyze, select important antecedents and consequences, and synthesize information across a number of episodes. That is, the therapist does not assume that the patient comes to therapy with good behavioral analysis skills already in place. When a targeted behavior or problem situation has occurred more than once during the preceding week or is currently evident in the session, a number of factors can influence which one is chosen for analysis. How severe or intense the instance was, how well remembered it is, how important it was in setting off other events, and the patient's own preference are all important. When severity and priority are equivalent, the therapist should select behaviors occurring within the session over those occurring between sessions for analysis. Over time and repeated analyses, a sample of behavioral instances will be chosen that represents the entire class of events.

At the third level, if no DBT high-priority behaviors are relevant for analysis or a crisis situation has developed demanding attention, the focus of the analysis is determined by the patient as noted earlier.

Attending to the Links of the Chain

Where to Start? Since maladaptive behavior is viewed as a solution to a problem, a good way to figure out the beginning of the chain is to ask the patient when the problem began. Maladaptive behavior is viewed as occurring within a context or an episode that for the purposes of analysis has a beginning, a middle (the behavior in question), and an end. In my experience, a patient can usually pinpoint, at least roughly, when that episode began. The idea, however, is to locate in the environment the event that precipitated the patient's chain of behavior. Although precipitating events may at times be difficult to pinpoint, this task is very important. The overall goal is to link the patient's behavior to environmental events, especially ones that she may not realize are having an effect on her behavior. For example, the patient may simply have woken up feeling hopeless and suicidal, or she may not be able to identify anything in the environment that set off a series of worries. Nonetheless, the therapist should get a good description of events co-occurring with the onset of the problem, even if these events at first appear unrelated to the patient's behavior. Rather than asking "What caused that?", the therapist should ask "What set that off?" or "What was going on at the moment the problem started?" Therapists not trained in behavioral therapies, as well as patients, may be tempted to give up this search too easily. With persistence and the passage of time, however, a pattern of events associated with problem initiation may emerge.

Filling in the Links. The key here is that the therapist has to think in terms of very small units of behavior—the links in the chain, so to speak. A common problem is that many therapists assume they understand the link between one behavioral response and the next, and thus fail to identify many links in the chain that may turn out to be important. Once the therapist and patient identify the start of the chain, the therapist should get very detailed information about what was going on both in the environment and behaviorally with the patient at that point. By "behaviorally," I mean what the patient was doing, feeling (emotions and sensations), thinking (both explicitly and implicitly, as in expectations and assumptions), and imagining.

Once one link is described, the therapist should ask, "What next?" Behavioral and environmental events should be described for each link in the chain. Both patient and therapist may be inclined at times to jump over a number of links. To fill in links, the therapist can ask questions of the "How did you get from here to there?" type—for example, "How did you get from feeling like you wanted to talk to me to calling me on the phone?" When one patient and I were analyzing a suicide attempt, the patient told me that before she attempted suicide she decided to kill herself. I asked what had led up to this decision. She said that it was her feeling that life was too painful to live any longer. From the patient's point of view, the link between feeling that life was unendurable and deciding to kill herself was self-evident, but it was not to me. Indeed, it seemed to me that one could decide life was too painful to live any longer and then decide to change life. Or one could believe that death would be even more painful and decide to tolerate life despite its pain. As it turned out upon questioning, the patient actually assumed that she would be happier dead than alive. Challenging this assumption then became one of the solutions to stopping her persistent attempts at suicide.

The strategy here is almost exactly the opposite of the validation strategy of reading the patient's emotions, behavior, or mind, described in Chapter 8. Rather than understanding the links in the chain, the therapist must play the role of naive observer, understanding nothing and questioning everything. This is not to suggest that figuring out the links in the chain independently of the patient is never helpful. It can be when the patient skips over parts of the chain of events. At these points, the therapist can question whether a particular event, thought, or feeling might not be an important link.

The goals here are several. First, the therapist wants to identify events that may automatically elicit maladaptive behaviors or are precursors to them. Emotional responses in particular, but also other behaviors, may be controlled primarily through their conditioned associations with events. Second, the therapist wants to identify behavioral deficits that may have set up the problematic responses. If parasuicide is a "cry for help," it may be that alternative help-seeking behaviors are unavailable to the person. Third, the therapist wants to pinpoint events, either in the environment or in the person's prior responses (fears, beliefs, incompatible behaviors), that might have interfered with more appropriate behaviors. Finally, the therapist wants to get a general idea of how the person arrives at dysfunctional responses, as well as of possible alternative paths she could have taken.

Where to Stop? A chain analysis requires information concerning events that led up to the problem behavior (antecedents), as well as information about the consequences of the behavior. The most important consequences are those that may be influencing the problem behavior by maintaining, strengthening, or increasing it (reinforcers). These may include the occurrence of preferable events, the nonoccurrence or cessation of aversive events, or opportunities to engage in preferable behaviors. Similarly, the therapist wants to identify consequences that may be important in weakening or decreasing the problem behavior.

As with events preceding the behavior, the therapist should obtain information about external events (the effects of the behavior on the external context or relationships) as well as internal events (emotions, somatic sensations, actions, images, thoughts, assumptions, and expectations). It is important to get information both about the events that occur and about their valence or attraction to the patient. The therapist needs some knowledge of rudimentary principles of reinforcement. For example, immediate effects are more likely to influence behavior over effects that are temporally distant from the behavior. Intermittent reinforcement can be a powerful method of making a behavior very resistant to extinction. Punishment will suppress behavior, but if another potentially reinforcing response is not available, the behavior will typically reappear once the punishment is removed.

The goal here is to ascertain the function of the behavior, or, in other words, to determine what problem the behavior has solved. A most important point to keep in mind is that the patient may not be aware of what function the behavior has, nor of which of many consequences are important in maintaining the behavior. This is true of most behavior for most people; most behavioral learning occurs outside of awareness. (Or, from another point of view, most learning is implicit rather than explicit.) It is equally important to keep in mind that saying that consequences maintain behavior is not the same thing as saying that an individual does something "in order to" get the consequences. For example, students can influence where a professor stands in a classroom or what he or she says, simply by nodding and smiling when the professor moves in the targeted direction or makes certain comments. Inevitably, this effect occurs without the professor's awareness. Does this mean that the professor changes his or her behavior in order to get the nods or smiles of the students? A computer can be programmed to vary its "behavior," depending on consequences; does this mean that the computer acts in order to get certain consequences? Yet it is this very imputation of "in order to" that often gets in the way of patients' willingness to explore the effects of consequences on their behavior—primarily because the "in order to" is often inferred, is inaccurate, is not in accord with their phenomenological experiences, and imputes pejorative motives. Explaining these points, as I indicate later in the discussion of didactic strategies, is a very important part of the therapy.

Conducting Brief Chain Analyses of In-Session Behaviors

When currently targeted behaviors occur within a therapy session, they should be analyzed immediately. When the focus is on an in-session behavior, however, a chain analysis will often be shortened, consisting of perhaps only a few questions. For example, if the patient threatens suicide, the therapist might stop and ask several questions to determine what led up to the threat, comment on other alternative responses the patient could have made at each point, and then return to the previous discussion topic. Such a digression may take only a few minutes, but can have very powerful effects if done consistently. This technique blends conceptually with insight strategies (see below).

Maintaining Cooperation

Getting the patient to cooperate with chain analyses is one of the essential tasks of therapy. In my experience, both therapists and patients often resist this work. Patients have any number of reasons for avoiding it. First, it involves a great deal of effort, often when they are exhausted, want nurturing, or have settled into active-passivity responding. Analyzing past dysfunctional behavior also commonly elicits intensely painful shame. Furthermore, it interferes with patients' current interpretations of their behavior—interpretations that the patients may be motivated to hold on to. Finally, since the behavior is past, patients often want to forget it and attend to the crises of the moment. Even when old problems are attended to, patients want to focus on the situation (which can be either the environment, their own behavior, or a blend of the two) that set off the chain rather than on their maladaptive solutions. Therapists must remember that much of the time, dysfunctional behaviors are viewed as problems by therapists but as solutions by patients. Reminding patients of the problematic aspects of their behaviors and their commitment to work on these behaviors may be necessary, sometimes over and over.

Therapists also may prefer to avoid these analyses. As for the patients, they involve a lot of active work. It is often easier and frequently more interesting just to sit and listen to the patients talk. For many therapists, it is difficult to direct patients or to get them to do things in therapy they don't want to do. Some are afraid that if they make the patients go through chain analyses, the patients may get suicidal. Or the intense resistance and hostility directed at the therapists are simply too aversive. In my experience, the tendency to avoid behavioral analysis in general and chain analysis in particular is one of the major impediments to conducting DBT. The most helpful antidote is the case consultation team.

Using Previous Analyses to Guide the Current Analysis

After a number of chain analyses of a particular behavior pattern, the therapist should work collaboratively with the patient to generate several hypotheses about usual or typical controlling variables. These hypotheses may relate to the situations in which the problem behavior occurs; other behaviors (thoughts, feelings, sensations, and overt actions) that ordinarily lead to the problem behavior; reinforcers that may be maintaining the problem behavior; beliefs and expectancies about the utility of the problem behavior; and so on. The therapist and patient should discuss and generate these hypotheses together. Hypotheses formulated should, in turn, guide the information explored during the next chain analysis. That is, once a hypothesis is formed, subsequent chain analyses can be used to test its validity. In this manner, the information searched for becomes more fine-tuned over time.

Helping the Patient to Monitor Her Behavior

As noted earlier in this chapter, there is ample experimental evidence to demonstrate that current mood can have a powerful effect on memory and on how information is organized, retrieved, and processed (Williams, 1993). This is a particular problem in treating borderline patients, since variable mood and affect regulation is a defining characteristic of the population. In DBT, emphasis is given not only to behaviors occurring within the treatment session, but also to behaviors and events occurring since the last session. In order to assess and treat these behaviors properly, more or less accurate information is essential.

Reliance on unaided memory is the least acceptable way of obtaining information. Thus, in DBT, as in most types of behavior therapy, there is an emphasis on having patients monitor their own behavior on a daily basis. Use of the diary cards described in Chapter 6 is an essential component of DBT, at least during the first two phases of therapy, where very specific behaviors are targeted. These cards provide a record of frequency and intensity of problem behaviors during the interval between individual sessions. They do not, however, record information about events surrounding the problem behaviors. Thus, these cards are best used as signals of problems that need tracking and assessment.

Whether a patient should be requested to keep more detailed diary records depends on the patient's ability to remember events, the current phase of problem assessment, and the patient's ability and willingness to monitor behavior in writing. Some patients are quite good at verbally reconstructing events surrounding problem behaviors. Although a week or two of daily monitoring might be a good idea to check the validity of these patients' recall, ongoing daily monitoring is often not needed. Other patients seem to have great difficulty recalling the specific details surrounding stressful behaviors. In-session chain analyses of behavior with these patients can be quite helpful in teaching them how to organize and recall events. In my experience, after a number of such analyses, most patients improve in their ability to attend to, organize, and recall specific details of both problem behaviors and the events surrounding them. There is some evidence to suggest that this improvement in specific recall ability may be one of the therapeutic mechanisms of DBT (Williams, 1991).

In a comprehensive behavioral log, the therapist should include space for recording a brief description of the problem behavior; the date, duration, and frequency of the behavior, the place or context of the behavior (where and who with); thoughts, feelings, and other behaviors preceding the problem behavior (antecedents); and what happened afterwards (consequences). Depending on the task, one or more of these categories may be dropped or collapsed into another. The use of such a log provides an opportunity for the therapist to help the patient learn to observe and describe the who, what, when, where, and how of events; to discriminate inferences from observations; and to structure and organize recall to maximum benefit of behavior change.

When daily monitoring is used, therapist and patient should collaborate on the form of the monitoring system. The importance of this cannot be overemphasized. Patients almost always have definite opinions and preferences about how to structure this task; it is pointless and unnecessary to impose a particular format on them.

Some patients love to keep diaries, and will arrive at each session with copious notes and records of the preceding week or will send daily diaries through the mail. With these patients, the task usually is to structure their record keeping so that data can be easily and quickly extracted and organized. Other patients are very unwilling or are actually unable to do comprehensive daily monitoring. Although filling out DBT diary cards is required (and so far I have never had a patient who was unable to fill out a card), other monitoring should be at the discretion of each therapist and patient. Dyslexic patients, for example, often have great difficulty with any writing task. Other patients report that their problems interfere with their ability to focus on a monitoring task.

Whether a refusal or inability to undertake self-monitoring is viewed as therapy-interfering behavior depends on the importance of the information to the conduct of the therapy. For example, if cognitive modification procedures are being used to change ongoing or frequent thoughts and assumptions, it is next to impossible for a patient to recall accurately and specifically during a therapy session her sequence of thoughts during the previous week, or the way in which these thoughts were related to problem behaviors. Daily monitoring here may be essential, and the therapist should be very careful not to drop it just because the patient does not want to do it or finds it difficult. At other times, monitoring may be useful but is not really essential. For example, in my experience, most patients can (with help) learn to remember reasonably accurately the events leading up to, surrounding, and following parasuicidal behavior. A therapist should not insist on monitoring just because it seems like a good idea.

3. GENERATING HYPOTHESES ABOUT FACTORS CONTROLLING BEHAVIOR

Using Theory to Guide Analysis

DBT assumes that each individual has a unique pattern of variables controlling her "borderline" behaviors, and, in addition, that the variables controlling behavior in one instance may be different from those guiding it in another.

Also, as noted in Chapter 2, DBT does not assume that any particular behavioral system, such as actions, cognitions, physiological/biological responses, or sensory responses, is intrinsically more important than another in the elicitation or maintenance of problematic behavior. In this sense, DBT is based on neither pure cognitive nor pure behavioral theory. Although reference is always made to the environmental context of behavior, DBT assumes that proximal causes of behavior may be behavioral or environmental, depending on the specific instance.

This does not mean, however, that DBT has no theoretical preferences; it does, and they are very important. With respect to antecedent or eliciting variables, DBT focuses most closely on intense or aversive emotional states. Maladaptive behavior, to a large extent, is viewed as resulting from emotion dysregulation. The amelioration of unendurable emotional pain is always suspected as one of the primary motivational factors in borderline dysfunctional behavior. Thus, in any chain analysis antecedent emotional behaviors should be explored in particular depth. DBT also suggests typical patterns or chains of events that are likely to lead to these aversive emotional states. That is, DBT suggests various sets of environmental events and patient behaviors that are probably instrumental in producing and maintaining borderline behaviors. Behavioral deficits in dialectical thinking and the ability to synthesize polarities, as well as deficits in the behavioral skills of mindfulness, interpersonal effectiveness (especially in conflict resolution), affect regulation, distress tolerance, and self-management, are theoretically important to assess.

From a somewhat different perspective, DBT suggests that particular sets of extreme behavior patterns are also likely both to be instrumental in the generation and maintenance of borderline behavior, and with the process of change. These patterns include deficits in emotional modulation, self-validation, realistic reasoning and judgment, emotional experiencing, active problem solving, and accurate expressions of emotional states and competence. Corresponding to these deficits, and usually co-occurring with them, are excesses in emotional reactivity, self-invalidation, crisis-generating behaviors, grief inhibition, active-passivity behaviors, and mood dependency. These patterns and their relationship to BPD and therapy are discussed extensively in the first three chapters of this book. The interested reader should review these chapters carefully before initiating DBT assessments with borderline patients.

INSIGHT (INTERPRETATION) STRATEGIES

The goal of insight strategies, as the label suggests, is to help the patient notice patterns and achieve insight into functional interrelationships. Although this is a fundamental goal of behavioral analysis as described above, the therapist may also offer his or her own "insights" at many other points in therapy, independently of a formal behavioral analysis. Offering therapeutic insights (typically labeled "interpretations" in more traditional psychothera-pies) can be very powerful in both a positive and a negative sense. Thus, it is essential that they be offered as hypotheses to be tested rather than as im-mutable facts. Furthermore, the therapist should be careful to recognize that the insights offered are products of his or her own cognitive processes, and thus are not necessarily accurate representations of events external to the therapist.

Therapeutic behaviors that come under the rubric of insight include com-menting on the patient's behavior; summarizing what a patient has said or done in such a way as to coordinate and emphasize certain aspects; noticing and commenting on an observed interrelationship; and commenting on the implications of a particular patient behavior, such as an attitude or emotion that is implied. Offering such insights or interpretations is a fundamental part of all psychotherapy (Frank, 1973) as well as DBT. Insight is often used when the main focus of therapy is on another topic but the therapist wants to note a particular behavior or pattern for later reference. At other times, it may be the prelude to refocusing a session on topics the patient is avoiding or hop-ing the therapist will not notice. Insights can be brief and subtle, as when the therapist wants to cue the patient to a behavior or pattern but wants the patient to arrive at the conclusion on her own, or confrontational, as when the therapist is trying to push the patient to a more active or more flexible stance. In contrast to behavioral analysis, insight strategies focus more often on behaviors occurring within the therapeutic interaction.

Insight strategies do not take the place of behavioral analysis. Insights are formulations of various theories about what the patient is doing and why she is doing it. In behavioral analysis, patient and therapist attempt to verify these insights. It is important to keep in mind, however, that interpretations, like others theories, cannot be evaluated in terms of "truth" but only in terms of utility. They either help in the change process or do not help, and at times they can actually be detrimental. Kohlenberg and Tsai (1991) note that "every form of psychotherapy seems to include teaching the client to give reasons [for behavior] that are acceptable to the therapist." They go on to summarize Woolfolk and Messer (1988), who have suggested that psychoanalysis can be described as a process in which the patient tells what happened and gives reasons. The therapist then interprets, giving different reasons, and therapy is complete when the client's reasons are the same as the therapist's. Insight strategies are summarized in Table 9.2.

What and How to Interpret: Guidelines for Insight

Theorists differ markedly in regard to what behaviors should be interpreted with borderline patients and how these interpretations should be carried out. For example, Kernberg (1975) suggests focusing on the negative features of "transference." Masterson (1990) recommends keeping the focus on maladap-tive behavior outside the session. Many clinicians support challenging and

TABLE 9.2. Insight (Interpretation) Strategies Checklist

_____ T focuses insights on DBT target behaviors and their precursors.
_____ T explores current, observable, public behaviors and events.
    _____ T comments on in-session behaviors, with a special emphasis on behaviors obeservable to T.
_____ T uses DBT assumptions about patients and biosocial theory to structure insights.
_____ T favors nonpejorative, empathetic interpretations.
_____ T interprets behavior in terms of current eliciting and maintaining variables.
_____ T observes effects of insights, and changes pattern or type of insights offered accordingly.
_____ T uses insights sparingly and surrounds them with validation.
_____ T HIGHLIGHTS or comments on P's behavior.
    _____ T interjects a behavioral observation in an ongoing discussion with P.
    _____ T makes comments about P's behavior such as "Have you noticed that. . .?" or "Don't you think it's interesting that. . .?"
    _____ T balances highlighting of negative behavior with that of positive behavior.
_____ T helps P OBSERVE AND DESCRIBE recurrent patterns (behavioral, environmental, or both) in the context of constructing meaning out of the events of P's life.
    _____ T identifies recurring thoughts.
    _____ T identifies recurring affective responses.
    _____ T identifies recurring behavioral sequences.
    _____ T helps P observe and describe patterns of stimuli and their associative relationships that elicit (classical conditioning model) or reinforce/punish (operant conditioning model) P's response patterns.
_____ T comments on possible IMPLICATIONS of P's behavior.
_____ T EXPLORES DIFFICULTIES in accepting or rejecting hypotheses about behavior, in an open flexible manner.
    _____ T is open to possibility of P's interpretations being correct.

Anti-DBT tactics

_____ T imputes motives to P independently of P's perceptions of her own wishes, desires, or goals.
_____ T maintains insights according to theoretical bias, instead of basing them on observations of P's behavior and surrounding events.
_____ T insists on interpretations and operates in a noncollaborative manner.
_____ T offers pejorative interpretations when nonpejorative ones are available for the same behaviors and facts.
_____ T engages in circular reasoning, insisting that outcomes of behavior prove motives.
_____ T uses interpretations to attack, blame, or punish P.

confronting the patients' own interpretations (Kernberg, 1975; Masterson, 1990; Gunderson, 1984), while others point out the hazards of confrontations (Sederer & Thorbeck, 1986; Schaffer, 1986). Both Gunderson (1984) and Schaffer (1986) stress the importance of empathetic or affirmative interpretations. How does insight or interpretation in DBT differ from that offered in other types of therapies? The main differences are in the emphasis on observable, targeted behavior (what to interpret), as well as the assumptions that guide insight formulation (how to interpret).

What to Interpret

There are three general guidelines about what patient behaviors can or should be interpreted. The first guideline is that the majority of comments should focus directly on behaviors within the DBT hierarchy of targets or on behaviors functionally related to them. For example, suicidal behaviors or behaviors that commonly lead to them would take first priority; behaviors that either interfere with ongoing therapy or are predictive of upcoming problems would take second priority; and so on. The second guideline is that, all other things being equal, insights should focus on observable or public behaviors and events as opposed to private ones. Behaviors become public (to the therapist) under two conditions: Either the therapist observes them, or the patient reports private behaviors of her own that she has observed (e.g., what she is thinking or feeling or sensing). The third guideline is that insights should focus on events and behaviors in the present as opposed to those in the past.

All these points taken together suggest that the most effective insights are those pertaining to the patient's behaviors as they occur in interactions with the therapist (by phone or in person). Data presented by Marziali (1984) suggest that the greater the extent to which interpretations are focused on in-session behaviors, the more positive the treatment outcome. This approach works best when the patient's problematic behaviors occur spontaneously or can be elicited during interactions with the therapist. As Kohlenberg and Tsai (1991) have pointed out, the ideal therapeutic relationship is one that evokes the patient's problematic or clinically relevant behaviors, while at the same time providing opportunities for developing more effective alternative behaviors. Problematic interpersonal styles and behavior patterns that interfere with therapy are the behaviors most likely to occur in a borderline patient's interactions with her therapist, and thus the best candidates for insight. However, many other important problematic behaviors will occur in therapy interactions, including suicidal ideation and threats, emotional dysregulation, intolerance of distress and agitation, failures in self-management and impulsive behaviors, difficulties with mindfulness (especially with observing and describing nonjudgmentally), and the full range of posttraumatic stress responses. Similarly, improvements in each of these areas are also likely to be demonstrated within therapeutic interactions. Thus, the therapist should attend closely for opportunities to observe and comment on instances of patient behaviors that are relevant to clinical progress.

This constant but intermittent focus on behaviors occurring during the therapeutic session sets DBT apart from many other types of behavior therapy, where the usual focus is on behaviors occurring between sessions. The one exception to this guideline has to do with parasuicidal behavior and with planning and preparing for suicide, which rarely occur in the presence of the therapist. Since these are high-priority behaviors, the therapist must attempt to build insight relevant to the factors eliciting and maintaining these behaviors. Once the precursors are identified, however, the therapist should watch for their emergence in therapeutic interactions. For example, Mary was a patient of mine who characteristically cut her wrists whenever she felt intense emotions and believed that others were not taking her feelings seriously. In sessions, I noticed that Mary often communicated intense emotions in a bland, unemotional style, which made it difficult to take her seriously. I frequently commented that her verbal and nonverbal expressions conveyed different information, and that this made it hard for me to know how intensely she was actually feeling. At times, this comment would refocus the discussion on a behavioral analysis of factors controlling her verbal and nonverbal expressions, there and then in the session.

How to Interpret

How one interprets can be just as important as what behaviors to focus on. Commenting on a person's behavior within an interaction and offering ideas about factors to which those behaviors may be related, have the potential to increase the intensity of the interaction markedly. If the person disagrees with a comment or interpretation, the attempts at insight not only may fail, but may create further problems that must be sorted out. Insight, especially when directed at current behavior, should be used with great care.

There are three guidelines for the content and manner of interpretations in DBT that parallel to some extent the guidelines for what to interpret. The first guideline in that interpretations should be based on the biosocial theory described in Chapter 2, as well as on the DBT assumptions about patients outlined in Chapter 4. Indeed, one of the primary functions of any clinical theory or set of assumptions is to guide the therapist in constructing hypothetical interpretations of patient behaviors. The therapist should focus comments on rules that govern the patient's behavior, as well as the ways in which her behavior is functionally related to immediate behavioral precursors and outcomes, known psychological processes common to all people, biological influences, and situational events or contexts. Guidelines for formulating hypotheses about behavior during analysis, discussed above, are used in offering insights.

The second guideline is that efforts must be made to find nonpejorative language for offering insights. All other things being equal, nonpejorative insights should be entertained before pejorative ones. Similarly, insights that are congruent with the patient's phenomenological experience should be weighted more heavily than those that are incongruent. The exception here, as Chapter 12 indicates, is when the therapist uses irreverent communication strategies to effect change. In these instances, used strategically, interpretations may be both outrageous and anything but nonpejorative. (For example, the therapist may say, "Are you trying again to get this therapy not to work and to drive me crazy?" to a patient who engages in an already high-lighted therapy-interfering behavior for what feels like the millionth time.)

The third guideline is that interpretations should attempt to link current behaviors to current events. Borderline patients are often desperate to know how they came to be the way they are; they often want to discuss early childhood events and to determine the role of their early learning history in the development of their problems. The therapist should not avoid such discussions completely, as the goal is obviously legitimate. But the point needs to be made that an understanding of the factors contributing to the development of a pattern of behavior does not necessarily provide information about the factors responsible for the maintainance of the behavior. Nor does such an analysis always point to how a patient can change. (Indeed, the patient may respond by saying, "How can I ever get better having been through my life?") The peace of mind a patient sometimes obtains from such discussions can be well worth the time if they are properly handled; however, they should not take the place of attempts to understand the patient's behavior in the present context.

Timing of Interpretations

There are no guidelines applicable to all patients for when to offer which interpretations in DBT. Three points are important. First, when and how much to interpret should be determined empirically and idiographically. That is, the therapist should observe the effect of an insight on the patient and should modify his or her behavior accordingly. Second, the DBT therapist does not ordinarily treat the borderline patient as fragile or unable to tolerate hearing the therapist's actual interpretation of something. Third, principles of shaping guide which behaviors to ignore, until later, in favor of other behaviors to focus on now. (See Chapter 10.)

The four insight strategies are described next.

I. HIGHLIGHTING

In highlighting, the therapist gives the patient feedback about some aspect of what she is doing as a means of mirroring, highlighting, or bringing to the fore the patient's patterns of behavior. Often the highlighting is very brief, perhaps only a succinct comment (e.g. "very interesting"), and the topic may not be discussed at great length until some time later. Highlighting can often be phrased as a question (e.g., "Have you noticed that you have switched topics three times this session?").

Highlighting of negative behaviors is usually construed as criticism by everyone, and thus the therapist must be careful not to use this strategy as a cover for venting hostility or engaging in veiled criticism. Borderline patients are very quick to pick up on this. Generally, it is a good idea to try to balance highlighting of a patient's strengths with a focus on problematic responses.

2. OBSERVING AND DESCRIBING RECURRENT PATTERNS

An important part of any therapy is the construction of meaning out of life's events through observing recurrent, reliable patterns and relationships. In ongoing discussions of the patient's life as well as observations of behaviors occuring within the relationship, the therapist should be alert to recurrent relationships either among various patient behaviors or between behaviors and environmental events. In particular, the therapist should look for those relationships that will throw light on causal patterns. Thus, as in behavioral analysis, the focus is on noticing events that either elicit or reinforce behavior. At times, it is most useful for the therapist to ask the patient first whether she sees any interesting patterns. Or the therapist can convey his or her point indirectly by summarizing either what the patient has just said or a sequence of events in such a way as to highlight the pattern observed. At other times, it is most helpful for the therapist to communicate directly his or her observations and to discuss the validity of these observations with the patient.

3. COMMENTING ON IMPLICATIONS OF BEHAVIOR

As noted earlier, DBT does not assume that people (including borderline patients) are ordinarily aware of the variables controlling or influencing their own behavior. Although some rules guiding human behavior may be explicit, much of the time behavior is under the control of implicit rules and assumptions. Events that regularly elicit certain patterns of behavior, as well as events that function as reinforcers for behavior, also frequently function out of awareness. DBT does not assume that this lack of awareness is necessarily the result of repression (i.e., that it is motivated nonawareness). Instead, it is assumed that most people most of the time have difficulty accurately identifying the factors that control their own behavior. Most of the time, indeed, such identification is not necessary.

Generally, implications of behavior are based on "if–then" rules or relationships of which the patient may not be aware. By commenting, the therapist is saying, "If your reaction is X, then Y is probably the case also." (In contrast, when observing and describing patterns the therapist is saying "Isn't it interesting that X and Y always go together.") For example, if a patient says she wants to hit the therapist, a reasonable implication is that she is feeling angry or threatened. If she avoids or escapes a situation, then she may be afraid or may believe that the situation is hopeless. Deciding to go back to school implies that she has some confidence that she will pass her courses. The therapist should be particularly careful about suggesting that consequences of behavior are intended, especially when the consequences are painful or socially unacceptable. The theory and assumptions outlined in Chapters 2 and 4 are especially important to keep in mind here.

4. ASSESSING DIFFICULTIES IN ACCEPTING OR REJECTING HYPOTHESES

A recurrent pattern or implication may not be recognized by the patient. At other times, the pattern or implication may be recognized, but the patient may have difficulty either acknowledging it to the therapist or accepting it reality. Each of these alternatives should be explored with the patient when the therapist and the patient disagree on the presence or implication of a behavioral pattern. At the same time, the therapist should be alert to his or her own biases and difficulties in relinquishing "insights." It is possible that the proffered insight is simply incorrect. In these discussions, it is critical that the therapist respect the patient's point of view; furthermore, the therapist should communicate both directly and indirectly to the patient that she and the therapist are involved in a mutual, collaborative effort. Thus, disagreements between patient and therapist should be approached nonevaluatively, and possible difficulties the patient may be having in recognizing patterns should be discussed in a matter-of-fact and accepting manner.

In ongoing therapy, a patient will often offer her own insights and interpretations of both the therapist's behavior and the pattern of interactions between the two (or, in group therapy, between the therapist and other group members). The therapist should be open to recognizing these patterns and to validating the patient's insights where appropriate. Searching for the validity should precede searching for the patient's projections, defensiveness, lack of skill in offering insights, or ulterior motives in directing the discussion toward the therapist's behavior. Especially when the patterns are less than admirable behaviors on the therapist's part, this situation provides an opportunity both to reinforce valid observations and to model nondefensive, non-self-evaluative self-exploration. This topic is discussed more extensively in Chapters 12 and 15.

DIDACTIC STRATEGIES

The essence of the didactic strategies is the imparting of information about factors known to influence behavior in general, and of psychological, biological, and sociological theories that might cast light on particular behavior patterns. Information about borderline behaviors (including parasuicidal behaviors) and BPD, empirical data on various treatment strategies, and theoretical points of view are conveyed to the patient, and at times to her family or social network as well. The specific information imparted here is discussed in more detail in Chapter 14. The strategies are summarized in Table 9.3.

A basic didactic strategy is the direct teaching of the following principles of learning and development; biological consequences of various behavior patterns (including drug ingestion); and basic emotional, cognitive, and behavioral processes. Usually didactic information is imparted as it relates to effective methods of behavior change and self-control relevant to the patient's own problems. However, at times such information is also useful in understanding the behavior of others related to the patient. This didactic strategy is used to help the patient focus on relevant information during behavioral analysis, to generate solutions, and to make decisions and commitments to

TABLE 9.3. Didactic Strategies Checklist

_____ T provides INFORMATION to P about the development, maintenance, and change of behavior in general.
  _____ T presents empirical findings.
  _____ T presents learning-based and other current theories of behavior.
  _____ T discusses psychobiology of behavior.
  _____ T discusses interrelations and functions of behavior patterns.
  _____ T challenges P's self-blaming, moral, or "mental illness" explanations of current status or behavior.
  _____ T provides alternate explanations based on empirical findings.
  _____ T provides P with "problematic fit" overview of her problem.
_____ T presents parasuicidal and impulsive behaviors (e.g., drinking, drug use, child abuse, avoidant behavior) as problem-solving behavior.
  _____ T discusses relationship of behaviors to problem-solving skill deficits.
  _____ T discusses relationship of behaviors to funtional outcomes.
_____ T provides P with READINGS on behavior, treatments, BPD.
_____ T presents information about behavior and BPD to P's FAMILY, as necessary.

Anti-DBT tactics

_____ T overloads P with information.

_____ T insists on one version of reality.

specific goals in treatment. Information given didactically is meant to counteract overly moralistic, superstitious, and unrealistic views of behavior and change. The assumption is that borderline patients are often woefully lacking in such knowledge; they frequently have inadequate information about factors that typically influence behavior and about normative responses to situations in which they find themselves. This lack may be due to a variety of factors, including the deficient or faulty teaching and learning typical of invalidating environments.

I. PROVIDING INFORMATION

As noted previously, borderline and suicidal individuals quite often trace their problems to uncontrollable negative personal attributes; they often believe they are "going crazy," are "losing control," or are "terrible" persons because of their problems. A patient frequently has only two explanations for her own behavior and state of life: She is either crazy or evil (i.e., "mad or bad"). An alternative or rival conceptualization—namely, that the patient's behavior is a result of problematic learning histories or ordinary psychological processes—can often be quite helpful. Thus, whenever possible, learning-based explanations or other current, empirically based psychological theories should be offered, and attempts on the part of the patient to explain her behavior as a result of "mental illness" or "sin" should be refuted directly.

The emphasis on psychological explanations certainly does not rule out biological or genetic explanations of behavior when these are appropriate.

For example, it is appropriate to explain a borderline individual's extreme emotional lability as attributable in part to genetic or biological factors and dispositions. Distorted perceptions, cognitive biases (especially in memory), and rigid thinking can in turn be explained as ordinary and typical consequences of high emotional arousal. Problems in concentrating or attending may be attributed to depression, which may additionally be explained as stemming in part from physiological factors or genetic predisposition. Other problems may be chemically induced (e.g., lethargy and lack of motivation may be the result of poor nutrition, overeating, drug use, etc). At all times, the therapist must walk the fine line between indicating to the patient that problems may be due to faulty learning histories and suggesting that the problems result from more immutable characteristics of the patient. Here the dialectic of change versus acceptance is most important, and the therapist must be careful to synthesize these two points of view rather than to maintain either side of the coin as an independent truth.

2. GIVING READING MATERIALS

Some patients are willing and eager to read information relevant to their problems. Patients can be given this book; the accompanying skills training manual; articles and research papers on BPD as well as other diagnostic criteria that they meet; outcome studies pertaining to psychosocial and pharmacological treatments; textbooks or readings on introductory psychology, social psychology, behavior therapy, or other procedures the therapist may be using; self-help books that contain accurate and sound information on topics the therapist would like the patient to understand better (such as principles of learning, or sexual abuse and its effects on people); and so on. Generally, I try to teach patients as much as I know. Thus, any materials I am reading may be given to the patient. Most patients will not read long-winded or academically dry books, but many will read brief articles or book chapters. Unfortunately, most popular books on BPD present a theoretical formulation of the disorder that differs from the DBT formulation. In particular, many convey an idea that the individual's disordered behavior is caused by a "mental illness" from which the individual must recover before real changes can be made. DBT is not based on a mental illness conception of BPD; if it did accept one, it would suggest that making real changes is likely to cure it rather than vice versa.

3. GIVING INFORMATION TO FAMILY MEMBERS

The family of a borderline or suicidal individual often blames the patient for her difficulties. This blame is usually based on faulty information about behavior and BPD, and grows out of the family's frustration in trying to understand and help the patient. Whatever the reason, the family's inability to develop a theory of the patient's behavior that is compassionate and nonpejorative can be especially painful for both the patient and the family. Many of the patient's maladaptive behaviors are misguided attempts to change the family's negative and judgmental views of her. One of the most important tasks of family therapy sessions is for the therapist to impart to the family didactic information about the formation and maintenance of BPD and borderline behaviors. They are given the same information as that given to patients (for a fuller discussion, see Chapter 14). The therapist must remember, of course, that attempts to change the point of view of a patient's family must also be surrounded by the judicious use of validating strategies.

SOLUTION ANALYSIS STRATEGIES

DBT and behavior therapy in general assume that conducting behavioral analyses and achieving insight into the origin, pattern, and maintenance of one's problems are rarely sufficient to effect permanent behavioral change. Instead, once understanding and insight are achieved, therapist and patient must proceed with an active attempt to generate adaptive behavior patterns that can replace maladaptive behaviors and to develop a plan for making change come about. Aversive life situations presented by the patient are treated by the therapist as problems that can be solved, even if the solution only means a new way of adapting to life as it is (i.e., problem acceptance rather than problem solving and change). In solution analysis, the therapist actively models solving problems and, over the course of therapy, elicits and reinforces the generation and use of active problem solutions by the patient. The steps discussed below can be utilized in any order and combination to suit the particular situation. They are also summarized in Table 9.4.

Levels of Analysis

At the first level of analysis, in the beginning of therapy, the therapist and patient must decide whether their goals are compatible. The goal of DBT is to reduce borderline and suicidal behaviors as methods of coping with problems by working collaboratively with the patient to build a life worth living. If this is not a goal of the patient, however tentative, then problem solving cannot progress. At the second level, the therapist is examining whether the patient wants to improve other behaviors targeted in DBT. Beyond reducing parasuicidal behaviors and therapy-interfering behaviors, all other goals are dependent on the patient. The exception here is an instance when the therapist believes that a particular goal is essential to any further therapeutic progress. At the third level, the net is cast much wider, although the focus should remain on the problem situation under consideration. Basically, the question is "What would have to change for the problem to be solved or the situation to improve?" At this third level, it is also important for the therapist

TABLE 9.4. Solution Analysis Strategies Checklist

____ T helps P IDENTIFY WANTS, NEEDS, AND GOALS.
    ____ T helps P redefine wishes to engage in parasuicidal behavior or to be dead as expressions of desire to decrease pain and improve quality of life.
    ____ T helps P redefine lack of desire to change or inability to generate goals as an expression of hopelessness and powerlessness.
____ T and P GENERATE SOLUTIONS.
    ____ T pushes P to brainstorm as may solutions as possible.
    ____ T helps P develop specific coping strategies and practices to short-circuit impulsive, self-damaging behaviors.
____ T helps P EVALUATE solutions generated.
    ____ T focuses on consequences, both short- and long-term, of various strategies.
    ____ If necessary, T confronts P directly about probable negative outcomes of her behavioral choices.
    ____ T and P discuss problem solution criteria.
    ____ T helps P identify factors that might interfere with problem solutions.
____ T helps P CHOOSE a solution.
    ____ T gives advice, or at least an opinion, when necessary.
    ____ T implements specific DBT procedures as needed.
        ____ Case management strategies.
        ____ Skills training strategies.
        ____ Exposure strategies.
        ____ Cognitive modification strategies.
        ____ Contingency management strategies.
____ T reviews with P ways in which attempts to solve problem can go wrong (TROUBLESHOOTING).

to be sure that the patient does want to work on solving the problem at hand. Sometimes the patient (like anyone else) just wants to tell someone about her problem, have the other person understand and commiserate with her, and let it go at that. Insisting on continuing to "solve" the problem can be counterproductive in such instances. At other times, if wishing to stop at problem definition is a characteristic form of avoiding problem solving, the therapist may need to skip to the commitment strategies (see below) first, in order to obtain an initial agreement even to work on the problem.

I. IDENTIFYING GOALS, NEEDS, AND DESIRES

Impediments to the Patient's Knowing What She Wants

Suicidal individuals often suggest that their goal in life is to be dead, or that what they desire is to cut or otherwise hurt themselves or to engage in some other impulsive behavior. In essence, such an individual is representing self-destructive behavior as the solution to her problems. The first task of the therapist is to point out that it is very unlikely that the patient actually *wants* to engage in suicidal behavior; rather, she probably wants to solve the problem that she is experiencing, to feel better, and to be more satisfied with her life. Such a statement should then be followed by a comment that there are probably other ways of obtaining these goals. The patient may continue to insist that what she really wants is to be dead or to hurt herself; the therapist may feel that what is really wanted is the therapist's permission to engage in self-destructive behavior. The patient may actually be attempting to get the therapist to recognize how bad she is feeling. A useful technique here is simply to validate the patient's pain, and to follow such statements up with a refocusing of the conversation on alternative solutions. At times, this circular process may be required 10 or 20 times within a single interaction. At other times, (even in the same interaction), the patient will state that she does not want to change anything and that everything is fine. Such statements generally come from feelings of hopelessness and lack of control.

A fundamental dialectical tension in setting goals is that it is almost impossible for the patient to know what she wants if she is not free to choose and get what she wishes for. Often, it is simply not useful to engage in lengthy discussions regarding what the patient wants in particular situations. The therapy time is better used in first increasing the patient's ability to attain a range of goals. For example, I had a borderline patient who could not decide what she wanted from coworkers, or whether she wanted to be promoted, to stay on the current job, or to quit. After a number of lengthy discussions, it became apparent to me that the patient's extreme lack of assertive behavior actually prevented her from ever standing up for herself at work, from going for the promotion, or from searching for a different job. When I suggested that we work on learning to stand up for herself and handle conflict directly, she complained that she couldn't because she never knew what she wanted in conflict situations. My strategy was to teach her how to stand up for a variety of issues and ask for any number of things, reasoning with her that she might as well learn how to ask for the "sun and the moon"; she could decide *what* to ask for later. By the time she was competent at assertion, we did not need the discussion on goals and wishes. She knew what she wanted.

At times, especially when devising new reponses to crisis situations, the therapist should generate possible goals or objectives, describing them together with any means by which the patient might attain them. The therapist should make repeated attempts if necessary to engage the patient in a discussion of these therapist-generated goals, taking care to focus on short-term, realistic goals rather than long-term, seemingly unattainable goals. It may be useful to generate with the patient a list of possible goals or objectives for a particular problem and then rank-order them from most desirable to least desirable.

A final major impediment to the identification of goals, needs, and desires is the consistent tendency of suicidal and borderline individuals to believe that they do not actually deserve happiness, the good life, love, or the like.

This belief in their utter worthlessness must be countered at every turn. Techniques and strategies for changing such dysfunctional beliefs are described more fully in Chapter 11.

2. GENERATING SOLUTIONS

Levels of Solutions

As I have noted, at the initial level one possible solution to the patient's problems is getting into and staying in DBT. Other solution strategies—in particular, combining DBT with pharmacotherapy or other ancillary therapies—should also be explored. At the second level, the solution may be one or more of the specific problem-solving procedures making up DBT. Once a particular pattern of behavior is identified as an appropriate solution, new problems may emerge that must be responded to first. That is, the patient may not be able to utilize the solutions in her present state. At the third level, therapist and patient simply generate solutions to specific problems as they arise, or they may generate new, more effective ways to handle old problems. Once a solution is generated and chosen, the patient may be able to implement it, or may at least make a good attempt. In day-to-day individual DBT, these two latter approaches are typically interwoven.

Day-to-day Solution Generation

During the conduct of the behavioral analysis, the therapist will have noted along the chain possible alternative responses the individual could have made to solve the problem at hand. Conducting a chain analysis is a bit like constructing a road map to see how the patient got from one point to the next. Like all road maps, however, a chain often also indicates other "roads" the patient could have taken. These other roads, or solutions, should be pointed out as the analysis is constructed. However, it is usually not advisable at this time to go into lengthy discussions at each juncture about all the possible alternative solutions. Such a discussion often diverts both therapist and patient from the task of constructing the complete chain. At times, this pointing out of alternative solutions is all that is done by way of solution analysis.

At other times, a more complete solution analysis is conducted. This may be done in a phone conversation during a crisis, when the patient is attempting to cope with a problem in a more adaptive way. Or it may be done during a therapy session in which the point is to generate solutions to a current crisis situation. Alternatively, much of therapy can be viewed as attempting to generate and implement new solutions to chronic problems faced by the patient. The first task in these cases is to "brainstorm" solutions. The therapist should ask the patient whether she can think of any other ways to solve her problem. It is important to elicit as many alternative solutions as she can possibly think of. The patient's tendency will be to reject many solutions out of hand; thus, much urging and encouraging will be needed to get her to stop evaluating and simply to generate alternatives. The therapist should teach and model the "quantity breeds quality" principle underlying brainstorming tactics.

If the patient generates a list of solutions, one or more of which seem effective, than there is no need for the therapist to contribute other solutions. At the beginning of therapy, however, this is not likely to happen. At this point the therapist must not be fooled by the "apparent competence" of the patient into believing that she actually knows how to solve the problem but simply is not motivated or is too lazy to generate a good alternative. This is rarely the case. The eventual goal here is for the patient to generate, remember, and implement new behaviors independently of the therapist. Therefore, prompting should be faded over time, with an increasing emphasis on drawing from the patient specific behavioral plans for how to solve specific problems.

Because suicidal and borderline patients are unusually rigid and dichotomous in their thinking, a patient will often present the therapist with only one solution to a problem. If this solution is adaptive (or at least better than the patient's usual solutions), the therapist should, of course, reinforce her. However, quite often the solution presented is inadequate, is maladaptive, or otherwise is not the best solution possible (at least in the opinion of the therapist). New solutions must be generated.

Often, the patient cannot generate an effective action plan or is hampered from suggesting effective alternatives by emotional inhibitions or faulty beliefs and expectations about the outcomes she perceives as associated with such alternatives. In these instances, it is helpful for the therapist to suggest various action plans for solving the problem. The therapist may also need to help the patient develop specific strategies for coping with self-damaging behaviors that might sabotage the implementation of a solution.

3. EVALUATING SOLUTIONS

Solutions must be evaluated in terms of both their potential effectiveness and possible obstacles to carry them out.

Analyzing Potential Effectiveness of Solutions

The therapist should carefully assess the patient's expectancies regarding the utility of the outcomes (both short-term and long-term) associated with various solutions. During these discussions, the therapist can help the patient assess how realistic these expectancies are. The therapist should not automatically assume that negative expectancies on the part of the patient are unrealistic; she may indeed be functioning in an aversive environmental situation where the range of possible negative outcomes may be substantial. When a patient reports negative expectancies, it may be preferable for the therapist to respond by asking how such expected outcomes might be overcome or mitigated.

At other times, the therapist will feel that the patient is engaging in the "Yes, but. . ." syndrome: Every solution proposed by the therapist is discussed as inadequate. In these cases, the therapist should identify his or her sense of what is happening within the therapy interaction and ask the patient for suggestions to resolve the impasse. It may be helpful to discuss the patient's expectations of the therapy process. Once again, it is important to validate the patient's probable frustration and despair rather than to accuse the patient (directly or indirectly) of throwing roadblocks into the therapy.

Analyzing Possible Obstacles to Effective Solutions

A particular solution may be effective if employed, but for one reason or another the patient may not be able to use it in everyday life. Careful analysis of factors that may interfere with solution implementation is, therefore, a very important part of problem solving.

The analysis of possible obstacles in DBT is based on the behavior deficit and response inhibition models I have proposed previously for the analysis of failures in assertive behavior (Linehan, 1979). The behavior deficit model assumes that failure to use effective behavior when it is needed is the result of a deficiency; that is, relevant, effective behaviors (i.e., actions plus knowledge of how and when to use them) are absent from the individual's behavioral repertoire. The response inhibition model assumes that the person has the requisite behaviors but is inhibited from performing. There are two hypotheses about the determinants of inhibition. The first hypothesis is that it is due to conditioned negative affective responses; the second is that it results from maladaptive beliefs, self-statements, and expectations. A variant of the response inhibition approach assumes that the person has the requisite behaviors, but that performance of these behaviors is interfered with. Once again, there are two major sources of interference. First, a response may be precluded by the prior emission of incompatible behaviors; that is, inappropriate, incompatible behaviors are higher in the individual's response hierarchy than are appropriate, effective responses. Second, the contingencies operating in the current environment may favor ineffective over effective behavior. Effective behaviors may be punished and ineffective behaviors rewarded.

In analyzing solutions to a particular problem situation or life pattern, the therapist must be careful to assess the variables influencing the patient's behavior in that particular area, instead of blindly applying a preformulated theory. Once the therapist and patient have figured out what is interfering with the use of effective problem-solving behaviors, they can jointly consider how to proceed. If there is a skill deficit, skills training may be in order. Inhibition stemming from conditioned fears or guilt usually indicates the need for exposure-based techniques. Faulty beliefs may be remedied with formal cognitive modification procedures. Problematic contingencies in the environment suggest contingency management procedures. These procedures are described in detail in Chapters 10 and 11.

4. CHOOSING A SOLUTION TO IMPLEMENT

Generating, evaluating, and discussing potential solutions to problems are means to an end. They do not constitute the end itself, although the patient would often like this to be the case. The goal is to implement a solution that has some likelihood of working or of improving the situation. Thus, during the course of evaluation, the therapist should guide the patient in choosing a particular solution as the one to proceed with. Although there are many ways to organize criteria for this choice, the therapist should pay particular attention to long-term over short-term value, and to the effects of various solutions on meeting the patient's wishes or goals (objective effectiveness), maintaining or enhancing interpersonal relationships (interpersonal effectiveness), and maintaining or enhancing the patient's respect for herself (self-respect effectiveness). (A fuller description of these types of effectiveness is given in the accompanying skills training manual.) Working together on this step is an important means of helping the patient improve her abilities to make decisions according to appropriate judgmental criteria.

When the solution involves implementation of specific DBT procedures, the role of the therapist in helping the patient make the choice is much greater. For example, when skills training, exposure, or cognitive modification techniques are chosen to attack a problem, consensus between patient and therapist is essential, as these procedures require close cooperation. In contrast, contingency management can be implemented unilaterally by either the patient (through reinforcing or punishing therapist behaviors) or the therapist. The key here, however, is that the therapist must remain flexible, willing to entertain the idea that there are many roads to Rome.

5. TROUBLESHOOTING THE SOLUTION

In troubleshooting a solution, therapist and patient discuss all the ways implementation of the solution can go wrong and what the patient can do about it. The idea here is to prepare the patient for difficulties and to think ahead of time about ways to solve new problems that come up. At the beginning of therapy and in crisis management, the therapist should be very active here. Troubleshooting is often combined with the rehearsal of new solutions, discussed below in connection with orienting. The most important thing about troubleshooting is to remember to do it.

ORIENTING STRATEGIES

Orienting and commitment strategies are always interwoven and are pulled apart here for the sake of exposition. Orienting involves giving patients task information about the process and requirements of DBT as a whole (at the first level, where DBT is a general case of problem solving); about a treat-

ment procedure that will be employed (e.g., behavioral skills training to provide alternatives to suicidal behaviors); or about what is required in implementing a specific solution selected during the solution analysis of a particular
problem situation. Specifics on orienting the patient to therapy as a whole
are outlined in Chapter 14. Before each instance of new learning, however,
a similar orientation or task overview should be presented directly and deliberately to the patient in order to provide precise information about what has
to be learned, as well as a clarification of the conceptual model within which
the learning will take place.

Many apparent failures to learn stem from failures to understand what
has to be learned, rather than problems with acquisition or memory. Comprehension of the task is improved if requirements of the task are clarified
before practice begins; adequate learning can be assured only if the patient
knows exactly what has to be learned. Other failures in teaching skills may
result from inadequate clarification of the conceptual model or rationale underlying the procedure. The importance of the treatment rationale in affecting therapeutic gain has been demonstrated by Rosen (1974) as well as by
others.

Task reorienting will have to be conducted repeatedly during treatment
as a general first step in repeated recommitments to therapy, to specific therapeutic procedures, and to implemention of previouslly agreed-upon behavioral solutions. The general idea is that progress will be smoother and
faster if the patient has as much information as possible about the requirements for change, the rationale for the treatment strategies selected, and the
relationship of treatment process to outcome. Orienting strategies are summarized in Table 9.5 and are described below.

I. PROVIDING ROLE INDUCTION

Role induction involves clarifying for the patient what she may realistically
anticipate from the treatment or treatment procedure itself and from the therapist. The focus here is on what the patient and therapist will actually do,
both during therapy as a whole and in implementing a specific procedure;
what the therapist can expect from the patient, as well as what the patient
can expect from the therapist, is clarified. When a specific intervention is discussed, its targets and their relation to the patient's needs and desires are emphasized. Role induction is important because negative feelings toward both
the therapist and the treatment can result from misinformation or lack of information about what the patient can realistically expect during the course
of therapy. Conversely, events that confirm the patient's early-established expectancies are likely to increase her sense of attraction toward and trust of
the therapist.

The clarification of mutual expectations should be discussed throughout therapy. In particular, the therapist should be alert to picking up unver-

TABLE 9.5. Orienting Strategies Checklist

_____ T orients P to DBT and to her role in therapy (ROLE INDUCTION).
_____ To DBT as a whole.
_____ To specific treatment task.
　　　_____ T discusses goals (targets) of specific intervention and their relationship to overall outcomes desired by P.
　　　_____ T clarifies for P what both P's and T's roles will be in intervention.
_____ T REHEARSES with P exactly what she is to do in trying to respond to the problem.
　　　_____ T commiserates with P about how difficult P's treatment tasks are.
　　　_____ T points out that T did not create laws of learning/change and does not (at times) like them any better that P.

balized, unrealistic expectancies on the part of the patient. Such expectations should be reflected and summarized back to the patient in a nonjudgmental fashion, and clarifying discussions should follow. It is important that the therapist communicate understanding of how the patient may have arrived at such unrealistic expectancies. As always, a balance between acceptance and change should be maintained.

2. REHEARSING NEW EXPECTATIONS

In helping a patient prepare to implement a new behavioral response to an old or new problem, the therapist should go over with the patient in detail just what is expected of her—that is, exactly what she is to do. With a highly agitated patient, in particular, there simply is no substitute for a detailed, step-by-step review of the actions the patient is to try. Generally, this review should be carried out as the solution is discussed and chosen. It can be briefly run through again just before the session or phone interaction ends. Some patients may need to write down each step; others may need to write down the rationale for implementing the solution so they can "cheerlead" themselves when necessary. This cognitive rehearsal is itself an instance of new learning and an aid to memory that will enhance performance in the problem situation.

　　By the time therapist and patient finish reviewing what the patient is expected to do, the patient may be too discouraged to make the attempt if the therapist fails to interweave a heavy amount of validation along the way. I usually first commiserate with the patient about how hard it is going to be. Then I point out that I did not make up the laws of learning and I don't like them any better than she does. I think of this as the "Yes, but. . ." strategy in reverse.

COMMITMENT STRATEGIES

The final problem-solving step is eliciting and maintaining a commitment from the patient to implement the solution chosen. An enormous amount of evidence indicates that the commitment to behave in a particular way—or, more generally, commitment to a behavioral project such as a task, job, or relationship—is strongly related to future performance (e.g., Wang & Katzev, 1990; Hall, Havassy, & Wasserman, 1990). People are more likely to do what they agree to do. They are more likely to stay in jobs and relationships to which they have made strong commitments.

Levels of Commitment

At the initial stages of therapy, the commitment sought from a patient is to participate in DBT with this particular therapist for a specified period of time and to keep the patient agreements outlined in Chapter 4. At a very minimum at the beginning of therapy, the patient must agree to work toward eliminating suicidal behavior and building a more worthwhile life. In-session behaviors that may be addressed as inconsistent with this degree of commitment and collaboration include refusing to work in therapy; avoiding or refusing to talk about feelings and events connected with target behaviors; and rejecting all input from the therapist or attempts to generate alternative solutions. At these moments, the commitment to therapy itself should be analyzed and discussed, with the goal of eliciting a recommitment. The moments (sometimes very rare in the beginning) when a patient does display a committed and collaborative attitude call for alert reinforcement by the therapist.

At the second level, the commitment sought is for the patient is to collaborate in the specific treatment procedures selected. If skills training procedures are implemented, the commitment is for her to work on learning and applying new, more skillful behavior in problem situations. With exposure, the commitment is for her to enter the feared or otherwise stressful situation, to experience rather than avoid emotions, or to think or do things that she is afraid to try. With cognitive modification, the commitment is for her to examine and attempt to modify when necessary her assumptions, beliefs, and characteristic patterns of thought related to problem behaviors. Contingency management strategies differ from the others, in that the type and degree of collaboration needed are somewhat different. In contingency management, the therapist applies contingencies based on observations or reports of the patient's behavior. The assumption is that exposure to new contingencies will change behavior. Thus, the requisite commitment on the part of the patient is both to expose herself to the contingencies and to be honest in reporting her own behavior. For most patients in DBT, each of these commitments will be necessary.

At the third level, the commitment is to implement whatever behavioral solution the patient and therapist have selected in a solution analysis. The idea here is that the therapist should directly elicit the patient's agreement to try a new behavior, to work on a specific problem, or the like.

Commitment and Recommitment

In my experience, one of the chief reasons for many therapy failures and early terminations is inadequate commitment by either the patient, the therapist, or both. There may be insufficient or glib commitment in the initial stages of the change process, or more likely, events both within and without therapy may conspire to reduce strong commitments made previously. Patient commitment in DBT is both an important prerequisite for effective therapy and a goal of the therapy. Thus, a commitment to change or to implement new behavioral solutions to old problems is not assumed. Commitment is viewed as itself a behavior, which can be elicited, learned, and reinforced. The task of the therapist is to figure out ways to help this process along.

Throughout treatment, the therapist can expect that the patient will need reminding of the commitments she has made, as well as assistance in refining, expanding, and remaking behavioral commitments (sometimes over and over). In some cases, a patient and I have had to go back to the original commitment several times within a single (very difficult) session, making and remaking it. On other occasions, one or more whole sessions may be needed to readdress issues of commitment to change, to DBT, or to particular procedures. A failure in commitment should be one of the first things assessed (but not assumed) when a problem in therapy arises. Before moving to solve the problem, the therapist should first go back with the patient to the commitment strategy. Once recommitment is made, both can proceed with addressing the problem at hand.

Sometimes the uncommitted partner is the therapist, not the patient. This can happen under a number of circumstances. The patient may have been demanding resources that the therapist does not have available, or may have failed to make progress for a long time. Or progress that is being made may be so slow that it is imperceptible to the therapist. Sometimes, after a lot of progress, when the patient is reorganizing or integrating changes, the therapist simply loses interest in the patient. There may be value clashes, or after the crises that were so consuming at the beginning of therapy have passed, the therapist may find that he or she simply does not like the patient. Circumstances in the therapist's life may have changed in such a way that treating this particular patient is no longer a priority or no longer rewarding. I suspect that many therapeutic failures in commitment that have been laid at the feet of borderline patients could more properly be laid at the feet of their therapists. Therefore, the therapist must analyze his or her level of commitment to the patient and develop new, more vigorous commitments as needed. The most appropriate arena for this work is the DBT case consultation team, although loss of commitment is also an important clue that a patient therapy-interfering behavior may be on the scene.

The Need for Flexibility

It perhaps goes without saying, but flexibility and respect for the patient's own wishes, goals, and ideas about "how to get from here to there" are needed. Thus, the therapist should avoid being judgmental about the patient's choice of goals and/or commitments. The therapist should be careful not to impose his or her own goals or treatment procedures on the patient when such goals or procedures are not dictated by DBT or the therapist's own limits. Although it is tempting to present arbitrary therapist choices or preferences as necessary, such a tendency must somehow be averted or corrected when noticed. The case consultation team can be particularly useful here.

Eliciting a commitment from a patient may involve a number of steps. The therapist is often functioning like a good salesperson. The product being sold is DBT, new behavior, a renewed effort to change, or sometimes life itself. All or most of the steps discussed below and outlined in Table 9.6 may be needed when the task requires great effort on the part of the patient; when effort must be sustained over a long period or in the face of adversity or attempts by others to dissuade the patient; when the patient feels hopeless about her capacity to change; or when what is required is something the patient fears greatly. The best example here is making the commitment to therapy in the first place, which is discussed in Chapter 14. At other times, only a request for a verbal commitment may be needed, and other tactics can be discarded. The therapist should feel free to move back and forth among the various strategies as needed.

I. SELLING COMMITMENT: EVALUATING THE PROS AND CONS

People keep commitments they believe in better than those they do not believe in. Thus, once one or more action plans have been proposed, the therapist should engage the patient in a discussion of the pros and cons of actually making a commitment to a specific plan or solution. The idea here is twofold: (1) to rehearse the good points of the solution already evaluated and chosen in the solution analysis; and (2) to develop counterarguments to reservations that will almost certainly come up later, usually when the patient is alone and without help in combating doubts. The therapist should make an effort to relate commitments to change to the patient's own life patterns, to realistic expectations for the future, and to the rationale and expected outcomes for therapy.

2. PLAYING THE DEVIL'S ADVOCATE

At times, a patient will make a facile commitment that will not be strong enough to stand up during future adversity. Thus, once a tentative commitment is made, the therapist should try to increase the commitment if at all

TABLE 9.6. Commitment Strategies Checklist

_____ T highlights and discusses PROS AND CONS of a commitment to change.

     _____ T "sells" commitment.

     _____ T relates commitments to change to P's own life patterns, to realistic expectations for the future, and to therapy rationale and expected outcome.

_____ T uses the DEVIL'S ADVOCATE technique to strengthen P's commitment and build sense of control.

_____ T uses "FOOT-IN-THE-DOOR" and "DOOR-IN-THE-FACE" techniques to obtain P's commitments to DBT goals and procedures.

     _____ T presents goals somewhat vaguely and in a favorable light, omitting discussion of how hard goals will be to reach, so that almost anyone would agree.

     _____ T elicits P's commitment to reach goals.

     _____ T redescribes goals, presenting more specifics and highlighting difficulties a bit more.

     _____ T elicits another commitment to reach goals.

     _____ T "ups the ante," presenting goals as very difficult to reach, perhaps more difficult than anything P has ever attempted—but attainable if P wants to try.

     _____ T elicits another commitment to reach goals.

_____ T highlights PRIOR COMMITMENTS P has made ("But I thought we/you had agreed...").

     _____ T discusses with P whether she still has a commitment made previously.

     _____ T helps P clarify her commitments.

     _____ T focuses on recommitment if goal is essential to DBT or to T's limits.

     _____ T renegotiates commitments if changes do not conflict with DBT or T's limits.

_____ T presents P with CHOICE stressing P's freedom to choose while at the same time presenting realistic consequences of choices clearly.

     _____ T highlights that P is free to choose to continue a life of coping by parasuicide, but if that choice is made another therapy will need to be found, since DBT requires reduction of parasuicide as a goal.

     _____ T highlights that P is free to continue therapy-interfering behaviors, but also clarifies T's limits if that choice is made.

_____ T uses principles of SHAPING in eliciting commitment from P.

_____ T generates hope in P by CHEERLEADING.

_____ T and P agree specifically on HOMEWORK.

Anti-DBT tactics

_____ T is judgmental about P's choice of goals and/or commitments.

_____ T is rigid about goals or procedures to reach goals, when rigidity is not imposed by DBT or T's limits.

_____ T imposes his or her own goals or treatment procedures on P when such goals or procedures are not dictated by DBT or T's limits, presenting them as necessary rather than arbitrary.

possible. The discussion of pros and cons (see above) is one way; another is the "devil's advocate" technique discussed in Chapter 7. In this case, the therapist poses arguments against making a commitment. The secret here is to make sure that the counterarguments are slightly weaker than the patient's arguments for commitment. If the counterarguments are too strong, the patient may capitulate and retract her initial commitment. When this happens, the therapist should back down slightly and reinforce the arguments for commitment, and then revert back once more to the devil's advocate position. This tactic is also helpful in enhancing the patient's sense of choice and "illusion" of control.

3. "FOOT-IN-THE-DOOR/DOOR-IN-THE-FACE" TECHNIQUES

The "foot-in-the-door" (Freedman & Fraser, 1966) and "door-in-the face" (Cialdini et al., 1975) techniques are well-known social-psychological procedures for enhancing compliance with requests and previously made commitments. (The terms come from the initial research on door-to-door canvassing for donations to charities.) In the foot-in-the-door technique, the therapist increases compliance by making an easier first request followed by a more difficult request (e.g., first getting the patient to agree to make a difficult phone call, and then obtaining her subsequent agreement to try to use her new interpersonal skills on the phone). In the door-in-the-face technique, the procedure is reversed: The therapist first requests something much larger than he or she actually expects, and then requests something easier (e.g., first requesting the patient to agree not to harm herself during the upcoming week, and then requesting her to call the therapist before harming herself). A combined procedure—asking first for something very hard, then moving to something very easy, and progressing up to a more difficult request—may at times be the most effective strategy (Goldman, 1986). All three strategies are likely to be more effective than simply asking directly for a commitment.

When the therapist is obtaining commitment to therapy itself or to a particular treatment procedure, a variation of the combined strategy may be used as follows. First, the therapist presents goals (of therapy or of the procedure) somewhat vaguely and in a favorable light, omitting discussion of how hard goals will be to reach, so that almost anyone would agree. Second, the therapist elicits the patient's commitment to reach these goals. Third, the therapist redescribes the goals, presenting more specifics and highlighting the difficulties a bit more. Fourth, the therapist elicits another commitment to reach goals. Fifth, the therapist "ups the ante," presenting goals as very difficult to reach, perhaps more difficult than anything the patient has ever attempted (and more difficult than they may actually be)—but attainable if the patient wants to try. Finally, the therapist elicits another commitment to reach goals.

In eliciting commitments to engage in homework practice or to try new behaviors, the door-in-the-face procedure is often most successful. For example, I may first ask a patient to practice a new skill every day, and then scale the request back to once or twice between now and the next session. Once the patient agrees to this, and if I think successful compliance is likely, I may raise the request slightly to three times before the next session.

4. CONNECTING PRESENT COMMITMENTS TO PRIOR COMMITMENTS

A variation on the foot-in-the-door tactic is to remind the patient of previous commitments. This should always be done when the strength of a commitment seems to be fading or when the patient's behavior is incongruent with her previous commitments ("But I thought we/you had agreed. . ."). It can be particularly useful in a crisis situation, especially when the patient is threatening suicide or some other destructive response; developing new commitments during a crisis can be exceptionally difficult. This tactic can also be quite satisfying for the therapist and is preferable to attacking the patient or threatening immediate counterbehaviors. For example, a new patient once called me (as director of the clinic) in a crisis over the humiliation she felt at having to go to group skills training. When I did not give her permission to quit the group and still continue in our program, she said, "OK, then I'll just have to hurt myself." I immediately said, "But I thought you were going to try your best not to do that? That's one of the commitments you made on entering therapy with us."

In reminding the patient of previous commitments, the therapist should also discuss whether the patient still has a commitment made previously, and should then help the patient clarify her commitments. If a commitment or goal is essential to DBT (such as committing to working on parasuicidal behavior in the example above) or to the therapist's own limits, the therapist should next focus on establishing a recommitment. If changes do not conflict with DBT or the therapist's limits, then renegotiation of commitments may be in order.

5. HIGHLIGHTING FREEDOM TO CHOOSE AND ABSENCE OF ALTERNATIVES

Commitment and compliance are enhanced both when people believe that they have chosen a commitment freely and when they believe that there are no alternative paths to their goals. Thus, the therapist should try to enhance the feeling of choice, while at the same time stressing the lack of alternative ways to achieve the patient's goals. The way to do this is to stress the fact that the patient can simply change her goals. That is, although there may not be many choices about how to achieve a goal, she can choose her own life goals. The catch is that in choosing her goals, she also has to be prepared to accept what goes along with those goals. That is, she has to accept the natural consequences of her choices.

Thus, the therapist should stress the patient's freedom to choose, while at the same time presenting realistic consequences of choices clearly. For example, in developing (or redeveloping) a patient's commitment to stop attempting suicide, the therapist may emphasize that the patient is free to choose a life of coping by parasuicide, but that if this choice is made another therapy will need to be found, since DBT requires reduction of parasuicide as a goal. Similarly, the therapist may note that the patient is free to continue therapy-interfering behaviors, but should also clarify the therapist's own limits if that choice is made. For example, I once told a patient who persisted in a particularly aversive (to me) behavior pattern that she could continue the pattern, but that if she did I wouldn't want to work with her. She immediately asked whether I was threatening to terminate therapy if she didn't stop. "No," I said, "I'm going to stay in therapy with you; I just won't like it, that's all."

The reader may notice that both consequences have to do with the therapy relationship. These are usually the most powerful consequences for this particular strategy, since they are the ones the therapist can be most sure about. As I discuss in Chapter 10, however, therapeutic contingencies depend on a strong relationship. Thus, they must be used with caution if the relationship is not yet formed.

The therapist can look to the previous discussions of pros and cons or to previous analyses of outcomes of dysfunctional behaviors to get other ideas about likely and realistic consequences for dysfunctional behaviors. The point is that both therapist and patient must accept that the patient is free to choose these behaviors and their consequences. Highlighting this freedom while simultaneously stressing the negative consequences of failure to make a particular commitment can strengthen both a commitment and the likelihood of follow-through on the agreement.

6. USING PRINCIPLES OF SHAPING

It is important to keep in mind that commitments often have to be shaped. In the initial stages of change, commitments may be to limited goals that can be expanded over time. At other times, the patient may simply be tired or demoralized, and previous large commitments may have to be reduced for a time. Often the therapist will want larger commitments than the patient can give. The therapist must be flexible and creative in obtaining at times a just-noticeable difference in commitment. The ability to reduce requests or use the door-in-the-face technique, without at the same time making the patient look like a failure, is essential here.

7. GENERATING HOPE: CHEERLEADING

One of the major problems confronting suicidal and borderline individuals is their lack of any hope that they can put solutions generated into practice, or that their attempts will not end in failure and humiliation. Commitment without hope of keeping the commitment is extremely difficult. The use of cheerleading strategies is nowhere more important than in problem solving. During each problem-solving interaction (particularly as the interaction nears to an end and a commitment is needed), the therapist needs to encourage the patient, reinforce even minimal progress on her part, and consistently point out that she has within her everything it will take to overcome her problems in the end.

8. AGREEING ON HOMEWORK

Assigned, structured practice of new problem solutions or new behavioral skills is an integral part of the psychoeducational skills training groups. Structured homework assignments are not typical of individual therapy. However, the patient and therapist may often agree on specific behaviors that the patient will try between one session and the next. In such an instance, the therapist should be sure to write down the behavioral "assignment." It is also very important not to forget to ask about it during the next session. At times it may be useful for the patient to write down what she is going to do as well. If a task is very difficult, the therapist may ask the patient to check in during the week to report on progress or unexpected difficulties.

Concluding Comments

The problem-solving strategies in DBT are no different from those used in most forms of cognitive–behavioral therapy. If they were sufficient unto themselves, of course, there would be little need to develop a specific treatment for BPD. A major difference between these strategies with borderline patients and applying them with other patients is that with the former, the therapist must be prepared to repeat each step many times. Commitments made must be remade. The same insight may need to be repeated almost endlessly before it sinks in. Behavioral analysis can be time-consuming and tedious, especially when the process is punctuated by repeated therapy-interfering behaviors. Alternative behaviors and soloutions that seem possible to the therapist can seem impossible to the patient. Generally, skills training, application of contingencies, cognitive modification, and exposure-based procedures aimed at reducing interfering emotionality are needed, singly or in combination, to help the patient put into practice problem solutions that the therapist and patient have developed together. These procedures are discussed in detail in the next two chapters.

10

Change Procedures:
Part I. Contingency Procedures
(Managing Contingencies and
Observing Limits)

Change procedures—contingency procedures, behavioral skills training, exposure-based procedures, and cognitive modification—are interwoven throughout DBT. They are used by all therapists, although the mix will vary with treatment modality and phase of therapy. Application of the procedures is linked to four main groups of questions addressed in behavioral analysis. The relationship of these groups of questions to particular procedures can be seen in Table 10.1. Each type of procedure is used briefly and informally in almost every therapeutic interaction; they can also be used in a structured and formal way.

Examples of formal contingency procedures include such things as implementing a self-conscious treatment plan that specifies consequences for particular behaviors (e.g., the DBT rule that a patient cannot call the therapist for 24 hours following parasuicide, or a decision that if a patient phones over x times one week she loses the opportunity to call the therapist the next week); implementing level and privilege systems on inpatient units; or using "canned" or organized self-management programs between sessions. More informally, and often with little reflection, every therapist response observed or experienced by the patient (i.e., public behaviors of the therapist) can be either neutral, punishing, or reinforcing. Thus, every contingent response is an informal contingency procedure, skillful or not. Making direct changes in the environment to support new or more effective behavior is also an example of using contingency procedures.

An important point in the application of change procedures is that

TABLE 10.1. Relationship of Questions Addressed in Behavioral Analysis to Change Procedures.

Questions	Procedures
1. Are the requisite behaviors in the person's behavior repertoire? Does she know how to do the following:	Behavioral skills training
a. Regulate her emotions?	Emotion regulation
b. Tolerate distress?	Distress tolerance
c. Respond skillfully to conflict?	Interpersonal effectiveness
d. Observe, describe, and participate without judging, with awareness and focusing on effectiveness?	Mindfulness
e. Manage her own behavior?	Self-management
2. Are ineffective behaviors being reinforced? Do they lead to positive or preferred outcomes, or give the opportunity for other preferred behaviors or emotional states? Are effective behaviors followed by neutral or punishing outcomes, or are rewarding outcomes delayed? Are behaviors approximating the goal behaviors available for reinforcement?	Contingency procedures
3. Are effective behaviors inhibited by unwarranted fears or guilt? Is the person "emotion-phobic"? Are there patterns of avoidance or escape behaviors?	Exposure
4. Are effective behaviors inhibited by faulty beliefs and assumptions? Do these beliefs and assumptions reliably precede ineffective behaviors? Is the person unaware of the contingencies or rules operating in their environment? In therapy?	Cognitive modification

whenever possible, learning should occur in the context in which new behaviors are needed. For instance, learning to inhibit suicidal behavior on an inpatient unit and to replace it with distress tolerance and emotion regulation skills is not very useful if the new skills do not generalize to other environments and situations, particularly crisis situations. Similarly, learning to interact appropriately with a therapist is not a useful skill if it does not generalize to interactions in other relationships. In DBT, the emphasis is on keeping patients in problem or crisis situations while simultaneously teaching them new problem solutions and trauma coping strategies. Learning crisis survival skills (an important focus of distress tolerance training), for example, is difficult if the patient is removed from a crisis whenever the situation appears overwhelming to the therapist. This topic is discussed extensively in Chapter 15 in connection with the DBT telephone strategies and hospital protocol. Here, the therapist simply needs to keep in mind that either learning has to take place in the context where new behaviors are needed, or, if not, special efforts must be made to insure that learning generalizes to those situations.

The Rationale for Contingency Procedures

Although DBT theory emphasizes skill deficits, motivational factors are clearly important in the application of skills a patient does have. Thus, DBT balances a deficit model such as that of Kohut (1977, 1984) or Adler (1985, 1989) with a motivational model such as that of Kernberg (1984) or Masterson (1976). Even when borderline patients have the requisite skills for a particular situation, they often do not employ them. The difference here is between skill acquisition and skill performance. In DBT, motivational issues are analyzed in terms of environmental and person factors currently influencing and controlling the behaviors in question. Identifying these factors is a major focus of behavioral analysis.

Contingency procedures in DBT are based on a simple premise: The consequences of a behavior affect the probability of the behavior's occurring again. The aim is to harness the power of therapeutic contingencies to benefit the patient. At a minimum, contingency procedures require the therapist to carefully monitor and organize his or her own interpersonal behavior with the patient, so that behaviors targeted for change are not inadvertently reinforced while positive, adaptive behaviors are punished. "First, do no harm." Furthermore, when possible, the therapist should arrange outcomes so that skillful behaviors are reinforced and unskillful or maladaptive behaviors are replaced or extinguished. This is necessarily a delicate and somewhat hazardous balance in the case of suicidal behaviors, as the therapist attempts neither to reinforce suicidal responses excessively nor to ignore them in such a manner that the patient escalates these responses to a life-threatening level. This approach requires the therapist to take some short-term risks to achieve long-term gains.

"Reinforcement" here is defined in its technical sense as referring to all consequences or contingencies that increase or strengthen the probability of behavior. The definition is actually a functional one, that is, an event is only a reinforcer if it functions as one; thus, separate identification of concrete reinforcers is necessary for each person. This point cannot be overemphasized and is discussed in more detail later. Although reinforcers are typically thought of as positive, desirable, or rewarding events, they need not be. Kohlenberg and Tsai (1991), for example, point out that a dentist's being available for appointments strengthens the behavior of making a dental appointment (over going for dental work without an appointment), even for the person who hates to go to the dentist. In contrast to reinforcement procedures, extinction and punishment weaken or decrease the probability of behavior. "Extinction" is the cessation of reinforcement for a behavior that was previously reinforced. "Punishment" is the application of consequences that suppress the probability of behavior; any consequence that functions as a punishment is, by definition, "aversive." Although both procedures weaken or eliminate behavior, the way each works is markedly different. These differences are very important for the therapeutic enterprise.

In principle, DBT favors the use of reinforcement procedures, or reinforcement plus extinction, over either punishment or extinction used alone. Ideally, as noted above, the therapist tries to arrange things so that unskilled and maladaptive behaviors are replaced by incompatible skillful behaviors that have become more reinforcing for the individual. Ideal conditions, however, are not usual with borderline patients; as a result, either extinction or aversive consequences are necessary at times.

Contingency procedures in DBT, especially the use of aversive consequences, are very similar to procedures for setting limits in other therapeutic approaches. As usually defined, "setting limits" refers to the therapist's activities that punish or threaten loss of reinforcers for behaviors the therapist believes are harmful to the patient. "Limits" refers in this context to the limits of acceptable behavior. Usually, but not always, the behaviors limited are those that the therapist believes are maladaptive and out of the patient's control, or those that seriously interfere with therapy. DBT defines "limits" more narrowly and makes a distinction between limit-relevant and target-relevant behaviors (see below); however, again, the actual procedures used in DBT are quite similar to limit-setting procedures used in other types of therapy.

The Distinction Between Managing Contingencies and Observing Limits

There are two types of contingency procedures in DBT, addressing two types of behaviors. The first category. "contingency management," address the behaviors on the DBT priority target list as well as behaviors functionally related to them. Taken together, these can be considered "target-relevant behaviors"—a term very close in meaning to the term "clinically relevant behaviors," coined by Kohlenberg and Tsai (1991). Although including functionally related behaviors certainly can open Pandora's box, the targeted behaviors are clearly specified at the beginning of therapy (in principle, at least). The patient chooses to work on these behaviors by choosing to enter DBT. In long-term therapy, once behavioral patterns high in the hierarchy of targets have been remediated, target-relevant behaviors may consist primarily of patterns of behavior chosen by the patient. That is, they may reflect the seventh DBT target, the patient's individual goals. The sole factors deciding target-relevant behaviors are the welfare and long-range goals of the patient.

The second category, "observing limits," addresses all patient behaviors that push or cross the therapist's own personal limits. Taken together, these behaviors can be considered "limit-relevant behaviors." The patient's welfare and wishes are not the primary and deciding factors in this instance. Instead, the deciding factor is the relationship of the patient's behaviors to the therapist's own personal limits. Thus, limit-relevant behaviors will differ across therapists; behaviors targeted by one therapist will not necessarily be targeted by another.

DBT strongly emphasizes differentiating these two types of behaviors in using contingency procedures. Observing limits is a special category of DBT contingency procedures, in which the focus is on therapists' limits and patients' behaviors relevant to them. Limits, both for borderline patients and for their therapists, are often enormously controversial. The observing-limits approach has been developed to deal equitably and effectively with problems in this area; it differs somewhat from limit-setting approaches in many other therapies, however.

The Therapeutic Relationship as Contingency

For most borderline patients, the most powerful reinforcers usually have to do with the quality of the therapeutic relationship. With some patients, little else is powerful enough to counteract the reinforcing effects already in place for destructive and maladaptive behavior. Thus, contingency procedures are almost impossible to use before a strong relationship has developed between patient and therapist. A strong relationship enhances the valence of the therapist's behaviors, which are then used unabashedly in DBT to reinforce patient behavior. In sum, development of a strong and intense interpersonal relationship with the patient is essential. It is not that other reinforcers are unavailable, but that most other ones are either too weak or counter the reinforcing outcomes of patients' problem behaviors or not under the control of the therapist.

Once a strong positive relationship has been developed the most effective reinforcer available to the therapist is expression and continuation of the positive relationship. The most effective punishment is withdrawal of the therapist's warmth, good will, and/or approval (or, at times, withdrawal of therapy altogether). The relationship is used in the service of the patient's long-term goals. (In the vernacular used in Chapter 4, the therapist first develops a strong positive relationship and then uses it to "blackmail" the patient into making targeted, but excruciatingly difficult, changes in her behavior.) Two points are very important here. First, the therapist cannot use relationship contingencies before a strong, positive relationship is formed. "You have to get the money in the bank before you can spend it," so to speak. Second, since DBT also stresses natural over arbitrary contingencies (discussed below), the strength, if not the intensity, of the relationship has to be mutual. That is, a phony or less than genuine attachment of the therapist to the patient leads necessarily to arbitrary or less than genuine responses. (Maintaining a genuine liking for the patient is one target of the therapist supervision/consultation strategies discussed in Chapter 13.) Far from ignoring or downplaying the therapeutic relationship, DBT stresses the strength of the relationship.

For many therapists, the notion of using interpersonal warmth, attachment, and so forth as reinforcers may seem incompatible with genuinely caring for a patient. For some, the very idea feels manipulative. For others, genuine caring means staying warm and attached no matter what the other person does. As with most controversies, there is truth to both sides. On the one hand, in most relationships people naturally reinforce prosocial, adaptive behaviors and withhold reinforcement following negative or disliked behaviors. When a husband lies or steals, for instance, a loving wife does not immediately express approval and warmth. A person does not usually respond to a hostile verbal attack by spending more time with the attacker. Other types of human relationships differ from a therapeutic relationship not in how positive behaviors are responded to, but rather in who is benefiting from the positive behavior and the explicitness of the use of contingencies. In the therapy relationship, behaviors that benefit the patient are reinforced, and the use of contingencies is intentional and self-conscious. In most other relationships (particularly peer relationships), the benefit of both parties is equally important in determining what behaviors will be reinforced, and contingencies are used in an un-self-conscious way.

On the other hand, use of interpersonal contingencies should not be an excuse for withholding warmth, attachment, intimacy, approval, and validation from a relationship-deprived patient. Minute for minute, even the most difficult patient is usually engaging in far more positive, adaptive behaviors than problematic behaviors. Simply coming to a therapy session and sticking it out constitute an accomplishment for many. Indeed, the deprived lives of many borderline individuals suggest that therapists should attempt to provide as much interpersonal dependability, nurturance, and care as possible. That is, they should search for opportunities to reinforce the patients; more simply put, therapists must love their patients, giving them what they need to flourish and grow, and perhaps a bit more. Nor should the criteria for warmth and approval be set too high. The slightest misstep cannot occasion catastrophic loss. I discuss this point more fully below in connection with principles of shaping.

CONTINGENCY MANAGEMENT PROCEDURES

Every response within an interpersonal interaction is a potential form of reinforcement, punishment, or extinction. This is no less true in psychotherapy than in any other relationship, and holds true whether the therapist and patient intend it or not. How the therapist responds to the patient from moment to moment, affects what the patient subsequently does, feels, thinks, and senses. Contingency management strategies are ways to manage the contingent relationships between the patient's behavior and the therapist's responses so that the ultimate outcomes are beneficial instead of iatrogenic. The most important are reviewed in this section and summarized in Table 10.2.

Orienting to Contingency Management: Task Overview

The therapist should orient the patient to the use of contingency management in psychotherapy. The enormous confusion, among patients and profes-

TABLE 10.2. Contingency Management Procedures Checklist

____ T orients P to contingency management
    ____ T explains how learning, including reinforcement, takes place.
    ____ T discusses difference between "intending" an outcome and an outcome's being "functionally related" to behavior.
____ T REINFORCES target-relevant adaptive behaviors.
    ____ T makes reinforcement immediate.
    ____ T adapts schedule of reinforcement to fit strength of P's adaptive response.
        ____ When response is weak, T reinforces P every time (or almost) P emits desired behavior.
        ____ As response gets stronger, T gradually fades frequency and intensity of reinforcement to an intermittent schedule.
        ____ As environmental and self-managed contingencies become increasingly effective, T gradually phases out reinforcement completely.
    ____ T uses the therapeutic relationship as a reinforcer.
____ T EXTINGUISHES target-relevant maladaptive behaviors.
    ____ T assesses whether behavior is being maintained by reinforcing consequences.
    ____ T does not appease.
    ____ T holds to the extinction schedule during behavioral bursts.
    ____ T engages P in problem solving to help her find another behavior that can be reinforced.
        ____ T rapidly reinforces alternate adaptive behavior.
    ____ T soothes P during extinction.
        ____ T is solicitous and validating of P's suffering.
        ____ T warmly reminds P of extinction rationale.
____ T uses AVERSIVE CONTINGENCIES when necessary:
    ____ When the reinforcing consequences of high-priority target-relevant, maladaptive behavior are not under T's control.
    ____ When the maladaptive behavior interferes with all other adaptive behaviors.
    ____ T uses disapproval, confrontation, or withdrawal of warmth (cautiously).
    ____ T uses correction–overcorrection.
    ____ T uses vacations from therapy when necessary.
    ____ T terminates therapy as a last resort *only*.
____ T determines potency of consequences.
    ____ T identifies reinforcers and aversive consequences empirically; T does not assume that a particular event, item, or response (especially praise) is necessarily reinforcing or aversive for a particular P.
    ____ T uses a variety of different consequences.
____ T uses natural consequences over arbitrary consequences whenever possible.
    ____ T pairs arbitrary consequences with natural consequences, fading arbitrary ones over time to strengthen effectiveness of natural consequences.
____ T uses principles of shaping in reinforcing P's behavior. (T adjusts reinforcement contingencies to balance requirements of situation with current capabilities of P.)

(cont.)

Table 10.2 (cont.)

_____ T uses a reinforcement schedule that gradually and progressively shapes P's responses toward desired goal behavior.

_____ T reinforces behaviors already in P's repertoire that are in the direction of a target behavior.

_____ T pushes P to just below the limit of her capability; task difficulty required for reinforcement is just a little bit more difficult than what P has already accomplished.

_____ When P behaves near the limit of her capability, T reinforces behavior.

_____ T does not reinforce (T extinguishes) behaviors far from the goal behavior when behaviors more similar to it are within P's capability.

_____ T uses information about all variables in a situation (including those that impinge on P's current vulnerability) to grade difficulty of task.

Anti-DBT tactics

_____ T "gives in" to P's demands and reinforces behaviors well below P's capabilities when more capable behavior is required in the situation at hand.

_____ T is inconsistent in use of contingency management procedures.

_____ T is punitive in use of aversive consequences.

_____ T requires behaviors beyond P's capabilities before reinforcing behavioral attempt.

---

sionals alike, about principles of reinforcement and their effects on behavior makes this task both extra important and extra difficult. Getting across accurate information about how learning works is crucial if the patient is to collaborate in discovering the forces controlling her own behavior. It goes without saying that the therapist has to be fully familiar with principles of learning; most general textbooks on behavior modification or behavior therapy will have a summary of these principles (e.g., Martin & Pear, 1992; Masters et al., 1987; Millenson & Leslie, 1979; O'Leary & Wilson, 1987). The therapist also has to work at reducing the stigma of socially unacceptable patterns of reinforcement. In my experience, the following points (in any order) are the most helpful ones to make.

First, the therapist should discuss the differences among intentions, behavioral planning, purpose, and consequences as they influence how individuals respond or act in the world. With borderline patients, this is a particularly sensitive point. The intent of their behaviors is frequently unrelated to at least some of the outcomes, including outcomes that reinforce the behaviors. The therapist should point out to the patient (as I have pointed out throughout this book) that is it an error in logic to assume that the consequences of behavior necessarily prove intent. Many consequences are in fact unintended. Moreover, the fact that a consequence strengthens behavior (i.e., is a reinforcer) does not mean that the consequence was intended or wanted; unintended consequences can and frequently do reinforce behavior.

Second, the therapist should discuss the automatic nature of most learning. Examples that can be used include infant and animal learning, in which conscious or unconscious intent is usually not ascribed. The physical effects of reinforcement on the brain, independent of what a person may intend or want, can also be discussed. Reinforcing consequences cause chemical changes in the brain; neural circuits are changed.

Third, the therapist should point out that consequences can affect behavior without a person's awareness. In fact, most of us are not aware of how and when behavioral consequences influence our behavior. Thus, the fact that we "feel" as if we are doing something for one reason or purpose does not necessarily mean that this reason or purpose is actually influencing our behavior. All humans (not just "mental patients") tend to construct reasons for their own behavior when "causes" are not apparent (Nisbett & Wilson, 1977). An example of this would be as follows. In animals, research has shown that stimulating certain reward centers in the brain increases the frequency of any behavior immediately preceding the stimulation. In fact, the effect is so powerful that an animal can be made to engage in a "rewarded" behavior so frequently that it will not stop to eat even when food-deprived. (This research is summarized in Millenson & Leslie, 1979.) In humans, if there were a way to contingently stimulate the reward center in the brain, it would also increase the immediately preceding behaviors. If a person knew that this was being done, he or she would, of course, explain the increased behavior as due to the stimulation. But what if there were a way to stimulate a person's reward center in the brain without his or her knowledge? If this stimulation could be made contingent on some particular behavior, the behavior would increase, but the person would not know that the stimulation was influencing it. In this circumstance, normal people will make up a rational reason, unrelated to brain stimulation (e.g., "I like doing it"), to explain their own behavior. The therapist can give an example of when he or she has "constructed" a reason for behavior that was later found to be influenced by something else entirely, and then solicit examples from the patient.

Fourth, the therapist should note that when a person figures out what is influencing his or her behavior, this is called "insight." It is unlikely that insight into socially unacceptable behavior reinforcement patterns will be achieved if therapist and patient collude in assuming that intent, consequences, and reinforcement go necessarily hand in hand, or that "feelings" or beliefs about causes (without supporting data) are always the best information about what is really influencing behavior. When both patient and therapist formulate reinforcement principles in this manner, they work against observing and identifying the contingent relationships that influence behavior.

Fifth, it is very helpful to give a lesson on the effects of extinction on behavior. If necessary, the therapist can explain to the patient how maladaptive behaviors may temporarily increase in frequency or intensity after removal of reinforcement. Understanding these effects sometimes mitigates the pain associated with removal of usual reinforcers. The foot-in-the-door technique, described in Chapter 9, can be used to help the patient make a commitment to tolerating the painful aspects of changing contingencies.

Finally, principles of punishment, discussed below, should be reviewed with the patient. This information serves several purposes besides simple orientation. It provides a rationale for the patient's deciding to drop punishment as a self-control technique. As I have mentioned several times previously, self-punishment is sometimes the only self-control procedures used by borderline individuals. In addition, providing information on the time-limited and negative effects of punishment increases that patient's power in the therapeutic relationship, and gives her a "weapon" to use in trying to stop unwise use of coercion by the therapist.

The classes of behavior targeted for reinforcement (e.g., distress tolerance, mindfulness) and for extinction and punishment (e.g., threatening suicide, attacking the therapist) will have been discussed as part of the initial and continuing assessment and treatment planning. The principles discussed above, and others discussed more fully later in this chapter, should ordinarily be reviewed with the patient during the initial orientation to therapy. Reorientation may also be needed when patient and therapist are attempting to figure out what is maintaining a particular pattern of behavior. The principles may need further review when major new contingencies are being applied to the patient's behavior. However, it is not necessary or particularly helpful for the therapist to explain why, what, or how contingencies are being implemented in every single instance. To do this would so remove the pattern of contingencies from that used in everyday life that generalization might be seriously compromised. This is a particularly important issue when extinction and punishment are being used; it is discussed in more detail below.

I. REINFORCING TARGET-RELEVANT ADAPTIVE BEHAVIORS

A central principle of DBT is that therapists should reinforce target-relevant adaptive behaviors when they occur. The therapist must at all times pay attention to (1) what the patient is doing; (2) whether the patient's behavior is targeted for increase, is targeted for decrease, or is irrelevant to current aims (i.e., whether the behavior is target-relevant); and (3) how he or she responds to the patient behaviors. In Kohlenberg and Tsai's (1991) terms, the therapist must observe clinically relevant behaviors and reinforce those behaviors that represent progress. Two important principles of reinforcement are proper timing and proper scheduling.

Timing of Reinforcement

Immediate reinforcement is far more powerful than delayed reinforcement. This is why so many behaviors are extraordinarily difficult to decrease: They result in short-term, immediate reinforcement. Often, however, these same behaviors lead to long-term negative or punishing outcomes. Addictive behaviors are a good example here. The immediate reinforcing effects of drugs, alcohol, gambling, food, and often suicidal behaviors as well, strengthen the behaviors far more effectively than long-term aversive consequences weaken them. Thus, it is important for the therapist to reinforce improved behavior as soon as possible. Behaviors occurring in the therapist's presence, or during telephone conversations are much more available for immediate reinforcement. Thus, it is important to be alert to improvement during therapy interactions.

Scheduling of Reinforcement

At the beginning of therapy, continuous reinforcement may be needed. If positive behaviors occur at a low rate, almost every instance should be reinforced in some manner. Once the patient is emitting skilled behaviors at a high rate, the therapist can begin to fade the reinforcement schedule gradually, and can then phase it out altogether. Behaviors that are intermittently reinforced are far more resistant to extinction. However, the therapist should be alert to precipitous drops in reinforcement frequency and to long periods of little or no reinforcement. In such instances, the therapist should examine his or her own attentiveness to positive events or attitudes toward the patient.

Validation, Responsiveness, and Nondemanding Attentiveness as Reinforcers

How to reinforce a borderline patient can be exceptionally complex. For some patients, expressions of warmth and closeness are very effective; for others, such expressions are so threatening that their effect is just the opposite of that intended. Although a central procedure in DBT is to develop a positive relationship and then use that relationship to reinforce progress, how close the therapist and patient are to actually having such a relationship determines which therapist behaviors are likely to reinforce and which are likely to punish. How to determine the potency of consequences is discussed below.

For most (but certainly not all) borderline patients, the following relationship behaviors are reinforcing: (1) expressions of the therapist's approval, care, concern, and interest; (2) behaviors that communicate liking or admiring the patient (see cautions below on use of praise), wanting to work with her, and wanting to interact with her; (3) behaviors that reassure the patient that the therapist is dependable and the therapy is secure; (4) almost any validating response (except, at times, cheerleading); (5) behaviors that are responsive to the patient's requests and inputs; and (6) attention from or contact with the therapist (e.g., getting regular or extra appointments, being able to phone the therapist between sessions, having longer or shorter sessions as the patient desires).

2. EXTINGUISHING TARGET-RELEVANT MALADAPTIVE BEHAVIORS

Behavioral responses are extinguished when the reinforcers that maintain the behavior are removed. The therapist must determine what reinforcers are in fact maintaining a particular maladaptive behavior pattern, and then systematically withhold those reinforcers following the behavior. All other things being equal, a therapist should not reinforce high-priority, maladaptive behaviors once they have been targeted for extinction. The therapist should keep in mind that specific priorities for contingency management are determined by the target hierarchy and by the principles of shaping discussed below. Once a behavior is put on an extinction schedule, however, the therapist should not abandon the extinction program even if higher-priority target behaviors emerge.

Because extinction procedures can be misused so easily, it can be useful to remember that not all behaviors are maintained by their consequences. Some behaviors are, instead, elicited automatically by prior events. For example, take the baby who cries when stuck by a pin and then stops crying when the pin is pulled out. Is it reasonable to assume that pulling pins out of babies maintains (reinforces) crying? Perhaps, but it is more reasonable to assume that crying is automatically elicited by the pinprick. Rather than leaving the pin stuck in the baby so as not to reinforce crying, the sensible thing to do is to remove the pin. (From the point of view of "contingencies of survival," however, it may be just this contingency that caused humans to develop automatic crying following painful events in the first place. Babies who cry or yelp when in pain or danger are more likely to be taken care of, and thus have an increased potential to survive infancy and pass on their genes.) There simply is no substitute for a good behavioral analysis to determine what is, in fact, maintaining the maladaptive behavior in question. (This point, especially as it applies to suicidal behavior, is discussed more fully in Chapter 15.)

Nonetheless, much of human behavior, including many maladaptive behaviors of borderline patients, are maintained by their consequences. The idea of withholding reinforcement following a behavior targeted for extinction may seem simple and obvious, but it can be enormously difficult to carry out in practice, especially with suicidal patients. The reason for the difficulty is that many behaviors targeted for extinction are under the control of two types of consequences relevant to therapy: They result in reinforcing interpersonal outcomes, and/or they provide escape from aversive situations. Interpersonally, such behaviors may function to communicate, to get help, to maintain closeness (or distance), to obtain resources the person needs or wants, to get revenge, and so on. In addition, the behaviors often distract the patient from or put an end to painful events or interactions. A borderline patient's problem behaviors often function quite effectively. Mental health professionals (including previous therapists), family members, and other intimates have often inadvertently reinforced, usually on an intermittent schedule, the very behaviors the current therapist and the patient are trying to eliminate.

For example, a patient may beg to be hospitalized because she feels too overwhelmed to cope. If the therapist refuses because he or she believes that the patient can cope, but then reconsiders when she threatens to kill herself if she is not hospitalized, this will inadvertently (and usually without awareness of either the patient or the therapist) increase the probability and intensity of future suicidal urges and threats. If a helpless stance or out-of-control emotionality leads the therapist to pay more attention or give more help to the patient than when she asks for what she wants directly and competently, this will reinforce the helplessness and emotionality the therapist is trying to reduce. If in the middle of discussing a difficult or painful topic the patient is trying to avoid, the therapist switches topics or becomes solicitous when the patient dissociates, depersonalizes, or engages in personal attacks, dissociating, depersonalizing, and personal attacks (all other things being equal) can be counted on to increase.

By contrast, if the therapist does not reinforce these behaviors, this effectively puts the patient on an extinction schedule. Doing so has several predictable consequences. First, although in time the behavior can be expected to decrease, there will be a "behavioral burst" near the beginning of extinction and intermittently thereafter. Extinction has the paradoxical effect of temporarily increasing the strength, intensity, and frequency of behavior. Second, if the behavior previously functioned to meet an important need of the person or to terminate very aversive states, and if the patient has no other behaviors that work as well, the therapist can expect the patient's general behavior to become somewhat disorganized or intense. The person may search for other equivalent behaviors that will work; if these fail also, the person may react with extreme emotion and thinking, and behavior may become chaotic.

How the therapist responds to these reactions is critical. When a behavior is noxious for the therapist, or the therapist fears irrevocable harm to the patient, it is very tempting to decide to stop the extinction procedure temporarily. In the examples given above, it is very difficult to maintain the positions of not hospitalizing the patient who threatens suicide; of not giving more attention, help, and concern when the patient is out of control; and of not withdrawing and reorienting the treatment session when the patient dissociates, depersonalizes, or attacks. Although these responses may at times be necessary, and may result in short-term gain, their effect on the patient's long-term welfare may be iatrogenic. If these responses are indeed reinforcers for that particular patient, the behavior targeted for extinction is made even more resistant to extinction, and thus more likely to show up in the future. In addition, if the timing of a reinforcing response follows a behavioral burst or disorganized, extreme, or chaotic behavior this also makes the behavior worse. When the behavior in question is suicidal behavior, this can indeed be unfortunate: The individual can escalate such behavior only so far before she ends up dead.

Various factors may increase the likelihood of the therapist's breaking the extinction schedule. When the patient has previously been rewarded for persistence and very extreme responses, the patient may simply wear out the therapist. This is most likely when a therapist is tired, is overextended, and has not observed his or own limits. Breaking the schedule and appeasement is also likely when the therapist is unsure of his or her treatment plan, has not properly assessed the behavior, or feels guilty about not giving the patient what she apparently wants and needs. Appeasement usually occurs when the extinction process leads to a greater display of pain than the therapist can handle, or the therapist feels threatened by the patient's behavior (e.g., when the therapist fears that the patient will commit suicide or otherwise substantially harm herself). Borderline patients frequently threaten suicide if a therapist does not do something to reduce their pain. "Giving in" reduces the threat and the pain display, and soothes therapist and patient alike.

The therapist can do a number of things to ease the extinction process for patient and therapist alike. It is important to do so, because otherwise, one or both parties may simply quit the enterprise. An extinction schedule should be aimed at the targeted behavior, not at the individual herself. The aim is to break the relationship between the targeted behavior and reinforcing consequences; this aim is not necessarily to deprive the individual of those consequences completely. Two strategies are useful here: finding other behaviors to reinforce, and soothing.

1. *Finding another response to reinforce.* The first strategy is to get the patient to engage in some behavior that can be reinforced in place of the behavior being extinguished. According to the principles of shaping (discussed below), the idea is to get the patient to do something just a little bit better than usual and then to move in quickly with reinforcement. With a borderline patient this may require much use of problem solving, and considerable patience, but usually some positive or improved behavior will result if therapist and patient persist. (At least, it will once the patient learns that the therapist is not a person likely to give in and reinforce behaviors that both have agreed must stop.) The long-term task is to associate adaptive problem-solving behaviors with more reinforcing outcomes than those linked to maladaptive behaviors.

2. *Soothing.* With a patient on an extinction schedule, it is crucial for the therapist to validate the importance of her getting what she wants and needs, and to acknowledge solicitously how difficult the therapy process is. The problem rarely is in what she wants or needs but in how she goes about getting it. Thus, the therapist must combine extinction with a heavy dose of soothing and kindness. This can be particularly difficult for therapists, especially those who feel guilty about not giving patients what they want. Some therapists cope with their own painful emotions by closing themselves off emotionally from their patients; that is, they behave in a somewhat borderline fashion themselves—all or none. One possible tactic is to come up with a way to suffer along with the patient, meanwhile continuing the extinction. (A father who tells a child he is spanking that the spanking hurts him more than the child is an example here.) Orienting, didactic, and commitment strategies can also be applied. A patient often experiences extinc-

tion as arbitrary and emotionally withholding; explaining why it is being used, and working on a recommitment to work on the targeted behavior, can be helpful.

The bottom line is threefold. First, once a patient is placed on an extinction schedule, the therapist has to find the courage and commitment to stick to it. Second, when extinguishing behaviors that are functional for the individual, the therapist must help the patient find other, more adaptive behaviors that will function as well or better and be sure to reinforce those behaviors. Third, when putting a patient on an extinction schedule, the therapist must soothe her through it. Extinction is not a means of punishing patients.

3. USING AVERSIVE CONSEQUENCES...WITH CARE

When to Use Aversive Consequences

As I have noted above, punishment is the pairing of a behavioral response with an aversive consequence. Doing something to the patient that she doesn't want and taking away something she does want, for example, are aversive consequences for most people. As with reinforcement, however, the effect of any specific consequence depends on the particular situation, the particular behavior targeted, and other contextual characteristics. An event that is aversive in one context or situation may not be aversive in another. Once again, as with reinforcement, the definition of punishment is a functional or procedural one, and an event or outcome is labeled "aversive" (and the whole procedure is labeled "punishment") only if it acts to suppress behaviors in the specific case.

The difference between extinction and punishment is sometimes subtle but important. In extinction, the consequence that is reinforcing the behavior is removed; in punishment, positive conditions previously unrelated to the response are removed (or aversive conditions are added). For example, if parasuicide on an inpatient unit is reinforced by staff attention, ignoring the patient after parasuicidal behavior is extinction; taking away desired privileges or publicly humiliating her is punishment.

At times, aversive consequences are the only way to eliminate targeted maladaptive behaviors. They are used in DBT in two instances. First, they are used when the consequences reinforcing a target-relevant, high-priority behavior are not under the control of the therapist and no other stronger reinforcers are available. That is, the behavior cannot be put on an extinction schedule, nor can incompatible alternative behavior be reinforced. For example, "borderline" behaviors may immediately and effectively reduce or terminate painful emotions, thoughts and situations or create pleasant ones; result in desired inpatient admissions (or discharges) or money from public assistance; provide a way out of a difficult task; or elicit validation and expressions of care or concern from others. When these reinforcers cannot be controlled by the therapist and are more powerful than any equivalent reinforcers the therapist has at his or her disposal, the application of aversive consequences may be necessary. Second, aversive consequences are used when a maladaptive behavior interferes with all other adaptive behaviors—in other words, when no other behaviors occur that can be reinforced. This is particularly likely when the situation elicits the problem behavior more or less automatically. For example, a patient in our program was at times so hostile toward her therapist that no therapeutic work could be accomplished. The behavior appeared to be an automatic, conditioned response to certain topics brought up in therapy. Once it began, however, the hostile behavior was so pervasive that little or no positive behavior was emitted that could be reinforced. In this instance, the therapist responded by ending sessions early if the patient could not control her hostile, attacking behavior within 20 minutes.

Disapproval, Confrontation, and Withdrawal of Warmth as Aversive Consequences

Criticism, confrontation, and withdrawal of therapist approval and warmth can be extremely aversive for the average borderline patient. (See below for further cautions in determining the potency of consequences). Indeed, they can be so aversive that the therapist has to use them not only with very great care, but also in very low doses and very briefly. Often what the therapist sees as a minor criticism, for example, is experienced by the patient as not only a criticism of her entire way of being, but also as a threat to the continuation of therapy itself. Thus, both intense shame and equally intense fears of abandonment may be immediate consequences. Although this may be the intended level of punishment some of the time, it is usually far too extreme for the behavior in question. Expressions of frustration or dismay can be far more effective than expressions of anger. The therapist's anger can be so intensely disturbing that the patient becomes emotionally disorganized and perhaps even more dysfunctional than before. (Conversely, for some patients the therapist's anger is actually reinforcing, since it communicates that the therapist "cares enough" to get angry.) In using aversive interpersonal consequences, a therapist must be cautious and analyze their effectiveness at every step.

Nonetheless, with proper consideration, just enough disapproval, confrontation, or emotional withdrawal can be effective. Sometimes no other effective response is available. There are a number of ways to present negative opinions and emotional reactions. The reciprocal and irreverent communication strategies, discussed at some length in Chapter 12, can be used. For example, the therapist may say, "When you do X, I feel or do Y" (where X is the problem behavior and Y is a response that the patient does not want). Or, more irreverently, the therapist may say to a patient who threatens to kill herself, "If you kill yourself I'm going to stop being your therapist."

When the therapist responds to target-relevant maladaptive behavior with disapproval, confrontation, or withdrawal of warmth, it is very important to restore a positive interpersonal atmosphere following any improvement the patient shows, even if the positive change is minimal and barely discernible. That is, approval, praise and interpersonal warmth should follow; otherwise, the patient is likely to feel (reasonably, if sometimes disproportionately) that no matter what she does she cannot please the therapist. At times, of course, a patient can engage in behaviors that are so aversive or frustrating to the therapist that emotional warmth simply is not immediately available, even though the patient attempts to repair the situation. In these cases, the natural consequence of the patient's behavior is longer-lasting than the patient, and sometimes the therapist, may wish. A good strategy here is to discuss the problem with the patient in an open and accepting manner. The very discussion is itself a step toward relationship repair, and thus will probably reinforce the patient's improvement.

Correction–Overcorrection as an Aversive Consequence

The first and most important guidelines in using aversive consequences are that a consequence should "fit the crime" and that the patient must have a way to avoid or terminate it. The "correction–overcorrection" technique meets both these criteria (see Cannon, 1983, and Mackenzie-Keating & McDonald, 1990, for reviews of this procedure). In addition, it is usually satisfying for the therapist.

There are three steps in correction–overcorrection. First, following the occurrence of a problem behavior, the therapist withdraws a positive condition, withholds something the patient wants, or adds an aversive consequence. The best consequence is one that expands a natural but undesirable (from the patient's point of view) effect of the behavior. Second, the therapist requires the patient to engage in a new behavior that both corrects the effects of the maladaptive behavior, and goes past that and *over*corrects the effects. Instructions are explicit; the rationale of correction–overcorrection is clearly stated; and positive consequences for engaging in the correction–overcorrection are laid out. The required corrective behavior, is thus dialectically related to the problem behavior. Third, once the new "correcting–overcorrecting" behavior occurs the therapist immediately stops the punishment — that is, undoes the negative conditions or stops withholding. Thus, the patient has a ready way to terminate the punishment. The challenge, of course, is to devise outcomes and overcorrection behaviors that are aversive enough while not at the same time trivial or unrelated to the behaviors the therapist wants to teach.

The insistence in DBT that patients who engage in parasuicide between sessions participate in detailed behavioral and solution analyses of the behavior before other topics are discussed is an example of correction–overcorrection. The negative consequence expanded is the therapist's very natural concern for the patient and eagerness to be sure that this very difficult behavior is stopped. If a person is so miserable that she actually commits a parasuicidal act, how can a responsible therapist ignore it? The therapist insists on addressing the problem. The correction–overcorrection procedures are the behavioral and solution analyses. Although many borderline patients like to discuss the problems that set off their parasuicidal behavior, very few like to discuss the events and behaviors leading up to the response; for almost all, this is an aversive consequence. On the other hand, they usually have topics they do want to talk about. The reinforcement is the ability to talk about other things. A patient of mine who used to attempt suicide, overdose, and mutilate herself on a regular basis suddenly, after 6 months of therapy, stopped completely. I asked her what happened. She said she had figured out that if she didn't stop, she would never get to talk about anything else.

A similar strategy is used in skills training. For example, when a patient has not done any homework, the therapist launches into a full-scale, very empathetic analysis of what factors inhibited or interfered with her practice. In a group setting, other members are encouraged to offer ideas about how to counteract these influences. If the patient absolutely refuses to go along, the therapist may switch to a full-scale, equally solicitous analysis of her resistance. One patient used to appear at skills training in an emotional fog, saying that she hadn't remembered or had been too overwhelmed to practice her skills. One week, after several frustrating months, she began to report and discuss attempts to practice. Her practice as well as group interactions increased, and before too long she was interacting at the level of other patients. Her individual therapist asked what happened. She said she got tired of using up group time to analyze why she hadn't practiced and figured it was easier just to do it.

Correction–overcorrection is an example of using both the carrot and the stick. Interaction with the therapist is often the carrot, and the correction–overcorrection is the stick. A patient leaving a late appointment not only tore things off the walls, but stole the belongings of people working at the clinic. She thus crossed the limits of both the therapist and clinic (a topic discussed further below), a clear case of therapy-interfering behavior. The consequence was that she was required not only to restore the clinic to its previous state and return the stolen property, but also to improve the after-hours security of the clinic by contributing to the cost of hiring an after-hours receptionist. The carrot was another appointment with her therapist. In a similar crossing of the limits, another patient repaired numerous holes she kicked in walls, repainting and sprucing up the rooms while she was at it. Once the holes were repaired, sessions resumed. A patient of mine (with my collusion) developed a pattern of calling me on the phone in the evenings, threatening suicide and acting in such an abusive fashion that I started dreading going home and wanted to terminate therapy with her. Instead, I limited my availability by phone to 20 minutes per week, divided between two calls. Furthermore, I told her that her task was not only to correct her phone interactions with me so that they would influence me to be willing to talk to her, but to overcorrect so that I would actually want to do so. At that point I would change my policy. It took her a year, but she finally succeeded.

Vacations from Therapy as Aversive Consequences

Another guideline in the use of punishment is that it should be just strong enough to work. The ultimate punishment is termination of therapy, a consequence many borderline patients have experienced more than once. Many inpatient units and therapists have clear rules that if particular behaviors occur even once, therapy is terminated. Parasuicidal acts, especially near-lethal ones, are typical behaviors that automatically lead to therapy termination. Other examples are seeing other therapists, obtaining unauthorized admissions to inpatient units, bringing weapons to therapy, attacking therapists, and so on.

DBT discourages unilateral termination. It is as if a therapist says, "If you actually have the problems you came to therapy for, I will terminate therapy." Termination of therapy also terminates any chance the therapist has of helping the patient make needed changes. Putting a patient on a "vacation from therapy" is a DBT fall-back strategy. Vacations are used for both target-relevant and limit-relevant behaviors. Two conditions are required: (1) All other contingencies have failed, and (2) the behavior or lack of behavior is so serious that it crosses the therapist's therapeutic or personal limits. "Therapeutic limits" are the limits within which the therapist can conduct effective therapy. A vacation can be used when the therapist believes that unless the patient changes her behavior, the therapist can no longer be of help; that is, the patient's behavior is interfering with therapy to such an extent that effective therapy is not possible. "Personal limits," as noted earlier in this chapter, are the limits within which the therapist is willing to work with the patient. A vacation can be instituted when the therapist is personally unwilling to continue unless things change. The conditions resulting in a vacation will differ for each therapist and patient.

A "vacation" is the cessation of therapy for a specified period of time, or until a particular condition is met or change is made. A number of steps are necessary in organizing a vacation. First, the therapist must identify the behavior that has to change; expectations should be clear. Second, the therapist must give the patient a reasonable chance to change the behavior and help her to do so. That is, the patient should be able to avoid the vacation. Third, the conditions should be presented as resulting from the therapist's limits as a therapist (see the discussion on observing limits, below). That is, the therapist needs to show some humility here, acknowledging that another therapist might be able to help the patient without these conditions. Fourth, the therapist must make it clear that once the condition or time requirement has been met, the patient can return to therapy. Fifth, while the patient is on vacation, the therapist should maintain intermittent contact by phone or letter, encouraging the patient to change and return. (In the vernacular, the therapist kicks the patient out and then pines for her return.) Finally, the therapist should provide a referral or backup therapist while the patient is on vacation.

Here is an example. After working with a patient for some time, I came to believe that if she did not agree to work on reducing her excessive alcohol consumption, we could go no further. I could not determine whether alcohol abuse was causing many of her remaining problems or was a result of them. She refused, believing that alcohol was helping more than hurting her. I gave her 3 months to come to a different decision — to choose between me and alcohol, so to speak. She had to work with me on substance abuse or enter an alcohol treatment program. If she refused, I could not continue treatment, *but* (and this is how a vacation differs from termination) I would take her back as soon as she was willing to meet my terms. She felt that she could not stop drinking under pressure from me. This seemed fair enough; I suggested that she see someone else to help her decide for herself, and she went on vacation. Following a driving while intoxicated conviction, she was ordered to participate in a certain number of hours a week of court-approved substance abuse therapy, so that she had no time to work with me. After completing the 2-year court-ordered program, she called me to resume therapy.

Another patient was put on vacation because I felt I could not help her further unless she engaged in some productive activities. Because of her severe dyslexia, epilepsy, and a degenerative nerve condition, not to mention her 15 years of frequent psychiatric hospitalizations, she was on public assistance. Her choices were at least 20 hours per week of school, a job or volunteer work, or a therapy vacation. I gave her 6 months to get into vocational counseling or school, and then 6 more months to start work or school. She met the first condition the day before the deadline. She did not meet the second one and went on vacation, with my suggestion that she see another therapist to help her decide about continuing therapy with me. She stayed in group therapy and found a case manager to see her individually. She was so angry at me that she refused to talk to me and ended up back in a psychiatric inpatient unit, where she tried to get the staff to call me and make me change my mind. Every several weeks or so, I would catch her before her group meeting and tell her how I missed her in individual therapy and couldn't wait until she organized some productive activities. She finally did, and therapy turned around.

The examples above involved the absence of patient behaviors that I believed were essential for the conduct of therapy. What does a therapist do when a patient is actively engaging in high-rate behaviors destructive to therapy, or the therapist's willingness to continue is exhausted (personal limits) and all other change procedures have failed? A patient of one of our therapists repeatedly called the therapist's home answering machine and left messages. The frequency and abusiveness of the messages had been a focus of contingency management for some time. In one call, the patient threatened not only the life of the therapist but also that of the therapist's 9-year-old son, who just happened to be listening when the message came in. The patient's behavior clearly crossed the therapist's limits. The patient was told that if the behavior recurred for any reason whatsoever, she would be on vacation from therapy. The patient repeated the behavior and was put on vacation. Another therapist stepped in to help with a referral. The terms were that she could return to therapy if she managed to go an entire 30 days without contacting the therapist or the therapist's associates in any way (by phone, message, letter, etc.). This was the condition required to reassure the therapist that the patient would be able to control her behavior in the future. The condition that had to be met was that the patient had to reassure the therapist by her behavior that continuation would not be harmful to the therapist's family.

Vacations following adverse behaviors should only be used when the behaviors actually interfere with the conduct of therapy. One way to remember this is that the patient's behavior and the punishment should, when possible, occur in the same system, arena, or context. If behaviors interfere with therapy, therapy should be stopped. As in the dialectical technique of extending, (see Chapter 7) the therapist extends or exaggerates the normal consequences of the patient's behavior. The therapist also needs to know how aversive a vacation will be. For some patients, having to miss a week or two of therapy following dysfunctional behaviors is actually reinforcing; they feel too ashamed to come anyway. Obviously, such patients should not be put on brief vacations. For others, even a 1 week vacation is highly aversive and is sufficient to affect their behavior. Or a partial vacation, such as no phone calls for a specified period of time (if, say, the patient is making abusive calls), may be sufficient. Generally, if the behavior pattern is extreme and all else has failed (including brief vacations), the therapist should consider putting the patient on vacation until the end of the contracted period. At that point, the patient should be allowed to return to renegotiate a new contract for therapy with the therapist. In DBT, only one situation *requires* a vacation until the end of the contract: missing 4 scheduled weeks of therapy in a row (see Chapter 4 for a discussion of this rule).

Termination from Therapy. . .as an Aversive Last Resort

As in a marriage or family relationship, any permanent breakup is regarded as a last resort in DBT. However, under some conditions termination is unavoidable or even advisable. At the beginning of therapy, before a strong relationship is formed, a therapist may terminate if he or she believes that another therapist would be more helpful. Obviously, this is only an option if another therapist is available. In later stages of the relationship, DBT should be terminated before the end of the contracted period only after every available option for saving the relationship has been pursued, including resolute attention to therapy-interfering behaviors, outside consultation or "couples" counseling, and vacations. The idea is to treat behaviors that cause burnout before burnout occurs. However, if burnout does occur, despite one's best efforts, the situation may be irretrievable; that is, the therapist may not be able to recover. In such a case, it is better to terminate and refer than to continue a possibly destructive relationship. The important point to remember is that termination by the therapist is viewed in DBT as a failure of therapy, not a failure of the patient.

Punishment versus Punitiveness

Treating borderline patients is extremely stressful; often, the behaviors targeted for change are the very ones that increase this stress. Vindictiveness and hostility toward patients are not uncommon feelings for therapists in this situation. Punishing the patients, however, is not an appropriate way to express these feelings. In my experience, it is extraordinarily easy for therapists to punish patients covertly, hiding the behavior under the guise of therapeutic responding. Involuntarily hospitalizing a patient (or refusing to hospitalize her), suggesting a referral, terminating therapy, medicating heavily, confronting a patient, making invalidating appeals to unconscious motivations, and writing pejorative case notes can all appear "therapeutic" even when they are used in decidedly nontherapeutic ways. With aversive consequences in particular, therapists must watch their own behavior with borderline patients very carefully. The consultation team can be extremely useful here.

There are a number of guidelines for evaluating the legitimacy of aversive responses. First, the behavior being punished should be target-relevant. With the exception of observing limits (see below), DBT ignores behaviors that are not targeted, even if the therapist privately or professionally disapproves of them. Second, behaviors lower on the DBT target hierarchy are ignored in favor of higher-priority behaviors. Thus, in DBT, therapists let many maladaptive behaviors go by the wayside. (Behaviors ignored in the early phases of therapy, however, may not be ignored in later phases.) Third, if extinction or reinforcing competing behaviors would work just as well, aversive consequences should be delayed. Finally, the gains should outweigh the risks, which I describe next.

Side Effects of Aversive Consequences.

Aversive consequences, even when conscientiously applied, have important side effects that the therapist must consider. First, punishment functions only to suppress behavior; it does not teach new behavior. Thus, punishment used alone does not teach the individual how to solve her problems and meet her needs in more adaptive ways. Once punishment is stopped—say, at the end of therapy or a patient's discharge from a treatment unit—the punished behavior is likely to come right back. Second, the effects of punishment usually only last while the individual meting out the punishment is nearby; thus, the punished behavior is likely to continue in secret. This can create serious therapy problems if the therapist is using punishment to control suicidal behaviors. Third, people usually withdraw from and/or avoid people who punish them. Thus, the use of aversive consequences as a therapeutic procedure is likely to weaken the positive interpersonal bond necessary in the treatment of borderline patients. With borderline patients in particular, aversive consequences can prompt alienation, emotional withdrawal and inability to talk, premature termination, and suicidal behaviors (including actual suicide). Iatrogenic effects often result from matching the wrong punishment to the behavior. For example, harsh confrontation of a withdrawn or disassociating patient during a session is unlikely to help her talk. Commenting on the effects of her withdrawal—"I know this is very difficult for you, but I can't help you if we can't figure out a way to get you back into the session"—may help. Taken together, these negative side effects suggest that aversive consequences should be the last contingency management procedure considered.

Determining the Potency of Consequences

A therapist simply cannot *assume* that a particular consequence will be reinforcing, neutral, or punishing for a patient. What works for one patient may not work for another. The only way to determine whether a consequence is working is to observe closely. Although the therapist can use his or her theory or assumptions as well as the patient's to suggest possible reinforcers or punishments, these cannot guarantee what will in fact work. There is no substitute for observation and experimentation in this situation. Potential reinforcers differ not only between people, but also by context within the same person. This pattern creates enormous difficulty and frustration for therapists. Praise, warmth, advice, nurturance, cheerleading, belief in the patient, contact, and availability, for example, may or may not be reinforcing, depending on the particular state of the patient and current events (i.e., the context). Thus, it is important for the therapist and patient together to learn not only what various consequences will reinforce or punish, but the conditions under which they will do so.

Praise as a Reinforcer

Borderline and suicidal individuals are often both eager for praise and very afraid of it. The fear may be expressed either directly or through indirect statements (requests not to praise, questions about the validity of the therapist's praise, etc.). They sometimes even revert to more dysfunctional behaviors following praise. There may be many reasons for this dislike of praise. A patient may be afraid that praise means she is doing well and therapy will be ended. Abandonment fears surface. Or the patient may interpret praise as the therapist's trying to "get rid" of her. Anger and/or panic may result. When praised, a borderline patient may also fear that the therapist will now expect more than she can deliver. Fears of failure and of disappointing the therapist are set off. At other times, praise may be experienced as a denial of the patient's very real difficulties and failures in other areas. The patient experiences a sense of invalidation. The common theme in all of these reactions is the patient's fear of being left on her own, having to be independent of the therapist and self-reliant before she is able or ready.

A patient's fears about praise may have been reinforced in several ways. In the past, praise may have been associated with withdrawal of further help and assistance, or with punishment for subsequent failure on the same task. If so, praise for succeeding or doing well on a task she is not sure she can succeed at again will signal an upcoming absence of needed help and a threat of punishment. A skills training client of mine almost never gave me an opportunity to praise her, always saying that she hadn't practiced any new behaviors, was more miserable now than ever, and wanted to kill herself. Any attempt at praise was met with claims that I obviously did not understand her. After about 6 months, I began to question whether the program was effective for her and should continue. At that point she demonstrated how much she had actually learned, stating that she had no intention of letting me know this before, because if I knew I might not let her continue with skills training.

A borderline patient often sets unrealistically high standards for herself. As a consequence, she often believes that praise is undeserved. Anybody should be able to do what the therapist has praised her for. Praise is experienced as a further reflection of her inadequacies. This is especially likely if the behavior praised is indeed trivial or if praise is given in a glib or insincere manner. Guilt and/or humiliation may result, often followed quickly by self-directed anger and, at times, parasuicidal episodes. The therapist must anticipate this and other negative effects of praise and move to counteract them. For example, the therapist may explore the patient's unrealistic expectations for herself. Analysis of "shoulds" (see Chapter 8) as well as cognitive modification strategies (see Chapter 11) can be employed.

Generally, the inability to accept appropriate praise should be viewed as a therapy-interfering behavior and analyzed and treated as such. The therapist should discuss the consequences of an inability to accept praise, both in therapy and outside of therapy. The strategy is to continue praising when appropriate—that is, to continue giving positive feedback following progress or positive change. But for this to work, the therapist must be careful not to pair praise with negative consequences for the patient. Thus, praise should not be followed with withdrawal of or limitations in contact. After praising a patient, I often reassure her that I know she still has many other problems and difficulties that need work. The therapist should also be especially vigilant about not raising expectations too high for the patient following praiseworthy behavior. For example, praising a patient for going through a particularly difficult experience without resorting to parasuicide, and then the next time she engages in parasuicide accusing her of not wanting to improve her behavior (since the therapist now knows she can), will reinforce the patient's own fears of praise.

The continued exposure to praise in an atmosphere that does not rein-force fear, shame, or anger should in the long run change the valence of praise from negative to neutral. Pairing praise with other positive therapeutic be-haviors should eventually lead to a positive valence. The reasoning behind this is that it is important for the patient to learn to be reinforced by praise. Praise is one of the most commonly used social reinforcers in everyday life. A person who is either punished by praise or neutral to it is at a distinct dis-advantage.

Further Comments on Relationship Contingencies

In Chapter 5 I have discussed the "attached" patient versus the "butterfly" patient. The attached patient is the one who has little difficulty establishing a close and intimate relationship with the therapist. With this patient, ther-apist warmth, approval, and intimacy are likely to be strongly reinforcing. In contrast, a close therapeutic relationship may not be a potent reinforcer for the butterfly patient. Indeed, for this patient, therapeutic closeness may be aversive. This may be due to circumscribed factors related specifically to the relationship with the therapist, or it may reflect more general issues re-lated to interpersonal closeness and intimacy. For example, the adolescent patient may be working to achieve automony from all adults, including an adult therapist. Therapist behaviors that signal too much intimacy or close-ness, therefore, may be counterproductive.

The key here, as in all contingency management, is to keep a close eye on the effects of interpersonal warmth and attachment on the patient's be-havior. I find it helpful to take set point theory from the field of weight regu-lation and apply it to the interpersonal domain. Set point theory suggests that each individual has a "set point" for weight regulation, such that the body will defend that weight (plus or minus 10 or so pounds). When over the set point range, the individual stops being hungry and finds it difficult to eat; body metabolism speeds up to reduce the person's body weight back to set point. When under the set point range, the individual is famished and finds it difficult to think of anything other than eating; body metabolism slows down to keep the person from losing any further weight. By analogy, in in-terpersonal relationships, each individual has a set point range of intimacy that he or she is comfortable with and will defend that range, so to speak. When over their set point, people will push others away, and attempts at greater intimacy will be experienced as aversive. Even small steps toward greater in-timacy will be experienced as threatening. When under their set point, peo-ple will reach out for intimacy; warmth and closeness from others will be experienced as reinforcing; coolness and distancing behaviors will be ex-perienced as aversive; and even large steps toward greater intimacy will be viewed as inadequate. The frequent comments of therapists that their bor-derline patients can never be "filled up" reflect this phenomenon. I suspect that this is rarely, if ever, true. From my perspective, the attached patient and the butterfly patient differ in their respective relationship set points. The attached patient, once placed in a secure, bonded, and warm relationship for long enough, will eventually relax and stop clinging (much as the thin person with a high weight set point will stop being insatiably hungry after he or she gains enough weight to enter the set point range). The butterfly patient, if given enough room to move, not punished for frequently flying out of the therapist's hand, and not punished when she returns, will in time become more attached.

Principles of Satiation

The set point analogy provides a second important point, which applies to the use of praise (discussed above) as well as to any other reinforcer: The potency of any reinforcer depends on whether the individual has already received the desired or needed level of the reinforcer. The question to ask is this: Is the person already sated on what is being offered? Food is not likely to be a good reinforcer for a person who has just finished a large meal. Too much praise, freedom, or warmth, too many phone calls, and so on will not work. The secret is "just enough." Unfortunately, there is no substitute (once again) for trial and error and close observation to determine "just enough" for any particular patient. The principle also suggests that if the therapist offers too much of a "good thing," the value of what is offered as a reinforcer is likely to be diminished.

Using Natural Over Arbitrary Consequences

Whenever possible, natural rather than arbitrary consequences should be applied. Natural consequences are those that flow from and are characteristic outcomes of a behavior in everyday life. The consequences are intrinsic, rather than extrinsic, to the situation and the behavior. Smiling, moving closer, and nodding are natural consequences of someone's saying something we like; giving the proverbial M&M is an example of arbitrary reinforcement. Giving a patient what she asks for is a natural consequence of skillful assertive behavior. Saying "good!" but not giving her what she wants is not only arbitrary reinforcement, but far less potent.

Natural consequences are used for two reasons: Patients prefer them, and they work better. With respect to preference, in my experience borderline individuals have a very keen eye for arbitrary consequences, and distrust and dislike them intensely. Many an argument between patient and therapist revolves around the reasonableness of consequences, especially aversive ones. The more arbitrary a consequence is, the more difficulty a patient will have in seeing it as a result of her behavior. Instead, she is likely to view it as resulting from characteristics of the therapist or the treatment setting that have little to do with her. She may see the therapist as autocratic, withholding, or simply paid to approve. The relationship of the consequence to the behavior— an essential part of learning—is lost.

Natural consequences also work better because they promote generalization. Behavior under the control of arbitrary consequences is less likely to generalize to other situations; thus, regression or loss of gains can be expected. The use of interpersonal consequences and the correction–overcorrection technique, described above, have been designed to meet this criterion. The interpersonal reactions of the therapist, both positive and negative, are likely to qualify as natural as long as the responses are genuine and are reasonably typical of or similar to other people's. Observing limits (see below) and reciprocal communication strategies (see Chapter 12), also reflect this preference for natural consequences.

At times, however, arbitrary reinforcers are the only effective ones available to the therapist. In these cases, the therapist should pair the arbitrary consequence with a more natural consequence. As the natural consequence becomes associated with the arbitrary one, the therapist can then gradually, over time, fade out use of the arbitrary reinforcer. The idea is to try to strengthen the effectiveness of natural consequences by pairing them with highly desirable arbitrary ones. (This point has also been made above in discussing praise.) To go back to the example of assertive behavior above, praising what the patient said that influenced the therapist while at the same time giving her what she asks for is an example of pairing an arbitrary and a natural reinforcer.

Principles of Shaping

In shaping, gradual approximations to the target (or goal) behaviors are reinforced. Shaping requires the therapist to break the desired behavior down into small steps and to teach theses steps sequentially. Shaping is essential with all patients, but particularly with borderline patients because of their past histories favoring hopelessness and passivity. Trying to extract an adaptive behavior from such a patient without reinforcing small steps on the way to the goal behavior simply does not work. It is like promising a hiker a sumptuous banquet if she can get to the other side of a high mountain, and then refusing to feed her during the 10-day journey.

Shaping has to do with what behaviors a therapist expects from a patient and is willing to reinforce. The failure of the patient's environment to teach more adaptive behaviors can be laid, at least partially, to a failure to use principles of shaping. That is, the expectations of the environment are too high for the abilities of the patient; as a result, progress is often punished because it does not come up to expectations, rather than reinforced because it represents an improvement over past behavior. The unrealistic standards of borderline patients, discussed throughout this book, are another result of this failure to apply shaping principles.

It may be helpful to think of a line starting where a patient was at the beginning of therapy and ending where the patient is trying to get to (goal behavior). Whether the therapist reinforces, punishes or ignores target-relevant behavior has to do with (1) the patient's present location on the continuum,

(2) her ability to produce behavior further along the continuum, and (3) the requirements of the situation. If the patient has moved along the continuum—that is, if a behavior represents progress—the therapist should reinforce it. If not, the therapist should ignore or punish it and, if necessary, teach new behavior. During each interaction, the therapist must continually match the patient's behaviors with her present status (including her vulnerabilities within the situation), her potential capabilities, and the nature of the situation. This information, in turn, is used to produce a therapeutic response. No wonder working with this population is so difficult. Because of the complexity and extensiveness of borderline patients' problems, as well as the changing nature of their deficits depending on context, therapists usually have to keep a large number of continua in their heads at the same time. Keeping so much information organized and available for use is difficult under the best of conditions. It is magnified with patients who put so much personal stress on their therapists, making flexible use of the information tenuous.

DBT approaches this problem in two ways. First, clear hierarchical targeting allows a therapist to compartmentalize information—to attend to some behaviors and ignore others. The therapist does not attend to all patient behaviors equally. Instead, the therapist checks behaviors against the target hierarchy and then attends to only those that are relevant to the highest-priority current target. Thus, the task is simplified. Second, the consultation-to-the-patient strategies, discussed in Chapter 13, are designed to limit the number of people the therapist is "treating." In contrast to most other treatment programs, DBT stipulates that the therapist only treats the patient. There is no need to organize and try to implement the treatment plans of other professionals; that is, each therapist only has to worry about his or her own responses to the patient. Thus, again, DBT copes by narrowing the focus of the therapist to a manageable amount of complexity.

OBSERVING-LIMITS PROCEDURES

The observing-limits approach is simple in theory and difficult in practice. It is the application of problem-solving strategies and contingency management procedures to patient behaviors that threaten or cross the therapist's personal limits. Observing limits is essential to DBT. The responsibility for taking care of the therapist's limits in DBT belongs to the therapist, not to the patient. The therapist must be aware of which patient behaviors he or she is able and willing to tolerate and which are unacceptable. This information should be given to the patient in a timely fashion, before it is too late. The therapist must also specify which behaviors he or she can accept only temporarily and which are acceptable over the long haul, as well as which patient behaviors are likely to lead to therapist burnout and which are not. Patient behaviors that cross the therapist's limits are a special type of therapy-interfering behaviors; thus, limit-relevant behaviors are second only to suicide crisis behaviors and parasuicide (or other life-threatening behaviors) as a target of therapy. They are therapy-threatening because they interfere with the therapist's ability or willingness to carry on with therapy. It is crucial for a therapist not to ignore such behaviors; otherwise the therapist will sooner or later burn out, terminate therapy, or otherwise harm the patient. In observing limits, the therapist takes care *for* the patient by taking care *of* himself or herself.

Rationale for Observing Limits

Limits and how to set them constitute a major concern in almost every discussion of borderline treatment. Such discussions are ordinarily framed in terms of containing or stopping the patient's maladaptive behaviors. Green, Goldberg, Goldstein, and Leibenluft (1988), for example, state: "Should these [standard psychotherapeutic techniques] fail to stem an individual's regressive acting out, then more vigorous measures, in the form of appropriate limit setting interventions, are required" (p. ix). Maladaptive behaviors are viewed as a result of the patient's having no boundaries or limits to her sense of self; the major goal of limit setting, therefore, is reinforcement of the patient's sense of identity through enhancing her personal boundaries. (See Green et al., 1988, for a review of this literature.)

Observing limits in DBT, by contrast, is concerned with preserving the personal limits of the therapist—the *therapist's* sense of self, as it were. The goal is to make sure that the contingencies operating in therapy do not punish the therapist's continued involvement. The focus is on the relationship between the therapist's limits and the patient's behavior. When a patient pushes a therapist's limits, the situation is examined in terms of the fit between the patient's needs or desires and the therapist's abilities or wishes. That is, the patient is not *assumed* to be disordered (e.g., too needy, too fluid). Nor is the therapist *assumed* to be disordered (e.g., manifesting countertransference problems). Instead, the assumption is that people, legitimately or otherwise, often want or need from other people what others are unable or unwilling to give. They push other's limits. The interpersonal fit is poor.

This is not to imply that patient behavior and therapist limits should not be examined for disorder. The ability to limit one's demands on others, independently of one's own needs, is itself a very important interpersonal skill; reciprocal relationships require the ability to observe and respect another person's limits. Many borderline patients are deficient in this ability. Conversely, the ability to know and observe one's own limits in a relationship is equally important, and many therapists are deficient in this ability. Although DBT, more so than many behavior therapies, emphasizes the therapist's impact on the patient's experiences and perceptions in therapy, it also sees the therapist as reciprocally influenced by the patient's behaviors. This does not mean that the roles of the therapist and patient are seen as symmetrical; the therapist is expected to generate more accurate hypotheses about factors influencing the relationship and to display greater interpersonal skill during therapeutic sessions. The therapist is also expected to control his or her own behavior, to insure that therapist actions at least cause the patient no harm. Despite these caveats, the therapist is seen as inevitably affected by the patient's behavior; depending upon the behavior, this may either interfere with or promote the therapist's motivation and ability to help the patient.

Natural versus Arbitrary Limits

With very few exceptions, there are no arbitrary limits in DBT. The only patient behavior that is arbitrarily limited in both individual therapy and skills training is dropping out: Therapy is suspended if the patient drops out of either. The only arbitrary limits on therapist behavior are those set forth by professional ethical guidelines. Sexual interactions with patients, for example, are not acceptable under any conditions.

Natural limits vary among therapists, and within the same therapist over time, as a result of any number of factors. These include personal events in a therapist's life and work setting, the current patient–therapist relationship, the therapist's goals for the patient, and the characteristics of a particular patient. Limits narrow when a therapist is sick or overworked, and broaden when he or she is rested and has a reasonable caseload. The very broad limits of one therapist on my team narrowed after he and his wife had a baby. Therapists with a supportive consultation team or supervision will presumably have broader limits than therapists working alone or in a hostile environment. My willingness to put up with a patient's screaming in sessions is far greater in my private office than in a clinic setting where it bothers others. My willingness to put up with suicide threats at the end of a session is greater if I don't have another patient waiting than if I do.

Moreover, each therapist on a team, including those working with the same patient, may have different limits. One therapist's limits may be very broad, another's very narrow. For example, one therapist may carefully read every letter a patient writes, no matter how long or frequently sent; another may not. One therapist may be willing to call a patient when on vacation; another may not. My limits on suicidal risk I am willing to tolerate among my outpatients are broader than those of many other therapists in Seattle. Some therapists are not bothered when patients fail to cancel sessions before missing them or are late in paying fees, others are. Patients' engaging in clinging and dependent behaviors or sitting in the waiting room all day bothers some therapists and not others. The list could be endless.

Generally, a strong therapeutic alliance leads to broader limits. People in general are usually willing to do more for and tolerate more from those they feel close to than those they feel distant from. Therapists' limits are ordinarily broader with patients who work hard at therapy and narrower with those who refuse to comply with or resist interventions. The ways in which limits are affected by patient behaviors, however, may vary among members of the same treatment team. For example, some therapists' limits narrow when patients are attacking and broaden when they are not; other therapists take attacks in their stride and are not affected much one way or the other. I am willing to give a fair amount of phone time, even at inconvenient times, to patients who call and seem to be helped by calling. Patients who characteristically say that they feel as bad at the end as they did at the beginning, and who criticize my inability to stay on the phone longer, are not patients I am willing to have long phone conversations with. Whether patients "Yes, but. . ." me or reject all of my suggestions doesn't affect my limits much; I see it as a challenge. Other therapists I work with are not as bothered by ingratitude as I am, but refuse to talk for long with patients who keep rejecting suggestions.

In DBT, there is no need for limits to be universal among team members or across patients. It is only important that each therapist understand his or her own limits and communicate these clearly to each patient. This variability of limits across therapists and within the same therapist, in turn, provides a greater similarity between the treatment environment and everyday life. Life and people simply are not consistent, nor are they always available to meet an individual's needs. Even a person's closest intimates at times are withdrawn or unable to meet all expectations. The goal of DBT is to teach patients how to interact productively and happily within these natural interpersonal limits.

Observing natural or personal limits requires far more openness and assertion than does observing arbitrary limits. The DBT therapist cannot fall back on a set of predetermined rules. There is no book to look up how to respond when a patient comes late for the 35th time. DBT does not provide a rule book on limits because arbitrary rules and limits do not take into account the individuality of the persons in a relationship. Thus, the therapist must take personal responsibility for his or her own limits. This can be a very difficult task at times, especially when a patient is suffering intensely and the limits add to the suffering. There are, however, several guidelines for effectively observing limits with borderline patients, which are discussed below and summarized in Table 10.3.

1. MONITORING LIMITS

Therapists are required to observe their own limits with respect to what is acceptable patient behavior in each therapeutic relationship, and to observe these limits in the conduct of therapy. In particular, a therapist must carefully and continually observe the relationship of a patient's behaviors to his or her own willingness and motivation to interact and work with the patient, sense of being overwhelmed, belief that he or she can be effective with the patient, and feelings of burnout. This process is much easier for experienced therapists than for new ones. As a therapist on my team once remarked, "It is very difficult to know your limits before they are crossed." Warning signs include feelings of discomfort, anger, and frustration, and a sense of "Oh,

TABLE 10.3. Observing-Limits Procedures Checklist

____ T MONITORS his or her own limits in conducting therapy:
   ____ On a continuing basis.
   ____ With each patient separately.

____ T communicates his or her own limits to P HONESTLY and directly, in terms of the realistic ability and/or desire of T to meet the needs and wishes of P.
   ____ With respect to phone call timing, duration, frequency.
   ____ With respect to violations of T's privacy.
   ____ With respect to infringements on T's property, time, etc.
   ____ With respect to aggressive behavior in sessions or directed at T.
   ____ With respect to type of treatment T is willing to carry out or be a part of.
   ____ With respect to T's willingness to risk P's suicide.

____ T EXTENDS limits temporarily when necessary.
   ____ T gets professional backup or help when T is at edge of limits and P needs more.
   ____ T helps P cope effectively with T's limits when P is not in danger because of limits.

____ T is CONSISTENTLY FIRM about own limits.
   ____ T uses contingency management visa-à-vis limits.

____ T combines SOOTHING VALIDATION, AND PROBLEM SOLVING with observing limits.

Anti-DBT tactics

____ T refuses to expand limits on a temporary basis when P clearly needs more than usual from T.

____ T's limits change or fluctuate in an arbitrary and/or unpredictable manner.

____ T presents limits as for the good of P rather than for the good of T.

---

no, not again." The idea is for the therapist to catch themselves before they cross their limits—that is, before they are suddenly unable or unwilling to interact with certain patient's any further. The consultation team can be quite useful here.

2. BEING HONEST ABOUT LIMITS

A therapist's limits are not presented as for the good of the patient, but rather for the good of the therapist. Although the distinction is artificial, since the good of both parties is essentially linked in any therapeutic relationship, the emphasis is very different from presenting limits as for the patient's own good. This different emphasis in turn leads to different effects. The main point is that although the patient can and should have the major say in what is ultimately for her own good (she is not a child), she does not have the major say in what is good for the therapist. An analogy can be drawn to the therapist's telling the patient not to smoke in the office because it is bad for her, as opposed to telling her this because the therapist dislikes inhaling the smoke. In the first instance, both can argue the point; at a minimum, the patient can reasonably assert that her physical health is her responsibility. In the second instance, there is little room for argument. In the first instance, the therapist is showing little respect for the individual's autonomy and sense of what is good or bad for herself. In the second instance, the therapist is modeling self-care. At times, the second instance is also the only honest one; that is, much of the time we all (therapists included) try to control others' behavior by telling them it is for their benefit, when it really is for our own benefit.

Honesty as a strategy can be extraordinarily effective. A borderline patient is often hungry for respect; honesty about the therapist's own limits is ultimately respecting the patient. It is treating the patient like an adult. The therapist may agree with the patient that the limits are not fair (when they are not), but should point out nonetheless that his or her going beyond these limits will probably hurt the patient in the end. If need be, the therapist can review with the patient the times she has been hurt by other therapists who did not take care of themselves properly.

Dishonesty and/or confusion about whose limits are being observed is a special lure for psychotherapists, for several reasons. First, some theories of psychotherapy suggest that pushing a therapist's limits is pathological by definition. The therapist who told me that all calls by a patient to a therapist at home are acts of aggression toward the therapist (see Chapter 3) is an example here. This or a similar theoretical perspective makes it is quite difficult to assess the interaction flexibly. A therapist may be unlikely even to examine the possibility that the trouble lies in his or her inability or unwillingness to extend limits for the welfare of the patient. Concepts such as countertransference wisely focus on the possible pathology of a therapist's own limits; however, they do not provide for the "difficult-fit" situation, where legitimate limits of the therapist lead to his or her not meeting equally legitimate needs of the patient. Second, being a therapist is a position of great power with regard to other people. It allows arrogance and dishonesty to go unchecked. This possibility is one of the reasons why supervision consultation plays such an important role in DBT.

Third, most therapists have been taught that therapy is solely for the benefit of the patient; in training programs, the benefit of the therapist is rarely if ever mentioned. Thus, therapists can easily feel guilty or somehow untherapeutic if they attend to their own desires and needs. Borderline patients often suffer terribly, and sometimes therapists feel that they really could make it better if they just had broader limits. The options for a therapist here are these: (1) to repeatedly cross his or her own limits; (2) to decide that the patient's needs are simply pathological; or (3) to allow the patient to continue suffering and accept responsibility for being unable to help. Difficulty in accepting that the therapist is the proximate cause of the patient's suffering often leads to one of the first two choices. Observing limits leads to the third choice. In my experience, it is this difficulty in accepting one's own impotence that causes the most trouble for new and inexperienced therapists; arrogance is often the problem for more experienced therapists.

3. TEMPORARILY EXTENDING LIMITS WHEN NEEDED

Observing limits is not a license to be uncaring or unresponsive to important patient needs. Nor is it permission to be chaotic in responses to patient requests and demands. It is necessary for therapists at times to push their own limits, extend themselves, and give what they do not want to give. This is particularly true with chronically suicidal and borderline patients. An analogy to surgeons may be useful here. When they are on call, surgeons cannot refuse to go into the hospital for an emergency because they would rather stay at home, saying that it crosses their limits. But even surgeons can only be on call periodically. A surgeon who has been up for five nights in a row, getting 1 or 2 hours of sleep per night, may reach his or her outer limits and need someone else to take calls for a day or two. No one can survive for long without sleep. Similarly, when a therapist is about to reach his or her limits and the patient's life is in danger, the appropriate strategy is to involve other professionals in the provision of care. When limits are an issue and the patient is not in danger, problem solving and other change procedures are the appropriate strategies. The dialectic here is between pushing limits when necessary, on the one hand, and observing limits when necessary, on the other.

4. BEING CONSISTENTLY FIRM

Patients often try to get therapists to extend their limits by arguing the validity of their own needs, criticizing the therapists for inadequacy, or at times threatening to find another therapist or commit suicide. They may engage repeatedly in parasuicide, or refuse to cooperate until the therapists "cooperate" with them. In clinic and inpatient settings, they may go to other staff members and try to elicit their assistance, complain vociferously to other patients, or go directly to your supervisor. As psychodynamic therapists put it, they may "act out."

The important point here is that observing limits often means placing patient behaviors on an extinction schedule. The answer to a patient's limit-extending efforts is simple: "I am who I am." Thus, in the end, the therapist has no option but to observe his or her own limits. It is tempting when a lot of pressure is applied to vacillate between expanding limits and attacking the patient, implying that her needs are excessive or inappropriate. The temptation must be resisted. Giving in and appeasing the patient following behavior escalations will only reinforce the behavior the therapist is trying to stop; responding punitively means risking the side effects of aversive consequences. The tactic here is to use the same "broken record" strategy patients are taught in interpersonal skills training: Over and over and over, the therapist states his or her position calmly, clearly, and firmly. It may also help to restate frequently that the observation of these limits will benefit the patient in the end. (The therapist will not precipitously terminate therapy or otherwise harm the patient.)

5. COMBINING SOOTHING, VALIDATING, AND PROBLEM SOLVING WITH OBSERVING LIMITS

The importance of soothing the patient while simultaneously observing limits cannot be overstated. Not giving the patient what she wants, or being unwilling to tolerate a certain behavior, does not mean that the therapist cannot comfort the patient at all. The therapist also needs to validate the patient's distress and help her find other ways to cope with the problem. Observing limits must be surrounded on all sides with interwoven validation and problem-solving strategies. Invalidating the patient's wishes and needs is rarely therapeutic.

Difficult Areas for Observing Limits with Borderline Patients

Phone Calls

Since DBT encourages rather than prohibits telephone contact, therapists must determine at what hours they can be available and how long phone calls can last. Therapists who cannot accept any after-hours telephone calls should probably not work with borderline patients. Beyond that, individual patient and therapist needs as well as short-term issues must be considered in determining an appropriate telephone policy. A therapist who has never placed some restrictions on telephone calls (if only that the patient cannot call just to chat at 2 A.M.) either has never had a needy patient or is headed for burnout and rejection of the patient.

The duration and frequency of allowable calls vary for different therapists and for different patients of the same therapist. Some therapists are willing to take calls at almost any time and do not seem bothered by many calls. A therapist who once worked with me did woodworking and painting in his basement in the evenings. Patients who called during the evening had almost unlimited time, as he continued to sand or paint while talking. Other therapists are unwilling to spend so much time on the phone and learn to end calls quickly or to call a patient back when convenient. Conditions for phone calls may also vary. For example, in our clinic I have had therapists who would (1) take calls only through an answering service and then call the patient back (the therapist needed time to get a glass of water and "get set"); (2) end calls immediately after a certain hour unless it was an emergency (the therapist in this case had to get up at dawn); (3) only return calls in the evenings, suggesting that the patient call the crisis clinic or emergency room for daytime emergencies (this therapist's daytime schedule was too packed to allow her to return calls); (4) end calls immediately unless the patient had already tried a certain number of skills (the therapist was tired of "doing for" this patient and believed it was untherapeutic); (5) end calls if a patient had consumed alcohol in the last 6 hours (drinking interfered with the patient's ability to be helped); or (6) refuse to take another call during the week if the patient called and then refused to engage in problem solving (the therapist always felt frustrated after these calls). The important point here is that each therapist must set his or her own limits, which in turn must be respected both by the therapist and the supervision/consultation team.

Suicidal Behaviors

Some therapists have more tolerance for suicide threats, especially serious ones, than others. Some are more willing than others to follow a well-thought-out, but high-risk treatment plan that puts them at risk of being sued if the patient commits suicide. Some therapists are philosophically opposed to involuntary confinement to prevent suicide; others are not. Every therapist has to examine his or her limits in these areas. In general, patients need to know that continuation of serious suicidal behavior, at least, is likely to strain the therapist's limits. In my clinic and my areas of clinical responsibility, patients who might engage in lethal behavior are not allowed to have lethal drugs. Some risks are not within my limits. I have also put patients in the hospital when I needed a rest from their crisis calls and suicide threats. However, when consequences of observing limits are extreme for the patient (e.g., involuntary commitment), it is essential that the therapist both give the patient proper warning and provide a way for the patient to avoid the aversive consequence. It is also essential for the therapist to observe his or her limits. The topic of suicidal behavior and limits is discussed more fully in Chapter 15.

Concluding Comments

It is very important for therapists to be aware of the contingencies they are applying in psychotherapy. It is equally important to be aware of the effect of contingencies on behavior, whether such effects are intended or not. Many therapists seem to feel that it is unacceptable to influence patients' behavior by applying contingencies. Positive contingencies are viewed as bribes, and negative contingencies are viewed as coercive, manipulative, or threatening. Often these therapists value autonomy and believe that behaviors under the control of external influence are not as "real" or as permanent as behaviors under the control of internal influences. In other words, these therapists value behaviors under the control of the individual's "choosing" or "intent." Therapists who hold to the idea of unconscious intent and choice, sometimes function as if they believe that *all* behavior is actually under the control of intent and choice; the intent and choice are simply conscious or unconscious. The goal of therapy in this case might be to bring all behavior under the control of conscious intent and choice. Cognitive–behavioral therapists would certainly agree to this goal, at least with respect to unwanted, maladaptive behaviors.

The difference between an approach based on "choice" or "intent" and a cognitive–behavioral approach is twofold. First, cognitive–behavioral therapists would ask what controls "choosing" and "intent." If this question is answered by saying that what one chooses is what one wants or prefers, no new information has really been added. The explanation is post hoc. Cognitive–behavioral therapists would assert that choosing and intent are controlled by outcomes, both behavioral and environmental. People make choices and form intents that have previously been reinforced; they avoid those that have been punished.

Second, cognitive–behavioral therapists would not suggest that when behaviors are not under the control of conscious choice or intent, they must be under the control of unconscious intent. Indeed this may be a tautological statement. Instead, the cognitive–behavioral view is that the absence of a connection between intent or choice, and action is the problem to be solved. Such a connection must be learned. It is learned when reinforcing outcomes follow actions that fit previous intent to act or choice. From this perspective, intent and choice are cognitive activities (even though there may be an emotional component, especially with intent). Thus, the relationship between intent or choice and action is a behavior–behavior connection. The connection is not assumed *a priori*. Indeed, with borderline patients the problem is often an inability to influence behavior by prior intent, choice, and commitment. Thus, therapists may set out to systematically reinforce such a behavior–behavior connection.

An overreliance on choice as a determinant of behavior ignores the role of behavior capability. The notion of choice assumes freedom to follow through on one's choices. One cannot do what one is unable to do, no matter how much or how often one chooses to do it. Borderline patients are often unable to control their behavior as they and their therapists want them to. Although contingencies at times create capabilities where few or none existed before, good intentions alone are not sufficient to effect behavioral control and change.

11

Change Procedures: Part II. Skills Training, Exposure, Cognitive Modification

SKILLS TRAINING PROCEDURES

Skills training procedures are necessary when a problem solution requires skills not currently in the individual's behavioral repertoire. That is, under ideal circumstances (where behavior is not interfered with by fears, conflicting motives, unrealistic beliefs, etc.), the individual cannot generate or produce the behaviors required. The term "skills" in DBT is used synonymously with "abilities," and includes in its broadest sense cognitive, emotional, and overt behavioral (or action) response repertoires together with their integration, which is necessary for effective performance. Effectiveness is gauged by both direct and indirect consequences of the behavior. Effective performance can be defined as those behaviors that lead to a maximum of positive outcomes with a minimum of negative outcomes. Thus, "skill" is used in the sense of "using skillful means," as well as in the sense of responding to situations adaptively or effectively.

The integration of skills is emphasized in DBT because often (indeed, usually) an individual has the component behaviors of a skill, but cannot put them together coherently when necessary. For example, everyone has the word "no" in his or her repertoire. But a person may not be able to put it together with other words in a skillful phrase to refuse an invitation while simultaneously not alienating the person giving the invitation. An interpersonally skillful response requires putting together words that one already knows into effective sentences, together with appropriate body language, intonation, eye contact, and so on. The component skills are rarely new; the combination, however, often is. In DBT, almost any desired behavior can be thought of as a skill. Thus, coping effectively with problems and avoiding maladaptive or ineffective responses are both considered using one's skills. The aim of DBT is to replace ineffective, maladaptive, or nonskilled behaviors with skillful responses.

During skills training, and more generally throughout DBT, the therapist insists at every opportunity that the patient engage actively in the acquisition and practice of the skills she needs to cope with her life. The therapist directly, forcefully, and repeatedly challenges the borderline individual's passive problem-solving style. The procedures described below can be applied informally by every therapist where appropriate. They are applied in a formal way in the structured skills training modules (described in the companion manual to this volume).

There are three types of skills training procedures: (1) skill acquisition (e.g., instructions, modeling); (2) skill strengthening (e.g., behavior rehearsal, feedback); and (3) skill generalization (e.g., homework assignments, discussion of similarities and differences in situations). In skill acquisition, the therapist is teaching new behaviors. In skill strengthening and generalization, the therapist is trying both to fine-tune skilled behavior and to increase the probability that the person will use the skilled behaviors already in her repertoire in relevant situations. Skill strengthening and generalization, in turn, require the application of contingency management, exposure, and/or cognitive modification procedures. That is, once the therapist is sure that a particular response pattern is within the patient's current repertoire, then other procedures are applied to increase the patient's use of this pattern in everyday life. It is this emphasis on active, self-conscious teaching, typical of behavioral and cognitive therapies, that differentiates DBT from many approaches to treating borderline patients. Some skills training procedures, however, are virtually identical to those used in supportive, dynamic psychotherapy.

The targets of skills training are determined by the parameters of DBT (e.g., mindfulness, interpersonal effectiveness, emotion regulation, distress tolerance, and self-management skills), as well as by behavioral analysis in the individual case. Almost any behavior pattern that the individual does not currently have in her repertoire but that would be helpful in improving her life can be a target of skills training. The choice of specific procedures (e.g., acquisition vs. strengthening procedures) depends on the skills the patient already has.

Orienting and Committing to Skills Training: Task Overview

Orienting is the therapist's chief means of selling both the new behaviors as worth learning and DBT procedures as likely to work. Skills training can only be accomplished if the person actively collaborates with the treatment program. Some patients both have skill deficits and are fearful about acquiring new skills. It can be useful to point out here that learning a new skill does not mean that a patient actually has to use the skill. That is, she can acquire a skill and then choose in each situation whether to use it or not. The patient's problem is much like that of persons who fear flying: They do not want to reduce their fears, because then they might have to fly. Sometimes a patient does not want to learn new skills because she has lost hope that anything will really help. I find it useful to point out that the skills I am teaching have helped either me or other people I know. However, a therapist cannot prove ahead of time that particular skills will actually help a given individual.

Before teaching any new skill, the therapist should give a rationale (or draw it in Socratic fashion from the patient) for why the particular skill or set of skills might be useful. At times this may only require a comment or two; at other times it may require extensive discussion. (Specific rationales for each set of DBT target skills are given in the companion manual to this volume.) In individual problem solving, this will ordinarily take place in the solution analysis phase. At some point, the therapist should also explain the general rationale for his or her methods of teaching—that is, the rationale for the DBT skills training procedures. The most important point to make here, and to repeat as often as necessary, is that learning new skills requires practice, practice, practice. Equally importantly, practice has to occur in situations where the skills are needed. If these points do not get through to the patient, there is not much hope that she will actually learn anything new.

SKILL ACQUISITION PROCEDURES

Skill acquisition procedures are concerned with remediating skill deficits. DBT does not assume that all, or even most, of a borderline person's problems are motivational in nature. Instead, the extent of the patient's abilities in a particular area is assessed; skill acquisition procedures are then used if skill deficits exist. At times, in lieu of other means of assessment, the therapist employs skill acquisition procedures and then observes any consequent change in behavior.

A Note on Assessing Abilities

It can be very difficult with borderline patients to know whether they are incapable of doing something or are capable but emotionally inhibited or constrained by environmental factors. Although this is a complex assessment question with any patient population, it can be particularly hard with borderline individuals because of their inability to analyze their own behavior and abilities. For example, they often confuse being *afraid* of doing something with not being *able* to do it. In addition, there are often powerful contingencies mitigating against their admitting having any behavioral capabilities, as I have discussed in Chapter 10. Of particular concern here are a patient's fears that if she admits to having capabilities the therapist will decide (prematurely) that therapy is completed. Or the patient may fear that if she is known to be able to do something in one context the therapist will think she can do it in all contexts, including those where she cannot. Thus, the therapist will withdraw assistance that is still needed, posing the possibility of failure (with all the associated losses and further problems that this would cause). Patients may also say that they do not know how they feel or what they think, or that they cannot find words, when in reality they are afraid of expressing their thoughts and feelings. As many patients say, they often do not want to be vulnerable. Finally, some patients have been taught by their families and therapists to view all of their problems as motivationally based. They have either bought this point of view entirely (they thus believe they can do anything, but just do not want to), or have rebelled completely and never entertain the possibility that motivational factors might be as important as ability-related factors (they believe they cannot do anything, and this includes learning more adaptive ways of behaving).

Some therapists respond to patients' statements that they can't do anything with an equally polarized statement that they can if only they want to. Failing to behave skillfully, and claiming not to know how to behave differently, are viewed as resistant (or at least as determined by motives outside awareness). Giving advice, coaching, making suggestions, or otherwise teaching new behaviors is viewed as encouraging dependency and need gratification that gets in the way of "real" therapy. Other therapists, of course, fall into the trap of believing that these patients can hardly do anything. At times they even go so far as to believe that the patients are incapable of learning new skills. Acceptance, nurturance, and environmental intervention constitute the armamentarium of these therapists. Not surprisingly, when these two orientations coexist within a patient's treatment team, conflict and "staff splitting" often arise. A dialectical approach would suggest looking for the synthesis. (I discuss this topic further in Chapter 13.)

To assess whether a behavioral pattern is within a patient's repertoire, the therapist has to figure out a way to create ideal circumstances for her to produce the behavior. For interpersonal behaviors, an approximation to this is role playing in the office—or, if the patient refuses, asking her to describe what she would say in a particular situation. I am frequently amazed to find that individuals who appear very interpersonally skilled cannot put together reasonable responses in certain role-play situations, whereas individuals who seem passive, meek, and unskilled are quite capable of responding skillfully in the comfort of the office. In analyzing distress tolerance, the therapist can ask the person to describe what techniques she uses or thinks helpful in tolerating difficult or stressful situations. Emotion regulation can sometimes be assessed by interrupting a session and asking the patient to see whether she can change her emotional state. Self-management and mindfulness skills can be analyzed by observing the patient's behavior in sessions and questioning her about her day-to-day behavior.

If the patient produces a behavior, the therapist knows she has it in her repertoire. However, if she does not, the therapist cannot be sure; as in statistics, there is no way to test the null hypothesis. When in doubt (which will usually be the case), it is safer to proceed with skill acquisition procedures. Generally, there is no harm in doing so, and most of the procedures also affect other factors related to skilled behavior. For example, both instructions and modeling (the principal skill acquisition procedures) may work because they give the individual "permission" to behave and thus reduce inhibitions, rather than because they add to the individual's behavioral repertoire. These two basic procedures are described below and outlined in Table 11.1.

I. INSTRUCTIONS

Instructions are verbal descriptions of the response components to be learned. According to a patient's needs, they can vary from general guidelines ("When restructuring your thinking, be sure to check out the probability that the dire consequences will occur," "Think reinforcement") to very specific suggestions as to what the patient should do ("The minute an urge hits, go get an ice cube and hold it in your hand for 10 minutes") or think ("Keep saying over and over to yourself, 'I can do it' "). They can be presented didactically in

---

TABLE 11.1. Skill Acquisition Procedures Checklist

____ T assesses target-relevant abilities.

    ____ T creates circumstances conducive to performance of skills P has.

    ____ T observes P's behavior in sessions and phone interactions.

    ____ T asks P how she would ideally handle a situation or problem.

    ____ T asks P to try new behaviors, such as changing emotions, during session or phone interactions.

    ____ T role-plays with P.

____ T INSTRUCTS P in skill to be learned.

    ____ T specifies necessary behaviors and their patterning in terms concrete enough for P to understand.

    ____ T breaks instructions down into easy-to-follow steps.

    ____ T begins with simple tasks relative to P's capabilities and fears and then proceeds to more difficult aspects of skill.

    ____ T provides P with examples of skill to be learned.

    ____ T gives P handouts describing skills.

____ T MODELS skilled behavior.

    ____ T role-plays with P.

    ____ T uses skilled behavior in interacting with P.

    ____ T thinks out loud, using self-talk to model adaptive thinking.

    ____ T discloses own previous use of skilled behavior in everyday life.

    ____ T tells stories illustrating skilled behaviors.

    ____ T points to models in the environment for P to observe.

        ____ Other people P knows with skilled behavior.

        ____ Public figures demonstrating skilled behavior.

        ____ Books (e.g., biographies), movies.

a lecture format with a blackboard as an aid. In standard DBT, written instructions are given in the handouts with each skill area (see companion manual to this volume); other self-help books can be given. Instructions can be suggested as hypotheses to be considered, can be presented as theses and antitheses to be synthesized, or can be drawn from the patient via the Socratic method. In all cases, the therapist must be careful not to oversimplify the ease of behaving effectively or of learning the skill.

2. MODELING

Modeling can be provided by the therapist, others in the patient's environment, audiotapes, videotapes, films, or printed material. Any procedure that provides the patient with examples of appropriate alternative responses is a form of modeling. The advantage of a therapist model is that the situation and materials can be tailored to fit the patient's needs.

There are a number of ways in which the therapist can model skilled behavior. In-session role playing can be used to demonstrate appropriate interpersonal behavior. When events between the patient and therapist arise that are similar to situations the patient encounters in her natural environment, the therapist can model handling such situations in effective ways. The therapist can also use self-talk (speaking aloud) to model coping self-statements, self-instructions, or restructuring of problematic expectations and beliefs. For example, the therapist may say, "OK, here's what I would say to myself: 'I'm overwhelmed. What's the first thing I do when overwhelmed? Break down the situation into steps and make a list. Do the first thing on the list.' " Telling stories, relating historical events, or providing allegorical examples (see Chapter 7) can often be useful in demonstrating alternative life strategies. Finally, therapist self-disclosure can be used to model adaptive behavior, especially if the therapist has encountered problems in living similar to those the patient is currently encountering. This tactic is discussed at length in Chapter 12.

In addition to in-session modeling, it can be useful to have a patient observe the behavior and responses of competent people in her own environment. The behaviors that she observes can then be discussed and practiced for eventual use by the patient herself. Written models for how to apply some of therapeutic suggestions are also useful. Biographies, autobiographies and novels about people who have coped with similar problems also give new ideas. It is always important to discuss with the patient any behaviors modeled by the therapist or presented as models outside of therapy, to be sure that the patient is observing the relevant responses.

SKILL STRENGTHENING PROCEDURES

Once skilled behavior has been acquired, skill strengthening is used to shape, refine, and increase the likelihood of their use. Without reinforced practice, a skill cannot be learned; this point cannot be emphasized too much, since

TABLE 11.2. Skill Strengthening Procedures Checklist

____ T uses BEHAVIORAL REHEARSAL.
    ____ T role-plays with P.
    ____ T guides P in in-session practice.
    ____ T guides P in imaginal (covert) practice.
    ____ T guides P in *in vivo* practice.
____ T REINFORCES skilled behavior.
____ T gives P behaviorally specific FEEDBACK.
____ T COACHES P.

Anti-DBT tactics

____ T punishes or ignores P's behaviors that represent improvement but make T feel uncomfortable.

____ T's feedback focuses on motives rather than on performance.

____ T provides no link between inferred motives and specific behaviors.

____ T gives P feedback on every detail instead of selecting out important points.

skill practice is effortful behavior and directly counteracts borderline patients' tendency to employ a passive behavior style. Skill strengthening procedures are outlined in Table 11.2.

1. BEHAVIORAL REHEARSAL

Behavioral rehearsal is any procedure in which the patient practices responses to be learned. This can be done in interactions with the therapist, in simulated situations, or *in vivo.* Any skilled behaviors—verbal sequences, nonverbal actions, patterns of thinking or cognitive problem solving, and some components of physiological and emotional responses—can, in principle, be practiced.

Practice can be either overt or covert. Various forms of overt behavioral rehearsal are possible. For example, the therapist and patient may role-play problematic situations together so that the patient can practice responding appropriately. Biofeedback is a method of practicing control of physiological responses, or the therapist can ask the patient to practice relaxing during a session. In learning cognitive skills, the patient may be asked to verbalize effective self-statements. In the specific case of cognitive restructuring, the patient may be asked first to examine and verbalize any dysfunctional beliefs, rules, or expectancies elicited by the problem situation, and then to restructure these beliefs by generating more useful coping statements, rules, or the like. Covert response practice—that is, the patient's practicing the requisite response in imagination—may also be an effective form of skill strengthening. It may be more effective than overt methods for teaching more complex cognitive skills, and it is also useful when the patient refuses to engage in overt rehearsal. A patient can be asked to practice emotion regulation; generally, however, "emotional behavior" cannot be practiced directly. That is, a patient cannot practice getting angry, feeling sad, or experiencing joy. Instead, she has to practice specific components of emotions (changing facial expressions, generating thoughts that elicit or inhibit emotions, changing muscle tension, etc.).

In my experience, patients rarely like behavioral rehearsal; thus, a fair amount of cajoling and shaping is needed. If a patient will not role-play an interpersonal situation, for example, the therapist can try talking her through a dialogue ("Then what could you say?"), or try practicing just part of a new skill so that the patient is not overwhelmed. The essence of the message here, though, is that in order to be different the patient must practice *acting* differently. Some therapists do not like behavioral rehearsal either, especially when it requires them to role-play with patients. When therapists feel shy or uncomfortable about role playing, the best solution is for them to practice it with other members of the consultation team. At other times, therapists resist role playing because they do not want to push rehearsal on their patients. Such therapists may not be aware of the wealth of data indicating that behavioral rehearsal is related to therapeutic improvement (e.g., Linehan et al., 1979).

2. REINFORCEMENT OF NEW SKILLS

Therapist reinforcement of patients' behavior is one of the most powerful means of shaping and strengthening skilled behavior in borderline and suicidal patients. Frequently, these patients have lived in environments that overuse punishment. They often expect negative, punishing feedback from the world in general and their therapists in particular, and apply self-punishing strategies almost exclusively in trying to shape their own behavior. Over the long run, skill reinforcement by a therapist can improve such a patient's self-image, increase her use of skilled behaviors, and enhance the patient's sense that she can control positive outcomes in her life.

The techniques of providing appropriate reinforcement have been discussed extensively in Chapter 10. Here, however, it is important to point out that the therapist has to stay alert and notice patient behaviors that represent improvement, even if these make the therapist somewhat uncomfortable. For instance, teaching a patient interpersonal skills to use with her parents, but then punishing or ignoring those same skills when she uses them in a therapy session, is not therapeutic. Encouraging a patient to think for herself, but then punishing or ignoring her when she disagrees with the therapist, is not therapeutic. Stressing that "not fitting in" in all circumstances is not a disaster and that distress can be tolerated, but then not tolerating the patient when she does not fit comfortably into the therapist's schedule or preconceived notions of how borderline patients act, is not therapeutic.

3. FEEDBACK AND COACHING

Response feedback is the provision of information to patients about their performance. I stress that the feedback should pertain to *performance,* not to the motives presumably leading to the performance. One of the unfortunate factors in the lives of many borderline individuals is that people rarely give them feedback about their behavior that is uncontaminated with interpretations about their presumed motives and intent. When the presumed motives do not fit, the individuals often discount or are distracted from the valuable feedback they may be getting about their behavior. A therapist's feedback should be behaviorally specific; that is, the therapist should tell the patient exactly what she is doing that seems indicative of either continuing problems or improvement. Telling the patient that she is manipulating, expressing a need to control, overreacting, clinging, or acting out is simply not helpful if there are no clear behavioral referents for the terms. This is, of course, especially true when the therapist has pinpointed a problem behavior correctly but is inferring motivations inaccurately. Many arguments between patient and therapist arise out of just such inaccuracy.

The therapist must attend closely to the patient's behavior (both behavior within sessions and self-reported behavior between sessions) and select those responses on which the patient should be given feedback. At the beginning of therapy, when the patient may do little that appears competent, the therapist is usually well advised to give feedback on a limited number of response components. For example, the therapist should limit feedback to only one or two of the responses needing improvement, even though other deficits could be commented upon. Feedback on more responses may lead to stimulus overload and/or discouragement about the rate of progress. A response shaping paradigm (discussed in Chapter 10) should be used with feedback, coaching, and reinforcement designed to encourage successive approximations to the goal of effective performance.

Borderline patients often desperately want feedback about their behavior, but at the same time are sensitive to negative feedback. The solution here is to surround negative feedback with positive feedback. Treating a patient as too fragile to deal with negative feedback does her no favor. An important part of feedback is giving information about the effects of the patient's behavior on the therapist. This is discussed more extensively in Chapter 12 in connection with reciprocal communication strategies.

Coaching is combining feedback with instructions. The therapist tells the patient how a response is discrepant from the criterion of skilled performance and how it might be improved. That is, coaching is telling the patient what to do or how to improve. Clinical practice suggests that the "permission" to behave in certain ways that is implicit in coaching may be all that is needed to accomplish changes in behavior.

SKILL GENERALIZATION PROCEDURES

DBT does not assume that skills learned in therapy will necessarily generalize to situations in everyday life outside of therapy. Therefore, it is very im-

TABLE 11.3. Skill Generalization Procedures Checklist

_____ T PROGRAMS GENERALIZATION of skills.
  _____ T teaches a variety of skilled responses to each situation.
  _____ T varies training situations that P practices skills in.
  _____ T duplicates within the therapeutic relationship important characteristics of interpersonal relationships P has outside of therapy.

_____ T CONSULTS with P between sessions to help P apply skills _in vivo._
  _____ T assists P in applying skills to problem situations via phone calls.

_____ T gives P AUDIOTAPE of session to listen to between sessions.

_____ T gives P _in vivo_ BEHAVIORAL REHEARSAL ASSIGNMENTS.
  _____ In standard DBT (with separate individual therapy and skills training therapists), individual T gives P specific tasks to practice with skills training therapists; skills training therapists give P tasks to practice with individual T.
  _____ T tailors assignments to needs and capabilities of P; T uses principles of shaping.

_____ T helps P to CREATE AN ENVIRONMENT that reinforces skilled behaviors.
  _____ T teaches P how to recruit reinforcement from the natural community.
  _____ T teaches behaviors that fit the natural contingencies in P's environment.
  _____ T teaches P in self-management skills, especially how to structure her environment.
  _____ T is explicit and firm regarding necessity of P's reinforcing or arranging for environmental reinforcement of desirable responding if P's life is to change.
  _____ In family and couples sessions, T highlights necessity of social reinforcement for adaptive behaviors and reduction of punishment for adaptive behaviors.
  _____ T fades reinforcement to an intermittent schedule, such that T's reinforcement is less frequent than environmental reinforcement.

portant that the therapist actively encourage this transfer of skills. A number of specific procedures for doing so are discussed below and outlined in Table 11.3.

1. GENERALIZATION PROGRAMMING

At every step of skills training, the therapist should actively program two types of generalization. In the first type, technically called "response generalization," the therapist is concerned that skills learned will be general and flexible, so that in most settings the patient will have a number of behavioral options to choose from. In applying the procedures described above, the therapist should be careful to model, instruct, reinforce, and prescribe a variety of skilled responses to each situation. For example, when generating skillful solutions to problem situations, the therapist should help the patient think up a number of different responses rather than stopping as soon as one skillful responses is produced. Similarly, a variety of different responses should be modeled and reinforced for the same type of situations. In the second type, technically called "stimulus generalization," the therapist is concerned that skills learned in one setting will generalize to other settings. Most of the procedures listed below are designed to enhance this type of generalization. The basic idea is that the therapist should get the patient to try out skills in as many types of situations as possible. It is particularly important that the therapist attempt to duplicate in the therapeutic relationship important characteristics of the patient's interpersonal relationship outside of therapy. One way to do this, and still stay genuine in the relationship, is to highlight similarities between situations outside of therapy and the problems and interactions that occur within therapy sessions.

2. BETWEEN-SESSION CONSULTATION

Patients should be encouraged to seek consultation between sessions if they are unable to apply new skills in their natural environment. In individual outpatient therapy, this consultation will usually be obtained through phone calls to the therapist. Another technique, developed by Charles Swenson at Cornell Medical Center/New York Hospital at White Plains and discussed in Chapter 6, is to provide a behavioral consultant with regular daily office hours whose task is to help patients apply their new skills to everyday life. On inpatient and day treatment units, patients can be encouraged to seek assistance from staff members when they are having difficulty.

During these interactions, the therapist and patient can discuss application of relevant skills to the patient's real-life situations. In general, the interactions should be conducted in a problem-solving manner, with the therapist being careful to help the patient arrive at effective solutions or ways to use her developing skills, rather than simply giving solutions to the patient. The temptation to give a solution rather than to work with the patient is most likely when the therapist is short on time or does not want to be bothered with the patient at that moment. In these cases, it is preferable for the therapist to ask the patient to phone again or come back at a more convenient time. Phone calls and other ad hoc consultation strategies are discussed in more detail in Chapter 15.

2. PROVIDING SESSION TAPES FOR REVIEW

All psychotherapy sessions should be audiotaped for both evaluation and supervision purposes. A second audiotape can be made of each session for the patient; the tape can then be listened to in its entirety by the patient between sessions. There are several reasons for the audiotape monitoring strategy. First, because of high emotional arousal during sessions, concentration difficulties accompanying depression and anxiety, or dissociative responses a patient is often unable to attend to much of what transpires during a therapy session. Thus, the patient may improve her retention of material offered during the session by listening to the tape. Second, listening to a tape may provide the patient with important insights about her own behavior, about the therapist's reactions to her, and about the interaction between the two of them. Such insights often help the patient understand and improve her own interpersonal behavior and the interpersonal relationship between the patient and therapist. Third, listening to the session at home can help the patient use and integrate this material in the natural environment. Essentially, she is relearning therapeutic insights outside of the therapy session. Finally, many patients report that listening to tapes can be very helpful when they are feeling overwhelmed, panicked, or unable to cope between sessions. Simply listening to a tape has an effect similar to that of having an additional session with the therapist. Such use of the tape is to be encouraged.

Several problems may come up in getting a patient to review tapes of sessions. One problem may be that the patient cannot afford a tape recorder or audiotapes. If indeed this is the case (and often it is), the patient should be given several blank audiotapes at the beginning of therapy for her use. She should be loaned a tape recorder, and the problem of obtaining money to buy a tape recorder or finding someone from whom to borrow a tape recorder should be the focus of a problem-solving session. If no other solution can be found, arrangements should be made for the patient to listen to the tapes at the therapist's office. At other times, the patient may forget to bring a tape with her to a session. If listening to tapes is an integral part of therapy, such forgetfulness should be analyzed and treated as a therapy-interfering behavior. Finally, a patient may state that she is unable to listen to sessions, usually because she finds it very uncomfortable to listen to herself. In these instances, the therapist can point out that most patients find it difficult to listen to tapes at the beginning, but with time listening not only becomes easier but is frequently quite beneficial. However, listening to tapes should not become a power issue in the therapy session. If a patient adamantly refuses to listen to tapes, her wishes should be respected. The topic should be reintroduced occasionally throughout treatment to see whether the patient can be persuaded to change her mind.

4. *IN VIVO* BEHAVIORAL REHEARSAL ASSIGNMENTS

Weekly behavioral assignments are an important part of the structured skills training modules and are the principal way of insuring generalization of skills to everyday life. It is essential, therefore, that both the skills trainer and the individual therapist support the assignments made, ask the patient how she is doing with them, and help her overcome obstacles to engaging in the assigned practice. There is often not sufficient time in structured skills training, especially when is conducted in groups, to give enough attention to individual problem. Patients are frequently reluctant to admit or discuss their difficulties with practice. "Standard" DBT combines skills training with individual psychotherapy. It is essential that the individual therapist focus closely on helping the patient apply the skills she is learning to the problems for which she is seeking help. It goes without saying that the therapist must keep track of what the patient is learning in structured skills training.

Homework assignments in structured skills training are keyed to the specific skills currently being taught. The individual therapist, however, may want to use some of the homework assignments and accompanying forms throughout therapy, or on an as-needed basis. In individual therapy, the use of homework forms can be tailored to the individual's needs. For example, one of these forms focuses on identifying and labeling emotions, and takes the patient through a series of steps to help her clarify what she is feeling. The individual therapist may suggest that the patient use this form whenever she is confused or overwhelmed by emotions. The companion manual to this volume contains a large number of homework assignment forms, covering each of the DBT behavioral skills. There is no reason, of course, why individual therapists cannot revise these forms to fit either their patients' or their own personal preferences and needs.

Using Consultation-to-the-Patient Strategies in Developing Assignments. In standard DBT, patients will often complain about one therapist while interacting with another therapist in the treatment program. Such complaints are also often heard in clinic, day treatment, and inpatient settings. Problems with another therapist in the treatment program provide a rich opportunity for patient and therapist to work on a variety of skills, which can then be practiced with the other therapist.

For example (as is often the case in my program), a patient in structured skills training may complain to her individual therapist that the skills training therapist is being unreasonable or is making some other mistake. The individual therapist should respond by helping the patient analyze the situation and determine which set(s) of skills might be most apropriate or useful to practice with the other therapist. The patient might practice her interpersonal skills to get the skills trainer to change his or her behavior. Or it might be an opportunity for distress tolerance practice — accepting both the skills training situation and the patient's own feelings about it just as they are. Or, if emotions are particularly intense or painful, it might be an opportunity for the patient to practice trying to modulalte or change emotional responses to this particular type of interpersonal problem. All the while, the individual therapist might pay particular attention to helping the patient practice her mindfulness skills (particularly a nonjudgmental stance) in the situation. At the next session, patient and therapist can review how the skills practice went. Just as often in my program, the complaints go in the other direction: Patients complain about their individual therapists during skills training sessions. The skills trainer can help such a patient figure out what new skills she can practice with her individual therapist.

With suicidal patients it can be useful to help them practice new skills, particularly in communicating about suicidal behaviors, with inpatient and emergency professional staff persons. For example, patients can practice interpersonal skills to get into hospitals, get out of hospitals, get more (or less) attention from hospital staff, ease the worries of emergency personnel, prevent involuntary detainment, and so on. Distress tolerance and emotion regulation skills can be practiced if rules are arbitary, restrictions are unreasonable, and demands are overwhelming. Teaching patients to use their behavioral skills with other health professionals is so important in DBT that an entire set of treatment strategies is devoted to it—the consultation-to-the-patient strategies (described in Chapter 13).

Using Dialectical Strategies and Shaping in Devising Assignments. From a DBT perspective, problematic *in vivo* and therapeutic situations can be viewed as opportunities for practicing behavioral skills. Changing the frame in this way (from problem to opportunity) is an example of the "making lemonade out of lemons" dialectical strategy described in Chapter 7. The overall dialectical tension here is usually between wanting the patient to practice new skills in difficult situations and wanting to patient to have success experiences so that new skills will be reinforced and strengthened. Principles of shaping (see Chapter 10) are likewise crucial in devising homework assignments and must be advocated strongly by the therapist. Patients who want to practice only in very safe situations should be pushed, and patients who want to practice in situations far above their ability level should be held back.

5. ENVIRONMENTAL CHANGE

As I have discussed previously, borderline individuals tend to have a passive style of personal regulation. On the continuum whose poles are internal self-regulation and external, environmental regulation, they are near the environmental pole. Many therapists seem to believe that the self-regulation pole of the continuum is inherently better or more mature, and spend a fair amount of therapy time trying to make borderline individuals more self-regulated. Although DBT does not suggest the converse—that environmental regulation styles are preferable—it does suggest that going with a patient's strength is likely to be easier and more beneficial in the long run. Thus, once behavioral skills are in place, the therapist should teach the patient how to maximize the tendency of the natural environment to reinforce skilled over unskilled behaviors. This may include teaching the patient how to create structure, how to make public instead of private commitments, how to find communities and lifestyles that support her new behaviors, and how to elicit reinforcement from others for skilled rather than unskilled behaviors. This is not to say that patients should not be taught self-regulation skills; rather, the types of self-regulation skills taught should be keyed to their strengths. Written self-monitoring with a prepared diary form, for example, is preferable over trying to observe behavior each day and make a mental note of it. Keeping alcohol out of the house is preferable to trying a self-talk strategy to inhibit getting out the bottle.

A final point needs to be made here. Sometimes patients' newly learned skills do not generalize because they themselves punish their own behavior out in the real world. This is usually because their behavioral expectations for themselves are so high that they simply never reach the criterion for reinforcement. This pattern must change if generalization and progress are to occur. Problems with self-reinforcement and self-punishment have been discussed more extensively in Chapters 8 and 10. Behavioral validation strategies, used to counteract these problems, should be used here also.

Family and Couples Sessions. One way to maximize generalization is to have individuals from the patient's social community come to sessions. Usually, these will be members of the patient's family or the patient's spouse or partner. Family and couples sessions promote generalization in a number of ways. Skills learned and practiced with the therapist can be practiced with important others. These sessions also allow the therapist to observe with the patient exactly what the difficulties are; sometimes both parties may find that the skills taught so far simply are not sufficient, and that new skills must be developed. These sessions also afford an opportunity to instruct the family, spouse, or partner in the need to reinforce skilled over unskilled behaviors. Often new skills do not generalize because they are punished rather than rewarded by the natural community. Assertion skills, for example, are a typical problem here, especially when the current social environment does not have the time, energy, or desire to respond to the individual's needs.

Principles of Fading. At the beginning of skills training, the therapist models, instructs, reinforces, gives feedback, and coaches the patient for using skills both within the therapy sessions and in her natural environment. If skillful behavior in the everyday environment is to become independent of the influence of the therapist, however, then the therapist must gradually fade out his or her use of these procedures, particularly instructions and reinforcement. The goal here is to fade skills training procedures to an intermittent schedule, such that the therapist is providing less frequent instructions and coaching than the patient can provide for herself, and less modeling, feedback, and reinforcement than the patient is obtaining from her natural environment.

EXPOSURE-BASED PROCEDURES

Exposure-based treatment procedures were designed originally to reduce unwanted, problematic fear and fear-related emotions.[1] In DBT, these procedures are extended and somewhat modified to treat other emotions, including guilt, shame, and anger. Four conditions prevalent among borderline individuals suggest that a direct focus on painful emotions is necessary in any therapy for these individuals. First, anxiety, fear, panic, shame, guilt, sadness, and anger are current major problems for many. The functional value of many dysfunctional borderline behavior patterns lies in their effectiveness at reducing these emotions. Second, although borderline individuals often have many of the behavioral skills they need in a particular situation, their ability to use the skills they have is often inhibited by anticipatory fear, shame, or guilt or is interfered with by excessive anger or sorrow. Third, many borderline patients have such a fear of experiencing and expressing emotions that they are often unable to discuss emotional topics in therapy. In other words, they are emotion-phobic. Finally, because of past traumatic events (including childhood sexual abuse), many borderline individuals suffer from unresolved, intrusive emotional reactions associated with the stress. Some borderline patterns may be directly related to these ongoing emotional responses. In DBT, exposure-based procedures, broadly conceived, are an important ingredient in the treatment of these difficulties.

There is little question that nonreinforced exposure to feared objects or situations is effective in treating anxiety based emotional disorders. Exposure to anxiety-related cues is important in the treatment of dysfunctional fears, panic, phobias, posttraumatic stress responses, agoraphobia, obsessive thinking, compulsive behaviors, and general anxiety (Barlow, 1988). Exposure-based treatments have not traditionally been applied to emotions such as shame, guilt, and anger, however. In DBT, modified versions of exposure-based procedures are used to reduce these emotions as well as fear-related emotions. In particular, the procedures as used in DBT include nonreinforced exposure to events that prompt fear, sorrow, guilt, shame, and anger, as well as simultaneous blocking or reversal of automatic, maladaptive emotional action and expressive tendencies. The emphasis is on both exposure and acting differently.

Exposure-based procedures are used somewhat informally in DBT. That is, there is no formal module in which whole sessions or a series of sessions are devoted to utilizing these procedures in an explicit manner. The exception here is the treatment of posttraumatic stress responses in the second stage of therapy. In the case of sexual abuse in particular, the strategy is to employ the DBT exposure-based procedures in a very focused fashion. Alternatively, any well-developed treatment module, especially one developed specifically for sexual abuse victims, can be either inserted or conducted concurrently.

Despite the informal nature of exposure in DBT, the process nonetheless runs through the whole of the therapy. Many of the strategies I have discussed previously can be reanalyzed in terms of their tendencies to expose the patient to emotionally conditioned stimuli and to block emotional action tendencies. The key steps in exposure are as follows: (1) Stimuli that match the problem situation and elicit the conditioned affective response are presented; (2) the affective response is not reinforced; (3) maladaptive coping responses, including escape responses and other action tendencies, are blocked; (4) the individual's sense of control over the situation or herself is enhanced; and (5) exposure lasts long enough (or occurs often enough) to work.

Orienting and Commitment to Exposure: Task Overview

The old advice "If you fall off a horse, get back on it" is an example of exposure as a treatment for fear. Most patients will have heard this adage or one similar to it. In orienting a patient to exposure, the therapist must emphasize the effectiveness of this advice. That is, the therapist must convince the patient that doing the opposite of what her emotions tell her to do will be helpful in the long run. Usually, she will agree in principle with the adage but will not see how it is relevant to her own problems. The therapist's task is to make it relevant. Dialectical strategies, such as storytelling and other uses of metaphor, can be quite helpful here.

Again, borderline patients are so fearful of emotions, especially negative ones, that they try to avoid them by blocking their experience of the emotions. That is, they avoid emotional cues and inhibit the experience of emotions; thus, they have no opportunity to learn that when unfettered, emotions come and go. The therapist's task is to convince such a patient that emotions are like waves of water coming in from the sea onto the beach. Left alone, the water comes in and goes out. The emotion-phobic patient tries to keep the waves from coming in by building a wall, but instead of keeping the water out, the wall actually traps the water inside the walls. Taking down the wall is the solution.

In most instances of exposure, the patient's collaboration is crucial. A patient can block exposure by disassociating, depersonalizing, distracting herself with other thoughts and images, leaving or walking out, digressing, or diverting the topic; in short, she can close her eyes and ears. Orienting and commitment strategies are therefore crucial. In particular, it is helpful to orient the patient to the fact that very brief exposures may create misery but not help it. That is, if she consistently shuts off exposure very rapidly, she may make herself feel worse instead of better. Validating the extreme difficulty of exposure to painful and threatening stimuli, and combining this with the foot-in-the-door strategy (see Chapter 9), are very important here.

Helping the patient understand the rationale of exposure-based treatments is often the key to gaining commitment and collaboration. Reviewing research results and the therapist's personal and clinical experience can also be quite helpful. Explaining in a clear way how emotions work and how emotions change can also be helpful. As with learning theory and contingency management, the therapist needs to have a reasonably clear grasp of the research in emotions in order to orient the patient to and use exposure-based procedures properly. A number of books are excellent here, including those by Barlow (1988) and Greenberg and Safran (1987). A number of competing theories on emotional change have been proposed. Depending on the patient's degree of resistance to exposure and sophistication, they may be discussed during orientation. The effectiveness of exposure-based treatment has been attributed to processes of extinction, habituation, and biological toughening up (see Barlow, 1988, for a review). Information-processing theorists have suggested that change is the result of emotional processing that leads to integration of new corrective information incompatible with existing threat-related cognitive structures (Foa & Kozak, 1986). The general idea is that learned or conditioned anxiety reactions can be unlearned,or unconditioned. Barlow (1988) and others (e.g., Izard, 1977), however, citing current emotion theory and research, have suggested that the effectiveness of these procedures is attributable to the fact that exposure-based procedures prevent the action tendencies associated with emotions. In all procedures targeting fear-related problems, for example, emotion-driven escape and avoidance are resolutely blocked. That is, the action tendency associated with fear (flight) is prevented. As Barlow puts it, in exposure procedures individuals "act themselves" into new feelings.

With the exception of blocking premature escape when treating fear, standard exposure-based procedures do not usually focus on changing emotional behavior during exposure to emotion provoking situations. In DBT, this emphasis is added, and it is very important to get across a clear and convincing rationale for it to the patient. Many patients believe that expressing an emotion different from the one they are feeling is invalidating. Indeed, the invalidating environment puts such a premium on hiding and "masking" negative emotions that a therapist's request to work on changing emotional behavior is likely to be experienced as one more invalidation. The therapist can make a number of points in discussing this request.

It is important to distinguish "masking emotions" from "changing emotional expressiveness." Masking usually involves the tensing of facial muscles. Expressing an opposite emotion, such as calmness in contrast to fear or satisfaction in contrast to guilt or shame, requires the relaxation of these very same muscles. Masking and tensing are very different from relaxing; for instance, grinning to mask anger feels very different from smiling as an expression of joy. Having the patient try the different facial expressions can be very effective.

The idea behind changing facial and postural expressions is that muscles, especially those in the face, send messages to the brain about what one is feeling. These messages in turn amplify and maintain the original emotion. In DBT exposure-based procedures, the idea is to try to get the face and body to send a different message to the brain—for example, that a feared situation is not frightening. Masking, in contrast to relaxing, sends the message "This is frightening and I can't show it." In a similar vein, actions also send messages to the brain about emotions. Changing an action changes the message. The research literature makes it reasonably clear that changing the message can change the duration and intensity of the emotion. Inhibiting emotional expression, modulating (reducing or increasing) the intensity or duration of expressions, and simulating emotional expressions can be used to regulate or even activate genuine emotions (Duncan & Laird, 1977; Laird, 1974; Laird, Wagener, Halal, & Szegda, 1982; Rhodewalt & Comer, 1979; Zuckerman, Klorman, Larrance, & Spiegel, 1981; Lanzetta, Cartwright-Smith, & Kleck, 1976; Lanzetta & Orr, 1980). Thus, modulating emotional expressions is one method of emotional regulation and control. This literature can be reviewed with the patient.

Changing expressions and action tendencies should be presented as a tactic to change those emotions that the patient herself wants to change. Thus, the tactic is used to reduce unwanted, dysfunctional aversive emotions in the situations that elicit them. It is not used to reduce all aversive emotions; indeed, a major tenet of DBT is that the inability to tolerate aversive emotions, rather than the aversive emotions themselves, is a source of many borderline behavior patterns. Thus, tolerating emotions rather than changing them is often the goal of DBT. Nor are exposure-based procedures directed at changing emotional expressiveness per se. On the contrary, a major focus of DBT is on reducing the fear associated with ordinary emotional expressiveness. Specific exposure-based strategies are discussed below and outlined in Table 11.4.

I. PROVIDING NONREINFORCED EXPOSURE

The first requirement is for the individual to be exposed to the cues that set off an aversive emotion in a manner that does not recondition the very emotion the therapist and patient are trying to decrease. That is, the person should not re-experience the same sort of conditions that produced the aversive emotional reaction in the first place. To put it more elegantly, the exposure situation does not reinforce the anxiety response. As Foa and Kozak (1986) put it, the exposure situation must contain "corrective information."

Criteria for Nonreinforcement

In the case of fear-related emotions, the person should be exposed to cues that currently set off anxiety or fear responses in such a way that new information is received and processed. The situation has to provide new information about the threatening qualities of the situation. For example, a student who has failed five exams in a row becomes test-anxious. Taking another exam, followed by yet another failure, is not likely to reduce test anxiety. Although the situation is matched and elicits fear, there is no corrective information; indeed, the fear associated with taking exams is reinforced. If a person fears that once an emotion starts she will lose complete control (e.g., faint), and then she does, the exposure has increased fear instead of reducing it. An important point to keep in mind, then, is that exposure-based procedures for aversive emotions, including fear, are only warranted when the emotional responses are overreactions to present circumstances—in the case of fear, when fear is out of proportion to actual threat.

In the case of guilt, the requirement that exposure be nonreinforced suggests that exposure-based procedures should only be used when the guilt is unsupported. Guilt can be supported either by a person's firm beliefs or moral code or by the social community. By "unsupported guilt" I mean that the individual in her calmer moments—using "wise mind," so to speak—does not

TABLE 11.4. Exposure-Based Procedures Checklist

_____ T orients P to exposure-based procedures and elicits commitment to collaborate.
    _____ T makes sure that P understands principles of exposure-based procedures so that P can cooperate better.
    _____ T distinguishes "masking emotions" from "changing emotional expressiveness."

_____ T provides NONREINFORCED EXPOSURE to cues that elicit problematic emotions.
    _____ T makes sure that new information about fear and anxiety-eliciting situations is received and processed.
    _____ For problematic guilt and shame, T uses exposure-based procedures only when guilt and shame are unsupported by the situation.
    _____ T presents anger-eliciting situations that eventually work out the way P wants, if P tolerates the frustration a bit.
    _____ T matches exposure situation to problem situation.
    _____ T insures that exposure actually takes place.
        _____ T is alert for diversion tactics.
        _____ In covert exposure, T has P describe scenes in detail and in present tense.
    _____ T graduates exposure intensity.
    _____ T makes sure that exposure lasts long enough for emotion to be elicited and for some reduction to occur, but not so long that P loses control.
    _____ T uses specific change strategies and procedures as exposure techniques, as appropriate:
        _____ Behavioral analysis.
        _____ Skills training.
        _____ Contingency procedures.
        _____ Withdrawal or fading of supportive activities.

_____ T BLOCKS ACTION TENDENCIES associated with P's problem emotions.
    _____ T blocks P's tendency to escape/avoid when feeling afraid.
    _____ T blocks P's tendency to hide or withdraw when feeling shame.
    _____ T blocks P's tendency to repair or self-punish when feeling unsupported guilt.
    _____ T blocks P's tendency to hostile and aggressive responses; or, if P is afraid of experiencing anger, T blocks avoidance of anger and helps P disinhibit experience of anger.

_____ T helps P EXPRESS CONVERSE EMOTIONS to those she is feeling.
    _____ T differentiates "masking" from expressing a different emotion.

_____ T ENHANCES P's SENSE OF CONTROL over aversive affect-arousing events.
    _____ T designs exposure treatment collaboratively with P.
    _____ T instructs P at beginning that she has ultimate control over stimuli and can end exposure at any time.
    _____ T gets P to collaborate in staying in emotional stimulus conditions as long as possible.
    _____T helps P leave or escape situations voluntarily instead of automatically.
    _____ T is vulnerable to P's influence.

_____ T makes use of more formal exposure-based procedures as necessary, especially in the treatment of posttraumatic stress responses (second stage of DBT).

(cont.)

Table 11.4 (cont.)

Anti-DBT tactics

____ T encourages P to mask emotions.

____ T reinforces highly maladaptive attempts by P to escape or avoid emotions.

____ T punishes adaptive styles of ending aversive situations.

____ T forgets principles of shaping.

____ T treats P as overly fragile.

herself believe that the actions in question are wrong or immoral. That is, the guilt is not supported by her own beliefs or moral code. Nor is she confronted with believable social condemnation or personal moral accusations during re-exposure; that is, she does not receive new information that changes her moral stance from acceptance to condemnation. Thus, exposure-based treatments to cues associated with childhood sexual abuse in the presence of an empathic therapist should reduce conditioned guilt. Exposure to cues associated with an act the individual believes firmly was wrong (e.g., stealing, cheating, or lying, hurting a friend), especially if the act is unrepaired, may intensify guilt rather than reduce it. An individual who feels guilty about standing up for her rights will probably feel more guilty if each time she practices her assertion skills she is told that she is selfish or overcontrolling.

Shame is a particularly vexing and difficult emotion, primarily because it is so pervasive among borderline individuals and because by its very nature shame interferes with the free flow of therapeutic discourse. The interpersonal event that reinforces shame is public censure or humiliation. The problems shame creates in conducting therapy with a borderline individual are that, first, it is often not expressed in a manner the therapist can understand; and, second, the patient often attempts to hide her feeling of shame. Thus, the therapist often does not even know that a problem with shame exists. The interpersonal events that reinforce shame are ostracism, rejection, and loss of the respect of others. Thus, it is particularly important when a patient is revealing shameful material that the therapist respond with validation as opposed to censure, with acceptance rather than rejection. In particular, the therapist should be alert to the fact that disclosing the shameful events is itself shaming. Thus, care is needed in responding to and validating the act of disclosing.

As in the case of guilt and shame, the efficacy of exposure in the reduction of anger is not explored in any detail in the emotion literature. Efficacy, however, is probably inextricably linked to the prevention of anger action and expressive tendencies and to the inducement of converse actions and thinking, which I discuss further below. With respect to the procedure of non-reinforced exposure, however, it seems reasonable to suppose that attention should be paid to altering how much the situation either actually or perceptually frustrates the individual's attainment of goals. For example, a patient may want to talk about topic A during a session, and may then respond with anger when the therapist wants to talk about her parasuicidal behavior during the previous week. Consistent exposure to sessions in which talking about previous parasuicide is followed by discussions of topic A is likely to reduce the automatic response of anger to the therapist's insistence on conducting behavioral analyses of previous parasuicidal acts. Consistent exposure to losing the opportunity to discuss topic A may (all other things being equal) enhance anger. Likewise, consistent exposure to the therapist's unavailability during crises resulting in unwanted events, such as intense suffering or hospitalization, is likely to increase the patient's anger when she is exposed again to the therapist's unavailability during a crisis. Consistent exposure to the therapist's unavailability, paired with the ability to get other help or to make use independently of behavioral skills to avert suffering or hospitalization, will defuse the situation.

A number of additional principles must be remembered. First, the therapist must be sure that the exposure situation or event matches the problem situation or event. Second, the therapist should not assume that exposure is occurring simply because the patient is in the situation. Third, the exposure should be intense enough that emotions are evoked, but not so intense that it interferes with information processing or produces avoidance of therapy. Fourth, the exposure should last long enough for emotions to build, but not so long that the patient loses control.

Matching the Exposure Situation to the Problem Situation

There is no substitute for assessing both the characteristics of the situation that elicit the problem emotion and the elements of the situation that further reinforce the emotional response. The exposure situation has to mimic the problem situation. Context is all-important here. For example, a person who is afraid to assert her needs with intimate friends may have no fears with strangers, or vice versa. A person who is unbothered by criticism at home may be very bothered at work. Shoplifting may elicit little guilt, whereas stealing from a friend may elicit considerable guilt. The therapist must be as careful in assessing the events that reinforce or recondition the emotion as in assessing the context that elicits the emotion. For example, the test-anxious student is probably afraid of both exam taking per se and failing exams. Fear of taking exams may be reinforced by failing exams; fear of failure may be reinforced by consequences of failure, such as being expelled from school; fear of being expelled may be reinforced by losing friends and social status; and so on. The parameters of context that make a difference will vary by patient, emotion, and problem; effective treatment may require exposure to each parameter in turn. Exposure carried out in the relative safety of therapy interactions must be supplemented by direct exposure in the day-to-day environment of the patient. The more practice exposure the patient gets in her everyday world, the better. The generalization procedures discussed above for skills training can do double duty as exposure procedures.

Insuring That Exposure Takes Place

Presentation of emotion-relevant cues can be direct or indirect. In direct exposure, the patient is exposed to actual situations or events that are emotion-related. The individual enters feared situations, does things she is afraid of doing, and thinks and talks about topics associated with feared emotion. She repeatedly re-enacts the very things she feels ashamed of or guilty about. The message here is simple: The only way out of emotions is through them. Depending on the problem situation, exposure during sessions can include verbal confrontation, structured discussion of avoided emotional topics, or instructions to the patient to practice mindful self-awareness during the interaction. For many borderline patients, simply going to a therapy session is an exposure condition. Practically anything in therapy that elicits unconditioned problem emotions can be the focus of direct exposure, *as long as* the therapist is careful to place new, corrective information side by side with the emotion-eliciting elements. Covert or indirect exposure involves having the patient imagine emotion-eliciting scenes. With imagined exposure, it is particularly important that the therapist guide the patient in "entering" into the imagery, rather than "watching" it as on a TV monitor. Between sessions, covert exposure can be practiced by listening to therapy tapes. With particularly difficult topics, the therapist might consider making up special exposure tapes for the patient's use in practice between sessions.

It is very important for the therapist to make sure that the exposure that is supposed to be occurring is actually taking place. The therapist must be alert for cognitive diversion tactics, such as dissociating, depersonalizing, focusing on unrelated thoughts or images, daydreaming, and so on. Sometimes these avoidance strategies are so automatic that the patient is not even aware of their occurrence. When using covert exposure, the therapist should ask the patient to describe the scene in minute moment-to-moment detail, in the present tense.

Graduating the Intensity of Exposure

Should the therapist have the patient wade into the pool from the shallow end or throw the patient into the deep end the first time out, so to speak? This question has been a controversial one for years. Exposure intensities vary from the very low intensity and graduated exposure of systematic desensitization to the very intense exposure of implosion and flooding procedures. The accumulated literature suggests that the exposure has to be, at least intense enough to elicit the conditioned emotion. There is no need, however, for exposure to extreme situations. Instead, graduated exposure to increasingly emotion-arousing cues is easier on the patient and just as effective.

Controlling the Length of Exposure

The question of exposure length has also been the subject of much theoretical controversy in the research literature on fear. The data are complex, but three points are important. First, the exposure should last long enough to elicit the aversive emotion at a relatively intense but still bearable level. Escaping or diverting attention before the emotion is elicited is unlikely to be beneficial. Second, the patient should end the exposure voluntarily instead of allowing automatic processes (dissociating, depersonalization, impulsive running away, attacking the therapist, etc.) to stop the exposure. With fear, in particular, the patient's learning that she can control the amount and degree of exposure may itself be therapeutic and render future exposure less frightening (this point is discussed further below). Third, when the problem emotion is fear (including fear of emotions), shame, or guilt, some reduction in the emotion should occur before the exposure is ended. Although it is not clear whether this is an essential ingredient, the tendency of borderline patients to believe that emotions are uncontrollable and unending suggests that the corrective information this tactic provides may be very important. The relationship of exposure length to efficacy may dictate longer-than-normal sessions at times. For example, with intense and complex fears (such as those typical of trauma victims), exposures may need to last 1 hour or more.

Specific Change Stategies and Procedures as Exposure Techniques

Behavior Analysis as Exposure.   As I have pointed out repeatedly and described in Chapter 9, if a patient engages in a high-priority target behavior between or within therapy sessions, a structured and minutely detailed behavioral analysis follows. That is, the patient is required by the therapist to talk publicly and in graphic detail about her own maladaptive behaviors and the surrounding circumstances. Borderline individuals often experience intense shame, humiliation, fear of disapproval, anxiety, and sometimes panic when asked to describe their own maladaptive actions and reactions. Some experience such intense sorrow or grief at the telling that they fear they will not survive the experience. Almost all try to avoid or short-circuit the analysis. More than one patient in our program has had to be "dragged kicking and screaming" through the process.

As we have seen, the behavioral analysis of targeted borderline behaviors is a major problem-solving strategy. It is both assessment and an avenue for developing behavioral insight and interpretations (Chapter 9). It is also a correction–overcorrection procedure within contingency management (Chapter 10). And it can be considered an instance of exposure as well. The individual is verbally and imaginally exposed not only to her own aversive behaviors and the events that surround them, but also to the circumstance of public disclosure. To the extent that the therapist is validating rather than judgmental, provides empathy rather than social censure, and understands and accepts rather than humiliates, this exposure does not reinforce further shame. As the individual repeatedly analyzes her behavior in the presence of the therapist, survives the experience, and does not lose the affection of the therapist, the exposure does not reinforce anxiety and fear.

Contingency and Skills Training Strategies as Exposure. Much of the behavioral practice linked to the skills training modules has, as one effect, the exposure of the individual to activities and situations associated with intense and aversive emotions. Patients are routinely asked to do things they are afraid of or feel unrealistically guilty about, to enter situations that set off anger or sorrow, and expose to the public eye events they are ashamed of. In contingency management and the observing of limits, the therapist confronts the patient about her problematic behavior. In both skills training and contingency procedures, in other words, a therapist gives a patient direct, evaluative feedback about her problematic behavior and the likely consequences. The patient is exposed to interpersonal disapproval or criticism and public highlighting of her negative or problematic behaviors. Like behavioral analysis, these procedures expose the patient to circumstances that elicit conditioned shame and fear-related emotions. However, in contrast to behavioral analysis, where the emotion is a response to the act of self-disclosure, the emotion is a response to the acts of the therapist. Indeed, these therapist acts (confrontation, disapproval) may be the very ones that the patient fears in self-disclosure. The patient may respond automatically (and sometimes with breathtaking speed), with fears of abandonment, shame related to dependency, intense anger, or all three in rapid succession. The oscillating action tendencies of escape, hiding, and attacking often confuse both the patient and the therapist.

Once the therapist realizes that contingency and skills training procedures contain elements of exposure, a number of further guidelines about the use of these procedures follow. First, the therapist should not stop using the procedures simply because they make the patient uncomfortable. In particular, the therapist should not provide very brief exposure and stop in the middle of overarousal of the patient. The tactic here should be to back off slightly, soothe the patient, and stop as the patient's arousal (fear, shame, etc.) goes down, even if only slightly. Second, exposure should be graduated instead of massed or intense. A little bit of confrontation or disapproval can sometimes go a long way with borderline patients. Third, as with any other form of exposure, the therapist should take care that a procedure does not further reinforce shame- and fear-related responses. When a procedure elicits anger, the therapist should maintain the exposure while simultaneously providing information that decreases the actual frustration of important goals or needs. Finally, contingency and skills training procedures should always be combined with validation of the patient's responses. The fact that she needs to change does not mean that her reactions are not understandable, nor does it mean that everything associated with a problem behavior is problematic.

Unlinking behavioral feedback from inferred motives can be an especially beneficial tactic here.

Mindfulness Practice as Exposure.   In mindfulness practice (described in detail the companion skills training manual), patients are instructed to "experience" exactly what is happening in the moment, without either pushing any of it away or grabbing onto it. They are also instructed to "step back from" and observe judgmental responses to their own behaviors. Mindfulness practice may be particularly helpful for individuals who are afraid or ashamed of their own thoughts and emotions. The idea is to let thoughts, feelings, and sensations come and go, rise and fall away, without attempting to exert control (although it is important to point out that, in reality, the individual is in control and can stop the process at any point). In its entirety, mindfulness is an instance of exposure to naturally arising thoughts, feelings, and sensations. It may be particularly useful as a way to encourage exposure to somatic cues associated with emotions. The reconditioning lies in the fact that if a person does pull back, so to speak, and simply observes sensations, thoughts, and feelings, they will do just that—come and go. For many borderline individuals, this is an entirely new experience and is important in reducing their fears of emotions.

Withdrawal of Therapist Supportive Activities as Exposure.   During the last phase of therapy, the therapist withdraws or fades some of the previous validating and supportive activities. Generally, this withdrawal will cue intense anxiety and sometimes anger. The patient is being exposed to situations where she is bereft of help and must help herself unaided. Therapists often collaborate with patients in short-circuiting this exposure; it is painful for both. However, with proper timing and orienting, the exposure can lead to reductions in anxieties about independence and aloneness. The secret, of course, is not to withdraw validation and support before the patient can adequately fend for herself. To do so reinforces and reconditions the aversive emotions.

2. BLOCKING ACTION TENDENCIES ASSOCIATED WITH PROBLEM EMOTIONS

During exposure procedures, it is essential for the therapist to block the patient's emotional action tendencies associated with the problem emotion. In a way, all of DBT is an instance of this strategy; DBT focuses on changing emotion-related behavior before changing the emotions these behaviors control. The basic idea here is to follow the advice of Barlow (1988) and try to get the patient to "act her way" into feeling different.

The most important response to block is avoidance. The fundamental action tendency in fear-related emotions is escape or avoidance. Borderline patients (and many other patient populations as well) consistently try to avoid situations that create aversive emotions. During sessions, they resist behavioral analysis and discussions of emotion-provoking situations. Once they are persuaded to participate, they continually divert the discussion to more comfortable topics. During imaginal procedures, they start thinking about something else. Most patients avoid homework practice and are reluctant to do role playing in sessions. At times, the avoidance comes so early in the emotional chain that the patient never even experiences the aversive emotion. The fundamental action tendency associated with shame is hiding. In therapy, hiding is accomplished by clamming up, failing to disclose important information or events, not bringing in diary cards or failing to fill them out, withdrawing emotionally and verbally, or not coming to sessions or terminating prematurely. Important action tendencies associated with guilt are attempts at repair or self-punishment. Excessive confessions and apologies, gifts, long letters begging forgiveness, and the doing of favors for the injured person, as well as pejorative and overly critical self-judgments and parasuicidal or suicidal acts, are typical responses here.

The therapist's task is to block the avoidance of fear, the hiding of shame, and the repairing of guilt. The aim is to expose the person to the emotional situation without letting the person change the situation by escaping, hiding, or repairing. The best way to do this, of course, is by enlisting the patient's cooperation. This can often be accomplished by proper orientation to the principles of exposure; sometimes, the patient will need to be reoriented many times in one session. At other times, escape responses must be blocked unilaterally by verbally pulling the patient's attention back to the cues, over and over. The secret is for the therapist to be persistent and soothing, and to avoid becoming demoralized himself or herself.

The case of anger deserves special comment Escaping from emotion-evoking situations actually goes against the action tendency of anger, in contrast to fear, shame and guilt. That is, anger naturally leads to the "fight" response, including approaching and attacking, fixing the situation or overcoming it, and so on. The opposite of this is withdrawing from the situation for some time (and thinking about something else) or changing the topic. When anger is the conditioned emotion the therapist and patient are trying to reduce, the responses to inhibit fall into a class that, as a group, can be considered hostile approach or attack responses. First, of course, the therapist wants to block actual aggression, including the self-destructive behaviors that often accompany self-directed anger. In addition, the therapist wants to block or inhibit the individual's tendency to respond with overt or covert verbal aggression (e.g., hostile dialogues and diatribes, yelling, aggressive threats, and sarcastic remarks). Verbal aggression, whether overt or covert, usually includes judgmental, one-sided, escalating verbal or mental reviews of the actual frustrating events and their deleterious consequences for attainment of the patient's goals. Sometimes, covert aggression takes the form of imaginary verbal attacks on the object of the anger. The person can be encouraged to replace these hostile responses with nonjudgmental, decatastrophizing responses. Replacing them with thinking or talking about unrelated topics (distraction), however, may be just as effective. One of the mindfulness practice exercises, having to do with empathizing with one's enemies, also has the effect of changing one's natural anger response. The evidence is reasonably strong that catharsis increases rather than decreases anger.

The problem for many borderline patients is not the overexperience and expression of anger, but rather the underexpression of it; that is, they are anger-phobic. In these cases, the goal is to disinhibit the experience and expression of anger. Paradoxically, learning to inhibit anger once it is aroused may be very important to learning to disinhibit the initial experience and expression of anger. Many patients are afraid that if they do get angry, they will lose control and possibly react violently. They also fear that if they engage in hostile behavior, overtly or covertly, they will be rejected. Many have indeed had these experiences in their past. With such a patient, the therapist must combine exposure to anger arousal and angry behavior with training in expressive control. The reduction of anger phobia will require a balance between accepting anger arousal and expression (so that shame and rejection anxieties about anger are not reinforced further) and helping the patient inhibit overexpression (so that fear of losing control is not reinforced further).

3. BLOCKING EXPRESSIVE TENDENCIES ASSOCIATED WITH PROBLEM EMOTIONS

As I have noted earlier, changing emotionally expressive behavior can be an effective means of changing the emotion one is experiencing. Thus, it is helpful to instruct a patient to try her best to physically express an emotion different from that elicited by the exposure cues—for example, to focus on relaxing her facial muscles, and then half smile. Patients often resist this procedure. They may be afraid that if they relax their faces they will cry; most borderline patients are very afraid and/or ashamed of crying. The therapist may have to take a gradual approach.

Working on postural expressions of emotion can also be effective. Positioning of the head, shoulders, arms, torso, and legs is important in expressing emotion. Often the therapist will need to give the patient very precise coaching on exactly what changes she needs to make. The patient may be advised to practice in front of a mirror. Problems with body image, especially discomfort with body size, have been a special problem with borderline patients I have worked with; thus the therapist must proceed here with great care and sensitivity. As noted earlier, it is also important to point out the difference between masking and actually relaxing and changing facial and postural expressions. A lot of orienting is usually necessary here.

It is important to know when to instruct a patient to change her emotionally expressive behavior and when not to. The rule is reasonably simple. If an emotion secondary to a primary emotion has been targeted for reduction (e.g., fear of fear, or shame about anger), the therapist wants to expose the patient to the primary emotion cues (fear and anger, respectively). The aim in this case is not to change expressions of the primary emotion, but instead to expose the patient to the primary emotional cues (including the somatic cues) associated with emotional expression. Changing primary emotional expressiveness in these cases is avoiding the exposure. Blocking and changing expressiveness should instead be associated with the secondary emotion. For fear of fear, avoidance of fear cues should be blocked; for shame elicited by anger, hiding the anger or apologizing for it should be blocked. In contrast, if a primary emotion (e.g., dysfunctional primary fear or anger), has been targeted for reduction, the therapist should suggest changing emotional expressiveness.

4. ENHANCING CONTROL OVER AVERSIVE EVENTS

The fact that the therapist blocks avoidance does not mean that the patient can never stop the exposure trial. Indeed, gaining a sense of control over aversive events appears to be important in regaining emotional control. Thus, while avoidance is blocked, the individual must also be taught how to control the event. At times leaving the situation and stopping exposure will actually be therapeutic. As noted above, the general idea is that the patient should end the exposure voluntarily—that is, control the ending—rather than end it through automatic or impulsive responses not under the patient's control. The structure of DBT as a whole is designed to enhance the individual's control over both her environment and herself. This enhanced control, together with exposure to emotion-relevant conditions, will presumably work together to enhance emotion regulation and decrease debilitating emotions.

Since so many of the ordinary therapy interactions in DBT can be construed as exposure trials, it is important to be aware that this principle dictates giving the patient some control over how session time is used. That is, she must be allowed to titrate or stop exposure when the emotions elicited are unendurable. Accordingly, the therapist and patient need to collaborate on positive and adaptive as opposed to negative and dysfunctional ways to end exposure. Throwing a tantrum or threatening suicide when the therapist confronts the patient or insists on behavioral analysis of parasuicide, for example, is not the type of controlling behavior to encourage. Negotiating on intensity or amount of confrontation during sessions (especially when the patient is more vulnerable than usual), setting agendas that include discussion of other topics along with the behavior analysis, and other similar tactics are behaviors to encourage. With respect to behavioral analysis in particular, I often negotiate both the amount of time allocated to it and the placement of the analysis within the session (beginning, middle, or end). In summary, when therapists' behaviors are the exposure conditions, patients must be given some control over what therapists do and how they do it. Therapists must be vulnerable to influence.

Structured Exposure Procedures

Although many DBT strategies enhance therapeutic exposure, the treatment of trauma following sexual abuse, in particular may need a more formal implementation of exposure procedures. Other traumatic events, such as death of a close family member or physical catastrophe, may also need structured attention. These targets are the focus of the second phase of DBT, in which the therapist combines the substance of DBT with a more organized approach to exposure. In this phase, almost every session should be devoted to implementation of exposure, usually by imaginal recreation of trauma cues associated with the abuse. To keep the patient oriented and attending, the therapist ordinarily asks her to describe the traumatic event detail by detail (including visual, kinesthetic, auditory, olfactory, and somatic cues, as well as what she was thinking and doing at each point). The exposure sessions may be audiotaped. Patients should also be instructed to practice exposure between sessions. Even when conducted in well-controlled doses, this treatment procedure creates such enormous and sometimes unpredictable stress that it is delayed until the first-phase targets are well under control. In some circumstances, hospitalizing a patient for the initial exposure sessions can be quite useful. Formal exposure-based procedures have been developed by Foa (Foa & Kozak, 1986; Foa, Steketee, & Grayson, 1985) and Horowitz (1986), and can be adapted for second-phase treatment.

COGNITIVE MODIFICATION PROCEDURES

The relationship among cognitive processing, emotions, and actions is complex and multi-directional. Clinical lore is rich in evidence that borderline individuals cognitively distort events, usually by engaging in selective attention, magnifying and exaggerating events, forming absolute conclusions, and viewing the world in a dichotomous, black-and-white fashion. Suicidal and borderline persons also tend to cognitive rigidity, which exacerbates any other cognitive problems they may have. Cognitive theories of emotions and emotional disorders (e.g., Arnold, 1960, 1970; Beck et al., 1979; Beck et al., 1990; Lazarus, 1966; Mandler, 1975; Schachter & Singer, 1962; Lang, 1984) suggest that an individual's cognitive appraisals of events are primary determinants of emotional responses. Young (Young, 1987; Young & Swift, 1988) has suggested that early maladaptive schemas underpin personality disorders; both the initial perception of a stimulus and cognitive elaborations of that perception are viewed as important. A large body of research and theory suggests that cognitive expectations and rules, or implicit and explicit beliefs about contingencies, are equally important determinants of action (see Hayes et al., 1989, for a review of this literature). Cognitive therapies, based on cognitive theories of emotion, aim at changing the individual's typical appraisals, rules, and cognitive style as a first step in remediating emotional and behavioral difficulties.

DBT differs from cognitive and many cognitive–behavioral therapies in the place that cognitive modification holds. As I have noted repeatedly, the first task in DBT is to find and reinforce the borderline individual's valid and functional beliefs, expectations, rules, and interpretations. That is, the aim is to validate aspects of the individual's characteristic cognitive content and cognitive style. However, once this is done, the therapist is often left with a patient who, while arriving at valid conclusions in some cases, is also simultaneously selecting, remembering, and processing information dysfunctionally in many other instances. This creates new problems instead of providing solutions to current problems.

For the sake of simplicity, I use the term "cognitive content" to refer to assumptions, beliefs, expectancies, rules, automatic thoughts, self-talk, and schemas. That is, content refers to both what the individual thinks and what the individual remembers. "Thinking," as used here, refers to verbal or propositional cognitive processing and can occurs at both the conscious and nonconscious levels (see Williams, in press, for a review of this point). "Cognitive style," as I use the term, refers to characteristic modes of information processing such as cognitive rigidity and flexibility, divergent and convergent thinking styles, dichotomous thinking, concentration, abstracting styles, and attentional deficits. The distinctions are not as clear-cut as I am making them seem, but are helpful for discussing the focus of cognitive procedures. Cognitive modification procedures in DBT help the patient assess and change cognitive content and modify cognitive styles. Like exposure, however, cognitive modification is more informal than formal. That is, DBT does not include a self-contained module consisting primarily of structured activities aimed at cognitive change. In contrast to cognitive therapies of personality disorders, the principal goal of treatment is not to identify and change pervasive schemas that are believed to underpin borderline patterns. Nonetheless, cognitive processes are not ignored in DBT. An important assessment task is to ascertain the role of cognitive content as well as cognitive style in the elicitation and maintenance of targeted behaviors, including emotions. Cognitive modification procedures are interwoven throughout DBT.

A very important point to remember with borderline patients is that cognitive procedures should always be blended with more validation than modification. Most borderline individuals have spent their entire lives listening to others accuse them of distorting and misperceiving. All too often, such criticisms have been a way to discount the patient's legitimate claims. Saying "It is all in your head" is a simple-minded approach to cognitive therapy, but one that most patients have encountered. Thus, when a therapist provides feedback that a patient could indeed profit from examining the utility of her perceptions, conclusions about events, and remembering of events, she is likely to interpret this in a typically all-or-none way as meaning, once again, that her problems are "all in her head." A particular problem that arises is difficulty with the idea that she can be "wrong" in one conclusion or belief without therefore being "wrong" in everything she has ever believed or thought. The problem is an understandable one. If she is distorting now, without knowing it, then how can she ever trust her perceptions, beliefs, and remembering? That is, what guidelines can she use to tell her when to trust herself and when not to? Helping the patient to develop these guidelines is an important part of cognitive modification in DBT.

There are two main types of cognitive modification procedures: cognitive restructuring and contingency clarification. Cognitive restructuring aims at changing the general or habitual content or form of the patient's thinking, as well as the patient's cognitive style. Contingency clarification is a special case of the more general cognitive restructuring. The focus is on modifying dysfunctional rules or "if–then" expectancies operating in specific instances. The relationship of contingency clarification to cognitive restructuring is similar to the relationship of behavioral analysis to insight (see Chapter 9). In both contingency clarification and behavioral analysis, the focus is on the specific case or event; the focus is on the here and now, concrete situations, and contingent relationships. In both cognitive restructuring and insight strategies, the focus is on patterns of events, thoughts, or personal rules over many events, instances, and times; the emphasis is on the general and habitual.

Contingency clarification is discussed here as a special procedure in order to focus the therapist's attention on its importance. In my experience, borderline individuals often have difficulty learning appropriate behavioral rules. By "rule," I mean a verbal proposition, either explicit or implicit, of contingent relationships between events. Behavioral rules concern contingent relationships between behaviors and outcomes. Borderline patients, especially those in their teens and 20s, sometimes appear remarkably naive for their age. For example, although they report feeling hopelessness, watching them in action suggests that they frequently trust inappropriately, expecting others to respond to them positively and altruistically when such outcomes are unrealistic. Borderline patients frequently respond well to very high levels of threat. In contrast, they may not respond to everyday communication of contingencies, especially when these communications are subtle or indirect. Sometimes only extreme threats work to modify their behavior. It is as if one has to threaten them to get their attention or to get a rule through to them. (To put this more positively, they sometimes do very well when, and if, they hit bottom.) Difficulties in learning contingencies may result from many factors, including the influence of mood on learning and attention; attentional problems per se; or more general difficulties in selecting, abstracting, and remembering relevant information. Contingency clarification is aimed at redressing these problems.

Orienting to Cognitive Modification Procedures

From a DBT perspective, dysfunctional cognitive content and style are both causes of emotional and behavioral dysfunctions and results of them. It is the emphasis on the latter that distinguishes DBT from many other cognitive–behavioral treatments, and constitutes an important part of the orienting given to patients. That is, the patients are told that many of their misappraisals and information-processing errors are normal results both of mood and of extreme emotional arousal. Failure to learn and remember appropriate rules may result from the interference of mood with learning and remembering. Distortions (or failures to distort normally) are viewed as results of their problems, not as fundamental causes. Once cognitive distortions and faulty information processing begin, however, they exacerbate rather than ameliorate problems. Failure to learn and remember, although understandable, must still be remediated.

In my experience of supervising and consulting with therapists, the idea that borderline patients may not always be distorting, exaggerating, magnifying, or simply "getting it wrong" seems extremely difficult for most therapists to put into practice. Because a patient so often uses information differently than her therapist does, observes parts of situations that the therapist ignores, and comes to conclusions different from those of the therapist, it is very difficult for the therapist to avoid dichotomous thinking himself or herself. Someone has got to be wrong; too often, a therapist assumes that it must be the patient. Even when the therapist is willing to explore the possibility that he or she is "wrong," there may be little to gain. The idea that both parties may be "right" is what is needed. It can be very helpful if both the therapist and the patient are acquainted with the literature on mood, behavior, and cognitive processing. The material in Chapter 2 regarding the influence of mood and emotion on cognition and attention control (see the "Emotional Vulnerability" section) is generally shared with the patient in small doses over the course of therapy as needed. It is crucial that the therapist understand this material and present it in language that the patient can comprehend and accept.

CONTINGENCY CLARIFICATION PROCEDURES

Contingency clarification is designed to help the individual observe and extract contingencies operating in her life. As noted above, borderline persons seem at times to have difficulty attending to relevant contingencies, and thus fail to behave in ways likely to lead to positive outcomes. At other times, they attend but fail to extract or remember important rules. There are two types of contingency clarification interventions. First, the therapist highlights natural rules operating in the patient's life; that is, the therapist helps the patient attend to and extract unfolding "if–then" relationships. In this sense contingency clarification is a part of behavioral analysis, insight, and reciprocal communication strategies. Second, the therapist tells the patient rules that will be operating in new situations the patient is entering, and highlights appropriate expectations. Contingency clarification in this sense is used mainly with respect to contingencies operating in therapy. The procedures are discussed below and summarized in Table 11.5.

TABLE 11.5. Contingency Clarification Procedures Checklist

_____ T HIGHLIGHTS CONTINGENCIES; T focuses P's attention on effects of behavior on current outcomes.

    _____ In everyday life.

    _____ With respect to P's problematic behavior.

    _____ With respect to effect of P's behaviors on other people and their responses to P.

    _____ With respect to effect of P's behavior on therapeutic relationship.

    _____ With respect to effect of P's behavior on treatment outcomes.

    _____ T is mindful of clarifying contingencies when using behavioral analysis, insight, and reciprocal communication strategies.

_____ T CLARIFIES FUTURE CONTINGENCIES IN THERAPY, especially when orienting P to DBT as a whole or to particular treatment procedures.

    _____ What T will do, given certain P behaviors (especially suicidal and therapy-interfering behaviors).

    _____ What P can reasonably expect from T and from treatment procedures.

1. HIGHLIGHTING CURRENT CONTINGENCIES

The first goal is to help the patient observe, abstract, and remember the contingencies operating in her everyday life. Knowing the rules and accurately predicting outcomes increase the probabilities of adaptive behavior. In particular, it is important that the patient understand the outcomes of her own behavior and the effects it has on others. Patients often attend to the wrong details of a situation, or, conversely, may be so sensitive to details that they cannot abstract the important "if–then" relationships. Clarifying the outcomes of maladaptive behaviors is particularly important in obtaining a commitment to change: If outcomes are not negative or painful, why change? Here attention must be paid to both immediate and long-term outcomes, and to effects on both the patient and others.

Clarifying the effects of situations, especially other people's behavior, on the patient's own responses—feelings, thinking, and action urges—is also important. Borderline individuals sometimes have a remarkable ability to keep forgetting that certain situations or people repeatedly have detrimental effects on them. Contrary to the evidence at hand, they keep expecting either the situation or their own responses to be different. Finally, the therapist also helps the patient identify general rules operating in the environment, especially social rules. As noted earlier, borderline individuals frequently have naive conceptions of how others will respond to various events. Although they are quite accurate at predicting people like themselves, they have a hard time predicting responses they have never experienced. That is, their empathy is strong with people who are experiencing circumstances similar to their own, but weak with people who are dissimilar.

Contingency Clarification in Behavioral Analysis and Insight Strategies.
The conduct of a moment-to moment chain analysis of behavior offers an

opportunity for the therapist to highlight contingent relationships. In examining the chain of events leading up to dysfunctional behaviors, the therapist helps the patient extract rules about what leads to what. In examining the functional utility of targeted behaviors, the therapist helps the patient extract rules about the outcomes of her own behavior. The therapist asks, and encourages the patient to ask herself, questions such as these: "What happened then?", "What was the effect of that on you?", "What was the effect of what you did?", and "How did others react?" The idea is to direct the patient's attention to the relationship between her behavior and others' responses. In insight strategies, the therapist helps the patient summarize information over a number of instances of behavior. The therapist should highlight rules (i.e., consistent "if–then" patterns) that have emerged over time. The idea is to articulate the rules in somewhat brief, propositional form and then to encourage the patient periodically to repeat them back to the therapist.

Contingency Clarification in Reciprocal Communication Strategies. I discuss reciprocal communication in the next chapter. However, an important part of these strategies is for the therapist frequently to give the patient information about the effect of the patient's behavior on the therapist. A statement such as "When you do X, I feel Y" is, strictly speaking, a statement of a contingent relationship between the patient's behavior and the therapist's behavior. The therapist should keep up a rather continuous verbal patter of the sort "When you do X, Y happens." The value of these statements in helping the patient learn the effects of her own behavior on another is one of the primary reasons for including reciprocal communication strategies in DBT.

2. COMMUNICATING FUTURE CONTINGENCIES IN THERAPY

Among the most important contingencies for a borderline patient are those having to do with therapy. Contingency clarification here has two aspects: (1) what the therapist will do, given certain behaviors on the patient's part; (2) what the patient can reasonably expect from the therapist and from therapy. DBT emphasizes therapist clarity and directness, at least in the beginning of therapy. In the final phase, such directness should be faded out to encourage the patient's abilities to read subtle and indirect relationship communications.

Orienting to DBT as a whole, and to treatment procedures as they are implemented, has been discussed extensively in this chapter and the previous two. Orienting is an instance of teaching the patient rules about therapy. The patient is told what behaviors on her part will lead to positive and negative outcomes, which expectations of hers are likely to be met and which not, and what the consequences of some of her behaviors are likely to be. Orienting not only occurs at the start of therapy (see Chapter 14 for specific rules to impart) and of each new procedure, but should form an ongoing backdrop to therapy. That is, the therapist should be continually teaching, assessing the patient's comprehension and memory, and coaching. It is this continuing clarification of contingencies, in many different contexts and mood states, that is essential to DBT. Especially during the initial stages of therapy, the therapist simply should not expect the patient to extract and remember all of the rules. Nor should failure to learn or remember contingencies always be interpreted in motivational terms.

COGNITIVE RESTRUCTURING PROCEDURES

Cognitive restructuring is a way of helping the patient change both the style and content of her thinking. Four aspects of thinking are of interest: (1) non-dialectical thinking (e.g., dichotomous, rigid, extreme thinking styles); (2) faulty general rules governing behavior (beliefs, underlying assumptions, ideas, expectations); (3) dysfunctional descriptions (e.g., automatic thoughts, evaluative name calling, exaggerated labels); and (4) dysfunctional allocations of attention. The procedure first requires the observation and analysis of these aspects of the patient's thinking, followed by an attempt to generate new and more functional styles, rules, descriptions, and attentional strategies to replace those that cause the patient trouble. Change can be initiated by verbally challenging current thinking and attentional biases; by offering alternative theories, explanations, and descriptions; and by examining available evidence (and obtaining new evidence where needed) pertaining to the accuracy of the patient's rules and labels. Changes are strengthened by relentless practice. Cognitive restructuring procedures are discussed below and summarized in Table 11.6.

I. TEACHING COGNITIVE SELF-OBSERVATION

If the patient is to succeed in monitoring and changing her cognitive patterns over time and across situations, it is crucial that she learn to observe her own thought patterns and style. For a variety of reasons, suicidal and borderline individuals rarely have this ability. Instead, their involvement in the process of appraising or thinking about an event or situation is so intense that they are unable to step outside of themselves, so to speak, and reflect on the actual thinking and appraisal processes independently of the activities themselves. The primary therapeutic strategy used is that of cognitive self-observation practice (i.e., behavioral rehearsal where the behavior rehearsed is self-observation of cognitive processes), with the therapist giving the patient instructions, feedback, coaching, and reinforcement. Practice methods can range from instructing the patient to try to stand imaginally outside herself and observe what is going on in a session, to giving her an assignment to monitor and write down her thought patterns during specific situations or under specified conditions. If a writing assignment is given, it is useful for the therapist to review in detail with the patient various methods of carrying out the assignment. Mindfulness practice (see the companion manual) and other medi-

TABLE 11.6. Cognitive Restructuring Procedures Checklist

____ T explicitly helps P OBSERVE AND DESCRIBE her own thinking style, rules, and verbal descriptions.

____ T IDENTIFIES, CONFRONTS, and challenges specific dysfunctional rules, labels, and styles, but does so in a dialectical manner.

____ T assists P in GENERATING more functional and/or accurate thinking styles, rules, and verbal descriptions.

    ____ T does not claim to have a lock on absolute truth.
    ____ T values intuitive sources of knowing.
    ____ T values getting data when none have been collected so far.
    ____ T focuses on functional, effective thinking rather than necessarily "true" or "accurate" thinking.
    ____ T pushes P to the limit of her ability in generating her own adaptive thinking styles, rules, and verbal descriptions.

T assists P in developing GUIDELINES on when to trust and when to suspect her own interpretations.

____ T applies contingency and skill training procedures in cognitive modifications.

____ T helps P integrate cognitive strategies used in skills training modules into everyday life.

____ T implements or refers P to a formal cognitive therapy program, as appropriate.

Anti-DBT tactics

____ T tells P her problems are "all in her head."

____ T oversimplifies P's problems, implying that all will be well if P can just change her "attitude," her thoughts, or her way of viewing things.

____ T gets into a power struggle with P about how to think.

---

tation disciplines can also support the learning of self-observation.

The key problem in teaching cognitive self-observation is that it is usually most needed when the patient is experiencing extreme negative affect. And it is just at those times that the patient is least likely to tolerate the emotion long enough to observe her thought and appraisal patterns accurately. Fears of what she will find if she ever looks "inside" closely can also lead to avoidance of the task. Thus, the therapist has to monitor the procedure carefully in order to keep requirements at a level that the patient can master. The principles of shaping must be remembered here.

2. IDENTIFYING AND CONFRONTING MALADAPTIVE COGNITIVE CONTENT AND STYLE

As noted repeatedly, DBT suggests that cognitive content and cognitive style are no less important than environmental or other behavioral factors in the development and maintenance of dysfunctional borderline patterns. Thus, when conducting behavioral analysis, the therapist should search for *cogni-*

tive precursors and effects of maladaptive actions and reactions just as carefully as for other precursors and outcomes.

Many of the DBT strategies require the therapist (implicitly, if not explicitly) to identify, challenge, and confront problematic beliefs, assumptions, theories, judgmental evaluations, and tendencies to think rigidly and in absolute and extreme terms (i.e, nondialectical thinking). Dialectical strategies, problem-solving strategies, irreverent communication strategies, and all of the skills training modules focus in whole or in part on how the patient organizes and uses information and what the patient thinks about herself, about therapy, and about the relationship between herself and her world. The therapist's ability to ferret out the cognitive problem in a specific instance, to present it to the patient in a persuasive manner, and to suggest a viable alternative are very important. A number of the strategies discussed in previous chapters (e.g., the devil's advocate dialectical strategy, the foot-in-the-door commitment strategy) are designed with this in mind. A dialectical style is very important, however, for the therapist must help the patient expand her cognitive options rather than prove her "wrong." Therefore, validation of existing viewpoints is important while suggesting that others are possible.

3. GENERATING ALTERNATIVE, ADAPTIVE COGNITIVE CONTENT AND STYLE

Once maladaptive patterns of thought, dysfunctional rules and expectations, and problematic cognitive styles have been identified, the next step is to find more adaptive ways of thinking that the patient can adopt. The most important DBT rule here is that the therapist should teach and reinforce dialectical thinking styles over purely "rational" or purely emotional-based thinking. Dialectical thinking (as well as dialectical dilemmas for borderline patients) has been discussed at length in Chapters 2, 3, 5, and 7; thus, I do not define and discuss it further her. In keeping with a dialectical approach however, the therapist must remember that he or she does not have a lock on absolute truth. Even dialectical thinking has its limits. One of the dialectical tensions in cognitive modification is that between rational and empirical thinking on the one hand, and intuitive and emotion-focused thinking on the other. On the one side, as in more purely cognitive therapies (e.g., Beck's cognitive therapy), the therapist should value "performing experiments" in the real world to test one's assumptions, beliefs, and rules. On the other, the therapist values intuitive knowing that cannot be proved in any conventional sense. Functional and effective thinking, rather than necessarily "true" or accurate thinking, is valued.

Like any other skill, learning how to think dialectically and functionally requires an active effort on the part of the patient. The therapist can aid this effort by judicious questioning within sessions, as well as by giving cognitive homework assignments. In the latter, the therapist has the patient keep track of dysfunctional thinking during the week, attempt to replace it with more functional thinking, keep a diary or notes, and discuss the efforts during the next session. (Forms for this practice are in the accompanying skills training manual.) In many cases, the therapist must at first more or less drag more appropriate thinking out of the patient. Borderline patients often say "I don't know" when requested to produce new ways of approaching old problems. Often, they are simply afraid to reveal more effective ways of thinking for fear of being punished or ridiculed. Thus, a fair amount of pushing, cheerleading, and shaping may be necessary to get a patient to generate her own adaptive thinking styles, rules, and verbal descriptions of events.

4. DEVELOPING GUIDELINES FOR WHEN TO TRUST AND WHEN TO SUSPECT INTERPRETATIONS

It is crucial that the therapist attend to the patient's tendencies to believe that if she is wrong, biased, or distorting in one instance, she must have been wrong all along—and will always be wrong in the future. This is, of course, an instance of almost pure nondialectical thinking. But what is the appropriate counter to it? The best solution is to help the patient develop guidelines that will assist her in determining when she probably should trust herself and let other opinions go, and when she might at least check out her perceptions and conclusions.

Some general guidelines of this sort apply to almost everyone. Social-cognitive and personality psychologists, for example, have spent years studying people's tendencies to be biased in their evaluations and judgments. A number of well-known biasing effects that influence people in general, and thus are relevant to the task here, are listed in Table 11.7. Each individual patient, in addition, will have particular areas in which biasing and distortion are most likely. Thus, besides identifying general areas that must be watched, guidelines should also cover the patient's specific biasing tendencies. For example, one patient may make characteristic errors when she is extremely angry, or with particular people. Another may be biased primarily when sad. Women who suffer from premenstrual syndrome may need to be especially careful during the days before their menstrual period. Borderline individuals often attend selectively to rejection cues. Feminists may attend selectively to cues that can be interpreted as sexual or sexist. One patient of mine who was single and wanted to be married almost never noticed people walking alone, but could provide almost an exact count from memory of how many couples she passed while walking.

The points are important here. First, the patient should be told that all people bias and distort; this does not mean that people can never trust themselves. Second, knowledge is power, or at least increases security. Knowing when and under what conditions one is most likely to bias and distort can be useful in catching and correcting errors. The idea is to normalize rather than pathologize information biasing.

TABLE 11.7. Judgmental Heuristics and Biases

1. People are influenced by the relative availability, or accessibility from memory, of events related to a judgment they are making ("availability heuristic"). (Example: Subjective estimates of the probability of death from a number of causes are related to disproportionate exposure to lethal events via media descriptions, as well as to their memorability and imaginability.)

2. People base judgments on the extent to which they believe that a specific event is prototypical of a larger group of events ("representativeness heuristic"). (Example: The tendency to overlook base rates when predicting what someone will do. For example, in most doctoral programs, over 90% of students admitted eventually get doctorates. Yet, many students would predict that a student who incurs the disapproval of his or her adviser will not finish. This overlooks the fact that many more students complete doctorates than do not, and that at least some of these must have incurred the wrath of their advisers.)

3. Initial positions taken continue to influence subsequent judgments even when their irrelevance should be obvious ("anchoring heuristic"). (Example: People cling to initial hypotheses, even when the evidence on which they were originally based has been totally discredited.)

4. People favor gathering information that confirms their beliefs, rather than information that challenges them ("confirmation bias"). (Example: When people try to determine whether another person has a particular personality characteristic or tendency, they will typically ask questions that tend to confirm rather than disconfirm the characteristic they are testing.)

5. People tend to adjust their remembered or reconstructed probability judgment to match present knowledge ("hindsight bias"). (Example: When presented with clinical case histories and required to explain a hypothetical outcome, such as suicide, likelihood estimates for this outcome's occurring in fact are systematically increased.)

6. Negative mood states produce a consistent negative bias in judgment and estimates of bias ("mood bias"). (Example: When in a positive mood [compared to a neutral or negative mood], people will report themselves as more satisfied with what they have and will rate their own performance more positively, even when performance is experimentally controlled by giving false feedback as to success and failure. When in a negative mood, people show a global increase in their estimates of the subjective probability that any of a range of disasters will occur.)

7. When people imagine an outcome's occurring, they increase their estimated likelihood that the outcome will actually happen ("imagined outcome bias"). (Example: People who have imagined being falsely accused of a crime become more accepting of the idea that they themselves could possibly be accused in this way.)

Note. Adapted from *The Psychologoical Treatment of Depression: A Guide to the Theory and Practice of Cognitive Behavior Therapy,* 2nd ed. by J. M. G. Williams, 1993, New York: Free Press. Copyright 1993 by Free Press. Adapted by permission.

Applying Contingency and Skills Training Procedures in Cognitive Modifications

As with all active DBT interventions, the therapist's role in confronting and challenging maladaptive thinking styles and content, and in generating new, more adaptive and dialectical patterns, should be faded out over time as the patient becomes more competent at observing and replacing her own cognitive errors and biases. At the beginning of therapy, it is often necessary for the therapist to "mind-read" (see Chapter 8 for an extensive discussion of this topic). During the middle of therapy, the therapist should be pushing the patient to observe and describe her own maladaptive assumptions, beliefs, or rules, and to generate new ways of thinking. At the end of therapy, the patient should be able to think more dialectically and catch her own problematic style and content, with little or no coaching from the therapist. Principles of contingency management and skills training, discussed in Chapter 10 and earlier in this chapter, should be applied to cognitive modification.

Integrating Cognitive Skills From Skill Modules

As noted above cognitive skills are taught in every skill modules. Specific self-statements are taught in the distress tolerance and interpersonal effectiveness modules; clarifying outcomes and appropriate outcomes expectancies is also an important part of interpersonal effectiveness training. Identifying and changing evaluative, judgmental descriptions are taught in the mindfulness module, as are skills in setting distance and observing. The emotion regulation module includes skills in identifying cognitive appraisals related to emotions. If these skills are taught in skills training, but the individual therapist either uses different terminology or simply ignores the skills, they are unlikely to be learned and will do the patient little good. Thus, it is essential to DBT that the individual therapist pay very close attention to the cognitive skills being taught in skills modules, and build upon and reinforce them.

Formal Cognitive Therapy Programs

There is nothing in DBT that prohibits implementing or referring patients to formal cognitive therapy programs. As adjunctive therapy programs, especially for patients who are ready and willing, they may have much to recommend them. Organized, structured cognitive change procedures are not included as a formal module in DBT for several reasons. First, in my experience, focusing primarily on changing how the individual thinks and uses information as a solution to her problems is frequently too similar to the invalidating environment. It is difficult to counter the message that if the patient would just think right, everything would be OK. Although this is an unintended and nondialectical response to well-carried-out cognitive therapy, I have found that it is an extraordinarily difficult objection to overcome.

Second, formal cognitive therapy generally requires at least some cognitive self-monitoring, writing down thoughts and assumptions, figuring out challenges or experiments to test thoughts and beliefs, and actually carrying out the experiments. These activities require a number of preliminary skills that many borderline patients simply do not have. A program that requires a fair amount of independent work at the beginning is not appropriate for severely disturbed patients. As cognitive treatment is modified, such that change procedures are carried out with the therapist in therapy sessions, the difference between DBT change procedures and many other types of cognitive and cognitive–behavioral therapy lessen.

Concluding Comments

In this chapter and Chapter 10, I have reviewed basic cognitive–behavioral change procedures and discussed how they can be applied to the problems of borderline patients. These four sets of procedures—application of contingencies, skills training, exposure-based techniques, and cognitive modification—make up the bulk of current behavior therapy. That is, DBT does not include much that is new in this respect. It is important for you, the reader, to keep in mind, that you can and should add any techniques that you believe are effective change procedures or that have been shown in research to be effective. That is, you or I could write additional chapters for therapy procedures I have not included. For example, if you are a Gestalt therapist, there is no reason not to add Gestalt techniques. In the second and third stages of treatment in particular, procedures such as the two-chair technique may be very useful.

When working on specific behavioral problems (e.g., marital or sexual dysfunction, substance abuse, eating disorders, or other Axis I disorders), you might consider adding procedures that have been demonstrated to be effective with those problems. If you are working with an individual who meets criteria for multiple personality disorder, you might add some of the techniques that experts in that area have developed to enhance personality integration or "merging." It is important, however, to integrate other procedures in a thoughtful, theoretical consistent manner. The prescription here is not for switching tactics whenever you get discouraged or immediately trying every new technique you hear about.

Note

1. Many of the guidelines and much of the structure in this section were provided by Edna Foa (personal communication, 1991), who has developed a number of effective exposure-based treatment programs.

12

Stylistic Strategies: Balancing Communication

Stylistic strategies, as the label implies, have to do with the style and form of therapist communication. They focus on *how* the therapist uses other treatment strategies, rather than on the content of communication. Style has to do with tone (warm vs. cool or confrontational), with edge (soft and flowing vs. hard and abrupt), with intensity (light or humorous vs. very serious), with speed (fast, quick-moving, or interruptive vs. slow, thoughtful, and reflective), and with responsiveness (vulnerable vs. impervious). A therapist's style can communicate attitudes such as condescension and arrogance versus respect and affection.

There are two primary communication styles in DBT. The reciprocal communication style is defined by responsiveness, self-disclosure, warmth, and genuineness. By contrast, the irreverent communication style is unhallowed, impertinent, and incongruous, Reciprocity is vulnerable; irreverence may be confrontational. The two styles constitute the poles of a dialectic. They not only balance each other, but must be synthesized. The therapist must be able to move back and forth between the two with such rapidity that the blending itself constitutes a stylistic strategy.

Borderline persons are remarkably sensitive to differences in interpersonal power and to "games" that therapists play. Often, the majority of their life experience has been in a "one-down" position. Many of their interpersonal problems are a result of somewhat clumsy attempts to rectify power imbalances. The intent of reciprocal communication is to rectify such imbalances more skillfully, and to provide an environment that holds the patient within the therapeutic enterprise. It is also intended to model for the patient how to interact as an equal within an important relationship.

Borderline persons have great difficulty getting enough psychological distance to observe and describe the ongoing events and processes of their lives.

Such observation, however, is essential to change. The intent of irreverent communication is to help provide this distance by keeping the individual just off balance enough to shake up her typically rigid, narrow-bounded approach to life, to herself, and to problem solving. The idea is to highlight both poles of the dialectic without denying either.

RECIPROCAL COMMUNICATION STRATEGIES

Responsiveness, self-disclosure, warm engagement, and genuineness are the four basic reciprocal communication strategies. Reciprocity is important in any good interpersonal relationship. It is particularly important within an intimate relationship, such as psychotherapy; it is essential in a therapeutic relationship with a borderline individual. Reciprocal communication is the usual communication mode in DBT.

Power and Psychotherapy: Who Makes the Rules?

Patients in psychotherapy often complain that while they can be emotionally touched and deeply hurt by their therapists, they feel unable to influence their therapists in a similar manner. They are vulnerable; the therapists are invulnerable. Patients strip naked while therapists keep their clothes on, so to speak. Risk is unevenly divided. Patients also hold a sense of their therapists' impenetrability—namely, that while the therapists have infinite boundaries, they have none. In short, the power in a therapeutic relationship is not only unequal; by the very nature of psychotherapy, it is unequal in just those areas of a patient's life that count the most. Many of the battles that go on in psychotherapy have to do with this maldistribution of power and patients' attempts to rectify it.

Although therapists are not nearly as invulnerable as patients often believe, there is much in the current mores of psychotherapy to account for patients' dissatisfaction on this topic and for their confusion. That is, although therapists might prefer it to be otherwise, patients' complaints are often valid. Rules guiding a therapist's behavior and interpersonal style are often arbitrary, known to the therapist but not to the patient; as a result, the behavior of the therapist is not only incomprehensible to the patient but also unpredictable. The therapist encourages emotional intimacy within the relationship, but the ordinary rules of intimate relationships do not apply. Rules of intimacy designed for a person engaged simultaneously in many patient–therapist relationships (the therapist) may be completely inappropriate for a person who is engaged in only one (the patient). A therapist is often uncomfortable with or theoretically opposed to self-disclosure on his or her own part, while insisting on self-disclosure by the patient. Although the therapeutic relationship is presented as a nurturing and helping one, the availability and flexibility inherent in almost all other nurturing relationships are frequently nonexistent or severely diminished.

The borderline patient in therapy is treated similarly in some respects to a child in a parent–child relationship: She is frequently treated as less qualified than the therapist to make decisions about her own welfare. A child, however, eventually becomes an equal of a parent; by contrast, as the patient "grows up," her power in the therapy relationship does not necessarily change. When that event (equality) appears likely in psychotherapy, the relationship may be terminated.

There is a saying in academia that students stand on their teachers' shoulders. Lineage from teacher to student is traced to show influence. In psychotherapy, however, the mores of the culture conspire to keep the relationship secret—something to be ashamed of rather than proud of. Even therapists who have been psychotherapy patients themselves often do not disclose this information to their own patients.

Borderline patients in particular are quick to pick up on power differences and intolerant of arbitrariness in the therapeutic relationship. This may be the case because they have suffered so in the past from unequal distributions of interpersonal power. In addition, they often do not have other intimate relationships, in which power is more nearly equal, to balance the therapeutic relationship. Many of the problems in psychotherapy with borderline patients have to do with this fundamental inequality. Unable to equalize relational power or give up the relationship, they often oscillate between behavior that is subservient, needy, and clinging and behavior that is domineering, dismissing, and rejecting. They go back and forth between overdependence and overindependence. Very few adults are willing to stay for long within intimate relationships where their own position of power and influence is so limited. The need for a long-term therapeutic relationship places a borderline individual in a particularly vulnerable position; effective therapy requires that the therapist be particularly sensitive to this dilemma.

Reciprocal communication strategies are designed to reduce the perceived power differential between therapist and patient; to increase the vulnerability of the therapist to the patient, and thereby communicate trust and respect for the patient; and to deepen the attachment and intimacy of the relationship (see Derlega & Berg, 1987, for reviews of the literature on responsiveness and self-disclosure). The strategies are discussed below and outlined in Table 12.1.

I. RESPONSIVENESS

"Responsiveness," broadly defined, is the degree to which the therapist addresses the patient's communications in a manner that indicates interest in what the patient is saying, doing, and understanding, as well as concern with the substance of the patient's communication, wishes, and needs. It is a style indicating that the therapist is listening to the patient and taking her seriously, instead of discounting, ignoring, or overriding what she says and wants. Characteristics of a responsive style include the following.

TABLE 12.1. Reciprocal Communication Strategies Checklist

___ T is RESPONSIVE to P.

   ___ T attends to P in a mindful manner; T is "awake" during interactions with P

      ___ T attends to small changes in P's behavior during interactions.

      ___ T varies affect expression and nonverbal responses (posture, eye contact, smiles, head nods) according to content of P's communication, expressing interest and active involvement.

      ___ T matches P's intensity.

      ___ The timing of T's response conveys understanding and interest.

   ___ T takes P's agenda seriously.

      ___ T responds to the content of P's communications.

         ___ T responds to P's questions with relevant answers.

         ___ The content of T's response is directly relevant to P's communication.

      ___ T elaborates P's content.

___ T SELF-DISCLOSES.

   ___ T orients P to role of self-disclosure in DBT.

   ___ T engages in self-involving self-disclosure.

   ___ T provides P with ongoing reactions to P and to her behavior using "I" statements of the form "When you do X, I feel [or think or want to do] Y."

   ___ T discloses T's own experience of the interaction and ongoing relationship; T has "heart-to-hearts."

      ___ T focuses on the process of the interaction.

      ___ T tells P where she stands with T.

   ___ T blends self-involvement and responsiveness.

      ___ T stays clear about P's behavior and T's own, differentiating the two.

      ___ T tracks the effects of self-disclosure and responsiveness on P's behavior.

   ___ T discloses others' reactions to himself or herself.

   ___ T engages in personal self-disclosure.

      ___ T uses self-disclosure as modeling.

         ___ T self-discloses personal efforts (and successes or failures) at coping with problems similar to P's.

         ___ T models normative behaviors and problems.

         ___ T models coping with one's own problems in living.

         ___ T models coping with failure.

      ___ T discloses professional information about himself or herself.

         ___ Professional training, degrees.

         ___ Therapy orientation.

         ___ Experience with borderline/suicidal patients.

      ___ T discloses personal information about himself or herself (age, marital status, etc.), to the extent that T is comfortable in doing so and it seems helpful to P.

   ___ T uses consultation team to manage self-disclosure.

___ T expresses WARM ENGAGEMENT (as opposed to reluctance to interact with and work with P).

   ___ T is honest when momentarily unwilling.

(Cont.)

Table 12.1 (cont.)

_____ If T is interpersonally reserved by nature, T expresses caring in other ways.

_____ When P evokes rage in T, T copes with it.

_____ T uses touch therapeutically.

　　_____ The role of touch in T's treatment plan is very clear.

　　_____ A hug or touch is brief.

　　_____ A hug or touch expresses the current level of closeness in the therapeutic relationship.

　　_____ T is very sensitive to P's wishes and comfort.

　　_____ T is honest about own personal limits on touch.

　　_____ T strictly avoids sexual touch.

　　_____ T treats inappropriate initiation of touch or hugs as therapy-interfering behavior.

　　_____ T keeps physical contact potentially public.

_____ T is GENUINE.

_____ T's behavior is natural rather than arbitrary.

_____ T's helpfulness is role-independent.

_____ T observes natural limits to relationship.

<u>Anti-DBT tactics</u>

_____ T's self-disclosures are relevant to T's needs, not P's.

_____ T does not observe limits on responsiveness and self-disclosure.

_____ T gets into "heart-to-hearts" with P instead of working on relevant problem behaviors.

_____ T is phony.

_____ T engages in sexual behavior with P or is sexually inviting or flirtatious with P.

Staying Awake

Staying awake means keeping attention focused on the patient without engaging in distracting ruminations or daydreams, scribbling while listening (unless it is necessary to keep notes), allowing interruptions for phone calls, or keeping an eye on the clock. The therapist must be particularly awake to changes in the patient's mood or emotional response within the interaction. As I have repeatedly noted, a borderline patient's nonverbal emotional expression is often very subtle and hard to pick up. Thus, the therapist should note small changes and should check periodically with the patient on what is happening or changing. "What are you feeling right now?" can often be useful. Sometimes a few minutes may be needed to explore the effect of the current interaction on the patient; changes in therapeutic style or focus may or may not be necessary. Although this may momentarily distract from the content of what is happening, it is relatively easy to get back on track. Staying awake is the quality of not missing anything.

Staying awake also requires an engaged, reciprocal interaction pattern. Verbal expressions of emotion, and the intensity of these expressions, as well as nonverbal responses (posture, eye contact, smiles, head nods), should vary according to what the patient is saying and doing in a manner that conveys active involvement in the interaction.

Taking the Patient's Agenda Seriously

Responsiveness requires taking the patient's wishes and needs about session agenda into account—that is, taking them seriously. Taking the patient's agenda seriously, however, does not necessarily mean following her agenda instead of the therapist's. It does mean recognizing her wishes openly rather than ignoring them, negotiating a compromise when possible, putting her agenda ahead of the therapist's if it really is more important, and validating the legitimacy of her wishes if the therapist chooses to insist on his or her own agenda.

Responding to the Content of the Patient's Communications

Responsiveness requires the therapist to follow the patient's questions with relevant answers, to make remarks that relate to what the patient has just said or done, and to elaborate or extend the content of what the patient has just said. Responding to a patient's question with the counterquestion "Why do you ask?" may be therapeutic, but it is not responsive.

2. SELF-DISCLOSURE

"Self-disclosure" involves the therapist's communicating his or her own attitudes, opinions, and emotional reactions to the patient, as well as reactions to the therapy situation or information about pertinent life experiences. In the psychotherapy literature, therapist self-disclosure is a topic of much professional controversy. It can also become a point of controversy between patient and therapist. Usually, but not always, a patient wants more therapeutic self-disclosure than the therapist is comfortable with; at times, however, she may want less. DBT encourages therapeutic self-disclosure in some instances and discourages it in others. Decisions about self-disclosure should always be made from the point of view of helpfulness to the patient and relevance to the topic under consideration at the moment.

Two main types of self-disclosure are used in DBT: (1) self-involving self-disclosure and (2) personal self-disclosure. "Self-involving self-disclosure" is a somewhat technical term for the therapist's statements to the patient about his or her immediate, personal reactions to the patient. In the counseling literature, this is sometimes referred to as "immediacy." In psychodynamic terminology, one might refer to it as a focus on the countertransference. "Personal self-disclosure" refers to the therapist's giving the patient information about himself or herself, such as information about professional qualifications, social relationships outside of therapy (e.g., marital status), past or current experiences, opinions, or plans that may not relate necessarily to therapy or the patient.

Self-disclosure can be used effectively as part of almost every DBT strategy.

It is part of (1) validation when it normalizes the patient's experience or responses by disclosing agreement with the patient's perceptions or interpretations of a situation, understanding of her emotions, or valuing of her decisions; (2) problem solving when it discloses ways of analyzing a problem or solutions the therapist has tried for similar problems; (3) skills training when the therapist offers new ways of handling a situation drawn from his or her own personal experience; (4) contingency management and clarification if it is used to disclose the therapist's reactions to the patient's behavior; (5) exposure when the therapist's reactions are ones the patient fears or finds frustrating. In addition, self-disclosure enhances the strength of the therapeutic relationship by increasing intimacy and warmth. As with all strategies, there are a number of guidelines for using self-disclosure wisely.

Orienting the Patient to Therapist Self-Disclosure

The utility of self-disclosure often depends on whether the patient expects therapist self-disclosure as part of a helping relationship. Patients who have been told that professionals and effective therapists do not self-disclose are likely to be put off by a therapist's self-disclosure and may view such a therapist as ineffective and incompetent. A patient of mine was referred to me after her previous therapist unilaterally terminated therapy. Some time later I was going out of town and the patient asked me where I was going. My informative response was met with anger and derision: If I was willing to tell her where I was going, I was obviously not a good therapist. Her former therapist would never have told her! I had not prepared her for the differences between DBT and psychoanalysis. Although careful preparation may not have solved the problem in this case, the therapist should orient the patient at the beginning of therapy to the role of therapist self-disclosure in DBT. It is useful to find out and discuss the patient's expectations and beliefs about it.

Self-Involving Self-Disclosure

Disclosing Reactions to the Patient and to Her Behavior. In DBT, the therapist presents in an ongoing manner, as part of the dialogue of therapy, his or her immediate reactions to the patient and her behavior. The form of self-disclosure here is "When you do X, I feel [or think or want to do] Y." For example, a therapist might say, "When you call me at home and then criticize all of my efforts to help you, I feel frustrated," or ". . . I don't want to talk to you any longer," or ". . . I start thinking you don't really want me to help you." Following a week when the patient's phone behavior improved, the therapist might say, "When you criticized me less on the phone this week, I found it much easier to help you." A therapist in my clinic whose patient complained about his coolness said, "When you demand warmth from me, it pushes me away and makes it harder to be warm." When my patient kept begging me to help her but wouldn't fill out the self-monitoring diary cards,

I said, "You keep asking me for help but won't do the things I believe are necessary to help you. I feel very frustrated, because I want to help you but feel you won't let me." "I'm pleased" is a common disclosure of mine when patients show improvement, confront something particularly difficult, or do something nice for me (e.g., send me a birthday card). "I'm demoralized" might be my disclosure to the patient who admits herself to an inpatient unit against my advice for the 10th time.

Self-disclosure of reactions to the patient serves both to validate and to challenge. It is a principal method of contingency management, observing limits, and contingency clarification, targeting the patient's behavior in relationship to the therapist. It is contingency management because a therapist's reactions to a patient's behaviors are almost never neutral to the patient. They are either positive and reinforce the "X" behavior, or they are negative and punish it. As I have discussed in Chapter 10, the therapist's relationship with the patient is one of the most important contingencies in working with a borderline patient. Self-involving self-disclosure is the means of communicating the momentary state of the relationship.

Self-disclosure of individual limits, both of ability and of preference, is essential to using the observing-limits procedures. Here, indeed, the therapist is careful to disclose limits as a property of the therapist, of the "self," and not as a property of the therapy or of some therapy rule book. Self-disclosure is itself a form of observing limits.

Disclosing reactions to the patient and her behavior is also a means of contingency clarification, since it gives the patient information about the effects of her own behavior. To the extent that the therapist's reactions are reasonably normative, this information can be extremely important in helping the patient change her interpersonal behaviors. Borderline individuals were often raised in families where reactions to their behavior were either not communicated or not normative. Thus, a patient is often unaware of how her behavior affects others until it is too late to repair the damage. It is particularly important to give the patient feedback on her behavior early in the chain of detrimental interpersonal behaviors, rather than waiting until a reaction is so strong that the relationship will be difficult to repair.

"*Heart-to-hearts.*" Self-involving self-disclosure also includes discussing with the patient the therapist's experience of what is going on in the immediate interaction, whether on the phone or in a therapy session. Although this is not really very different from disclosing reactions to the patient's behavior, the focus here is on the back-and-forth interaction between the two parties. The therapist discloses his or her perceptions of the current interaction, along with his or her own response to it. The form is "It seems to me that X is happening between us. What do you think?" For instance, "I'm feeling like our interaction is getting more and more tense. Are you feeling it too?" The therapist switches the focus of the dialogue to the here-and-now interactional process. The switch can be very brief (just a passing comment), or can lead to an in-depth discussion of the interaction.

When asked, the therapist should be willing to discuss with the patient where he or she stands in relationship to the patient. In this instance, the therapist reviews with the patient how he or she sees the relationship as a whole, instead of focusing on a specific interaction. For example, one of my patients missed her therapy session (again) without calling because she had failed to take her antiseizure medications (again), resulting in an admission to the seizure clinic (again). At the next session, she asked whether I was going to get upset with her (again). I replied (in essence), "Well, yes, I guess I will. But I've noticed that when you do these sorts of things, I get distressed, we work it out, and then we go on again. We seem to have a pretty good relationship, and both of us can tolerate these ups and downs pretty well. So let's get to work figuring this out, and then we can go on to other things." A borderline patient often asks directly, "How do you feel about me?" or "Do you like working with me?" Such questions should be answered directly and clearly. In the case above, I might have said, "Right now you drive me crazy, but I like you anyway."

Process discussions are often needed when the patient is engaging in therapy-interfering behavior during an interaction. Deciding whether to stick to the agenda and ignore interfering behavior or to stop and attend to the process can be very difficult. In my experience, if one always stops to discuss interfering behavior, almost no other therapy will get done. If such behavior is never discussed, however, the same outcome occurs—little or no therapy. Interfering behaviors are often avoidance behaviors that function to deflect therapy from the task at hand. The therapist has to be very careful not to collude in the diversion. Process discussions, in contrast, are usually very reinforcing to both patient and therapist and constitute what can be loosely called "heart-to-heart" discussions.

Effective use of heart-to-hearts requires that the therapist have a firm grasp of their function at a given moment with a given patient. The general idea is to use them to advance problem solving or reinforce therapeutic activities, and to avoid them when they serve to divert attention from an important topic at hand. This said, there are several occasions when heart-to-hearts are appropriate.

First, brief heart-to-hearts can be used to break up in-session patient behaviors that interfere with work on higher-priority problems. Used in this manner, the heart-to-heart is an instance of highlighting (an insight strategy; see Chapter 9) and, depending on the level of confrontation, may also serve as an aversive contingency (see Chapter 10). For example, a patient may come to therapy in a hostile but passive mood and reject all of my ideas and attempts to solve a problem in therapy. I may ask, "I'm feeling like we are in a power struggle, with you trying to get me to be responsible for this problem and me trying to get you to be responsible. How are you feeling?" Or I may say, "What's going on here? I'm doing the best I can to help with this problem, and I feel like you are just sitting back and making me do all the work. So I'm trying harder and harder to get you involved. But it doesn't seem to be working very well. What do you think? Is that your perception too?" After a brief interaction on the topic (taking care to keep it from digressing to a general discussions of our relationship), I then return to the original problem at hand. This tactic may be repeated several times during the session ("We're getting in a power struggle again"). Always returning to the topic, however, is crucial. Otherwise, instigating heart-to-hearts will be an effective way for the patient to avoid difficult topics.

Second, elaborated heart-to-hearts are used as reinforcers. In this instance, their timing should be such that they immediately follow some improved patient behavior, or at least some exposure to the avoided task. For example, I may drag a patient through a behavioral analysis and then have a heart-to-heart about how hard it was.

Third, elaborated "heart-to-hearts" are used to repair the relationship when the therapist has made an error. They can also be used to repair the relationship when the patient has made an error and wants to work on repairing it. Relationship problem-solving strategies, discussed at length in Chapter 15, are in some respects elaborated versions of a "heart-to-heart." It is important here, however, to keep in mind the reinforcing value of heart-to-hearts for most patients. The therapist must not allow "heart-to-hearts" to divert the therapy focus from difficult topics. The balance between heart-to-hearts and focusing on topics the patient is attempting to avoid is similar to the balance the therapist must strike between validation and active problem solving.

Blending Self-Involvement and Responsiveness. As this discussion has indicated, self-involving self-disclosure requires the therapist to be alert both to the patient and to himself or herself. It requires a certain ability to be clear about one's own feelings and reactions, as well as an ability to put those reactions into words that the patient can hear. Two points are important. First, when presenting the situation, the therapist should keep to the "observables" rather than presenting inferences about the patient's motives, fantasies, or wishes as part of the situation. Such interpretations are part of the therapist's own reaction to the situation; they are not part of the situation per se. Saying "I feel as if you are playing games with me" is very different from saying "You are playing games with me." Second, when presenting reactions, the therapist should be careful not to make the intensity too high or too low. For example, telling a new patient who is fearful of rejection "I am very frustrated" may be better than saying "I am angry." Matching the intensity (though not necessarily the emotion) to the patient's is a good way to start.

As with all therapist behavior, it is essential to track the effect of self-disclosing behavior on the individual patient. The goal is for the therapist to be able to share with the patient—verbally and behaviorally, openly and spontaneously—his or her reactions to the patient. This may not be possible at the beginning of therapy. Disclosure has to be titrated.

Self-Disclosure of Others' Reactions to the Therapist. Self-disclosure about how others react to the therapist can also be important in helping the patient accept her own reactions to the therapist and the therapist's to her. The emotionally cool therapist mentioned above responded to complaints about his lack of warmth by saying (in essence), "You are not the only one who feels that way. Other people in my life, in and out of work, have said the same thing. I know it would be easier for you if I were warmer, but I am doing my best." Such a self-disclosing and vulnerable response made it very difficult for the patient to continue her demanding behavior. She had no further need to validate her experience of the therapist or prove her point that she needed more warmth. Instead, she and the therapist could focus on how to manage a relationship in which the other person could not give her the warmth she wanted and perhaps needed. My patients have complained about many of my own interpersonal weaknesses that others also pick up on. Sharing the fact that others also complain is immensely validating and refreshing to these patients. Sharing the fact that I am working on the characteristic (if it really is detrimental and if it is changeable), but doing so without undue guilt or shame, suggests a degree of self-acceptance that the patients can imitate.

Personal Self-Disclosure

Self-Disclosure as Modeling. DBT encourages personal self-disclosure to model either normative responses to situations or ways of handling difficult situations. The therapist may disclose opinions or reactions to situations, either to validate the patient's own responses or to challenge them: "I agree" or "I disagree." This modeling can be especially powerful for patients raised in chaotic or "perfect" families, where the opinions and reactions to which they were exposed were not normative for the culture. Often they are unaware that other reactions to events and opinions about the world are not only possible but acceptable.

Similarly, therapist self-disclosure can be useful when the patient's reactions are discrepant from normative reactions, but nonetheless, are valid, are admirable, or are otherwise to be encouraged. If both the therapist and the patient don't "fit into" to the culture in similar ways, self-disclosure can be extremely validating for the patient. The feminist woman in a sexist culture, the member of an ethnic minority living within the majority culture, and the relational person in an individuated culture are examples. In these cases, it is equally important that the therapist disclose how he or she copes with not fitting in, such that both self-validation and positive relationships with the majority are maintained.

In teaching behavioral skills, it can be extremely useful to present a coping model (rather than a mastery model) of skill application. The therapist here shares with the patients his or her efforts, including failures as well as successes, in using the skills being taught. Including failures can be important especially when the therapist goes on to describe the handling of a failure. The important point to remember, however, is that although the therapist's situation may be similar to the patient's, it is never identical.

Self-Disclosure of Professional Information. The therapist should be clear with the patient about his or her professional background, training, therapy orientation, and views about professional issues. A patient will sometimes ask about a therapist's experience in treating BPD and about successes or failures in such treatment. This information should be disclosed, along with information about supervision and consultation arrangements.

Self-Disclosure of Personal Information. Patients are often interested in personal details about their therapists, such as age, marital status, children, friendship patterns, religion or religious beliefs, work habits, whether the therapists have themselves been in therapy, and so on. Therapists should disclose information they are comfortable sharing. The principle here is that as long as a disclosure is in a patient's best interest, there are no rules (other than common sense and the guidelines above) limiting information given to the patient. Some therapists are more private than others; the important point is for therapists to observe and disclose their own privacy limits. Unless a patient's behavior would be clearly inappropriate in any intimate relationship, a therapist should not communicate to the patient that her wishes for more disclosure are pathological.

A patient will, at times, ask whether the therapist has ever experienced personal problems similar to hers. How to respond depends on the therapist's actual experiences, how willing the therapist is to be open about his or her own life, and whether the information can be used effectively by the patient. In some treatment programs, such as many aimed at substance abusers, therapists are selected because they have experienced the same problems as their patients; sharing this information is thus an important part of the treatment program. Women's groups are based on the same notion—that there is a commonality of experience between therapist and group members. In DBT such sharing is not definitional to the therapy, but it is not proscribed.

Several points should be kept in mind about this type of self-disclosure. First, no matter how similar the situations, the differences between the therapist and the patient may be far greater than the similarities; both the differences and the similarities should be respected. Second, the therapist should be very careful about sharing current problems. Burdening the patient, or putting the patient in the role of "therapist to the therapist" should be avoided. These points are discussed in more detail below.

Using Supervision/Consultation

Managing self-disclosure is a very difficult task and is one reason why many schools of therapy suggest that therapists themselves undergo individual psychotherapy. In DBT, the individual supervisor or the case consultation team can be essential in helping therapists track their ongoing self-disclosing behavior.

3. WARM ENGAGEMENT

Interpersonal warmth and therapeutic friendliness are related to positive out-come in the research literature on psychotherapy (see Morris & Magrath, 1983, for a review of this literature in behavior therapy). This is at least as true with borderline patients as with other populations (Woollcott, 1985). Paradoxically, these patients can elicit both very strong positive and very strong negative affect in therapists. On the one hand, the tendency to unchecked empathy, warmth, and friendliness (i.e., overly strong positive affect) can lead therapists to break the therapeutic contract in favor of nontherapeutic friend-liness, emotional and physical closeness, and at times role reversal. On the other hand, as I have discussed in Chapter 1, borderline patients can be par-ticularly difficult to like at times. The tendency of many therapists to get an-gry and hostile, and to invalidate and "blame the victim," is so great that DBT actively works to foster liking and motivation to work with borderline pa-tients. Often, the same therapist vacillates between overinvolvement and ag-gressively pushing the patient away. (This topic is discussed in much more detail in Chapter 13.)

The middle way, expressing warm engagement, is the usual therapeutic stance in DBT. "Warmth" can be defined as the active communication of a postive response to the patient. Warm engagement couples the positive response to the patient with a positive interest in working with her in the therapeutic enterprise. Both voice tone and conversational style should reflect warmth and engagement in the therapeutic interaction, as opposed to reluc-tance and withdrawal. On the phone in particular, the therapist should en-gage fully in the conversation, being careful that voice tone does not un-intentionally communicate impatience or annoyance at being interrupted. Posture should reflect interest and care. For many reasons (some very valid), a borderline patient often believes that her therapist is angry at her, wants to get rid of her, finds her boring, or the like. Such a patient may dread com-ing to sessions, fearing a cold, disapproving, or uninterested welcome. One of the more therapeutic aspects of this particular guideline is the communi-cation of warmth and of looking forward to seeing the patient each week. A friendly, affectionate style, rather than a cool, business-like approach is the goal here.

Limits on Warmth

Warm engagement can be difficult at times, especially when the patient seeks additional therapeutic contact, either by phone or through an unscheduled office visit. If the therapist is unwilling to talk to the patient at a particular point (and there is no immediate crisis requiring attention), he or she can offer to talk to her at a later point. Or the therapist can be open about his or her reservations, negotiate a brief interaction, and then engage with the patient as fully and warmly as possible during this brief period. A therapist who repeatedly feels cool, distant, uninterested, or bored with the patient during regular sessions may be sure that something is wrong—with the therapist, the patient, or both. The strategies here are to discuss the topic with the consultation team, analyze the interactions with the patient, and employ a relationship problem solving. Often, a therapist's unwillingness is a sign that the patient is engaging in therapy-interfering behaviors or the therapist is not observing his or her limits.

Some therapists are just not "the warm type"; that is, they are interpersonally reserved by nature. Of course, this is no problem with patients who do just as well with some distance in the relationship. In contrast, with patients who prefer or need more warmth, or who misinterpret reserve for lack of affection, it can be a stumbling block to therapy. The first thing is to remember the observing-limits procedures (see Chapter 10). In this case, the strategy is for a reserved therapist to be honest with the patient about his or her ability to express affection obviously or directly. Second, the therapist should help the patient interpret (and, ideally, experience) other characteristics of the relationship as indications of his or her friendliness and affection. That is, the therapist should try to mitigate the effects of his or her reserve by highlighting other positive aspects of the relationship. For example, a therapist who is exceptionally dependable may note that this is a sign of care and affection. Third, the therapist can rely on words to communicate feelings—for example, "I like working with you," "I find you interesting," "I'm looking forward to seeing you next week," or "You can call me and I don't mind talking to you" (when this is true).

Coping with Rage at the Patient

Telling therapists to express warm engagement is all well and good when the patient is not questioning the therapist's competence, credibility, and genuineness during every interaction; is not overwhelming the therapist with unwanted phone calls at all hours; is not threatening to kill herself whenever the therapist makes the slightest misstep or when the therapist is overloaded with other concerns; is not threatening to quit therapy every single week; is not complaining about the therapist (in ways that feel exaggerated) to anyone who will listen; is not rigidly rephrasing what the therapist has just said in a manner that feels distorted and extreme (saying also, "Well, if that is the case, I might as well . . ."); is not responding with protracted silence whenever an insensitive remark is made; and is not simultaneously failing to improve or is even deteriorating despite the therapist's best efforts. But what about when the patient is engaging in some or all of these activities, or even worse? Not only is it hard to be warmly engaged at these points, but it can also be difficult not to retaliate by attacking the patient. I have never experienced or observed in other therapists as much rage at patients as with borderline patients. The rage is especially intense when the patient is communicating intense suffering and seems not to be improving. Main (1957), in a beautifully empathetic analysis of staff difficulties with recalcitrant distress, has captured the essence of the problem as follows:

With recalcitrant distress, one might almost say recalcitrant *patients,* treatments tend, as ever, to become desperate and to be used increasingly in the service of hatred as well as love; to deaden, placate, and silence, as well as to vivify. . . . there can never be certain guarantee that the therapist facing great and resistant distress will be immune from using interpretations in the way nurses use sedatives — to soothe themselves when desparate, and to escape from their own distressing ailment of ambivalence and hatred. The temptation to conceal from ourselves and our patients increasing hatred [with] frantic goodness is the greater the more worried we become. Perhaps we need to remind ourselves regularly that the word "worried" has two meanings, and that if the patient worries us too savagely, friendly objectivity is difficult or impossible to maintain.

The first step in overcoming rage is the willingness to "let it come and go." That is, the therapist must cultivate a mindful stance of seeing his or her own emotional reactions, including rage at the patient, as simply that — emotional reactions that come and go. Although any emotional reaction can give the therapist important clues to understanding the patient and her difficulties better, little is gained if rage persists. Persistent or very frequent rage is usually a clue that some personal issues of the therapist has been tapped by the patient's behavior. In agency and group practice settings, persistent rage may indicate institutional problems as well. Honest self-analyses and use of the therapist supervision/consultation strategies (discussed in Chapter 13) are essential here. Individual supervision and/or therapy, or consultation outside the institution, may also be indicated .

Rage is invariably based on some sort of pejorative judgment or "should" statement about the events eliciting the anger. The person engaging in the disliked behavior is viewed as responsible, free, and able to act better if she only wanted to: "She should not have done that," "She is manipulating me," "She just doesn't want to get better," and so on. The biosocial theory of DBT was developed in part to counter just these attitudes. Thus, the second step in countering rage is to try to change perspective, seeing the patient's behavior as a result of biosocial factors that have as yet not been remediated. The therapist must move to a phenomenological perspective, seeing events from the point of view of the patient. It is when the therapist can hold down both points of view at once — the "My response is the only one possible, given my life history" view of the patient, and the "Your response is unacceptable nonetheless, and must change" view of the therapist — that progress can be made in therapy. I have had periods with particular patients when I have had to make this shift many times within the space of one interaction with a patient. Thus, the therapist must have virtually inexhaustible patience in repeating the process over and over.

Third, the therapist should closely examine his or her own limits with respect to the patient's behavior, and question whether these are being adequately observed and communicated to the patient. The observing-limits procedures, outlined in Chapter 10, were developed primarily to moderate therapist frustration and rage. It is rarely useful to communicate these limits in the middle of a rageful reaction; however, once the therapist calms down, such a discussion may be fruitful. Unfortunately, with many borderline patients, the therapist must expand his or her limits for some time until the patients' behavior improves. Principles of shaping are essential to keep in mind here (see Chapter 10 for a review). In fact, reminding oneself of these principles can be helpful in reducing anger.

Finally, it is important to keep in mind that perfect control and perfect therapy are simply not possible. It is not a catastrophe if the therapist occasionally blows up or engages in hostile or angry behavior. That is, it is not catastrophic if the therapist repairs the relationship well. This topic is discussed more fully in Chapter 15, so I do not go into it further here. But it can be useful to remember that unrelenting warmth is not a characteristic of any relationship, no matter how positive it is.

Warm Engagement and Touch in Psychotherapy

A problem with borderline patients is that it is easy to go overboard—to be *too* warm and *too* engaged. In an effort to avoid that, some therapists go the opposite direction and withdraw too far, both physically and emotionally, from their patients. This is nowhere more true than in the area of physical touch in therapy. Many therapists (especially in this era of litigation), have an arbitrary rule that they never touch a patient, no matter what the circumstances. When it is responsive to an individual's need or request, however, touch can be healing in any interpersonal relationship, including the therapeutic relationship. A borderline patient often asks for or initiates physical contact or a hug. When this is appropriate, it seems unreasonable to deny the request or push the patient away for arbitrary reasons. A good-bye hug can be particularly soothing for some borderline patients. The value of touch in these instances, at least with some patients, should not be underestimated. Even when a session has been appropriately wound down, parting is very difficult for many.

I suspect that the problem here is that the rules are murky but the penalties for violating the rules (whether advertently or inadvertently) are very high. If the rules were clearer, things would be easier. So what are the rules in DBT?

1. *Physical touch should be careful.* Its role in the context of the therapeutic relationship with each specific patient should be clear in the therapist's mind. The relationship of touch to the treatment plan should be conscious and explicit. In sum, touch should be thoughtful rather than careless.

2. *Physical touch should be brief.* Patting the patient on the shoulder as she goes to her chair in the therapy room, hugging her when saying good-bye or when meeting after some time, briefly putting a hand on the patient's hand during a particularly difficult disclosure, and firmly gripping the patient's hand or arm when she is out of control can all be appropriate and therapeutic in certain circumstances.

3. *Physical touch should express an existing therapeutic relationship.* It is a communication strategy; it should not be used as a change procedure. Thus, physical contact should be appropriate to the level of therapeutic intimacy in the relationship. Within close relationships, touch (e.g., a good-bye hug) should reflect the current state of the relationship. It should not be used to create a different relationship state. For example, if the relationship is strained, touch should not be used to try to repair it. A hug reflects repair already accomplished (for both parties); it is not a means of repair. Massaging a patient's neck to relax her it not appropriate in DBT. Nor is physical contact a validation procedure surrounding a change procedure. Thus, holding the patient within a therapy session, even during particularly difficult disclosures, is not a DBT strategy. The only exceptions here are those rare situations where firm physical contact may be helpful or necessary to restrain or control a very agitated patient.

A patient sometimes asks for a hug in farewell or for consolation when a therapist does not feel close enough in the relationship to be comfortable with touch. This is especially likely with new patients and in therapeutic relationships marked by patient hostility or nonattachment (e.g., the "butterfly" patients discussed in Chapter 5). In such a case, the discussion should focus on helping the patient learn to monitor when such requests or initiation of touch are appropriate and to act accordingly. Individuals with sexual abuse histories often have problems in this area.

If a patient persists in asking for a good-bye hug that the therapist does not feel comfortable giving, he or she should examine how sessions are ending. The therapist may not be giving the patient enough wind-down time before parting. (See Chapter 14 for a further discussion of this topic.) If the patient is forced to leave the interaction when she is too vulnerable emotionally, a good-bye hug may become especially important. Many battles concerning touch center around just this problem. The patient's problem should not be ignored, but a hug should not be substituted for appropriate session wind-down.

4. *Physical touch should be sensitive to the patient's wishes and comfort.* The therapist should ask permission before hugging a patient or touching her hand, and should not touch a patient who does not want to be touched. The therapist must be alert to changes in comfort level and act accordingly. It should not be assumed that a patient does not care simply because she does not protest. Nonverbal communication is important here.

5. *Physical touch should be within a therapist's own personal limits.* For example, a therapist who is not the "hugging" type with anyone should make this clear to the patient, without implying that her wish for physical contact is somehow pathological or problematic in principle (see above). As I have discussed in Chapter 10, learning to observe others' limits is an important social skill. Or a therapist may not feel safe touching a patient (even when it is apparently safe to do so), especially if friends or colleagues have been sued or reprimanded for sexual involvement with patients. This concern is

most likely in male–female dyads, but can be an equal consideration in same-sex dyads when one or both parties are lesbian or gay. The therapist may want to confine a good-bye hug to open, public places (such as the hallway or the office with the door open). Discussing the ethical issues surrounding touch with the borderline patient can be very important.

6. It should go without saying that *sexual touch is never acceptable.* Nor is the expression of sexual willingness, by touch, word, tone, or invitation, ever appropriate. Borderline patients and their therapists, in particular, tend to get into inappropriate sexual relationships; the risks or mistakes of touch are higher here than with many other patient populations. Thus, great care is needed. The therapist should be particularly careful about how the patient construes touch. There is no substitute for talking about how the patient interprets a hug or pat on the shoulder. The therapist should not simply assume on the basis of gender and sexual orientation that touch is experienced as nonsexual.

If there is no way for a therapist to touch the patient without its becoming somewhat sexual for either party, no touch should take place. If a therapist is sexually attracted to a patient (more than briefly), I would recommend not only avoiding physical touch but getting a consultation immediately. The secret here is not to trust oneself too much.

7. *When inappropriate touch or a sexual overture is initiated by the patient, the therapist should "talk it to death."* Such behavior is therapy-interfering behavior and should be treated as such. The therapist should also be willing to examine his or her own behavior for inadvertent encouragement or reinforcement of such behavior.

8. *Physical touch should be potentially public.* This does not mean that all touch has to occur in public. Nor does it mean that a therapist should discuss it publicly with any or all of his or her professional colleagues. It means simply that the therapist should not try to keep the fact of hugging a patient good-bye, for example, a secret. The topic should be periodically discussed at supervision/consultation meetings. A therapist who videotapes sessions should not move out of the camera range when hugging a patient. The purposes of this rule are honesty and self-protection. A therapist who keeps discussing the topic is much less likely to drift into mistakes.

4. GENUINENESS

Almost all experienced psychotherapists and therapy schools value genuineness as an important characteristic of therapists; DBT is no exception. Borderline patients, in particular, often demand a genuineness from therapists that can be exhausting to maintain. These patients can pick up subtle communications, and it is extraordinarily difficult for their therapists to hide behind a role. Having a borderline patient is like having a supervisor for a patient: Every artificial response, unartful intervention, inconsistent comment, or attempt to use power inappropriately is noted and commented upon.

Borderline patients often express a need for their therapists to be "real." They are frequently uncomfortable with the ambiguity of meaning imposed by the therapeutic role. Does a therapist "really care," or is caring behavior a reflection of the role? Most other patients tolerate artificial limits and barriers imposed by the therapeutic role; borderline individuals do not tolerate them well; in part because their lives have been full of arbitrary rules, limits, and distinctions. This does not mean that a therapist should have no barriers. Having no barriers would also be arbitrary. A genuine relationship within the context of therapy allows the patient to learn that even in a good relationship there are natural limits and barriers as well as arbitrary ones.

DBT places a strong emphasis on therapy as a "real" as opposed to a transferential relationship. Rather than acting as a mirror in order for the patient to work out transference problems, the therapist is just himself or herself. The therapist develops a real relationship with the patient and helps the patient change within the relationship; the idea is that within this genuine relationship, healing takes place. The genuineness of the therapist provides a vehicle to contain the therapy procedures that bring about change. It also provides a counterfoil for the patient to react against and with in order to improve her interpersonal behavior. Finally, the therapist's genuineness provides an intimacy and connectedness that enhance the lives of both patient and therapist. This quality of being oneself has been described as follows:

> He [sic] is without front or facade, openly being the feelings and attitudes which at the moment are flowing in him. It involves the element of self-awareness, meaning that the feelings the therapist is experiencing are available to him, available to his awareness, and also that he is able to live these feelings, to be them in the relationship, and able to communicate them if appropriate. It means that he comes into a direct personal encounter with his client, meeting him on a person-to-person basis. It means he is *being* himself, not denying himself. (Rogers & Truax, 1967, p. 101)

In a similar vein, Safran and Segal (1990) discuss the relationship in cognitive therapy as follows:

> Ultimately, however, it must be remembered that all theoretical concepts and techniques. . . are merely tools; they are tools designed to help the therapist overcome the obstacles to having an I–Thou relationship with the patient. These tools themselves, however, can become obstacles if they are used to avoid authentic human encounters, rather than to facilitate them. As an old Zen saying puts it: *"The right tools in the hands of the wrong man become the wrong tools."* The wise therapist will thus not confuse the particular vehicle for change. . .with the underlying essence of change.
>   Therapists who let concepts blind them to the reality of what is truly happening for their patients in the moment are relating to the patient as an object, or in Buber's phraseology, an *"It"* rather than a *"Thou."* Therapists who hide behind the security of the conceptual framework provided here rather than risking authentic human encounters, which could lead to therapists' transcending all roles and preconceptions about how they themselves should be, rule out the possibility of the very experiences in human relatedness that will be healing for their patients. (pp. 249–250).

A most important characteristic of genuineness has to do with arbitrary, role-defined behavior versus natural, congruent, role-free behavior. In DBT, the therapist does not overemphasize his or her role; that is, effectiveness and natural limits rather than arbitrary role definitions determine the therapist's response. This naturalness can be quite difficult for therapists trained in schools that emphasize strict boundaries and "professional" behaviors. As with observing limits, there is no rule book in DBT to indicate what behaviors reflect being one self in therapy. Instead, therapists must look to their own natural helping style.

The Need for Therapist Invulnerability

Some therapeutic approaches take it as accepted fact that the levels of vulnerability and self-disclosure for patient versus therapist not only are not but *should* not be equal. In these approaches, the therapist–patient relationship is similar to any high-power–low-power relationship. The hallmark of such relationships is that one person (the low-power person) is more vulnerable than the other. As I have noted previously, however, borderline individuals are very sensitive to power differences in relationships. They often dislike intensely the quasi-parental nature of many therapeutic relationships, asserting quite rightly that they are not children themselves. They ask why vulnerability is not shared more equally. DBT is not based on a medical model and actively works against a quasi-parental relationship, or one that treats the patient as a child. It is most similar in its relationship model to feminist therapy, where the goal is to "empower" the patient. Yet, even in DBT, vulnerability and reciprocity are not shared equally between therapist and patient. Thus, the following question is a very good one: How should the therapist respond when the patient contends that reciprocal vulnerability and disclosure would enhance treatment, not interfere with it? As one patient said to a colleague, "The less you act like a therapist, the more helpful you are."

There are many answers. In DBT, paradoxically, each answer revolves around the therapist's willingness to be natural rather than arbitrary within the relationship. Three important reasons have to do with the therapist's personal limits, particular characteristics of the patient, and the interaction of vulnerability with the therapist's ability to conduct effective therapy.

Therapist Limits on Vulnerability

A primary reason why levels of vulnerability and self-disclosure are not equal between patient and therapist is that a therapist can't endure it if they are. There is just so much reciprocity any person can tolerate, and no one is completely vulnerable and open in every relationship he or she in. None of us really could sustain that. Most of us are open and vulnerable with one or two, or at the most three or four, people in our lives (usually members of our families). People without families have one or two close friends they are vulnerable and self-disclosing with. In general, humans are not reciprocally vulnerable with everyone. If therapists were vulnerable in this way with all of their patients each day, they would not be able to crawl home at the end of the day.

When a therapist forces vulnerability and self-disclosure for the sake of therapy, the interaction is not genuine or authentic. A patient's complaints that caring behavior is simply part of the role as therapist are then correct. Although the patient may want reciprocal vulnerability, expecting or demanding it may be unrealistic. A relationship that is authentically reciprocal, self-disclosing, and genuine can only occur in the context of what the therapist is willing and able to do or be. It is not necessary to make up rules or come up with stories of how reciprocal disclosure and vulnerability would be harmful to a patient, even though it may indeed be harmful. It is not necessary to convince the patient that the therapist's inability or unwillingness to interact as she wishes is in her best interest. Nor is it necessary to assume that the patient's needs and wishes for more reciprocity are somehow pathological. What is required here is honesty on the therapist's part. When I talk about "reciprocal communication," I am not talking about a therapist's disclosing everything that is going on in his or her life or sharing every reaction with the patient. Instead, I am referring to an openness in the moment, to the moment.

Patient Characteristics That Limit Vulnerability

In DBT, the therapist does not build interpersonal boundaries or barriers. This does not mean, however, that no barriers and boundaries exist between the therapist and the patient; it means that the therapist does not purposely build them as a part of the therapy. Observing limits includes observing such boundaries, including barriers to vulnerability and self-disclosure.

A number of patient characteristics and behavior patterns may create barriers to intimacy and reciprocity. Borderline patients not infrequently push, impinge upon, or demand intimacy and vulnerability from other's including their therapists. When this happens, the persons being pushed, impinged upon, or demanded pull away and build barriers. It is a natural reaction. It is hard to be relaxed and spontaneous with a person who threatens suicide if one makes an interpersonal mistake. It is difficult to be intimate with an individual who responds warmly one day and engages in bitter attacks the next. Reciprocal communication requires the observation of these barriers and the reasons for them. The therapist discusses the barriers with the patient, including describing how the patient is contributing to them.

Sometimes there is simply not a good match between patient and therapist. Differences in personality and communication style, social class, gender, religion, politics, education, or age, for example, may decrease the therapist's comfort as well as the utility of self-disclosure. Reciprocal communication is not the tearing down of those barriers but the open acknowledgment of them. It is a natural event in life that cultural and stylistic barriers exist between people for various reasons. The therapeutic value is that the patient can learn about natural barriers in a nonmoralistic, nonjudgmental context. It is not in the patient's best interest to learn that there are no barriers ever. It is in the patient's best interest to learn about the world as it is. Barriers exist.

DBT therapists should be open to the fact that much of psychotherapy training advocates creating boundaries between patient and therapist. Most therapists have undergone such training. Thus, therapists in DBT should constantly explore within themselves how many of the barriers and boundaries that exist are artificial and how many are natural, and should work on lowering the artificial ones and acknowledging the natural ones.

Limits of Effective Therapy

The degree of therapist vulnerability and self-disclosure must also be limited by the boundaries between effective and ineffective therapy. There are two sources of limits: the therapist's previous experience with vulnerability and disclosure, and the focus in DBT on the patient. With respect to the first of these, DBT requires a sometimes difficult balance between personal experience with different patients and appreciation of the individuality of the current patient. What is effective with one patient may not be with another. What was once effective with a particular patient may no longer be. Some patients do well within a close and intimate relationship; others become frightened and may do better with some distance built in. As with all strategies, there is no substitute for ongoing assessment.

Second, in DBT the focus of therapy should be kept on the patient. Therapists must be careful not to talk about their own feelings or life history in a manner that shifts the focus to themselves. Such a shift can be particularly tempting with borderline patients, who often make persuasive arguments against the inequality and role-dependent norms inherent in psychotherapy. Frequently, their desire for greater intimacy, their ability to be nurturing and to reinforce therapist self-disclosure, and their tendency to punish interpersonal distance lead therapists down a dangerous path to abandoning the therapeutic relationship. A borderline patient's discomfort with the patient role sometimes leads to a complete role reversal: The therapist, in effect, becomes the patient. At other times, the reversal is partial and the relationship becomes one of cocounseling. Although role reversal or a cocounseling relationship may not always be detrimental to a patient, both are problematic for a number of reasons. Neither one was the type of relationship agreed to in the first place; that is, each violates the therapy contract. When such a change takes place, a patient often finds it extremely difficult to complain, even when she wants more attention directed to her own problems. The patient may also find the therapist's problems or life story burdensome. In DBT, self-disclosure must be used strategically—that is, within the framework of a treatment plan.

Irreverent Communication Strategies

Irreverent communication strategies are used to provoke the patient to "jump the track," so to speak. The main idea here is to push the patient "off balance" so that rebalancing can occur. Irreverent communication is used (1) to get the patient's attention, (2) to shift the patient's affective response, and (3) to get the patient to see a completely different point of view. It is used whenever the patient, or both patient and therapist, are "stuck" in a dysfunctional emotional, thought, or behavior pattern. The style is offbeat.

Irreverent communication indicates to the patient that any idea or belief held by either the therapist or the patient is ultimately open to question, exploration, and change. Logic is used to weave a web that the patient cannot get out of. To be effective, irreverence must have two components: (1) It must come from the therapist's "center" (i.e., it must be genuine), and (2) it must be built on a bedrock of compassion, caring, and warmth. Otherwise, there is the possibility for misuse when it is used out of context. Irreverent communication balances reciprocal communication.

Irreverent communication is difficult to define or explain behaviorally and is easier to learn by example or observation. In many instances, it requires a matter-of-fact, almost deadpan style: The therapist takes the patient's underlying assumption and maximizes or minimizes it in an unemotional manner (similar to that of a straight man in a comedy team), to make a point the patient may not have considered before. By contrast, if the patient is herself matter-of-fact or deadpan, high intensity and emotionality or the making of extreme statements can also be effectively irreverent. Whether deadpan or intense, the style is in sharp contrast to the warm responsiveness of the reciprocal style.[1] Specific irreverent communication strategies are discussed below and outlined in Table 12.2

Dialectical Strategies and Irreverence

Many (if not most) of the dialectical strategies described in Chapter 7 have an irreverent flavor. Indeed, their success often depends on the therapist's presenting paradoxical or unorthodox positions as believable and reasonable. Entering the paradox, playing the devil's advocate, extending, allowing change, and making lemonade out of lemons are only effective if the therapist presents them with confidence and as completely matter-of-course. The therapist uses a "but of course" style, perhaps slightly incredulous that the point is not seen immediately by the patient. For example, in extending, the therapist incredulously reframes the patient's position: "How could you expect me to respond to your unhappiness over being fired when you are thinking of suicide? Why, of course we have to deal with the suicide first! What good is a job if you are dead?" In allowing change, the therapist responds to the patient's questions, "Last week you said I have everything I need; this week you are saying I don't have the skills I need?" with a simple "Right."

TABLE 12.2. Irreverent Communication Strategies Checklist

_____ T's voice tone is matter-of-fact with respect to maladaptive behaviors.

_____ T uses logic irreverently to weave a web.

_____ T employs a deadpan or a highly intense style, as appropriate, to contrast with P's style.

_____ T uses dialectical strategies in an irreverent manner:
    _____ Entering the paradox.
    _____ Playing the devil's advocate.
    _____ Extending.
    _____ Allowing change.
    _____ Making lemonade out of lemons.

_____ In a matter-of-fact way, T REFRAMES P's communication in an unorthodox manner, or picks up on an unintended aspect of P's communication.

_____ T PLUNGES into sensitive areas.
    _____ T's style is straightforward, direct, and clear; T "calls a spade a spade."
    _____ T uses humor.
    _____ T discusses dysfunctional behaviors in a matter-of-course manner.
    _____ T surrounds irreverence with validation.

_____ T uses DIRECT CONFRONTATION of dysfunctional behavior.
    _____ T communicates "bullshit" to responses other than targeted adaptive behavior.
    _____ T prevents escape into diversionary dysfunctional traumas.

_____ T CALLS P's BLUFF.

_____ T OSCILLATES INTENSITY of emotions, voice, and posture; T also uses SILENCE to encounter P.

_____ T assumes OMNIPOTENCE or admits IMPOTENCE, as seems appropriate.

Anti-DBT tactics

_____ T uses irreverent communication in a mean-spirited way.

_____ T uses irreverent communication without awareness of effects on P.

_____ T uses irreverent communication in a stilted or rigid manner.

And then the therapist goes on, leaving the patient to find the synthesis. Or the therapist changes techniques or strategies abruptly, with no warning, no apology, and no explanation. If the patient says, "Have you changed treatments again?" the therapist says "Yes" and continues on matter-of-factly.

I. REFRAMING IN AN UNORTHODOX MANNER

An irreverent response is almost never the reaction the patient expects. Although responsive to the patient's communication, it is nonresponsive to the patient's expectations (and, perhaps, immediate wishes). The therapist reframes the patient's communication in an unorthodox manner, or picks up on an unintended aspect of the patient's communication. For example, if the patient says, "I am going to kill myself," the therapist might reply "I thought you agreed not to drop out of therapy."

A patient of mine was failing again in her attempts to keep a job. Figuring (rather realistically) that she might be fired during the next week, she tried to convince me that the stress of such constant failure was reason enough to kill herself. She then implied that I didn't know or appreciate how stressful it was, since I was obviously a very successful professional. In the center of a very intense and emotional discussion, I replied calmly, matter-of-factly, and irreverently, "Oh! But I do understand. I have to live with a similar amount of stress much of the time. You can just imagine how stressful it is for me to have a patient constantly threatening to kill herself. Both of us have to worry about being fired!" Used judiciously, irreverent reframing facilitates problem solving and at the same time does not reinforce suicidal behavior.

2. PLUNGING IN WHERE ANGELS FEAR TO TREAD

Borderline individuals are often interpersonally direct and intense. As I have said previously, they are not good at social manipulation. They frequently relate better to people with a similar style—those who communicate in a straightforward, direct, and clear manner. Such a style is part of irreverent communication. DBT assumes that borderline patients are both fragile and not fragile; irreverence is directed at patients' nonfragile aspects. Irreverence assumes that timing of "interpretations" or hypotheses is not ordinarily crucial. The style of the therapist is direct, clear, concrete, candid, and open. The therapist "calls a spade a spade"; he or she plunges in where angels fear to tread. Humor and a certain apparent naiveté and guilelessness are also characteristic of the style. The rationale for this irreverence is the same as that for the firefighter who, dispensing with social niceties, throws a fire victim out the window into the safety net, or for the lifeguard who grabs hold of a drowning swimmer to bring her to safety. When pain is intense, time is of the essence. Time is saved by taking the direct route.

Dysfunctional attempts at problem solving and other sensitive topics, including suicidal behaviors, therapy-interfering behaviors, and other escape behaviors, are accepted as normal consequences of the individual's learning history and of factors currently operating her life. The behaviors are treated as normal consequences of aberrant contexts. The therapist does not step back from discussing them or approach them gingerly, but rather plunges ahead calmly and resolutely. In particular, suicidal ideation, suicide threats, and parasuicide are discussed in a manner similar to the manner of discussing any other behavior. The possibility that the patient could indeed kill herself is acknowledged openly (though not encouraged). This matter-of-factness regularly comes as a surprise to the patient, for whom the behaviors have usually elicited a significant community response in the past. The matter-of-fact style distracts her somewhat from the intensity of the topic and her usual strong emotions. The idea is for the therapist to move quickly and naturally enough to pull the patient along. In essence, the response to suicidal behavior is to treat it lightly and matter-of-factly, and at the same time to take it completely seriously.

Finally, irreverence is surrounded with validation. Thus, if a therapist tells a patient that she should not kill herself because it will interfere with therapy, this statement is followed immediately with a communication that she must be feeling terribly frustrated, hopeless, or the like. An irreverent strategy should not be confused with being unemotional. Drama and emotional expressiveness are encouraged.

3. USING A CONFRONTATIONAL TONE

The irreverent therapist confronts dysfunctional behavior directly, and at times blatantly (e.g., "Are you getting irrational on me again?" or "Are you out of your mind?" or "You weren't for a second actually believing I would think that this is a good idea, were you?"). The therapist communicates "bullshit" to responses other than the targeted adaptive response. The therapist may also use an irreverent style to prevent escape into diversionary dysfunctional traumas. For instance, when the patient responds to anxiety-provoking topics by diverging into (and persisting in) discussion of another irrelevant trauma or "soap opera," the therapist may say, "Do you want help with your real problems or not?" or "Oh, no! Another soap opera." As these examples indicate, confrontation depends on a very strong and positive relationship. Nor can it stand alone without surrounding validation.

4. CALLING THE PATIENT'S BLUFF

The irreverent therapist calls the patient's bluff. For example, if the patient says, "I'm quitting therapy," the therapist responds, "Would you like a referral?" The dialectical strategy of extending—taking the patient more seriously than she wants to be taken—is usually an instance of calling the patient's bluff. The therapist, however, must be careful to leave or provide the patient with a way out when her bluff is called. The secret here is in the timing of calling the bluff and of providing the safety net. The meek therapist provides both at once (bluff and net); the cruel, insensitive, or angry therapist forgets the net.

5. OSCILLATING INTENSITY AND USING SILENCE

Deliberately oscillating the intensity of emotions, voice, and posture can be irreverent when it cuts across the grain of the patient's own intensity. Here the therapist quickly moves from high intensity to relaxed calmness and back again, or from between dead seriousness to playfulness and back again. The irreverence is in the oscillation itself, as well as in the incongruity between the patient's apparent mood and that of the therapist.

Silence can also be used either to escalate or to reduce intensity, to withdraw from or to move closer to the patient. For example, the therapist may be trying to get a commitment from the patient, a change in affect, or movement from an unreasonable position. After arguing back and forth, the therapist may use silence to encounter the patient and produce a vacuum of initiative that the patient may fill. The therapist does not speak, smile, or move at all, but gazes at the patient, into space, or at a fixed point. The therapist waits for the targeted response (e.g., one with affect, a commitment, a "reasonable" comment) from the patient. Then the therapist responds.

6. EXPRESSING OMNIPOTENCE AND IMPOTENCE

It can be very effective and irreverent at times for the therapist to assume omnipotence, suggesting that only by working with the therapist or following the therapist's suggestions can the patient make progress. For example, the therapist may say, "The problem with suicide, of course, is that if you are dead you won't have me to help you." Or if the patient says, "How do you know I have a 'wise mind'?", the therapist says, "How do I know? Take it from me. I know these things." Just as effective is the opposite — admitting impotence. For example, in response to therapy-interfering behavior the therapist may say, "You have won. Maybe this therapy doesn't work for you." Or in discussing the treatment relationship, the therapist, may admit, "You can beat me if you wish. It isn't difficult. All you have to do is lie." When the patient has complained once again about the therapist's behavior or her own hopelessness, the response may be "Perhaps you need a better therapist than me." A certain element of calling the patient's bluff is evident in these examples. Like the cup of sand that contains a nugget of gold, the comment must include an element of truth. Irreverence is not a substitute for genuineness.

Concluding Comments

Reciprocity and irreverence must be woven together into a single stylistic fabric. Used exclusively or in an unbalanced manner, neither represents DBT. Reciprocity by itself is in danger of being too "sweet"; irreverence used alone is in danger of being too "mean." Reciprocity can be overused by the meek or guilty therapist; irreverence can be overused by the arrogant or angry therapist. In DBT, the styles must balance each other. Unfortunately, knowing this does not give precise guidelines for how to accomplish this blend. Although dialectical theory can guide you, only practice and a certain amount of certainty or self-confidence can produce the rapid movement and blending that DBT communication requires. Timing of your movements from style to style must be based on what is happening in the here and now of the therapy interaction. You need to keep an eye both on what is happening and what is needed — where you are now and where you are going.

Irreverence is usually riskier in the short term. It can produce fireworks, sometimes when you least expect them. At other times, irreverence can produce a breakthrough after a long period of little progress. Reciprocity, while usually safer in the short run, can be risky in the long run. Like validation without change, it can fail to take the patient's dire situation seriously. In the same way that validation is blended with change strategies, reciprocity must be blended with irreverence. During some sessions, irreverence will predominate; during others, reciprocity will take precedence. As with any skill (including those you teach a patient), the craft is frequently in the timing. This can only be learned though experience.

Note

1. The irreverent communication style in DBT is very similar to the style of Carl Whitaker (see Whitaker, Felder, Malone, & Warkentin, 1962/1982, for a description; for an introduction to Whitaker's work in general, see Neill & Kniskern, 1982). Whitaker's style, at least as represented on the written page, is quite a bit stronger than that recommended here. The style is also similar to the use of paradoxical intention by some therapists.

13

Case Management Strategies: Interacting with the Community

Case management strategies have to do with how the therapist reacts to and interacts with the environment outside the patient–therapist relationship. These strategies focus on how the therapist responds to other professionals (including other consultants to the patient, as well as consultants to the therapist); family members and significant others of the patient; and other individuals making day-to-day environmental demands on the patient. Case management strategies do not involve any brand-new treatment strategies. Instead, they provide guidelines for how to apply dialectical, validation, and problem-solving strategies to case management problems. There are three sets of case management strategies that balance one another: consultation-to-the-patient strategies, environmental intervention strategies, and therapist supervision/consultation strategies.

"Case management" refers to helping the patient manage her physical and social environment so that her overall life functioning and well-being are enhanced, her progress toward life goals is facilitated, and her treatment progress is expedited. Thus, whenever problems or obstacles in the environment interfere with the patient's functioning or progress, the therapist moves to the case management strategies. With a borderline patient, problems often arise when other professionals or agencies are engaged in ancillary medical or psychological treatment with the patient. The therapist as case manager helps the patient manage interactions with other professionals or agencies, as well as cope with problems of survival in the everyday world.

Within the case manager role, issues of autonomy versus dependence, freedom versus security, control versus helplessness are central. Generally, the emphasis in traditional case management (and in DBT's environmental intervention strategies) is on interventions by the therapist in the patient's environment. The case manager from this point of view is the systems coordinator and service broker. In DBT, the bias is toward teaching the patient to be her own case manager (the consultation-to-the-patient strategies). Thus, consultation to the patient is the dominant form of case management, balanced when necessary by traditional intervention oriented case management strategies. The environmental intervention strategies are used when, because of characteristics of the environment or the patient's abilities, the consultation strategies are clearly unworkable and inappropriate.

From the perspective of managing the therapist, case management has to do with helping the therapist apply the DBT protocol in a skillful and effective manner. Supervision and consultation in DBT are designed to keep the therapist in the DBT frame, so to speak, no matter how strong the temptation to break the frame may be. In settings with multiple caregivers, the supervision/consultation team meets to coordinate and exchange information. The team provides the therapeutic community within which the treatment is delivered, and balances the therapist in his or her interactions with the patient.

Put most simply, the environmental intervention strategies involve taking care of the patient, conveying information about the patient to others on the patient's behalf, giving others advice on how to treat the patient, and intervening in her environment to make changes. The consultation-to-the-patient strategies involve assisting the patient in accomplishing these same tasks for herself—taking care of herself, conveying information about herself to others, advising others on what she needs and wants, and making changes in her own environment. The therapist supervision/consultation strategies involve exchanging information about patients therapists are treating jointly, taking care of one another, giving one another advice on treatment planning, and consulting with one another in how to make beneficial changes in the treatment environment.

In each set of strategies, treatment coordination across settings and providers is valued. In each set of strategies, inclusion of the family and social network in the therapeutic work is welcomed and encouraged. In each set of strategies, the safety, welfare, and long-term progress of the patient are paramount. What differs is the way the therapist goes about reaching these goals in each case.

It is extremely important to keep in mind the spirit of the case management strategies—teaching the patient to manage her own life (including her social and health care network) effectively in an environment that is not unnecessarily risky or unsafe. Decisions about how the therapist should interact with others flow from the spirit rather than the letter of the law. It is especially difficult to ascertain ahead of time all of the potential difficulties in situations where they might come up. Indeed, a significant function of the therapist supervision/consultation strategies is to assist the therapist in the balance of the other two sets of strategies in each particular instance.

ENVIRONMENTAL INTERVENTION STRATEGIES

Although the main goal of DBT is to get the patient active in solving her own life problems (the basis of the consultation-to-the-patient strategies), at times an issue is so important and/or the patient's ability to intervene on her own behalf is so limited that intervention by the therapist is necessary. Environmental intervention strategies are used instead of consultation-to-the-patient strategies when (1) the outcome is essential and (2) the patient clearly does not have the power or the capability to produce the outcome. "Essential" in this context generally means avoiding substantial harm to the patient. The environmental intervention strategies are also sometimes needed when the environment has high power relative to the patient; in such a case, the therapist may step in to equalize the power distribution.

The rule in DBT is that direct or unilateral interventions by the therapist should be kept to the absolute minimum consistent with the well-being of the patient. The therapist intervenes *only* when the harm to the patient of not intervening outweighs the harm (short- and long-term) of intervening on her behalf. Furthermore, when the therapist does actively intervene, the degree of unilateral intervention should be at the lowest level possible. Thus, when the therapist is consulting with other professionals or family members, the patient not only should be present but should be encouraged to be as active as possible in the consultation. If the patient cannot be present but the intervention is nonetheless absolutely necessary, a complete summary of the intervention should be given to her as soon as possible. It goes without saying that whenever possible, the patient should be informed about the intervention before it takes place. Indeed, except in emergencies where there is a risk of suicide, serious self-injury, or violence to others, the patient *must* give informed consent before interventions take place.

Case Management and Observing Limits

In many settings, it is usual for patients to have both a case manager and a psychotherapist. In these settings, most of the case management interventions can and should be conducted by the case manager rather than by other therapists on the treatment team. If a large amount of such assistance is necessary in other settings, the therapist might want to consider with the patient the possibilities for obtaining a case manager. When the patient has a designated case manager, the role of other therapists, including the primary therapist, is to assist the patient in using those services appropriately. Although it is appropriate in DBT for the individual therapist also to perform tasks traditionally associated with case management, the personal limits on time and energy of the therapist will probably constrict the therapist's own abilities here.

Conditions Mandating Environmental Intervention

Intervening When the Patient Is Unable to Act on Her
Own Behalf and the Outcome Is Very Important

At times the patient is unable to act in her own best interest, no matter how well she is coached. The patient who is in a transient psychotic state or unconscious from a drug overdose is an example. Or a problem situation may require so many new behaviors, that principles of shaping dictate that the patient act for herself and the therapist act for her also. An adolescent patient in our program had been making very slow but very steady progress. She was suddenly accused of a particularly humiliating crime—which as far as we could tell, she did not commit. When her foster parents, whom she depended on, believed that she committed the crime and asked her to move out, she dissociated, depersonalized, and became extremely suicidal. Her history in such situations was to cope by cutting herself, sometimes to such an extent that she needed up to 100 sutures. She agreed to go onto a psychiatric inpatient unit rather than harm herself, but otherwise was in apparent psychological shock. To assure timely admission, the therapist consulted directly with the admissions coordinator, giving needed information for a decision about admission and placement. The plan was that the patient would use the hospital stay to integrate the crisis and find a residential treatment home to move to. Once admitted, however, the patient withdrew and would not talk at all to the staff members, who did not know about the events leading up to the crisis. They were at a loss as to how to help her. The therapist intervened and consulted by phone (with the patient's permission, but not in her presence) with the staff about the patient. The therapist continued to interact intermittently with inpatient staff by phone until the patient could begin intervening on her own behalf.

At times a patient may be admitted to an emergency room in a coma, or in substantial medical danger or risk. Knowing the patient's medications can be crucial. The therapist provides needed information if the patient cannot, and validates (or corrects) information the patient has given about herself, her medications, and her treatment course.

Intervening When the Environment Is Intransigent and High in Power

At times the problem is an intransigent, high-power environment. For example, mental health professionals are often unwilling to modify their treatment of a patient unless a high-power person intervenes, no matter how skilled the patient may be at interacting with them. At the beginning of our treatment program, I had to call most hospitals in the metropolitan Seattle area to let them know that yes, what the patients said was true. I did expect patients to get a pass to come to therapy even when they were on an inpatient unit. And, yes, it was true that if they missed 4 weeks of scheduled therapy in a row they were out of our treatment program.

Similarly, insurance companies may be unwilling to pay for therapy without a diagnosis and treatment plan from a therapist, no matter how skilled the patient is in her interactions with the insurance company. Public assistance programs may require therapist reports to maintain benefits. Therapist referral phone calls, and consultations with the admitting officer, can be very useful (and sometimes necessary), in getting a patient admitted to an acute psychiatric unit. A scared inpatient staff may be ready to commit a suicidal patient involuntarily to the state hospital even when it is not in the best interest of the patient, unless the therapist intervenes.

Intervening to Save the Life of the Patient or Avoid Substantial Risk to Others

Closely related to a patient's inability to intervene on her own behalf is a patient's unwillingness to do so. Although a therapist does not usually intervene in these cases, when there is substantial risk of harm to the patient (such as high risk for suicide), the therapist may actively intervene to safeguard the patient. Similarly, as in all therapies, the therapist must intervene if the patient poses significant risk to the welfare of a child or another person. State laws, and professional guidelines and ethical standards, must be adhered to. Interventions to prevent suicide are discussed in greater detail in Chapter 15 and are not discussed further here.

Intervening When It Is the Humane Thing to Do and Will Cause No Harm

At times a problem is a blend of a intransigent environment and temporary patient inability. For instance, a patient is on her way to therapy and her car unexpectedly breaks down. The car problem cannot be fixed immediately. The patient has no money with her for a bus or cab. She is unable to find alternative transportation in time to make her appointment. She calls the therapist, who has time and goes and picks her up. The rule here is that the therapist does for the patient what he or she might do for any friend in a similar situation, as long as this does not entail helping the patient substitute passive for active problem-solving behaviors. In contrast to typical psychotherapy, but similar to most forms of case management, DBT does not dictate that interventions be confined to a therapist's office. Instead, the therapist may intervene by going to a patient's home during a crisis, the roadside if her car breaks down, or the housing authority if she needs a coach to guide her through the administrative complexity of this agency.

However, when the problem is a lack of abilities the patient needs to learn, the therapist only intervenes in exceptional circumstances (not everyday crises). That is, the therapist does not intervene on a regular basis. An ability to tolerate the patient's distress and mishaps until she acquires requisite skills is, therefore, necessary. When the problem is the patient's lack of abilities that are either not possible to obtain (such as learning to get insurance companies to pay without a therapist's report) or not reasonable or necessary (such as learning to get broken down cars going), the therapist intervenes.

Intervening When the Patient Is a Minor

DBT has not been used by my treatment team for treating patients younger than 15 years. For a minor, both legal and practical considerations can require that the therapist suspend the role of consultant to the patient under certain circumstances. In particular, it may be very important to work with parents, guardians, or teachers of a minor patient. Although the usual policy in DBT is to intervene with the patient present, this may not be practical or always useful with a very young adolescent. Even when the minor is present, it may be necessary for the therapist to be far more active than the patient. Finally, legal requirements for reporting child abuse generally require that the therapist intervene and contact authorities in all instances of such abuse.

Specific environmental intervention strategies are described below and listed in Table 13.1.

1. PROVIDING INFORMATION INDEPENDENTLY OF THE PATIENT

Providing information to others is one of the most common forms of environmental intervention in the mental health community. Medical records, intake and discharge summaries, and test results are routinely sent to other professionals treating a patient. Phone consultations to plan therapy, to coordinate benefits, or to get advice in a crisis are more or less routine in most treatment settings. the crucial thing to remember in any therapy, including DBT is that information should be given on a need-to-know bases only. Confidential and personal details of therapy, private confidences, and information that would embarrass or humiliate a patient if made public should be kept confidential. Pejorative descriptions, motivational inferences without supporting data, and other characterizations of the patient that might have a negative influence on others' attitudes towards the patient should be strictly avoided.

2. PATIENT ADVOCACY

In patient advocacy, the therapist acts on behalf of the patient to arrange an outcome favorable to the patient or to influence others' treatment of the patient. Examples include sending required treatment rationales and progress reports to maintain the patient's medical benefits; calling insurance companies to work out billing problems; advocating the patient's acceptance into a treatment or residential program; working to keep the patient off involuntary treatment status (or on such status); getting her released from an inpatient program; and the like. Advocacy is done only when absolutely necessary.

TABLE 13.1. Environmental Intervention Strategies Checklist

____ T intervenes when P is unable to act for herself and outcome is very important.

     ____ T arranges psychiatric hospitalization for P when necessary.

     ____ T gives necessary information to inpatient staff to support immediate hospitalization and to implement treatment plan congruent with DBT outpatient treatment.

____ T intervenes when environment is intransigent and high in power.

     ____ T writes letters, makes phone calls required to maintain insurance, disability benefits, admission to collateral treatment programs, etc.

     ____ T intervenes to keep P from being involuntarily committed to alternative treatment or inpatient treatment.

____ T intervenes to save P's life or avoid high risk to others.

     ____ When appropriate, T notifies P's family when P is at risk for suicide, T does not keep suicidal risk confidential.

     ____ T notifies appropriate agency if P is abusing or neglecting children or elderly individuals, or is threatening bodily harm to a specific individual; T complies with laws concerning protection of other individuals.

     ____ T intervenes when it is the humane thing to do (e.g., goes and picks P up for a session when P's car breaks down) and will cause no harm.

____ T intervenes as above if P is a minor, but with due regard for parent's or guardian's rights.

____ T PROVIDES INFORMATION about P to other professionals on a need-to-know basis.

     ____ T keeps information that would unnecessarily embarrass or humiliate P confidential.

____ T ADVOCATES for P.

____ T ENTERS into P's environment to assist her.

     ____ T observes own limits on case management duties.

Anti-DBT tactics

____ T intervenes only because it is easier or to save time.

____ T fails to assess actual capabilities of P.

____ T fails to assess environmental demands.

____ T uses pejorative descriptions, motivational inferences without supporting data, and other negative characterizations of P when communicating to others about P.

3. ENTERING THE PATIENT'S ENVIRONMENT TO GIVE HER ASSISTANCE

Many borderline individuals live very isolated lives; they often have difficulty building and sustaining a supportive interpersonal network. They may not have family members nearby, or relationships with nearby family members may be severely strained. Friends may be few or unable to provide useful assistance when needed. Not uncommonly, a patient is unable to find anyone other than the therapist to call on for help in a crisis. In these cases, the therapist can reach out and directly help the patient if conditions discussed above are met. For example, the therapist may at times take the patient to the emergency room or hospital if she is severely suicidal; may go with her to assist with specific tasks when the patient is so phobic of the task that she cannot do it alone; or may give her a ride home after therapy if she misses the last bus.

At times the patient needs more than advice and coaching from afar, but is not incapable of working on her own behalf. As Kanter (1988) has put it, the case manager (here, the DBT therapist) sometimes functions not only as a "travel guide" but also as a "travel companion" to ease the loneliness of the patient. The loneliness that DBT seeks to ease is the loneliness of active problem solving without ready access to help should the need arise. Thus, the therapist sometimes goes with the patient to give moral support. The model for this approach in behavior therapy is in vivo exposure treatment, where the therapist ordinarily accompanies the patient in her attempts to enter fearful situations within her everyday environment. As I have noted earlier in this book, the DBT therapist often sticks to the patient like glue, whispering encouragement and advice in her ear. It is important, however, to keep clear the difference between coaching and giving moral support, and taking over for the patient. The latter is done only in exceptional circumstances.

CONSULTATION-TO-THE-PATIENT STRATEGIES

Consultation-to-the-patient strategies are simple in concept and very hard to carry out. The concept is this: The primary role of the DBT therapist is to consult with the patient about how to interact effectively with her environment, rather than to consult with the environment on how to interact effectively with the patient. The borderline individual is the patient, not the system or network. The therapist therefore functions as a *consultant to the patient* rather than to the patient's network. For problems the patient has with her network, the therapist engages in problem solving with the patient; the network is then left for the patient to manage.

With some exceptions, health professionals providing ancillary treatment to DBT patients are viewed much as other persons in the patient's life are viewed. In my experience, this aspect of DBT—the style of interactions with ancillary professionals—is one of the most innovative aspects of the treatment. It can be difficult to implement because it is counter to how health professionals are trained to treat health problems. Most communities devote a fair amount of their health care resources to trying to coordinate and integrate treatment for individuals in the health care system. DBT is not opposed to this view; in general, coordinated care is probably better care. The difference is in how DBT views its own role in coordinating care.

In this section, I first discuss the rationale or spirit of the consultation-to-the-patient strategies in general. Next, I outline specific consultation strategies. Finally, I discuss more explicitly the arguments against the consultation approach and the reasons why this approach was chosen nonetheless over the more standard approach to consulting with the medical and mental health community. I hope to convince you to give this approach a try.

Rationale and Spirit of Consultation to the Patient

The consultation-to-the-patient approach was chosen with three objectives in mind: (1) to teach patients to manage their own lives; (2) to decrease instances of "splitting" between DBT therapists and other individuals interacting with the patients; and (3) to encourage respect for the patients.

Teaching Effective Self-Care

The first consideration was to have a policy that would function as the opposite pole to borderline patients' preference for avoidance of problem solving. Frequently, these patients use indirect over direct means of interpersonal influence. They not infrequently try to get their therapists to intervene for them in interpersonal difficulties. The consultation strategies are geared toward consistently requiring active solutions by patients. This seems essential, since therapists cannot solve all environmental problems encountered now or in the future by their patients.

There are two competing needs here. On the one side is the need for information by all individuals treating or interacting with a patient. Health professionals, as well as family members, work associates, and friends, will all respond more effectively to a patient they know and understand. The therapist's providing of information increases understanding of the patient. On the other side is the patient's need to learn to interact effectively with other individuals (including health professionals), to take care of and for herself, and to increase her own abilities and self-confidence. The consultation strategies target this. Thus, in DBT the therapist is willing to let the patient suffer some of the short-term negative consequences of ineffective self-care for the sake of long-term improvement in self-care. When the immediate consequences of the consultation strategies would be too severe, the therapist switches to the environmental intervention strategies.

Implicit in this approach is a belief in the patient's capacities to learn to interact effectively. In DBT, the patient is the responsible party in interactions with others. The approach is based on the belief that the therapist's job is to help the patient cope with the world *as it is,* with all its problems and inequities—not to change it for the patient. Rather than intervening for the patient in solving problems or getting what the patient needs or wants, the therapist teaches and coaches the patient in how to resolve problems and get what she wants and needs. Adversity and "bad" treatment of the patient by the environment are viewed as opportunities for practice and learning: in other words, lemons are used for making lemonade. The patient is taught to "manage" the environment, not to submit passively to it.

Decreasing "Splitting"

The phenomenon of "splitting" occurs with regularity in the lives of borderline patients. Splitting occurs when different individuals in a patient's network are at odds over how to interact with or respond to her. Parents may be split; for example, one parent may want to continue giving the patient free room and board, while the other insists that the patient start paying her share of household expenses. Friends may be split, with some believing that others are behaving in mean-spirited or destructive ways. The patient's women friends may blame her spouse or partner for her troubles, and vice versa. In "staff splitting," health professionals treating the same patient not only disagree about treatment methods and priorities, but do so vehemently. (This is discussed in more detail later in the chapter.)

The consultation-to-the-patient approach was developed to reduce splitting. By remaining in the role of a consultant to the patient, the therapist avoids becoming entangled in the often contradictory positions taken by others involved with the patient. Disagreements on how to respond to the patient are viewed as opportunities for the patient to learn how to stand up for and think for herself, to integrate divergent advice, and generally to take responsibility for her own life and welfare. By staying out of arguments about how others should respond to the patient, the DBT therapist avoids taking part in and contributing to splitting.

Promoting Respect for the Patient

Finally, the consultation approach promotes respect for the patient and her capabilities, which is consistent with the stance of DBT in general. The message sent to the patient is that she is a credible source of information and can intervene effectively in her own behalf within her own social and health network. Although it is not unusual for "experts" to consult with one another about cases they are working on (whether the area is education, law, medicine or psychotherapy), such consultation, when conducted in the absence of the person involved in the case, sends one of several messages. It may imply that the means of achieving the individual's goal is too complex for her to understand, that the individual's opinions and wishes are not necessarily important, or that the individual's input is not trusted. The consultation strategies consistently suggest that the patient's wishes and opinions about her own welfare are to be trusted. The approach includes teaching, with one aim being to demystify the process of behavioral and psychological change so that the patient can become a better advocate in her own behalf.

The "Treatment Team" versus "Everyone Else"

There are several variations on the consultation-to-the-patient approach. The variations depend primarily on whether the person needing information or consultation is a part of the therapy team or not. In principle, all ancillary therapists can become part of the DBT treatment team. The only requirements for a therapist's being on the DBT team are these: (1) The patient agrees; (2) the therapist agrees to apply DBT principles to treatment; and (3) the therapist attends regular DBT supervision/consultation meetings. DBT was developed as an outpatient treatment provided in a research clinic where all therapists were committed to providing DBT. This setting is duplicated in inpatient and outpatient units where a special DBT treatment program (or program within a program) is instituted. It is duplicated when a small group of practitioners provides joint treatment for a number of borderline patients (e.g., one or more therapists provide individual psychotherapy but then coordinate with one or more other therapists who provide skills training). And, it is duplicated in settings where solo practitioners treat borderline patients but then meet regularly with colleagues for DBT supervision/consultation. In settings where a patient is treated by a team, but only one or a few of the team members are applying DBT, the consultation strategies probably cannot be applied as strictly as I describe them here unless all members of the team can be persuaded to go along with the DBT case management philosophy, at least.

By definition, members of the treatment team consult among themselves on a regular basis, exchanging information about the patient, as well as their reactions to and interactions with the patient. By definition, people outside of the team (i.e., everyone else) do not share information on a regular basis. Members of the team are treated like family members. All have agreed to confidentiality rules, and all are interested in applying the same treatment principles to patients and therapists alike. Information given will be interpreted in a reasonably predictable way. Nonmembers of the team are treated like friends. They are not assumed to be applying the same rules to the patient as the DBT team, nor is it clear how shared information will be interpreted and used. Although the general principles and philosophy of the consultation-to-the-patient approach are the same for the DBT team and everyone else, the specific strategies differ. These differences are important.

Specific consultation strategies are listed in Table 13.2 and are described below.

I. ORIENTING THE PATIENT AND THE NETWORK TO THE APPROACH

When first introduced in Seattle, the consultation-to-the-patient approach was quite controversial within the local community. A fair amount of community orientation was needed, and the idea took some getting used to. Both a patient and members of her network must be oriented to the consultation approach. The first time the therapist refuses to intervene for the patient, the therapist and patient should discuss why this is being done and how treating the patient like a competent person will, in the long run, be in her best interest. An irreverent style—irreverence about the patient's presumed fragility or incompetence to manage—can be very useful here. A patient is often afraid

TABLE 13.2. Consultation-to-the-Patient Strategies Checklist

____ T ORIENTS P and other professionals to consultation approach.

____ T CONSULTS with P about how to interact with OTHER PROFESSIONALS; T does not intervene to adjust P's treatment environment (see Table 13.1 for exceptions).

    ____ T gives other general information about treatment program, philosophy of treatment, program limits, and so on.

        ____ T speaks for himself or herself, not for P.

____ Outside of the treatment team, T discusses P only when P is present.

    ____ T asks P to arrange phone or in-person consultations when necessary.

    ____ T coaches P at case conferences; T encourages and helps P to arrange such conferences.

    ____ T collaborates with P in writing reports and letters about P.

____ Within the treatment team, T obtains and gives information about P to guide treatment planning.

    ____ Even though P is not present at team meetings, T keeps the spirit of the strategy and does not do for P what she can do for herself.

____ T actively refrains from telling other professionals how to treat P.

    ____ T tells other professionals or agencies to "Follow your usual policies" and then consults with P.

____ T helps P act as her own agent in handling treatment planning issues with professionals outside the DBT team (as well as agencies and with persons in authority):

    ____ Making appointments with ancillary caregivers.

    ____ Getting appropriate medications, getting medication consultations, getting inappropriate medications changed, getting refills, etc.

    ____ Interacting effectively with psychiatric inpatient staff in order to be admitted, be discharged, get passes to come to skills training and individual DBT, get treatment plans changed.

    ____ Avoiding involuntary commitment.

    ____ Getting emergency care when T is unavailable.

____ T does not intervene or solve interpersonal problems for P with other professionals.

    ____ T consults with P about how to solve problems with other members of DBT treatment team and with ancillary professionals.

____ T does not defend (or unjustly accuse) other professionals.

    ____ T accepts responsibility for his or her own behavior, not for behavior of other members of the team; T does not stand in for other therapists with P.

    ____ T accepts that all therapists make mistakes.

____ T helps P to intervene in her own treatment community when other treatments prove ineffective or iatrogenic.

____ T handles calls from others concerning crises with P as a consultant, not as a case manager; T does not speak for P in P's absence.

    ____ T gives general information, obtains risk-related information from caller, and consults with P to develop effective response.

____ T coaches P at case conferences; T helps P to arrange such conferences.

(cont.)

Table 13.2. (cont.)

____ T CONSULTS with P about best way to respond to FAMILY AND FRIENDS, especially about therapy-related issues.

    ____ T gives family members or friends who call general information and obtains risk-related information from them, but does not give out information about P.

    ____ T holds family sessions with P, as appropriate.

        ____ T coaches P but does not speak for her.

        ____ T provides information to family members about treatment, theory of BPD, etc.

        ____ T helps family validate P.

Anti-DBT tactics

____ T defends other professionals working with P, or otherwise intervenes on *their* behalf.

____ T treats P as overly fragile.

____ T treats P as overly manipulative.

that she will be thrown to the wolves and left to fend for herself. Consultation is not that; the therapist will be right next to the patient every step of the way. This orientation may have to be repeated a number of times.

With other professionals, the best policy for the therapist is simply to attribute his or her stance to the rules of the therapy, and to explain to them the consultation approach. I generally say something like this: I am applying a specific therapy, which requires that whenever possible, I teach the patient to intervene for herself rather than doing it for her. I may point out that borderline patients often have enormous difficulty interacting effectively in the health system. Because of that, I am focusing my energy on teaching the patient how to be more effective. I point out that I am very willing (and, indeed, may be eager) to consult with another professional with the patient present.

The trick is to get the other professionals to see that it is in their long-term best interest for the therapist to work with the patient instead of with them. In my experience, once community professionals get used to this policy, they don't mind. It takes some getting used to, however, and the other professionals need a bit of validation along the way. With recalcitrant professionals, a therapist may occasionally have to abandon the consultation strategies and move to the environmental intervention strategies.

2. CONSULTATION TO THE PATIENT ABOUT HOW TO MANAGE OTHER PROFESSIONALS

The essence of consultation to the patient is this: The role of the therapist is to consult with the patient about how to manage other people, rather than to consult with others about how to manage or treat the patient. The task of each DBT therapist is to help the patient interact more effectively with all members of her interpersonal network, including other medical and mental health professionals—whether they are members of the DBT treatment team, or ancillary therapists treating the patient. As a general rule (and with the exceptions described earlier), a DBT therapist does not intervene to adjust the environment, including the treatment the patient received from other professionals, for the sake of the patient. In sum, this strategy is a prescription ("Tell the patient what to do with professionals") and a proscription ("Do not tell other professionals what to do with the patient") coupled together. There are several; corollary strategies or general rules that flow from this one strategy, as follows.

Corollary 1: Give other professionals general information about the treatment program. Consultation to the patient does not preclude the therapist from giving to other people general information about DBT, the therapist's philosophy of treatment, the therapist's individual or program limits, and behavioral principles underlying DBT. Although the therapist does not speak for the patient, the therapist can and does speak for himself or herself and for the program as a whole. On the phone, by letter, or in joint meetings with other professionals and the patient, the therapist explains his or her own point of view.

Corollary 2: Outside of the treatment team, do not discuss the patient or her treatment without the patient present. With the exceptions discussed above under environmental intervention strategies, the therapist does not interact independently of the patient with individuals not on the DBT treatment team. That is, the therapist takes no part in phone conferences, sends no reports, and attends no meetings or case conferences without the engagement of the patient. Even when the patient gives permission and interchange with professionals is necessary, information is not shared unilaterally; the therapist and patient compose letters and reports collaboratively and attend meetings together. Any necessary call to ancillary therapists or other persons involved with the patient is first discussed with the patient in the room during the consultation. A speaker phone is very useful here. When the therapist is coordinating backup care while he or she is out of town, the backup plan is developed with the patient, and the patient is given the task of calling the backup professional before the therapist leaves town to review the plan. Typically, of course, the therapist (after consulting with the patient) will have made prior arrangements with colleagues for backup coverage. Depending on the patient, the therapist may also want to double-check the backup plan with his or her colleague before leaving.

Therapists and staff members do not ordinarily write courtesy or referral letters introducing their patients. It is assumed that a patient can introduce and speak for herself. If such a letter is necessary or useful, the patient and therapist write the letter jointly. Information that needs to be given to the new professional is transmitted through the patient. It is presumed that the patient can summarize her problems, treatment to date, and current needs, at least with coaching from the DBT team. If she cannot speak for herself, a joint meeting with the patient present is arranged.

Corollary 3: Within the treatment team, share information but keep the spirit of the strategy. All DBT therapists working with a particular patient meet weekly in the supervision/consultation team to review and discuss the patient's progress. The patient is not present. A primary goal of these meetings is to share information that can then be used in working with the patient, and to obtain treatment consultation based on this shared information. In these instances, the entire team is considered the therapeutic unit (even if only one therapist is actually meeting with the patient). Information is gathered from all parts so that the unit as a whole can teach the patient. The consultation-to-the-patient approach is violated in this context when the therapist does for the patient what the patient can (or can learn to) do for herself. Information is shared to guide treatment planning, not to communicate for the patient.

Corollary 4: Do not tell other professionals how to treat the patient. Except as required by the environmental intervention strategies (see above), the patient serves as her own intermediary between the treatment team and ancillary professionals and other individuals in her network, as well as between the therapist and all other individuals. With ancillary professionals, the DBT therapist's usual response for treatment guidance is some variation of the comment "Follow your usual procedures." Within the treatment team, the therapist may assist other team members in thinking through various treatment options, and may provide information about the patient that will be useful in this planning, but in the final analysis, the advice is still the same: "Follow your usual DBT procedures."

This rule is followed even when the ancillary treatment may have a significant impact on the therapist's treatment. Here is an example. A patient in DBT is learning assertion skills in the interpersonal effectiveness skills training module. The patient has great difficulty standing up for herself; she is either very aggressive or very passive. Her individual therapist will not accept calls after 9 P.M. at home. The patient works until 8:30 P.M. and doesn't get home until after 9. She wants her therapist to change the cutoff time to 9:30. She has already tried demanding and verbal aggression, to no avail. She comes to skills training complaining about her therapist. The skills trainer works with her on developing a more skillful approach. The patient agrees to try it at her next therapy session. The trainer fervently wants her new, more skillful behavior to be reinforced. At a supervision/consultation meeting before the individual therapist's session with the patient, how does the skills trainer apply the consultation approach?

The most important factor here is the skills trainer's attitude toward the individual therapist. At the meeting, it would be appropriate to share with the team what is being covered in skills training. The skills trainer could even share the work with the individual patient and her homework assignment (although this might be a bit marginal). The trainer might also share his or her hopes that the patient will be reinforced if she uses new skills. But the key is in the attitude that no matter what happens, the skills trainer will assist the patient in coping with the situation. The individual therapist's job in this instance is to represent society. The skills trainer's job is to teach the patient to cope with society. If she asks skillfully and gets reinforced, she learns that skilled behavior is more useful than demanding and aggressive behavior. If she does not get reinforced, she has a chance to learn that even perfect behavior is not always reinforced in the everyday world. Which is the more important lesson? It is not clear, since both are crucial.

Let us say that the patient comes to the next skills training session and says that before she even completed her request, the individual therapist cut her off, said no abruptly, and refused to negotiate. The skills trainer's task now is to help the patient analyze her own behavior and the other person's as objectively as possible, and figure out how to cope with this turn of events. At the next team meeting, how does the trainer apply the consultation approach? The role of information exchange in this instance is to get the individual therapist's perspective—not in order to decide who is right, but in order to help the patient fine-tune her strategy. The objective is for the skills trainer to obtain the information he or she might have obtained from actually attending the individual session. It is an approximation of having a camera trained on the interaction, except (and this is very important) that instead of a camera the skills trainer has the prism of the individual therapist. DBT does not assume that patients distort and therapists do not.

In the next interaction with the patient, the skills trainer might share the information he or she has obtained about how the patient came across to the therapist or how the therapist saw it. Perhaps both saw the interaction similarly. Or maybe the therapist was having an "off" day, or perhaps the patient failed to realize that she made her request in the middle of discussing another important topic from which the therapist did not want to digress. Or perhaps the therapist felt that the patient once again presented her request in a very unskilled, demanding manner. Whatever the case, the skills trainer now has both sides of the story and can use that information (or not) in trying to help the patient improve her interactional style.

This rule can be particularly difficult, of course, when a therapist believes that another person's treatment of the patient is detrimental. But the belief in the patient in DBT is so strong that it dictates holding one's comments to another professional and assuming that the patient will be successful in modifying or stopping the detrimental treatment. For example, if another professional is inadvertently reinforcing maladaptive behaviors (a not infrequent occurrence), the DBT therapist teaches the patient to work with the other professional in making appropriate changes. Learning to be an informed and skillful consumer in the medical system is an important DBT goal. Because of its importance, this topic is discussed again below.

Corollary 5: Teach the patient to act as her own agent in obtaining appropriate care. An important role of the DBT therapist is to teach the patient how to obtain whatever professional care she may need. Thus, a therapist must teach the patient to evaluate her own needs, survey the available resources, contact those resources and ask for services, and evaluate the services she receives. For example, when a patient is admitted to an inpatient setting, it is her responsibility both to get a pass to come to individual and skills training sessions, and to keep enough control over her medication that she is not placed on medications she knows won't help (or are not allowed in her treatment program). The therapist should not call the inpatient staff (unless absolutely necessary, as described above), but should teach the patient how to be effective in that environment. The patient herself (perhaps with firm guidance from the DBT therapist) must work with the outpatient pharmacotherapist to limit undue access to potentially lethal drugs (see Chapter 15 for further discussion).

This principle appears deceptively simple. In practice, many of our cherished ways of treating patients must be rethought. Take the patient on an inpatient unit who cuts herself deeply. In DBT, the therapist or staff member does not call and arrange for a medical consultation (unless, of course, the patient is clearly unable to do so). Instead, the patient is instructed to call and make the appointment. The staff coaches; the patient calls. Therapists and staff members do not make appointments for patients with other professionals. It is assumed that adults are capable of making their own appointments. A therapist intervenes only when a patient is clearly unable to do so and the failure to make a timely appointment would lead to consequences more seriously negative than the positive learning the patient is engaged in.

Corollary 6: Do not intervene, solve problems, or act for the patient with other professionals. This corollary is the flip side of Corollary 5. If the patient serves as her own agent in resolving difficulties with other persons, including other medical and mental health professionals, then it stands to reason that the therapist should not intervene for her. If the patient is dissatisfied with an ancillary treatment she is receiving, or with another therapist, the therapist working with her at the moment helps her figure out how to communicate this effectively to the other professional. The therapist treats the patient as ultimately capable (with more or less skills training) of acting in her own behalf. For example, if a patient is having difficulties with one or more members of the treatment team, the therapist who knows about it does not go to the others and explain or try to solve the problem. Therapists do not serve as stand-ins for patients. For instance, "She is really angry at you, but is afraid to tell you. How could you have done that to her?" is not an acceptable communication. One can immediately see why this is easy in concept and difficult in practice. Humility is a requisite if this approach is not to go astray.

Corollary 7: Do not defend other professionals. Within the therapy team, consultation to the patient requires that each therapist accept responsibility only for his or her own behavior, and not for that of others. Thus, it is not the job of one therapist to defend another therapist to the patient. As in the real world, some people may interact with the patient better than others. All therapists make mistakes. Rules may change, depending on who is enforcing them. An assumption in DBT is that "bad" things patients think therapists do, they probably do. As noted earlier, the therapist does not intervene for the patient with other treatment professionals. The point here is that the therapist also does not intervene for other treatment professionals with the patient. That is, the therapist does not stand in for his or her professional colleagues.

The rule does not mean that one therapist cannot help the patient understand another better. Indeed, teaching the patient how to be effective with others often includes helping them develop an empathetic and understanding attitude. It also does not mean that one therapist cannot agree with another, even if the patient is furious at the other. For example, we had a patient in our clinic who had enormous difficulties with her skills training therapist, who in fact did make significant therapeutic mistakes. Once the mistakes were made, however, there seemed no way to repair the relationship. The patient not only became extremely abusive, but continued the abuse well after the end of skills training. The skills trainer finally cut off all contact. The patient then began calling me (as clinic director), imploring me to "make" her former skills trainer talk to her. My response was to validate the patient's distress, validate the trainer's right to observe her own limits, and assist the patient in problem-solving how she was going to handle this painful state of affairs.

Instances When Other Treatment Is Undermining Therapy

With the exceptions noted above under environmental intervention, the DBT therapist does not intervene with other professionals and try to get them to change ineffective or iatrogenic treatments or ones that don't fit with DBT. Instead, the response is to analyze the ancillary treatment situation with the patient and then set about teaching the patient how to intervene in her own treatment community. The first option should be to try to help the patient influence other professionals to change their treatment approach to her. If this fails, the option of terminating or changing to another professional or treatment program should be explored. Several examples may illustrate the point.

One patient in my clinic goes to emergency rooms whenever there is a crisis (which is often). Since she is usually threatening suicide, she almost always gets admitted. According to her, these admissions are against her wishes, although she admits that going into hospitals is a method of avoiding her problems. (Also, the food is very good.) Not only is the patient being reinforced for passive and suicidal behavior, but the frequent hospitalizations are so disruptive that she has lost three jobs and is now on public assistance. Her morale is decreasing further (along with ours), and therapy is going downhill. Can't I consult with the hospitals about developing new, more effective ways to handle her? No. Why not? Because even if I do get one hospital to adopt a more effective policy, in Seattle there are at least 10 reasonably good inpatient psychiatric units. If I "shape up" one, the patient may go to another. By the time I consult with all the hospitals, the patient may go back to the first, which will in all likelihood have a completely new staff; I will then have to go and consult there again. And what if the patient moves? Shall I follow her from city to city? No. It seems that it will be much easier if I just "shape up" the patient to manage ineffective hospital responses. The patient must learn how to consult with the hospital staff and how to refuse unnecessary hospital admissions. She and the hospital together need to work out a treatment plan—perhaps one in which she can go and talk to someone in an emergency, but cannot be reinforced for passive and suicidal behavior.

The consultation approach is also very effective at decreasing a therapist's own anger at other professionals, and at keeping attention and energy focused on helping the patient. I had an epileptic patient who was a long-time patient of a specialist in town. At times, the blood levels of her anticonvulsants would get too high or too low, and she would go to the emergency room. She was often admitted to a medical floor. Invariably the staff would start changing her medications from one to another, ignoring her statements that she did not do well on the new medication and her requests that they consult with her specialist. After discharge, it could take up to 3 weeks to get her back on her usual medications and stabilized again. It happened once more: She was admitted to a medical floor, and while talking to me on the phone told me that the staff was again changing her medications. My immediate emotional response was anger at the attending physician, primarily because I felt I was the one who had to "pick up the pieces" every time this happened. My first temptation was to call the attending physician and intervene. I was tired and impatient and wanted to stop the cycle. Calling, however, would have been a violation of the consultation approach. I soon realized that my task was not to change the people treating my patient (a task that felt overwhelming), but to change the patient (a task that felt much more manageable). My anger dropped to nothing. I called the patient back and told her (in a rather firm tone) that this time she simply had to refuse to let them change her medications without proper consultation. She was more of an expert on her own body at this point than they were. Although the consultation-to-the-patient approach took some time, it finally worked. The patient is now quite good at seeing that her medications are monitored correctly. The alert reader has probably noticed here that effective self-care for this patient meant that she needed to get one health professional to consult with another health professional. That is, she was trying to get her specialist to intervene with the attending physician—a good strategy.

What does the therapist do when it is a member of the DBT treatment team who is providing the nontherapeutic or destructive therapy? It is here that the therapist walks a delicate tightrope between the consultation-to-the-patient approach (not standing in for the patient or telling others how to treat the patient) and the therapist supervision/consultation approach (carrying out treatment planning and treatment modification as a group). The consultation-to-the-patient approach is biased toward exchanging with other therapists information about one's own treatment plan and goals, and the effects on the patient and your treatment goals of the other team members' treatment. The therapist supervision/consultation approach is biased toward searching for a synthesis between two or more treatment approaches.

Handling Crisis Calls

Calls from Professionals Outside the Treatment Team. Most health professionals are used to coordinating treatment for specific patients without the active involvement (although, of course, with the consent) of the patient. Crisis intervention teams, police and rescue squads, housing supervisors, residential counselors and case managers, and emergency room personnel sometimes take great pains to call an individual's psychotherapist to obtain guidance on how best to respond to the patient during a crisis. No matter what the situation, the DBT policy is the same: When professionals who are not members of the treatment team call, the therapist should (1) obtain as much information about the situation as they will give; (2) provide the callers with necessary information the patient cannot give, and verify (or correct) information the patient has given; (3) tell them to follow their normal procedures; and (4) ask to talk to the patient. The therapist then coaches the patient in how to best cope with the situation and interact with the professionals. (Again, the consultation approach is not applied if the patient is unable to cooperate and the outcome is important. For example, if the patient is unconscious or groggy, or too hostile to talk, the therapist gives necessary information about history, treatment, and medications.)

For example, my therapy unit sometimes uses space in a larger psychiatry clinic. One of our patients was constantly distracting the clinic staff members by engaging them in conversations they felt unable to break off and by occasionally acting in an overtly hostile manner in the waiting room, creating difficulties for other patients. The clinic director responded by sending me a series of notes complaining about "my" patient, indirectly suggesting that I should control the patient better. The clinic was not set up for this type of patient, and other patients were being harmed. I was more interested in keeping the patient alive, since suicide was a major risk at the time. Furthermore, I knew that the patient's behavior in the clinic was a considerable improvement over her previous behaviors in other clinics. The clinic responded to the patient by developing a series of (what seemed to me) repressive rules about permissible patient behavior. I responded by firing off my own series of complaining letters to the clinic director. Both of our tempers flared, and staff splitting emerged. Where was the mistake? The mistake was in my responding to the clinic director with anything other than "Follow your usual procedures and I will help the patient cope." I had protected the patient's fragility instead of strengthening her potential capability. Although a problem-solving meeting with the clinic director might have been useful, such a meeting should have been held with the patient present.

Calls from Members of the Treatment Team. Within the therapy team, the individual or primary therapist ordinarily handles crisis situations. Thus, all DBT collateral therapists should call the primary therapist for instructions on how to handle the patient if a crisis arises (unless clear procedures have already been worked out). In this instance, the primary therapist does not say, "Follow your usual procedures." Instead, the primary therapist gives instructions. Chapter 15 discusses this in greater detail.

Attending Case Conferences

The consultation-to-the-patient approach in no way proscribes coodinating treatment and attending case conferences about the patient. Treatment coordination with non-DBT ancillary therapists can sometimes be very useful, especially with therapists who will maintain a reasonably long-term relationship with the patient, such as case managers, inpatient attending physicians, or pharmacotherapists. It can also be extremely useful when therapy is "stuck," or when the patient is in crisis and is either on an inpatient unit or is going from therapist to therapist. The ideal situation is one in which the patient arranges for the case conference.

During the case conference, the therapist's primary tasks are to help the patient speak for herself and to share and obtain information. (This is usually not possible until after the therapist has oriented the network, however.) The therapist concentrates on helping the patient interact skillfully; unless absolutely necessary, he or she does not speak for the patient. The therapist is there as a coach, not a substitute player. The therapist does speak for himself or herself in explaining the treatment principles and plan, clarifying his or her own limits, and so on. The therapist at times must actively work to keep the patient collaboratively involved in the treatment discussion and planning. A patient's active passivity, and the traditional practices of many mental health professionals, can conspire to create an atmosphere where the patient can be present in body but left out in spirit.

3. CONSULTATION TO THE PATIENT ABOUT HOW TO HANDLE FAMILY AND FRIENDS

Family and friends can be important allies in treating borderline patients. Their support for the patient's staying in therapy is important. In my experience, invalidating families and friends often believe that people should be able to handle their problems, no matter how severe, without going to a therapist. In particular, parents are sometimes adamantly opposed to their children's participating in a treatment program. The acceptance of psychotherapy is quite different within different cultural and class backgrounds. Other families and friends may wish to be activelly involved in the treatment process. The therapist's primary role in each of these instances is to help the patient communicate effectively with her social network about her problems, her treatment, and her needs; to evaluate conflicting advice about treatment and problem solutions; and to make decisions for herself skillfully.

Calls from Family and Friends

An encounter that is often difficult for a therapist is a call of distress from family and friends (e.g., roommates) of the patient. Often they want advice from the therapist about what to do or how to handle general or specific problems with the patient. Sometimes they want a progress report on therapy or reassurance about the therapist's credentials. (This is especially likely when the person is a parent and/or is paying for the therapy.) Or they may be calling because of fears that the patient is going to commit suicide. The general principle here is that the therapist can get information (especially if the call is about suicide risk), can give information about himself or herself (e.g., credentials or experience), and can provide general information about DBT and BPD. However, the therapist does not give information about the patient or about therapy with the patient. The therapist can help callers cope with their own problems and feelings, but does not help them cope with the patient when the patient is not a party to the interaction.

Calls from family and friends must be handled with the utmost sensitivity. A cavalier or insensitive brushoff of family and friends by the therapist can harm rather than help a patient in her efforts to stay in therapy. Generally, it is best to make the point at the very beginning of each conversation that the therapist cannot share information about the patient. The therapist must make it clear that the refusal to share reflects on the nature of psychotherapy, not on characteristics of the caller.

Although the therapist may listen to the caller's difficulties, consultations with a patient's networks always include the patient. Thus, without the patient present the therapist can advise the caller how to get the consultation he or she needs, but not about how to help the patient. At times, the therapist may empathize with and reflect the emotional distress the family member or friend is communicating. The idea is to focus the conversation on the caller and on the therapist, not on the patient or on therapy.

The patient should be informed about the call, and the content of the conversation should be disclosed and discussed. The therapist's plan to do so, should have been disclosed to the caller.

Conducting Family Sessions

As noted earlier in this chapter, DBT has not been used in treating patients younger than 15. For an adolescent (especially an emancipated teenager), the patient's family is treated consistently with the consultation approach. If the therapist thinks that communication with the family might be helpful at times, it is advanced like any other solution to a problem — as something the patient must choose and implement. Family therapy sessions, however, are not inconsistent with DBT and may at times be prescribed (see Chapter 15). Sessions with family members without the patient present, however, are inconsistent with DBT. This means that although the therapist helps the patient understand the reactions of significant others, the therapist's contract is always with the patient, not with the others. During a meeting with family members or significant others, the therapist also helps the participants adopt a better understanding of and more validating attitude toward the patient. The DBT theory is advanced, and the need for validation and skill building is discussed.

Arguments Against the Consultation Approach

The consultation-to-the-patient approach in DBT is quite different from, and sometimes diametrically opposite to, the behaviors expected of mental health professionals. Furthermore, it is undeniably time-consuming. It also appears inconsistent, at least at face value, with a systems (including a dialectical systems) approach. These arguments are discussed below, together with my counterarguments for maintaining the consultation approach.

Mores of Psychotherapy

Psychotherapists are expected to exchange information routinely with their colleagues about patients' history, diagnoses, medications, treatment response, current status, and any other information that would help the professionals currently treating the patients. Even when patients are capable of speaking up for themselves and intervening on their own behalf, however, therapists are ordinarily still expected to provide information and consult with other health professionals treating the patients. Therapeutic mores are lightly disregarded in DBT. The divergence between DBT and usual practices is based on two lines of argument, one clinical and one empirical.

Clinical Argument. The mores of collegial behavior in psychotherapy are based on the model of medical treatment. Case consultation and provision of referral information are necessary in medicine because the average patient seeing a physician is not competent to convey complex medical information accurately to a new physician. When a patient with a history of heart ailments is taken to the emergency room, it may be of life-and-death importance that the physician know the individual's medical history and current medications.

The problem arises in transferring the rules of medical treatment for physical disorders to psychosocial treatment for behavioral disorders. Although patients may not be able to give a coherent review of their heart or liver functioning, most individuals, including borderline patients in psychotherapy, can give a quite coherent account of their behavioral functioning. To the extent that psychotherapy is collaborative, one would also expect psychotherapy patients to be able to give a reasonable account of their current treatment plan, although patients are rarely experts here. When the goal is enhancing an individual's abilities to control her own behavior and influence her own destiny, however, the situation is different: Either the patient is the best expert on her own behavior or she should be. The consultation-to-the-patient approach is designed to make sure that if the individual is not the expert on herself now, she becomes the expert.

Of course, at times a patient cannot give such an account and may even purposely distort information to obtain the treatment she wants. And, as noted above, when the immediate outcome is very important and the patient is unable or unwilling to intervene effectively for herself, the therapist should move from the consultation strategies to the environmental intervention strategies. In my clinical experience, however, many therapists and treatment settings underestimate the capabilities of patients and overestimate borderline individuals' tendency to distort and manipulate communications to meet their own wishes. Too often, too much is done for a patient. The borderline individual is often treated as more fragile or more manipulative than she is. A therapist intervenes when the patient can and should intervene effectively for herself. A consistent comment from the borderline patients in our program is that a very therapeutic part of the treatment is our belief in the patients' capabilities when others (including the patient) frequently do not believe. We trust them when many accuse them.

Empirical Argument. The strongest argument for adopting the consultation-to-the-patient strategies recommended in DBT is the empirical evidence that the DBT model of treatment, including this group of strategies, is an effective one. Although the consultation strategies may have been irrelevant to the treatment outcome, it is not inconsequential that the treatment as a whole has been found to be effective. At the moment, I know of no empirical data indicating that the strategies are detrimental or ineffective.

Time Demands on Health Professionals

The consultation approach can be quite time-consuming. Often it is easier to do something for another person than it is to walk her step by step through doing it for herself. A useful analogy is to compare the therapist to a parent in a hurry in the grocery store with a child just learning to walk: It is often easier to pick the child up and carry her than to wait for her every tentative step. Teaching sometimes requires infinite patience. Taking care *of* is often easier than taking care *for*. Although the DBT bias is toward taking the time necessary, at times the therapist has to be practical and pick the person up.

For example, a patient may go to an emergency room, threaten suicide, and say that she needs immediate hospitalization. Knowing that the patient has been repeatedly hospitalized under similar circumstances in the past without benefit can be important in deciding whether to hospitalize her now.

Taking an extensive history may be difficult in the emergency room setting; certainly, it is easier and quicker if the patient or the therapist can give such information. If the patient is desperate for hospitalization, she may not divulge accurate information about her past. Thus, the expedient thing to do is to call the patient's current therapist and ask both for information and for treatment recommendations. The expectation is that the therapist will provide such information. In DBT, the therapist does not provide such information in every case, but the therapist does not refuse every time either. To do so might alienate the very professional the patient needs on her side. The usual policy in such an instance is to review the situation with the patient, making it clear that the other professional does not have the time to evaluate her specific case, and then, with the patient's permission, to give the information necessary for the new professional to proceed. The therapist, however, does not generally tell the emergency room physician whether to hospitalize the patient or not, although the therapist may give information about his or her policies on hospitalization in general or in particular with this patient.

What about the System?

When an individual lives in an unsafe environment, how should a therapist target treatment? Should it focus on making the environment safer? Should the individual be taken out of the unsafe environment if it cannot be changed? Or should treatment focus on teaching the individual how to keep safe in an unsafe environment? Each approach has its merits; each is necessary at times. Within DBT, however, the philosophical emphasis is on the last of these—teaching the patient how to create safety for herself. As in feminist therapy, the focus is on "empowering" the individual.

Within DBT, the role of the therapist is to show the patient how to change the system (including the DBT system). The intervention approach is "bottom-up" rather than "top-down." When this is not possible—for example, the system is extraordinarily abusive, or unwilling or unable to change—the patient is helped out of the system. Although the therapist may try to change professional or other systems, these efforts are done on behalf of all patients, not a particular patient. Patients' aspirations to get themselves and their own lives under reasonable control, and then to work toward improving the system, are encouraged.

THERAPIST SUPERVISION/CONSULTATION STRATEGIES

Supervision/consultation with therapists is integral, rather than ancillary, to DBT. Consultation to the therapist, as a group of treatment strategies, balances the consultation-to-the-patient strategies discussed above. DBT, from this perspecitive, is defined as a treatment *system* in which (1) therapists apply DBT to the patients and (2) the supervisor and/or consultation team applies DBT

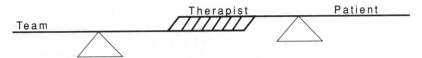

FIGURE 13.1. Relationship of supervision/consultation team to therapist and patient in DBT.

to the therapists. The supervisor and/or consultation team provides a dialectical balance for therapists in their interactions with patients.

There are three primary functions of consultation to the therapist in DBT. First, the supervisor or consultation team helps to keep each individual therapist in the therapeutic relationship. The role here is to cheerlead and support the therapist. Second, the supervisor or consultation team balances the therapist in his or her interactions with the patient (see Figure 13.1). In providing balance, consultants may move close to the therapist, helping him or her maintain a strong position. Or consultants may move back from the therapist, requiring the therapist to move closer to the patient to maintain balance. Third, within the programmatic applications of DBT, the supervision/consultation team provides the context for the treatment. At its purest, DBT is a transactional relationship between and among a community of borderline patients and a community of mental health professionals.

The Need for Supervision/Consultation

As I have noted previously, DBT was developed and first applied within a clinical research context. Extensive therapist training, close supervision of individual cases, and consultation among all therapists about applications of the treatment to emerging clinical problems are integral components of any clinical research program. Supervision and consultation, however, were originally viewed as ancillary to the treatment process itself. I believed that such extensive supervision/consultation would be unnecessary outside of a research context and/or once training of new therapists was completed. Feedback from therapists over the course of the research program and from patients with histories of therapy gone awry, however, persuaded me gradually that the role of supervision and consultation in nonresearch therapy applications is perhaps more important than I had first imagined.

I have come to believe that it is extraordinarily difficult to deliver effective treatment to most borderline patients without consultation or supervision. I have been amazed at how many very good therapists end up conducting ineffective therapy or making major mistakes with this patient population. In clinical settings, such as inpatient units and agencies, therapists at times seem to act almost as borderline as their patients. They are often extreme in their positions; invalidate one another and their patients; blame the patients as much as the patients blame themselves; are vulnerable to criticism or feedback from others about their manner of treatment; have chaotic relationships with one another, often marked by "staff splitting"; and vacillate among feeling alone, discouraged, hopeless, and depressed, feeling angry and hostile at the patients or other staff members, and feeling energetic, confident, encouraged, and hopeful. Although it is not difficult to understand why these patterns emerge, therapists often put unrealistic demands on themselves to be better in the absence of a context or community that supports change. Why do these patterns develop? There are a number of reasons.

First, the patients as a whole engage in the three most stressful patient behaviors (suicide attempts, suicide threats, and hostility) (Hellman, Morrison, & Abramowitz, 1986). They also communicate their intense suffering at every turn, adding to therapists' stress. Added to this, progress in therapy is much slower than with most patients, even when the most effective treatments are instituted. In sum, patients beg their therapist to help them immediately and threaten suicide if they fail. This would not be so stressful if the patient could be helped immediately, but they usually cannot. Therapists end up feeling incompetent, ineffective, and helpless in a situation where they very much care and want to succeed. The resulting tendencies are to "blame the victims," switch treatments impulsively, and/or engage in palliative activities that help the patients feel better now but harm their long-term prognosis. If all these fail, therapists often subtly push the patients out of therapy (perhaps by saying that the patients are not ready for therapy now) or precipitously terminate them.

Second, patients often inadvertently reinforce therapists for engaging in ineffective therapy and punish them for engaging in effective therapy. At least this is often the case when therapists are trying to implement DBT. In individual therapy, a patient usually does not want to discuss targeted behaviors, such as parasuicide, therapy-interfering behaviors of her own, or behavioral patterns seriously interfering with her life. If she does so, she wants to have a heart-to-heart discussion about her feelings or the therapist's behavior, rather than analyzing her behavior or engaging in more adaptive problem solving. The power struggle that ensues is usually very aversive to the therapist. It is much easier to let the patient control the agenda; frequently, it is also a lot more interesting. In skills training, patients want to discuss their current crises instead of concentrating on learning skills. When they are willing to focus on skills training, they criticize the skills for not being helpful enough. The skills trainer may begin to wonder, "Why bother?" If the trainer gets angry enough, it is easy to go overboard on the skills training structure, completely ignoring important process issues. If the trainer gets frustrated enough, it is easy just to drop skills training and "go with the flow," so to speak.

Third, patients present not only as needy but as very capable of nurturing the therapists. Patients often believe that being friends to the therapists is in their own therapeutic best interest; thus, it is easy for therapits to veer into discussing themselves and their own problems. This can then lead into a reversal of roles, where the patients become the therapists to the therapists. In my clinic, I have consulted on cases where patients have loaned therapists money for house mortgages, gone to therapists' homes to care for them when they are sick, accepted crisis calls from therapists who are getting divorces, and provided housekeeping and secretarial services for therapists. With borderline patients, it can be very easy for therapists to delude themselves into thinking that sexual contact and activity are somehow therapeutic for the patients.

The therapist consultation/supervision strategies are described below and are outlined in Table 13.3.

I. MEETING TO CONFER ON TREATMENT

Modes of Supervision/Consultation

How the therapist engages in supervision/consultation and who the community is depend almost completely on his or her work setting and borderline patient load. Therapists in private practice may contract for formal supervision with a more experienced therapist, may arrange with a colleague for peer supervision, or may attend peer consultation group. Such arrangements are usually not difficult in urban settings, but may require ingenuity (e.g., conference phone consultation) in rural settings. In agency, day treatment, and inpatient settings, the DBT supervision/consultation meeting may be the regular weekly team meeeeting or case conference, or there may be a special DBT consultation meeting.

The frequency and length of meetings depend on the number of therapists attending and the number of patients to be discussed. Meetings in my research clinic usually take place every week and last for 2 hours. When I have provided individual consultation for private practitioners, meetings have usually been 1-hour biweekly sessions. I myself usually discuss my own patients with a consultant or team at least twice a month. Although the minimum number of people required for a meeting is two, a dialectical approach is much easier to adhere to when there are three or more. Once a polarity develops, a third person can be very helpful in spotting the dialectic and encouraging a synthesis.

Meeting Agenda

In individual consultation, the agenda is, of course, set by the therapist seeking consultation. In peer consultation meetings and team meetings, or case conferences in institutional or programmatic settings, various formats for meetings are possible. The important items on the agenda are as follows:

1. Each therapist should have an opportunity to bring up any problems he or she is having with a particular patient. Problems might include determining which patient behaviors to focus treatment on at the moment; selecting or implementing treatment strategies; responding to problematic patient behaviors; or coping with the therapist's own feelings or attitudes toward the

TABLE 13.3. Therapist Supervision/Consultation Strategies Checklist

____ T attends regular supervision/consultation MEETINGS.

____ T makes and keeps supervision/consultation AGREEMENTS.

    ____ T takes a dialectical perspective, searching for syntheses of all views expressed in consultation meeting.

    ____ T consults with P on how to interact with other therapists, but does not tell other therapists how to interact with P.

    ____ T accepts other DBT therapists' behavior even when it presents different rules or expectations to P, seeing it as a lemon to help P make lemonade from.

    ____ T accepts other therapists' personal limits, even when they differ from T's, and helps other therapists observe their own limits.

    ____ T searches for nonpejorative, phenomenologically empathic interpretations of P's behavior.

    ____ T accepts that all therapists are falllible.

____ T CHEERLEADS other therapists.

    ____ T searches for unseen progress in patients.

    ____ T helps therapists find resources for their patients.

    ____ T helps other therapists make plans, repair difficulties with treatment and the relationship.

____ T assists other therapists in maintaining BALANCE in their attitudes and behaviors with patients; also T balances acceptance and change in reacting to therapists.

____ When involved in "staff splitting," T accepts a measure of responsibility; T helps to work out such problems as they arise.

____ T deals with another therapist's unethical or destructive behavior as necessary and in an appropriate manner.

____ T keeps information about therapists and/or patients confidential.

Anti-DBT tactics

____ T blames P for "staff splitting."

____ T searches for who is "right" and who is "wrong" when team members disagree.

____ T insists that he or she has "right" interpretation of P or a hold on absolute truth.

____ T tells other therapists how to respond to P, intervening for P.

____ T insists that everyone be consistent in how they interpret rules, set limits, and interact with P; T critcizes those who deviate.

____ T is judgmental of other therapists' limits.

____ T acts defensively, is oversensitive to critical feedback.

____ T is overcritical in giving feedback, forgets to validate other therapists.

patient or toward therapy. Each therapist should review at least one case (even if only briefly) at each meeting, and should give a brief progress report on all patients. The role of the team or consultant here is to help the therapist think clearly about how to conceptualize the patient, the relationship, and change in DBT theoretical terms, and how to apply the treatment skillfully.

    2. Skills trainers should have an opportunity both to tell the individual

therapists what skills are being taught at the moment and to highlight any problems individual patients are having in skills training. Individual therapists can provide information about patients' difficulties with skills and about specific areas of competence or incompetence. This is a chance for the individual and skills training therapists to exchange information about patients and discuss their respective treatment plans. Similar principles apply to the interactions with other modes of therapy (e.g., vocational rehabilitation, case management) that may be part of the DBT program. Because DBT does not require consistency, agreement among team members is not actually necessary here. However, the dialectical agreement argues for attempting to arrive at a synthesis if opposing positions are voiced. The entire team helps a skills trainer and an individual therapist in a particular case, or a case manager and individuall therapist in another, to do this.

3. In agency or clinic settings, or when therapy is part of a DBT program, institutional decisions that must be made are discussed. The goal is to reach a synthesis on how institutional problems should be responded to (although, once again, agreement is not strictly necessary). An example here is the patient who goes to skills training and kicks holes in the walls or acts in a way that disrupts other therapy sessions. What are the institutional limits? What is the clinic or unit director willing to put up with? Who should observe the limits? Who should communicate limits and consequences to the patient? Ordinarily, the patient's individual therapist will be responsible for day-to-day management of the case, including communication of any institutional limits. However, coordination (insofar as coordination is feasible or possible) is conducted at the DBT meeting. It is not at all unusual that patients will go directly to other members of the treatment team, including the unit director. These interactions are shared.

4. All therapists should have a chance to bring up any misunderstandings or problems they are having in implementing DBT. In this situation, the elements of DBT are like the U.S. Constitution, and the group as a whole operates like the Supreme Court. They try to figure out how to implement the elements in the specific case.

5. For therapists and other program staff members who are learning DBT, it is quite helpful if a segment of the meeting is set aside to review the DBT principles of treatment more generally. In my team meetings, during the first half hour of each meeting I review some aspect of DBT. This can be very important in developing a unit or team DBT culture. The task of developing and maintaining a shared treatment philosophy and approach to case conceptualization should not be put off or its importance minimized.

KEEPING SUPERVISION/CONSULTATION AGREEMENTS

The therapist supervision/consultation agreements have been discussed in Chapter 4 and are summarized in Table 13.3. The importance of these agreements cannot be overemphasized. They form the fundamental contract upon which meetings are based. The vulnerability and nondefensiveness that are requisite characteristics of those attending these meetings are simply not possible if there is no common basis of understanding.

In some institutional settings, this prescription may create a dilemma. Diverse theoretical orientations, treatment philosophies, time constraints, and institutional lethargy can interfere with a staff's willingness to agree upon and implement DBT supervision/consultation strategies. For example, on some inpatient units individual psychotherapists apply treatments based on other theoretical approaches, do not attend staff meetings, and are not part of the inpatient milieu. (Of course, when this is the case DBT is only being implemented partially, since the core of the treatment is the individual psychotherapy.) Or a borderline treatment program may be a subunit in a larger clinic that houses diverse treatment programs of many different orientations. When a small number of DBT therapists work within a larger institutional setting, the DBT-oriented staff should meet together, coordinate their treatments, and follow supervision/consultation agreements. Those applying other treatment programs—for example, the individual psychotherapists on inpatient units mentioned above—are viewed as ancillary (to DBT) treatment professionals. In some settings, the entire staff simply is not going to agree to trying DBT. Here, a synthesis must be searched for between the polarities of those implementing DBT and those not. The DBT therapists, at least, must attend to the DBT agreements. Polarizing between DBT and non-DBT is anti-DBT.

3. CHEERLEADING

It is all too easy to become demoralized when treating borderline patients. Sources of demoralization are numerous. It can at times be exceptionally difficult to see that a patient is making any progress. Sometimes a therapist is too close to the trees to see the forest. The role of supervisors and team members is to find and magnify that little bit of change or progress that the patient did in fact make. Reminding the therapist of the usual slow progress of borderline individuals and of other similar patients who were just as recalcitrant, but nonetheless proved successful, is also part of the consultants' task. These continuing reminders can sometimes be needed for quite some time. I once had a patient with whom I felt like a failure every week. Every week I went to the consultation meeting saying that we should refer her or send her back to the hospital; obviously I could not help her. And every week the skills training leader pointed out some very minor but nonetheless positive move the patient had made. Renewed and invigorated, I went back into the battle with energy. After a year of cumulative progress, even I could see it clearly, and demoralization became less of a problem for me.

Because of the extremely difficult environments within which they usually live, borderline patients often feel hopeless and helpless to change their situation, and therapists can easily fall into despair with them. A particular difficulty in our clinic is many patients' lack of financial resources. For example, patients lose the medical benefits of public assistance if they get employment. Recurrent medical problems then force them to quit their jobs in order to get medical care. Back on public assistance, they not only feel like failures, but must live on such low benefits that they may not be able to continue paying for therapy. If patients have educational aspirations, they may be unable to finance their education; very few borderline individuals can handle work and school at the same time. Or they may do better living alone, but may be unable to afford it. Many of our patients have difficulty paying for transportation to and from therapy, especially because rents are usually lower some distance from the city center. Moving to get away from abusive families or to take advantage of opportunities elsewhere may be impossible. The therapists of such patients must not only keep up hope, but must also be resourceful in the face of difficulties that would be daunting for even the best-adjusted individual. The task of the consultants is to help the therapists find the necessary resourcefulness.

At other times, therapists are in despair with themselves, not with their patients. As I have noted many times, therapists tend to make many mistakes with borderline patients. The emotional effect of such mistakes can be intense, and therapists can feel terrible. Although it is good to note one's own mistakes, feeling excessively bad about them is rarely helpful. Usually, what is happening is that such therapists are judging themselves (i.e., not using mindfulness skills) and comparing their own therapeutic behavior with that of mythical betters. The role of the consultants here is to use the validation and problem-solving strategies to help the therapists respond more reasonably to therapy mistakes. Usually, the best consultation strategy will be to make a concerted effort to help the therapists come up with a plan for making lemonade out of the lemons they have created. Being able to repair mistakes in this way can be extremely rewarding.

4. PROVIDING DIALECTICAL BALANCE

A fundamental goal of consultation to the therapist is to provide balance for each therapist so that he or she can stay within the dialectical frame of the therapy. When a patient is rigid, polarized, intense, and in great pain, it can be extraordinarily difficult for a therapist to remain flexible. When the patient attacks her therapist, refuses to cooperate, or goes backward instead of forward, it is not unusual for the therapist to move to the opposite extreme — withdrawing from the patient, wishing to attack back, or wanting to quit. It is not unusual on my team for a therapist to walk into a meeting saying, "I am ready to kill the patient; give me a DBT way to think!" The team is ready for the challenge, validates the therapist's position, and gets to work on solving the problem. The team members apply DBT strategies with one another.

When a patient is in a seemingly overwhelming crisis, believing herself to be too vulnerable to cope, it is also not unusual for the therapist to go to the patient's side of the therapeutic teeter-totter and become overly nurturing and solicitous. The therapist comes into the team meeting saying, "I am ready to kill every one of you who are being mean to my patient; give me a DBT way to think!" The job of the DBT team in this case is to validate the reasonableness of the therapist's response and provide a DBT interpretative counterpoint that will help him or her move to a more balanced position. The team uses DBT strategies to treat the therapist.

It is very important that consultants and supervisors remember the paradox of DBT: Change can only occur in the context of acceptance. Thus, an important role of consultants is to find the valid responses of the therapist and to reflect them within the consultation meeting. It is also the task of consultants to help the therapist make appropriate changes in treatment so that the patient is helped most effectively. At times consultants take the side of the patient, arguing her case to a recalcitrant and tough-minded therapist. At other times they take the long-term view, arguing that tough measures are needed.

A consultation team in a clinic or programmatic setting usually has two sources of information about a patient and her treatment. One source is the therapist's case review; the other is her interactions with other members of the program. On the basis of all the available information, the team applies DBT treatment strategies to help each therapist accept himself or herself in the moment and also change therapy strategies as needed to be more effective. To use my colleague Kelly Koerner's phrase, DBT team members are as "warmly ruthless" about maintaining fellow therapists within the DBT parameters as they are about helping the patients.

Working Out Problems of "Staff Splitting"

"Staff splitting," as mentioned earlier, is a much-discussed phenomenon in which professionals treating borderline patients begin arguing and fighting about a patient, the treatment plan, or the behavior of other professionals with the patient. The responsibility for the dissension among the staff is then attributed to the patient, who is said to have split the staff; hence the term "staff splitting."

For example, as part of discharge planning, an inpatient was referred to my treatment team. A member of our team was halfway through an assessment interview when a staff nurse interrupted, saying that the assessment should not continue. We later found that the attending physician did not believe a behavioral treatment would be appropriate for the patient. Both the patient and members of my treatment team got angry. The patient was then referred to an outpatient program in the same hospital, with instructions to the new unit that the patient should not be permitted to join my program. The head of the outpatient unit was now angry at the implication that she was not capable of making appropriate treatment plans. At a staff meeting, it was observed that it was clear that the patient was indeed borderline, since she had managed to split the staff before she even got to the unit.

In DBT, arguments among staff members and differences in points of view, traditionally associated with staff splitting, are seen as failures in synthesis and interpersonal process among the staff rather than as a patient's problem. The staff splits the staff. The belief that a patient does it runs perilously close to the type of thinking therapists try to change in their patients—blaming problems they are having on others or on external events. In DBT, staff members are encouraged to use their interpersonal skills to work these problems out as they arise. Therapists' disagreements over a patient are treated as potentially equally valid poles of a dialectic. Thus, the starting point for dialogue is the recognization that a polarity has arisen, together with an implicit (if not explicit) assumption that resolution will require working toward synthesis.

The precipitants of staff splitting are multiple, and a number of scenarios are possible. Much splitting has to do with the fact that therapists' attitudes toward patients follow a wave pattern similar to patients' vacillation between overidealization and devaluation of therapists. The wave fluctuates within a space anchored at one extreme by an attitude that the patient needs to try harder and the staff should be tougher, and at the other extreme by an attitude that the patient is fragile, the world is too tough on her and the staff should be gentler and more nurturing. In one common scenario, two factors are present. First, the intensity of the patient's pain communications evoke a reciprocal intense desire to care for the patient and cure the pain. The inability to do this leads to an intense sense of failure or anxiety, especially when suicide threats are part of the pain communication. Second, different therapists interacting with the same patient have attitudes toward the patient that are momentarily out of synchrony with each other; the attitudes are at opposite extremes of the wave pattern. Such a state is shown in Figure 13.2 between staff members A and B. The intensity of the "split" has to do with both the intensity of the patient's pain communications and the intensity of the therapists' discomfort with that pain. DBT handles this problem by searching for the synthesis between the tough and the gentle positions. In Figure 13.2, staff member C might be able to help members A and B arrive at a synthesis.

A second scenario has to do with a patient's complaints to one therapist (the "good guy") about the terrible behavior of another therapist (the "bad guy"). If the "good guy" is on the "patient-as-fragile" apex of the wave, it is particularly easy for him or her to get angry at the "bad guy." This tendency is exacerbated when the stakes are high (e.g., when the patient is suicidal) and the "bad guy" is at the "let's-get-tough" apex of the wave. Once again, DBT handles this by assuming that there is a synthesis to be found. The supervisor and/or consultation team searches for both the validity of the patient's complaints and the validity of the accused therapist's behavior. Defensiveness on the part of the "bad guy," of course, does not help matters.

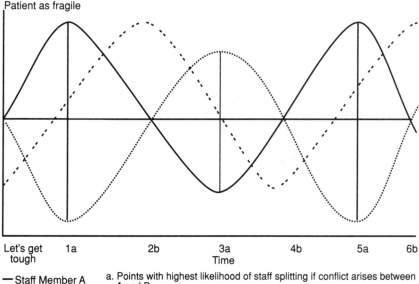

FIGURE 13.2. Illustration of a possible "staff splitting" scenario: Wave patterns of different staff members' attitudes toward a patient.

Here both the fallibility agreement (therapists usually make mistakes) and the phenomenological empathy agreement (therapists attempt to see life from the perspective of the patient) can be helpful.

Dealing with Unethical or Destructive Therapist Behavior

The therapist supervision/consultation approach is based on the assumption that all therapists working on a team meet at least minimum levels of competence, ethics, and nondefensiveness. The agreements are based on mutual respect. It is difficult for a therapist to validate the behavior of another therapist whom he or she does not respect, or to share opinions openly with another therapist who is overly sensitive to critical feedback. Occasionally, a therapist on the team or in the supervision/consultation group may have serious problems that intrude into the treatment, may engage in critical breaches of ethics, or may continue with a destructive treatment relationship. Patients may make serious accusations about one therapist to another. Generally, these problems are first dealt with privately, in individual supervision and outside of team meetings. The individual therapist may be confronted directly, or the unit director may be consulted. Serious accusations and therapeutic breaches are not ignored.

Keeping Information Confidential

With one exception, all consultation discussions are confidential. Information about patients is of course confidential, but, just as importantly, information therapists reveal about themselves is also confidential. The only exception is that patients are apprised of the fact that they are discussed at supervision/consultation meetings. When a patient requests it, an individual therapist may judiciously reveal some of the substance of the discussion if this information will have a positive effect on the patient's relationships with other therapists or when the feedback from others might help the patient enhance her skills. The potential for distorting the information must be kept in mind and freely admitted.

Concluding Comments

For some therapists, the case management strategies in DBT are the most difficult to implement. The DBT approach goes somewhat against the grain: Most of us have been taught principles that are just the opposite of some that I am advocating. My colleagues and I evolved these principles and strategies over a number of years of working with these patients in a clinical research setting. Some of the principles were first implemented because our research required them. For example, we could not easily use psychiatric inpatient days as an outcome measure for outpatient DBT if our treatment team controlled how long an individual stayed in the hospital. Caveats and exceptions were developed as we went to the limits of a strategy and found where we had to allow modification. I was surprised myself to find that many of the treatment strategies developed purely for research purposes turned out to be very effective clinically. Those that worked were kept and now are part of DBT.

The therapist supervision/consultation approach was at first a research necessity, because I had to be sure that all the therapists were actually conducting the treatment. But when we gave group skills training to a large number of patients receiving individual psychotherapy in the community, I got to know firsthand how many therapists were functioning without the support of a consultation group. I also consulted with a large number of therapists who contacted me for help with therapeutic problems; as noted earlier, I was surprised by the therapy mistakes that were being made among therapists who seemed otherwise to be very good therapists. As I have consulted further to inpatient units and public agencies, I have been struck over and over at the lack of supervisory and staff support in many institutional settings. I believe that the failure to obtain and give adequate consultation and support is based on a failure to recognize the importance of context and environmental events in shaping behavior, including therapeutic behavior. Therapeutic behavior requires a context that reinforces it. The laws of human behavior that apply to our patients apply equally to their therapists.

IV

Strategies for Specific Tasks

14

Structural Strategies

Structural strategies have to do with how both DBT as a whole and individual sessions are begun and ended. They also have to do with how the therapist structures time during the various phases of treatment and during individual sessions.

The primary task in beginning DBT is to develop a collaborative treatment contract. The primary task in ending DBT is to prepare the patient for life without DBT and to orient the patient to what she can expect from the therapist and treatment team after formal treatment ends.

The key emphasis in beginning and ending individual sessions is on creating an emotional atmosphere that will enable the patient to interact openly during the session and that will protect her as far as possible from uncontrollable negative emotions once the session is ended. Session time in individual therapy is structured according to the DBT target hierarchy (decreasing suicidal behaviors, decreasing therapy-interfering behaviors, decreasing quality-of-life-interfering behaviors, increasing behavioral skills, decreasing posttraumatic stress, increasing self-respect, and achieving individual goals). Session structure in other modes of therapy (e.g., skills training, phone calls, etc.) is determined by the target priorities of the particular mode of interaction. (Structuring of skills training is discussed in the accompanying skills training manual.)

There are no new acceptance or change strategies involved here. As in case management strategies, the focus in structural strategies is on the tasks to be accomplished; thus, structural strategies amplify and integrate old strategies rather than create new ones. Dialectical strategies and the core validating and problem-solving strategies form the backbone of the structural strategies.

CONTRACTING STRATEGIES: STARTING TREATMENT

The first task in meeting a potential patient is to orient the patient to DBT and develop an initial treatment contract with the patient. This contract then forms the basis of all future treatment.

Contracting strategies are used during the first several meetings with the patient to orient her to what DBT is about, what is expected of her, what she can expect of the therapist, and how and why the treatment is expected to work. The goal is to forge a commitment between patient and therapist to work together as a therapy team. Contracting is the application of the orienting and commitment strategies (from problem solving; see Chapter 9) to the initiation of therapy. Thereafter, these strategies are reapplied when the patient (1) is violating the therapy contract or is threatening to do so (e.g., says she is quitting skills training); (2) is threatening suicide or parasuicide; (3) appears to be making unrealistic demands or to have unrealistic expectations of the therapist; (4) is having difficulty using therapy appropriately (e.g., doesn't call the therapist when it would be appropriate to do so because of fear of imposing). In short, the treatment contract is remade over and over. Specific contracting strategies are summarized in Table 14.1 and are discussed below.

I. CONDUCTING A DIAGNOSTIC ASSESSMENT

If a structured diagnostic interview has not been conducted previously, a first task during the contracting phase is to conduct such an interview and obtain a detailed behavioral and psychiatric history, concentrating particularly on the patient's previous experiences in psychotherapy. In our clinic, we use the Structured Clinical Interview for DSM-III-R, Axis II (SCID-II; Spitzer & Williams, 1990), as well as the revised version of the Diagnostic Interview for Borderlines (DIB-R; Zanarini et al., 1989).

There are a number of requisite patient characteristics for DBT. The most important of these is voluntary participation. DBT requires at least the possibility of a collaborative relationship, continuing the relationship with the therapist can only be used as a positive contingency when a patient wants to be in the treatment program. Contingency management is thus seriously compromised with an involuntary patient. Court-ordered treatment is acceptable if the patient will agree to remain in therapy even if the therapist gets the court order lifted.

In my experience, a local residence is also desirable. Patients who do not live in the immediate area (i.e., transportation time of 1 hour or less) or who must move to the area for therapy will have difficulty finding the community social support and resources they need to tolerate the stress of therapy; thus, they will be more likely to terminate early. An additional patient characteristic needed for group therapy is the ability to control hostility toward others. Borderline groups with an overtly hostile member are greatly handicapped,

TABLE 14.1. Contracting Strategies Checklist

____ T conducts DIAGNOSTIC ASSESSMENT.
     ____ T uses a structured diagnostic interview (e.g., SCID-II, DIB-R).
     ____ T ascertains whether treatment is voluntary.
____ T presents a BIOSOCIAL APPROACH to problems in living in general, and to borderline behavioral patterns in particular.
     ____ T presents a functional, problem-solving approach to maladaptive (particularly parasuicidal) behavior.
     ____ T presents a skills deficit model of maladaptive behavior.
____ T ORIENTS P to DBT, with emphasis on DBT philosophy.
     ____ DBT is supportive.
     ____ DBT is behavioral.
     ____ DBT is cognitive.
     ____ DBT is skill-oriented.
     ____ DBT balances acceptance and change.
     ____ DBT requires a collaborative relationship.
____ T helps P ORIENT HER NETWORK to DBT.
____ T reviews TREATMENT AGREEMENTS AND LIMITS.
     ____ T discusses requisite patient agreements.
         ____ To stay in therapy an agreed-upon amount of time.
             ____ T negotiates length of initial treatment contract.
             ____ T clarifies for P requirements for contract renewal for another time period.
         ____ To attend therapy sessions.
             ____ T negotiates frequency and length of sessions with P, elicits P's preferences.
             ____ T communicates that P is expected to attend weekly individual and skills training sessions. Limit of four misses in a row is explained.
         ____ To work on reducing suicidal behaviors.
         ____ To work collaboratively with T.
             ____ T gives P information on what behaviors within a session and between sessions are appropriate (e.g., "It is not appropriate to miss sessions just because you are not in the mood").
             ____ To attend skills training.
         ____ To keep research and payment agreements.
             ____ T outlines any research requirements.
             ____ T negotiates fees and payment arrangements.
     ____ T discusses requisite therapist agreement:
         ____ To make every reasonable effort to be effective at helping P make changes she wants to make.
         ____ To obey standard ethical guidelines
         ____ To be reasonably available to P.
         ____ To respect P.
         ____ To maintain confidentiality.
             ____ T discusses nonconfidentiality of high-risk suicidal behavior.
         ____To obtain therapy consultation when needed.
     ____ T discusses availability of phone contact and recording/taping of sessions.
____ T uses COMMITMENT STRATEGIES to obtain P's commitment to DBT, and especially to goal of reducing parasuicidal behavior.
         ____ After careful consideration, T commits to working with P.

(cont.)

Table 14.1. (cont.)

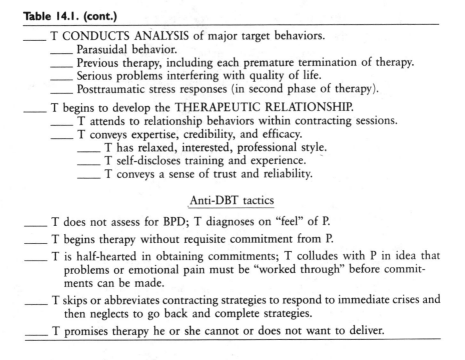

_____ T CONDUCTS ANALYSIS of major target behaviors.
  _____ Parasuidal behavior.
  _____ Previous therapy, including each premature termination of therapy.
  _____ Serious problems interfering with quality of life.
  _____ Posttraumatic stress responses (in second phase of therapy).
_____ T begins to develop the THERAPEUTIC RELATIONSHIP.
  _____ T attends to relationship behaviors within contracting sessions.
  _____ T conveys expertise, credibility, and efficacy.
    _____ T has relaxed, interested, professional style.
    _____ T self-discloses training and experience.
    _____ T conveys a sense of trust and reliability.

Anti-DBT tactics

_____ T does not assess for BPD; T diagnoses on "feel" of P.

_____ T begins therapy without requisite commitment from P.

_____ T is half-hearted in obtaining commitments; T colludes with P in idea that problems or emotional pain must be "worked through" before commitments can be made.

_____ T skips or abbreviates contracting strategies to respond to immediate crises and then neglects to go back and complete strategies.

_____ T promises therapy he or she cannot or does not want to deliver.

given the usual combination among the patients of high emotional sensitivity and behavioral passivity.

In the research demonstrating the efficacy of DBT, patients were screened for active psychosis and organic mental disorders. For a non-research-oriented application of DBT, such screening would be needed only to the degree that significant cognitive impairments such as inability to attend to or grasp skill concepts would prevent patients from benefiting from the skills training. The presence of substance dependence is not grounds for exclusion except in a case where the patient cannot benefit from other treatment before the dependence is eliminated. In principle, there is no reason why DBT cannot be modified to treat primary substance abuse problems. Several of our patients, however, were referred to short-term substance abuse inpatient programs before being admitted to DBT.

2. PRESENTING THE BIOSOCIAL THEORY OF BORDERLINE BEHAVIOR

During the first or several sessions, the therapist should present the dialectical/biosocial point of view on parasuicidal behavior and BPD (see Chapter 2). Suicidal behavior should be presented as an attempt by individuals in pain to solve problems in living. Thus, suicidal behavior does not differ in principle from other maladaptive behaviors, except that it has a high risk of being fatal. Although the function of parasuicide can vary over time, across situations, and among individuals, some functional characteristics of parasuicidal behavior are common to most suicidal persons. These characteristics should be described and discussed with the patient. It is best if this discussion can be a Socratic one, in which the patient herself generates many of the functions. The therapist should be careful to present the functions of parasuicide as common to many people, without implying that the particular patient is *necessarily* like other individuals.

In this context, it is also important that the nature of a functional relationship be described to the patient. As I have discussed in Chapters 9 and 10, it is not uncommon for a patient to understand a therapist's presentation of functional relationships as somehow implying that the person is consciously intending to achieve particular goals via parasuicide. Thus, the therapist should make clear to the patient that a particular behavior–outcome relationship does not necessarily mean that the person consciously (or unconsciously) intended such an outcome. On the other hand, the patient should be helped to see that such consequences can serve to reinforce parasuicidal behavior even if the patient does not wish this to be so. The therapist can do much to bolster the patient's confidence by specifically addressing this issue at the very beginning, since the patient no doubt has been told by significant others that her suicidal behavior is conscious and manipulative. This point has been discussed at some lengths in Chapters 1 and 9.

The patient should also be presented with the model of how borderline behaviors develop from a combination of emotional dysregulation and an invalidating environment (see Chapter 2). Once again, the therapist should present the model in a Socratic manner, eliciting confirmation or disconfirmation from the patient as the discussion goes along. Although DBT rests on a firm theoretical model, the task during the contracting phase (and throughout therapy) is to develop and modify the theory so that it fits the particular patient.

It is helpful at this time to draw on a blackboard a list of skills that borderline individuals are presumed to lack (see the companion manual to this volume for an outline of this material). Although this same material is presented in skills training, it benefits from repetition in each mode of treatment. After describing what each of the skills consists of, it is then useful to discuss the interdependence among the skills in a humorous or slightly dramatic fashion, to give the patient an appreciation and understanding of the origin of her own sense of frustration in trying to develop one set of skills when she doesn't have a second set of skills required for learning the first.

For example, because the individual can not tolerate aversive environments, she is unlikely to learn self-control. Any effective self-control program has to be conducted in small steps, and therefore requires a tolerance of the aversive state of affairs for a period of time. Of course, if the patient had self-control skills she would find tolerating aversive environments much easier, since the lack of such tolerance is often a result of the patient's sense that the situation will never improve because of her lack of skills at improving the situation. Similarly, learning to control emotions is contingent on having the self-control skills needed to carry out a program of learning the behaviors needed for emotion regulation. However, putting such a plan into action is hampered by the very lack of emotion regulation skills. Highly intense emotions make it difficult even to remember what steps to carry out, and inevitably tempt the patient to jettison the well-thought-out behavioral management plan in favor of trying to get rid of the painful affect by some quicker but maladaptive means.

As these examples indicate, it is quite easy to show the patient how interdependent the behavioral skills are. At this point, it is helpful to point out to the patient that it's just "luck of the draw" that she may be deficient in each of these areas. Although the patient must be given hope that she can remedy these deficits, such a description can also help her see why she is feeling frustrated. Such an understanding can presumably make it easier to tolerate the process of skill building that DBT involves.

3. ORIENTING THE PATIENT TO TREATMENT

The first several sessions of therapy involve orienting the patient to DBT and include a role induction aimed at giving the patient the appropriate information about her role as a patient and the therapist's role as a therapist. The following content should be covered during these sessions; the order of its presentation, however, can be individually tailored. Again, it is advisable to elicit in the context of discussion as much as possible of the material from the patient, so that a minimum of didactic presentation is necessary.

The therapy itself, as well as the number, form, and content of sessions, should be described clearly and in detail to the patient. In addition, these characteristics of DBT treatment philosophy should be described:

1. *DBT is supportive.* The orientation of the DBT therapist is to be supportive of the patient in her attempts both to decrease her suicidal behavior and to increase satisfaction with her life. In this regard, the DBT therapist will attempt to help the patient recognize her own positive attributes and strengths, and will encourage her both to develop these characteristics and to use them to enhance her life satisfaction. Now is the time to tell the patient that DBT is not a suicide prevention program; it is a life enhancement program.

2. *DBT is behavioral.* A major focus of the therapy will be on helping the patient (a) learn to analyze her characteristic problematic behavioral patterns, including the events that elicit them and their functional characteristics, and (b) learn to replace maladaptive behavior with skillful behavior.

3. *DBT is cognitive.* Therapy will also focus on helping the patient change beliefs, expectations, and assumptions that she has learned from her experience in previous settings but that are no longer effective or helpful. In addition, therapy will help her examine and change when necessary her style

of thinking, particularly her "all-or-none" thinking and tendencies to be over-judgmental (especially with respect to herself).

4. *DBT is skill-oriented.* Both structured skills training and individual therapy are designed to teach the patient new skills and enhance the capabilities she already possesses. At least within structured skills training, the focus will be on mindfulness, interpersonal effectiveness, distress tolerance, self-control, and emotion regulation skills. Individual therapy will focus on helping the patient integrate the skills she is learning in skills training into her daily life.

5. *DBT balances acceptance and change.* The therapy will focus on helping the patient gain greater tolerance for painful feelings, for aversive environments, for ambiguity, and for the slow pace of change in general. A constant theme of therapy will be resolving the contradictions that arise from focusing simultaneously on skill enhancement and reality tolerance. It is often useful to point out to the patient that she probably often vacillates between two seemingly contradictory positions; several examples of this may be elicited from the patient at this point. For example, the patient may note that she vacillates between feeling hopeful and feeling hopeless, between feeling in total control and independent and feeling totally out of control and dependent, and so on.

6. *DBT requires a collaborative relationship.* DBT requires the patient and therapist to function as a team to achieve the patient's goals. Toward this end, not only does the patient have to stay in the therapy, but both patient and therapist have to work constantly on their relationship behaviors so that they facilitate rather than hinder progress. Thus, a major focus of the treatment will be on helping both patient and therapist adapt their characteristic interpersonal styles to the needs of the current relationship.

4. ORIENTING THE NETWORK TO TREATMENT

During the initial assessment, the therapist will have gathered information about the patient's interpersonal network and about all other current medical and psychological treatments. It is the therapist's responsibility to see to it that the patient orients both her social and her medical/psychological treatment network to DBT and her participation in it. If the nature of the therapuetic relationship allows it, a therapist–patient joint meeting with one or more members of the patient's network may also be very useful. This can be particularly important with a highly suicidal patient, where communication of the high risk to the patient's entire network is almost always indicated. (Involvement of the network in management of suicidal behaviors is discussed more fully in Chapter 15.) These initial network meetings are also an opportunity for the therapist to orient the network to the consultation-to-the-patient strategies discussed in Chapter 13, to provide the network with the DBT theoretical formulation of BPD, and to gather further information about the patient and her network.

5. REVIEWING TREATMENT AGREEMENTS AND LIMITS

Patient and Therapist Agreements

The patient agreements and therapist agreements, presented in Chapter 4, should be thoroughly discussed. There are six patient agreements (to enter and stay in therapy, to attend therapy, to work on reducing suicidal behavior, to work on therapy-interfering behaviors, to attend skills training, and to abide by research and payment agreements) necessary for DBT. There are six therapist agreements (to make every reasonable effort to be effective, to act ethically, to be available to the patient, to show respect for the patient, to maintain confidentiality, and to obtain consultation when needed). These agreements operationalize the DBT treatment philosophy discussed above. Their rationale is discussed in Chapter 4, and I do not repeat it here.

Availability of Phone Contact

During the first session, the patient should be given phone numbers to contact the therapist and available emergency services in the community. The therapist's phone call limits should be discussed. If at this point the patient says that she could not possibly call a therapist, the therapist should discuss with her the DBT orientation to phone calls. In general, this is that not all of therapy can be done within the context of individual and skills training sessions. Thus, it is necessary for the patient to call the therapist at times for individual coaching, especially in crisis situations when she is very tempted to engage in suicidal or other seriously maladaptive behaviors. Further strategies regarding phone contact are discussed in Chapter 15.

Recording/Taping of Sessions

If sessions are recorded, the patient should be advised of this. DBT advises recording both individual therapy sessions and skills training sessions; the role of these tapes in her treatment should be discussed. If having the patient listen to sessions between sessions is part of the treatment plan, the therapist should make arrangements for the patient to have a tape recorder to listen to tapes between sessions. The role of tapes in DBT, and problems that may arise with this procedure, are discussed in Chapter 11.

6. COMMITTING TO THERAPY

Formal therapy cannot begin until the patient and therapist have arrived at an agreement to work together, the patient commits to the patient agreements, and the therapist commits to the therapist agreements. This point cannot be overemphasized. The commitment strategies outlined in Chapter 9 are the principal means of gathering and strengthening the borderline patient's com-

mitment to the process and goals of DBT. Until the necessary verbal commitments are made, the therapist should not proceed to discuss any other topic.
There should be no investigations of the patient's past to get clues about her
"resistance"; no discussions of the patient's emotional misery or life chaos
to get a better understanding of why she simply can't commit right now; no
extended heart-to-hearts about the patient's relationship with the therapist
(except as part of the initial orientation and mutual assessment) to see whether
the patient can work with this particular therapist. This point is cruicial because the patients sometimes balk at one or more of the DBT commitments,
saying that they aren't ready or able to make a commitment at that level right
now. At the same time, they present themselves as so desperate that therapists
become desperate to help as quickly as possible.

Despite a patient's (and sometimes a therapist's) desperation, if the patient refuses to make the six necessary patient agreements as noted above,
the therapist should accept the patient's statement, but remain firm nonetheless that therapy cannot proceed without these agreements. Starting therapy
without the requisite patient commitment is like being a train engineer who
is in such a hurry to get the train passengers somewhere that he or she starts
the engine car out of the station before the passenger cars are securely fastened.
No matter how fast that engine goes, those passengers left in the station are
not going to reach their destination any faster. Borderline patients typically
have great difficulty making a commitment to work on reducing parasuicide
and suicide risk. How to obtain this commitment is discussed in detail in
Chapters 9 and 15, so I do not go into it further here.

It is sometimes so easy to focus on getting a commitment from the patient that the therapist forgets to consider carefully whether his or her treatment can actually help the patient as much as or better than available
alternative treatments, and whether he or she actually wants to treat this particular patient. When individuals come to treatment in crisis, ready and willing to commit to anything, it is particularly easy to rush into treating them
without giving this the careful consideration such a commitment warrants.
Facile promises of therapy can readily inspire hope in a desperate patient, but
for just this reason they may be extremely difficult to break without serious
damage to the patient. In most cases, the therapist should not promise continuing treatment during the first session. I usually tell a potential patient
that we will use the first two or three sessions to assess whether we can work
together and whether the person's problems are the type that I am able to
treat. Between sessions, I consider whether I am able and willing to offer potentially effective treatment for this particular individual; if so, a firm commitment is made during the second or third session. If not, I help the person find alternative treatment. Occasionally, I have suggested that a patient
enter and complete an alternative treatment (e.g., a substance abuse program or a structured, long-term DBT inpatient program) and then return to
see me.

7. CONDUCTING ANALYSES OF MAJOR TARGET BEHAVIORS

During the first few sessions, the therapist should conduct a comprehensive behavioral analysis for each major instance of parasuicidal behavior that the patient can remember. Serious problems with previous treatments should also be examined. Generally, I do at least a detailed analysis of each premature termination of therapy. When treatment moves to the second phase of treatment (or if therapy begins here), a comprehensive analysis of posttraumatic stress responses should be conducted. Here, the therapist may need first to identify different patterns and then to select one or two instances in each pattern for more in-depth analysis. The focus should be on current rather than past stress responses. Guidelines for how to conduct such analyses are given in Chapter 9. If therapy is carried out in a research context, the research assessments can be used as guides to these analyses. But, in any case, they should not be skipped in the interest of getting to interventions quickly. Not only are they vital for obtaining information and clarifying patterns, but they help the patient to develop explanations for her behavior as neither "mad" nor "bad" (see Chapter 9 for further discussion).

8. BEGINNING TO DEVELOP THE THERAPEUTIC RELATIONSHIP

Observing Relationship Patterns in Contracting Sessions

An essential task of these initial contracting sessions is to begin establishing a positive interpersonal relationship. These sessions offer an opportunity for both patient and therapist to explore problems that may arise in establishing and maintaining a therapeutic alliance. The assessment and contracting sessions themselves serve as a sample of the patient–clinician interaction pattern, and may be useful in predicting future patterns. In-session patterns, response variability, and the like should therefore be carefully observed and documented for subsequent analysis.

Conveying Expertise, Credibility, and Efficacy

Expertise, credibility, and efficacy may be conveyed in a variety of ways. In general, many of the strategies and techniques of DBT are designed to enhance the efficacy of the therapist. Expertise can be communicated by interpersonal stylistic characteristics such as dressing professionally, being interested and relaxed, assuming a comfortable but attentive sitting position, speaking fluently with confidence and assurance, and being prepared for the therapy session. The therapist can also disclose his or her title, institutional affiliation, and academic and professional experience with cases similar to the patient's particular situation and experience, as well as with the treatment approach to be followed. Credibility is influenced by such characteristics as reliability, dependability, predictability, and consistency. Particularly important for the suicidal patient is her perception of the therapist's presumed motives and intentions in conducting the treatment. Therefore, it is important to attend to such factors as carrying out agreements, starting the sessions on time, and communicating a clear interest in the patient as a person rather than only as a customer or a research subject.

The credibility of the treatment and therapist can sometimes be enhanced if the therapist can arrange for the patient to undergo a positive, dramatic learning experience in the first several sessions. For example, teaching a patient briefly how to relax or how to let go of emotional arousal in a session can sometimes have a dramatic effect on the patient's belief in the therapist. The crisis survival strategies (see the accompanying skills training manual) can have much the same effect.

Caveats in the Real World

I have presented the contracting strategies in a very straightforward manner, which implies that therapy actually proceeds through the strategies much as I have outlined here. Often, however, this is not the case. This is particularly so when the patient enters therapy in a serious life crisis, is very serious about killing herself, or has such severe therapy-interfering behaviors that nothing can be accomplished until these behaviors are modified. The therapist may need to use a crisis intervention treatment model (see Chapter 15) for quite some time at the very beginning of treatment. In these cases, the therapist should add extra time at the beginning (usually one session is sufficient) to orient the patient to the basics of the treatment and obtain the rudimentary commitments necessary. These two things (orientation and commitment) simply have to be done before anything else. Formal diagnostic assessment may be best handled by a colleague or another therapist in the clinic. Presenting the DBT biosocial theory, assessing major target behaviors, taking a history, and orienting the social network may all have to be worked into the treatment later.

For example, a patient was referred to me for outpatient therapy following three near-lethal suicide attempts during the previous 9 months, all involving cuts to arteries in the throat. The patient had also drunk poison 12 times in the past year, and had so many self-inflicted burns that skin grafting had been required. After committing herself to work on these behaviors during the first session, the patient was immediately ambivalent about whether to live or kill herself, and could only commit to trying her best not to kill herself the next time she felt a strong urge to die. (Her dissociative states were a complicating factor, and she maintained that she was helpless during these states to control her own behavior.) Since almost overwhelming suicide urges were frequent and the desire to die almost continuous, therapy proceeded to concentrate on helping the patient stay alive and relatively uninjured. As I said to the patient repeatedly, we would get to work on her problems and on getting to know each other as soon as we had her suicidal behaviors under control. This took 3 months of nonstop effort, including several inpatient admissions and exploration of alternative treatment options. As the risk of immediate suicide, at least, receded, I began the history taking and assessment I would have ordinarily conducted much closer to the beginning of therapy.

A second example involved a patient seen in our clinic by a male therapist. (A female therapist, which the patient preferred, was not available; unfortunately, we could not find her any alternative treatment in the community.) This patient entered therapy, made the requisite agreements, and then almost immediately was seized by intense fears about being in therapy with a male. By the third week, a pattern had developed: The patient would leave five or six messages per week stating that she could not go through with therapy, could not see such an inexperienced therapist, could not be in such an ill-advised treatment program, could not continue a therapy where people were so insensitive, could not continue if we continued to require simultaneous skills training, and so on and so on. Requests for a call back would be canceled within an hour or two with a message that she was terminating therapy and the therapist should not blame himself. The patient would miss two or three sessions, repair her doubts over the phone or in a session, and then within hours of repair and recommitment (tentative though it was) would re-enter the cycle. Therapy focused on nothing but this pattern of therapy-interfering behavior (which was a step improved from her pattern in previous therapies of threatening suicide at the same rate) for the first 4 months. Diagnostic assessment was handled by a colleague. History taking and assessment of other target problems were put off.

SESSION-BEGINNING STRATEGIES

How a session begins is important in any psychotherapy. The beginning sets the tone for the remainder of the session. A patient often expects the therapist to approach her with a negative or rejecting attitude. She sometimes comes to sessions with dread, prepared to withdraw or flee; this is especially likely if the preceding interaction was intense and negative. Most borderline patients have not learned that negative emotions come and go, and that problems can be resolved. Without such experiences, negative encounters can take on catastrophic import. Meeting the patient repeatedly with a warm, inviting attitude can gradually teach her that anger, frustration, relationship problems, and mistakes on her part do not necessarily lead to abandonment or irreparable emotional strain. Self-soothing, which is necessary for keeping escalating emotions under some control, becomes considerably easier as a result.

A word on possible settings for therapy is in order her. In my clinic, the therapist's clinical practice office has routinely been the setting for individual DBT sessions and has generally been satisfactory. Another important setting for DBT is the telephone call, which has been discussed to some extent al-

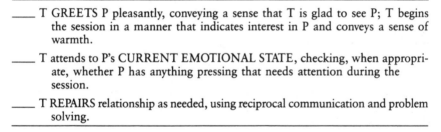

TABLE 14.2. Session-Beginning Strategies Checklist

____ T GREETS P pleasantly, conveying a sense that T is glad to see P; T begins the session in a manner that indicates interest in P and conveys a sense of warmth.

____ T attends to P's CURRENT EMOTIONAL STATE, checking, when appropriate, whether P has anything pressing that needs attention during the session.

____ T REPAIRS relationship as needed, using reciprocal communication and problem solving.

ready and is treated more extensively in the next chapter; environmental intervention strategies may occur *in vivo.* For some adolescent patients who are highly ambivalent about therapy, flexibility in setting can be extremely important for therapy retention. Out-of-office sessions in places such as bowling alleys and cars can be helpful in continuing contact through difficult phases. The same end might perhaps be accomplished by simply remaining in touch until the adolescent comes for an office appointment, but with a limit of four consecutive absences, this is not practical. It is also possible that such alternative meeting places are more natural environments for some adolescents and can be better tolerated in the midst of the traumas in their lives.

Strategies to keep in mind when beginning therapy are discussed below and are outlined in Table 14.2.

I. GREETING THE PATIENT

Generally the therapist should greet the patient warmly, in such a manner as to express obvious pleasure at seeing the patient again. This will usually involve smiling at the patient and, if she has missed one or more sessions, commenting on how good it is to see her again. The object is to communicate value and liking for the patient at the initial encounter.

2. RECOGNIZINGTHE PATIENT'S CURRENT EMOTIONAL STATE

It is important to recognize the patient's current emotional state when beginning the session. Hidden agendas on the patient's (or the therapist's) part should be brought out in the open. If topics are pressing to the patient, this should be noted. An informal agenda can be set at the beginning of the session so that both parties know what topics need to be discussed and in what order they will be discussed. The targeting strategies, discussed below, are crucial in this agenda setting.

3. REPAIRING THE RELATIONSHIP

With few exceptions, relationship repair, at least briefly, should precede other serious work within the session. However, a "heart-to-heart" should not be substituted for targeting high-priority behaviors within the session. The dangers of this temptation are discussed more extensively in Chapter 12.

A therapist who is ambivalent about meeting with the patient, anxious about difficult material that must be discussed, or still frustrated with the patient should examine carefully whether he or she actually wishes to resolve these conflicts with the patient. If the answer is no, the problem should be addressed in the next supervision/consultation team meeting; a certain amount of repair work, away from the patient, may be needed before the topic is broached with the patient. If the answer is yes, the therapist should use the reciprocal communication strategies (see Chapter 12) and therapeutic relationship strategies (see Chapter 15) to discuss the relationship with the patient and begin problem solving.

TARGETING STRATEGIES

Targeting strategues have to do with how the therapist structures the time during individual therapy sessions and what topics receive attention. They were developed to reflect the DBT emphasis on hierarchical organization of treatment targets and to insure that therapists would attend to the hierarchical ordering necessary in DBT. Implementing the targeting strategies requires integrating almost all of the previous treatment strategies. It can be extremely difficult in the first phase of DBT, because both patient and therapist often do not want to attend to targeted behaviors.

The rationale for the targeting strategies, and various objections to and difficulties with them (as well as potential solutions), have been discussed extensively in Chapters 5 and 6. It bears repeating here, however, that a therapist who ignores the targeting strategies is not doing DBT. That is, in DBT *what* is discussed is as important as *how* it is discussed. Difficulties in getting a patient to go along with the targeting strategies should be treated as any therapy-interfering behavior is treated; how to do this is discussed in the next chapter. A therapist who is having trouble following the targeting strategies (a not unlikely problem) should bring up the topic in the supervision/consultation meeting. Other therapists will almost certainly be having the same trouble.

Because I have already gone through the rationale for targeting at such length in other chapters, I do not go through it again here. It can be useful to look at targeting as setting an agenda. Although the agenda must remain flexible, depending on the patient's behavior during the week, it can nonetheless, be useful to review it before and after each session. The targeting strategies are described below and are summarized in Table 14.3. Although these strategies can be used in any order, all should be used every session.

TABLE 14.3. Targeting Strategies Checklist

_____ T REVIEWS P's PROGRESS since last contact.

    _____ During first and second phases of treatment, diary card is collected and scanned by T in an obvious way, so that its importance is clear to P.

        _____ If P does not bring the diary card, reasons are elicited; when appropriate, therapy-interfering behavior protocols (see Chapter 15) are utilized.

        _____ If P does not bring in the diary card, T asks P about any suicidal behaviors during the previous week (as well as other behaviors being tracked on the diary cards; T has P fill out card in session, if appropriate.

        _____ Any unusual or problematic responses are commented on; progress is reinforced.

    _____ T asks about progress on any behavioral assignments.

_____ T uses BEHAVIORAL TARGET PRIORITIES to organize session.

    _____ If suicidal behavior is reported (other than recurrent, low-level suicide ideation), T discusses this, using problem-solving strategies; T employs suicidal behavior protocols (see Chapter 15).

        _____ If misery is high and suicide ideation is low, and/or if self-harm urges are high and there is no parasuicide, T comments and attends to high misery/urges, validating that P's problems are important even when they are not accompanied by suicidal behaviors.

    _____ If therapy-interfering or quality-of-life-interfering behaviors are present, they are discussed and problem solving (general or in regard to the relationship) is used.

        _____ If P's phone calls are a current target, or if any unusual calls occurred during the previous week, they are reviewed during the session.

    _____ When required targets (suicidal behaviors, therapy-interfering behaviors, quality-of-life-interfering behaviors, posttraumatic stress) have been addressed, P allows T to control session content and direction.

_____ T ATTENDS TO P's STAGE of therapy; T does not jumb stages.

    _____ T returns to earlier stage of therapy if problems from that stage recur.

_____ T checks P's progress in OTHER MODES OF THERAPY.

    _____ T checks P's progress and attendance at skills training.

        _____ If P is not attending skills training sessions, is not completing homework for skills training, or expresses dissatisfaction with skills training, these issues are explored.

        _____ When appropriate, therapy-interfering behaviors protocol (see Chapter 15) is employed to improve compliance with skills training norms.

        _____ T conveys to P a value for the skills training.

        _____ T helps P relate skills learned in skills training to her current problems in living; where necessary T instructs P further in skills.

    _____ T helps P relate problems she is having in skills training, supportive group therapy, or other modes of DBT to other problems she is having in her life.

    _____ T helps P relate process issues in skills training or supportive group therapy to issues being examined in individual therapy.   _(cont.)_

Table 14.3. (cont.)

Anti-DBT tactics

_____ T does not ask to see diary cards.
     _____ T colludes with P in glossing over failure to bring card.
     _____ T does not ask for information that would have been on card if it
           were filled out.
     _____ T gives in or appeases P.
_____ T ignores or cursorily discusses suicidal behaviors.
_____ T ignores or cursorily discusses therapy-interfering behaviors.
_____ T ignores or cursorily discusses quality-of-life-interfering behaviors.
_____ T follows priority targeting rules but not spirit of the strategy.
_____ T pushes P to discuss childhood abuse while she is still in Stage 1.
_____ T communicates that skill training are someone else's responsibility.

---

1. REVIEWING TARGET BEHAVIORS SINCE THE LAST SESSION

The first therapeutic task in each session is to review with the patient her behavioral progress during the past week. In the first two stages of DBT, this inquiry is ordinarily structured by the therapist to obtain specific information about target behaviors.

Diary Cards

I begin every session with the simple question "Do you have your diary card?" (See Chapter 6 for a description of diary cards.) If the patient has it, I immediately scan it and from the card determine an initial agenda for the session. If the patient does not have the card, I ask whether she filled it out, what happened to it, and so on. If it was filled out but for one reason or another the patient did not bring it in, I quickly review the information orally. Specific questions depend on the stage of therapy and the current behavioral targets, although I usually try to get most of the card's information (on parasuicideal behavior and urges, suicide ideation and urges, substance use [including medications], daily misery, use of behavioral skills, and anything else we are monitoring). If she did not fill it out, I ordinarily give her a card to fill out while I wait during the session. As I have noted in Chapter 6, this type of consistent attention to diary cards tends to produce compliance sooner or later. (If not, it would be an instance of therapy-interfering behavior, and thus subject to even more attention.) The rationale for diary cards, as well as tactics for responding to both therapist and patient resistance to cards, is discussed in Chapter 6 and again in Chapter 15.

Homework Assignments

If homeworks assignments are given, the therapist must remember to ask about them during the session.

2. USING TARGET PRIORITIES TO ORGANIZE SESSIONS

As I discuss on a number of occasions, one of the distinctive characteristics of DBT is the use of behavioral target priorities to organize interactions. The basic rules are as follow. Individual psychotherapy time is oriented to current behaviors (since the last session), and priority for attention is determined by the target hierarchy. To remind the reader of that hierarchy (see Chapter 6), the highest priority in individual outpatient therapy is accorded to suicidal behaviors, followed by therapy-interfering behaviors, serious quality-of-life-interfering behaviors, skill deficits, posttraumatic stress behaviors, self-respect, and individual goals, in that order. In phone calls, the individual therapist also organizes the interaction according to a target hierarchy: decreasing suicide crisis behaviors, applying behavioral skills to the problem at hand, and resolving interpersonal crises or alienation between therapist and patient, in that order. Skills training sessions, supportive process groups, and all other modes of treatment have their own individual hierarchies. The task of each therapist is to use the order for the current interaction mode in guiding use of time. This particular strategy is one of the most difficult for new therapists and one of the most important to the overall progress of the therapy. (See Chapters 5 and 6 for a full discussion of using target priorities. Organizing time and coping with resistance are discussed extensively in Chapters 6 and 15.)

3. ATTENDING TO STAGES OF THERAPY

As also discussed in Chapter 6, DBT is organized into four stages: the pretreatment stage of orientation and commitment; Stage 1, attaining basic capacities; Stage 2, reducing posttraumatic stress; and Stage 3, increasing self-respect and meeting individual patient goals. It is important for the therapist to attend to these stages—not moving therapy to a higher stage before goals of the current stage have been met, and moving therapy back a stage when problems of a previous stage reappear. The necessity of completing orientation and commitment (pretreatment) before beginning therapy per se is discussed above. As I have discussed more fully in Chapter 6, it is equally important to make substantial progress in Stage 1 before moving to Stage 2. The stages strategy also informs the therapist that previous traumatic stress cannot be ignored in DBT. Thus, in the absence of a compelling rationale, skipping from attaining basic capacities to meeting individual goals (other than temporarily) would generally be a violation of this strategy.

4. CHECKING PROGRESS IN OTHER MODES OF THERAPY

In individual psychotherapy, when the patient is simultaneously engaged in other modes of DBT (such as skills training), the therapist should check progress in these other modes each session. The individual therapist must remember that he or she is the primary therapist, and thus is responsible for coordinating all treatment modes. It is difficult for most patients to believe that a particular mode of therapy is important if the individual therapist does not believe it is important enough even to ask about. Problems in attendence or cooperation with other modes of treatment are also the responsibility of the individual therapist and are treated as therapy-interfering behaviors.

SESSION-ENDING STRATEGIES

How a session with a borderline and suicidal patient ends can be extremely important. Borderline patients not infrequently leave therapy sessions with such intense negative emotions, including anger, frustration, panic, grief, hopelessness, despair, emptiness, and aloneness, that they have great difficulty tolerating the emotional pain without resorting to maladaptive behavior. It is very important to anticipate these emotions and work with them as "problems to be solved." It is equally important to conclude and summarize the "business" part of the session—that is, to review homework given and summarize the progress made in the session. Strategies for ending sessions are outlined in Table 14.4.

I. PROVIDING SUFFICIENT TIME FOR CLOSURE

When the ending of a session begins depends on the particular patient. For some patients, the ending begins at the beginning. That is, they are so anxious about leaving that their behavior from the very beginning of the session is influenced by the salient fact that the interaction is, in their words, "almost over before it begins." As I have noted previously, borderline patients often say that they cannot and will not "open up" emotionally during sessions because once they do so, there is insufficient time for "closing up." They are left with intense emotions that they cannot regulate. Although this problem cannot be completely averted no matter how long a session is, each therapist and patient should work out together how many minutes should be left at the end of sessions to do the important closure work. The time needed will certainly vary both across patients and within a patient, depending on the material discussed during the session.

2. AGREEING ON HOMEWORK FOR THE COMING WEEK

During the course of the session, the patient and therapist may discuss various activities that the patient should engage in during the coming week. At the end of each session, any suggestions for homework should be reviewed and clarified, and the patient's agreement to engage in the assignment should be reaffirmed. At this point, the therapist should ask the patient whether she sees any problems in completing the assignment during the coming week.

TABLE 14.4. Session-Ending Strategies Checklist

_____ T GIVES SUFFICIENT TIME for ending that P does not feel rushed and the session is not ended abruptly.
   _____ P is given notice that session is coming to an end.
   _____ T helps P cope with session's ending.
   _____ T helps P close up emotionally.

_____T REVIEWS HOMEWORK or tasks agreed upon for the coming week.

_____ When appropriate, T SUMMARIZES session.

_____ T gives P AUDIOTAPE of session.

_____ T encourages and CHEERLEADS, expressing faith in P's ability to progress and handle any difficulties she may be faced with, while at the same time validating the real difficulties P still confronts.

_____ T SOOTHES P and gives P sense of T's continued presence (e.g., arranges phone contact, reminds P of availability of phone contact or of phone plan, etc.).

_____ T TROUBLESHOOTS (if appropriate); problem-solving strategies for coping with difficulties expected following the session or during the coming week are utilized.

_____ T stands and parts with P in a manner that conveys warmth and expectation that they will meet again soon; other ENDING RITUALS are developed and employed that are comfortable for both T and P.

Anti-DBT tactics

_____ T ends early without warning P.

_____ T brings up sensitive material just before session ending.

_____ T invalidates P's difficulties with ending and leaving session.

Generally it should be assumed that there will be such problems, and the therapist should take this opportunity to help the patient troubleshoot these.

3. SUMMARIZING THE SESSION

When appropriate, the therapist should summarize at the end of a session the important points that have been covered. Generally, such a summary should be offered in an "upbeat" fashion. Important insights that the patient has gained during the preceding week or the session should be briefly mentioned. At times, only a sentence or two is needed here.

4. GIVING THE PATIENT A TAPE OF THE SESSION

At the end of each session (if this is part of the plan), the patient should be given a copy of the session audiotape, with instructions to listen to it at least once during the coming week. The tape can serve as a stimulus for the patient to cope when she is feeling overwhelmed, and is a way to make the therapist present, so to speak, in the patient's natural environment.

5. CHEERLEADING

At the end of each session, the therapist should directly and openly encourage the patient on progress that she is making, and should point out to the patient some positive attribute or praiseworthy behavior. Essentially, this is an opportunity for the therapist to validate the patient's behavior without the patient's having to ask for it. This is also an opportunity for the therapist to offer hope and encouragement to the patient. Encouragement from the therapist is especially important if a substantial part of the session has been devoted to helping the patient become more aware of self-defeating behaviors on her part. Quite often, the patient will feel discouraged and hopeless but will communicate competence to the therapist. It is important that the therapist not be fooled by such apparent competence. The therapist must be careful to combine praise with validation of how terribly hard and painful the patient's life still is, and should not overestimate the patient's ability to cope on her own. As therapy progresses, the therapist can usefully begin to elicit from the patient encouraging and self-validating statements. In the latter half of therapy, the therapist may ask the patient directly what progress she sees during the prior week or during the current session.

6. SOOTHING AND REASSURING THE PATIENT

A patient often feels bereft at leaving a therapy session. Her sense of desperation and aloneness resurges as the session draws to a close. The therapist should anticipate this and remind the patient that she can call the therapist if need be before the next session; that is, contact is not irrevocably ended. The therapist should remind her also that she can call emergency services at any time and can ask other people in her environment for help if need be. As noted previously, a parasuicidal and borderline patient often has great trouble asking for help appropriately. Although she may frequently call the therapist in the midst of a crisis, acting and feeling desperate and making inappropriate demands on the therapist, she very rarely calls the therapist to ask for help *before* a crisis is reached.

In the beginning of therapy, a main goal is to teach the patient how to ask for help appropriately. It is especially important for the patient to learn that she can call someone simply to discuss problems, ask for advice, or even just share what is going on with her. It is usually very difficult for the patient to do this, and in the first stages of therapy calling the therapist may need to become a homework assignment. Once the patient is comfortable calling the therapist during a crisis, she should be instructed at the end of sessions to try calling the therapist before a crisis arises. Once the patient is able to call the therapist appropriately, attention should be directed toward generalizing this skill to other people in her environment. At this point, the therapist may discover that the patient has very few supportive people whom she can call appropriately; this issue may then become an important focus of therapy. In any event, a major objective of therapy is to make the patient capable of calling on other people in her environment for appropriate help by the time the therapy is ended.

7. TROUBLESHOOTING

If the patient continues to have considerable emotional difficulty at the close of a session, the therapist should help the patient develop emotion regulation and distress tolerance strategies for use after leaving. Again, it is particularly important not to be fooled by the patient's apparent competence. Certainly at the beginning, almost all patients will have considerable difficulty handling session endings. Although the emotional pain will decrease over time on its own, both therapist and patient should attend actively to developing problem-solving solutions for alleviating the emotional pain and forestalling maladaptive patterns of coping.

8. DEVELOPING ENDING RITUALS

The development of ending rituals can be soothing for the patient and make parting easier. At a minimum, the therapist should accompany the patient to the door and convey the expectation that they will meet again soon. For some patients, a good-bye hug may become an important part of session ending (see Chapter 12 for guidelines).

TERMINATING STRATEGIES

It is essential to prepare the patient for termination of therapy from the very beginning. As in any strong and positive intimate relationship, ending can be extremely difficult. DBT does not advocate a complete rupture in the relationship; instead, the patient moves from the category of patient to that of ex-patient, and the therapist goes from the role of therapist to that of ex-therapist. "Ex-" roles are quite different from "non-" roles. In the former, the fact of a once intense and intense positive attachment is recognized and valued. The change is akin to the transformation from student to former student, or from dependent child to emancipated adult child. Successful termination also requires that the interpersonal skills the patient has learned with the therapist generalize to nontherapeutic situations. Specific strategies for attending to therapy termination are outlined in Table 14.5

I. BEGINNING DISCUSSION OF TERMINATING: TAPERING OFF SESSIONS

Although the focus on generalization and termination continues throughout therapy, active discussion of approaching termination must begin quite some

TABLE 14.5. Terminating Strategies Checklist

_____ T BEGINS DISCUSSING eventual termination of therapy with P during the first session; T begins TAPERING OFF sessions gradually as termination approaches.

_____ T REINFORCES SELF-RELIANCE AND RELIANCE ON OTHERS over reliance on T and stresses need for both dependence and independence as therapy draws to its conclusion.

_____ T begins ACTIVELY PLANNNING for termination at least 3 months before therapy ends (in a 1-year DBT treatment contract).

     _____ T uses problem-solvilng strategies to troubleshoot difficulties with terinating; T sets up periodic "booster" sessions with P on a fading schedule, if necessary.

     _____ T evaluates progress.

     _____ T and P set up ground rules for continued contact.

         _____ T clarifies for P the type of relationship that can be expected with T after DBT ends.

         _____ T discusses the difference among a therapy relationship, a relationship with an ex-therapist, and a friendship.

         _____ T helps P determine criteria for re-entering therapy, reviewing skills, or otherwise becoming more active in problem solving after therapy ends.

_____ If P wishes to continue in treatment with someone else beyond termination, T MAKES A REFERRAL and, if necessary, continues to see P until new T can begin treatment with P.

time before therapy ends. The timing, however, will depend on how long the therapy is continued. To make the transition out of therapy smoother, therapy sessions should be "tapered off" in frequency, rather than stopped abruptly. During this process of active termination, the therapist emphasizes and praises the progress of the patient; expresses clear confidence in her ability to live independently outside of therapy; and emphasizes that caring and concern for the patient will not stop simply because therapy is terminated, and that community and/or private resources remain available for the patient if the need arises.

2. GENERALIZING INTERPERSONAL RELIANCE TO THE SOCIAL NETWORK

The ordinary course of events in therapy with a parasuicidal and borderline patient is that the patient will initially have great difficulty in trusting the therapist, in asking the therapist for help, and in arriving at a optimum balance between independence and dependence; as discussed earlier. Exploration of these patterns will often indicate that they are also occurring with others in the patient's environment. Essentially, the ability to ask for help is a necessary skill for survival in what is often an aversive environment. Thus the ability to trust, to ask for help appropriately, and both to depend on someone and to be self-reliant will often be objectives of treatment.

As the patient begins to develop trust in the therapist, she will generally begin to be more honest with the therapist about her need for help. During the initial stages of therapy, strong emphasis is put on reinforcing the patient for calling the therapist for help when she is having trouble coping with a particular situation. However, if this ability to request help is not transferred to other people in the patient's environment, and if the patient is not also taught to render assistance to herself, termination of therapy will be extremely traumatic. Even in very short-term absences of the therapist (e.g., on out-of-town trips), a parasuicidal patient is quite likely to react with parasuicidal behavior. Thus, the transition from reliance on the therapist to self-reliance and reliance on others must begin almost immediately. Once again, the dialectic strategies should be employed; in this case, the therapist emphasizes being able to depend on other people while learning to be independent.

3. ACTIVELY PLANNING FOR TERMINATION

As noted above, the fact of therapy termination should be discussed during the very first sessions of DBT. Termination from therapy and termination from the therapist, however, should be clearly differentiated. Moreover, the role of ex-therapist and the role of friend should be equally well differentiated. With few exceptions, ex-therapists do not become personal friends with former patients, and such an expectation should not be created. If a friendship does emerge, it will be an unexpected delight rather than an expected right.

Troubleshooting

The therapist should discuss with the patient any difficulties that may be expected to arise during or immediately following termination. Problem-solving strategies should be used to develop solutions. Included among potential solutions should be the possibility of "booster sessions." It is sometimes a good idea to plan these sessions, perhaps at 6-month intervals, even when problems are not expected.

Evaluating Progress

Sufficient time should be given to a reasonably thorough review of how therapy has progressed, what gains have been achieved, and what further progress the patient would like to make in her life. Both the therapeutic relationship itself (from the therapist's and the patient's perspectives) and patient's changes in targeted behaviors should be reviewed. The therapist should present the idea that no one is ever completely "cured" of troubles, and that all of life involves growth and change.

Setting Up Ground Rules for Continued Contact

The roles of ex-therapist and ex-patient have been insufficiently explored in the psychotherapy literature. It is extremely important that the therapist have a clear idea of his or her own preferences about future interaction with the patient. This idea should be presented clearly to the patient; making vague promises that will not be kept does her no favor. In the normal course of events, ex-patients' contact with their ex-therapists may be quite frequent immediately following therapy termination and for a year or so thereafter, and then will gradually fade in frequency. Since I am almost always interested in keeping up with former patients over the long run, much as I am with former students, I encourage them to stay in touch periodically so that I will know how they are doing. This is the time for interweaving of reciprocal communication and observing limits.

The patient's wishes for continued interaction with the therapist should also be explored. Some want more contact than others; some may actually want a complete break in contact. Both parties should outline the criteria for re-entry into therapy. If re-entry is impossible, the therapist should be clear about that and help the patient apply problem-solving to the issue of how to find another therapist.

4. MAKING APPROPRIATE REFERRALS

In a perfect world, therapy with the borderline patient would progress through Stages 1, 2, and 3 and would end with a patient who is reasonably satisfied with her life and at peace with herself. For a patient entering at Stage 1, this can take a number of years. Indeed, for the seriously suicidal borderline patient, even progressing from Stage 1 to Stage 2 can take at least a year and often longer. Depending on the severity of previous trauma and tendencies to dissociate, Stage 2 therapy can also take a year or more. At least until we develop more effective and more efficient therapies, trying to hurry patients through these stages sometimes creates more problems than it solves.

Unfortunately, because of financial and insurance limitations, dictates of managed care, personal limitations of the therapist, and/or research restrictions, it is often not possible for a therapist and patient to remain as a team for the time necessary to achieve these goals. It is essential in these instances that the therapist not abandon the patient. That is, the therapist must assist the patient in making alternative treatment follow-up plans. For all the reasons cited above, making these plans can be extraordinarily difficult for the patient who lacks financial resources to pay for private therapy. An additional problem is the reluctance of many private therapists to see borderline and/or suicidal patients for therapy. The therapist may need to explore both public and low-cost private mental health resources, as well as peer counseling and support groups (e.g., Alcoholics Anonymous). If the therapist knows at the start that therapy will be time-limited, then planning for referral should start well before the end of therapy.

Concluding Comments

My patients often ask me whether they will ever get better, whether they will ever be happy. It is a difficult question to answer. Surely they can get better and happier than they are when they first come to see me. And, yes, I believe that life can be worth living even for a person who has at one time met criteria for BPD. I am less certain, however, whether anyone can ever completely overcome the effects of the extremely abusive environments many of my patients have experienced. Some amount of grieving may be necessary over their whole lives. The important thing here is not to catastrophize this reality. Many people over history have had to face and accept extraordinarily painful events; yet they have gone on and developed lives of reasonable quality or fulfillment. Of course, how to do this is not completely obvious, nor is it easy. Psychotherapy is only a small part of the attempts made by society to confront this dilemma. The limits of psychotherapy may be circumvented by involvement in religion, spiritual practices, study of literature, history or philosophy, community activities, and so on. That is, many answers will be found outside of psychotherapy.

Nor will all individuals find and maintain the loving, nurturing, and supportive interpersonal relationships they so frequently desire. At least, they may not find these qualities in one relationship; even if they do establish such a relationship, it may not be permanent. The relationship with the therapist may be the best one an individual ever finds — not necessarily because of deficiencies on her part, but because the ability of our society to provide community and companionship is limited, even for many of its best members. Supportive group therapy following termination of individual therapy may be a good option for many former borderline patients. Some may want to continue in such groups indefinitely; I think that this should be encouraged and supported. With others, ongoing if intermittent contact with their former therapists may be very important.

15

Special Treatment Strategies

This chapter covers strategies for responding to specific problems and issues in treatment with borderline patients. Like structural strategies, these strategies require the combination of standard strategies in new and unique ways. Integrative strategies for responding to the following are discussed here: (1) patient crises, (2) suicidal behaviors, (3) patient therapy-interfering behaviors, (4) telephone calls, (5) ancillary treatments, and (6) patient–therapist relationship issues.

CRISIS STRATEGIES

As noted throughout this book, borderline patients are often in a state of crisis. Such a state inevitably lessens a patient's ability to use behavioral skills she has been learning. Emotional arousal interferes with cognitive processing, thereby limiting the patient's ability to focus on anything other than the present crisis. In these instances, the therapist should employ the crisis response format described in this section.

In standard outpatient DBT, the responsibility for assisting a patient in crisis belongs to the individual or primary therapist. Other outpatient therapists and team members should (1) refer the patient to her primary therapist, assisting her in making contact if necessary; and (2) help the patient apply distress tolerance skills until she reaches her primary therapist. This division of labor can be very important in effectively treating the patient who calls other treatment staff members whenever she can't get hold of her primary therapist immediately, or who "shops around" for a sympathetic response when she doesn't like her primary therapist's response. Many of the crisis response strategies outlined in Table 15.1 and discussed below may prove useful in this limited task. DBT does not advocate, as a usual practice, an "on-call"

TABLE 15.1. Crisis Strategies Checklist

____ T attends to AFFECT rather than content.

____ T explores the problem NOW.
     ____ T focuses on time since last contact.
     ____ T identifies key events setting off current emotions.
     ____ T formulates and summarizes the problem.

____ T focuses on PROBLEM SOLVING.
     ____ T gives advice and makes suggestions.
     ____ T frames possible solutions in terms of behavioral skills P is learning.
     ____ T predicts future consequences of action plans.
     ____ T confronts P's maladaptive ideas or behavior directly.
     ____ T clarifies and reinforces P's adaptive responses.
     ____ T identifies factors interfering with productive plans of action.

____ T focuses on AFFECT TOLERANCE.

____ T helps P COMMIT herself to a plan of action.

____ T assess P's SUICIDE POTENTIAL.

____ T anticipates a RECURRENCE of the crisis response.

procedure in which patients in crisis can only talk to whichever team member is on call that day. (See the discussion of telephone strategies, below, for futher comments.) In other settings, such as inpatient or day treatment, responsibility for crisis intervention might be assigned to other members of the treatment team.

1. PAYING ATTENTION TO AFFECT RATHER THAN CONTENT

Paying attention to the patient's affect rather than to the content of a crisis is especially important when a patient is emotionally aroused. Techniques for validating emotional experiences are described in Chapter 8. In summary, a therapist should identify the patient's feelings, communicate to the patient the validity of her feelings, provide an opportunity for emotional ventilation, verbally reflect to the patient his or her own emotional responses to the patient's feelings, and offer reflective statements.

2. EXPLORING THE PROBLEM NOW

Focusing on Time Period since Last Contact

In a state of high emotional arousal, an individual quite often loses track of the event that precipitated the emotional response in the first place. She may attend not only to the precipitating event, but to all similar events that have occurred either in her whole life or in the past several weeks. Thus, one event may have set off the crisis, but the patient may rapidly switch from one topic to another in trying to communicate what is happening to her. A therapist should concentrate on helping the patient focus on what exactly has happened since the last contact, instead of drawn into a discussion of all the negative events in the patient's life.

Trying to Identify Key Precipitants of the Current Crisis

Frequently a very minor event will set off an overwhelming crisis response. In these instances, it is critical that the therapist help the patient identify this precipitating event. Often, the patient will list a whole series of unmanageable events and conditions in her life. The therapist should listen and respond selectively—that is, respond only to workable material and ignore irrelevant and/or unmanageable aspects of the story. In this context, the patient should be asked to be both concrete and specific in describing what is happening to her.

The therapist should select some portion of the patient's crisis response, such as her feeling overwhelmed, hopeless, desperate, suicidal, and so on, and ask the patient to pinpoint just exactly when that response first began, when it increased or decreased, and so on. For example, if the feeling is terror, the therapist might frequently ask, "Did you feel terror at that point?" If the answer is yes, the therapist might follow with "And did you feel terror right before he said 'X, Y, or Z'?" If the answer is yes, the therapist goes back in time moment by moment to find the exact comment or event that set off the terror. A bit later in the story, the therapist might say, "And did that increase or decrease the terror?" and so on. The idea is to constantly link a specific patient crisis response (or set of responses) to a specific event or series of events.

Formulating and Summarize the Problem Situation

Problem formulation and summary may be needed repeatedly during a crisis session; a therapist should focus on arriving at agreement as to the definition of the problem's main elements. Quite often, the patient will be focusing on solutions to the problem without adequately defining the problem. Of course, a main solution often put forward by the patient is suicidal behavior. The therapist should be very alert to a patient's tendency to state a suicidal behavior as a problem instead of as a solution.

Thus the patient may say, "The problem is that I want to kill myself." The therapist should emphatically and directly communicate that suicidal behavior is not a problem, but is rather a solution to a problem. The therapist may say, "OK. That's a solution to a problem. Let's figure out exactly when that first thought of killing yourself entered your mind. When did you first think of it? What set it off?" Once that moment is identified, the therapist can then explore what about that event is so problematic that it elicited the urge to commit suicide. For some individuals, thoughts of suicide are simply overlearned responses to any problematic event, or painful emotions or interpretations of the event may have intervened. As one can see, finding the precipitating event is usually the most direct route to figuring out the problem situation. Such an analysis should be followed by immediately reformulating the problem and by eliciting and reinforcing agreement from the patient when possible.

3. FOCUSING ON PROBLEM SOLVING

Once again, the therapist is faced with trying to synthesize contradictory points of view. The therapist must help the patient reduce the aversive, negative emotions while at the same time helping the patient see that the ability to put up with some unpleasant affect is necessary for arousal reduction. If problem-solving techniques are utilized here, it is almost always essential to select some small area of the current crisis for attention. The patient will often communicate an intense desire to "make everything OK right now"; the therapist should *model* breaking a problem down into small parts and dealing with one aspect at a time. In problem solving during a crisis, the procedure below should be followed, in addition to the standard problem-solving techniques described in Chapter 9.

Giving Advice and Making Direct Suggestions

In DBT, the therapist functions in multiple roles (consultant, teacher, cheerleader, etc.). Although it is preferable to adopt the consultant role in helping the patient choose from among several response alternatives she has generated, there are times when the patient simply does not know what to do or how to handle a given situation. In these instances, it is appropriate for the therapist to give the patient concrete advice and make direct suggestions about possible action plans. This is especially important in dealing with an "apparently competent patient. In such a case, it is very common for a therapist to assume that the patient actually could figure out what to do, but simply lacks confidence in her own ability. It is easy to make the mistake of refusing to give the patient advice under the mistaken theory that the patient does not need it. Thus, it is important to assess the patient's capabilities carefully and to respect the patient's knowledge of her own capabilities. A patient's passivity must not be unilaterally interpreted as lack of motivation, resistance, lack of confidence, or the like. Many times, passivity is a function of inadequate knowledge and/or skills.

Offering a Solution Based on the Behavioral Skills the Patient Is Learning

All problems can be solved in more than one way; it depends on one's perspective. The ability to employ the perspective of behavioral skills when generating problem solutions is crucial in DBT. Thus, when distress tolerance is the current treatment module (or a set of skills the therapist wishes the patient to practice), a crisis can be viewed as one in which distress tolerance is needed. If interpersonal effectiveness is the focus, the problem can be framed as related to interpersonal actions. Generally, events become "problems" because they are associated with aversive emotional responses; one solution might be for the patient to change her emotional response to the situation. An effective response might be cast in terms of mindfulness skills. The ability to apply any of the behavioral skills to any problematic situation is at once important and very difficult. Therapists must themselves know the behavioral skills inside and out, and be able to think about them quickly during a crises.

An example may be helpful here. Suppose a patient comes to a session and during the review of her week begins crying, saying that she simply cannot talk about her week because it is too upsetting. The therapist can take any of the following paths. First, the therapist can comment that the patient seems to be experiencing high distress, and can encourage her to focus on which skills she could use at this very moment to tolerate the pain she is feeling—indeed, to tolerate it well enough to plunge into a discussion of the week. Second, the therapist can focus the discussion on helping the patient evaluate her goals at this moment in interacting with the therapist. What interpersonal skills could she use right now to meet her objectives? What does she need to say or do so that she will feel good about herself when this interaction is over? How does she want the therapist to feel about her once this interaction is over and what could she now say or do to be effective here? Third, the therapist can focus the discussion on identifying the current emotion and generating ideas about how to feel better right now. Finally, depending on which mindfulness skill is being taught (or which the patient needs to practice), the therapist can suggest that she focus on observing or describing her current state or that she try to respond to herself in this moment in a nonjudgemental fashion; that she refocus her attention on just this moment and the task at hand; or that she consider right now what she needs to do to focus on what "works."

Predicting Future Consequences of Various Plans of Action

Suicidal and borderline patients often focus on short-term gain and ignore long-term consequences of their behavioral choices. A therapist should urge a patient to focus on long-term consequences of her behavior. The patient should be helped to examine the pros and cons of various action alternatives in terms of their effectiveness at achieving objectives, at maintaining interpersonal relationships, and at helping the patient respect and feel better about herself.

Confronting the Patient's Ideas or Behavior Directly

In the midst of a crisis and high emotional arousal, it is unusual for a patient to be able to examine the pros and cons of various action plans calmly. When the therapist believes that a given course of action will have detrimental effects, he or she should confront the patient directly about the outcomes of her behavioral choice. Frequently, choices will be linked to unrealistic beliefs on the part of the patient; in these instances, the patient's beliefs must also be confronted. When the therapist confronts a patient who is in a state of intense emotional arousal, the patient will frequently respond with statements indicating that the therapist does not really understand her situation. In these instances, it is helpful to express understanding and validation of the pain the patient is experiencing, and to follow this by indicating a belief that an alternative action choice, even though painful, would be preferable in the long term.

Clarifying and Reinforcing Adaptive Responses

As a patient begins to learn adaptive cognitive and behavioral responses, these responses must be reinforced. During a crisis, it is beneficial to attend carefully to any adaptive responses or ideas generated, to help clarify them, and then to reinforce these responses. At other times, the therapist can refer to other occasions when the patient has dealt with similar situations adaptively and can praise such behaviors.

Identifying Factors Interfering with Productive Plans of Action

Once the patient and therapist have identified a plan of action that appears productive, the therapist should help the patient identify factors that might interfere with the plan. If this step is neglected, the patient is likely to experience failure; consequently, problem solving in the future will be more difficult. The identification of factors interfering with productive plans should be followed, of course, by further discussion of how these problems can be solved.

4. FOCUSING ON AFFECT TOLERANCE

Generally, the patient will communicate to the therapist her inability to tolerate the crisis situation: Not only is the situation overwhelming, but she can't stand it. While validating the patient's pain, the therapist must also directly confront the patient with the necessity of tolerating the negative affect. It is frequently helpful to make a statement such as this: "If I could take away your pain, I would. But I can't. Nor, it appears, can you. I'm sorry for the pain you are in, but for the moment you have to tolerate it. Going through the pain is the only way out." The patient should not be expected to empathize with this point of view in the early stages of therapy. However, this should not deter the therapist from making these statements *repeatedly* throughout these stages.

5. OBTAINING COMMITMENT TO A PLAN OF ACTION

The therapist should make every effort to persuade the patient to agree to a plan of action that specifies what both the patient and the therapist will do between now and the next contact. An explicit, time-limited contract— one that includes demands or requirements the patient must fulfill before the next contact—should be negotiated. In other words, the therapist must communicate to the patient that she is expected to take the agreed-upon steps to begin to resolve her current crisis.

6. ASSESSING SUICIDE POTENTIAL

At the end of every crisis interaction, the therapist should reassess the patient's suicide risk. The patient may begin such an interaction by saying she is going to kill herself, injure herself, or engage in some other destructive action. Despite a therapist's best efforts, the patient may still maintain this point of view at the end of the interaction. The therapist should check whether the crisis has been alleviated sufficiently that the patient believes she can refrain from killing herself between this interaction and the next contact. If the patient cannot agree to this, the therapist should move to the suicidal behavior strategies, described next.

7. ANTICIPATING A RECURRENCE OF THE CRISIS RESPONSE

Together, the therapist and patient will often formulate an action plan that promises to reduce the patient's current feelings of being overwhelmed. Although these plans may in fact be quite helpful, the patient will commonly experience a resurgence of the overwhelming affect (after a short period of time). Thus, during a crisis the therapist should take responsibility for helping the patient plan or structure her time between the current contact and the next contact. The patient should be warned that the aversive feelings are very likely to recur and that several strategies for coping with such feelings should be planned.

SUICIDAL BEHAVIOR STRATEGIES

Treatment of suicidal individuals requires a structured protocol for responding to suicidal behaviors, including suicide crisis behaviors, parasuicide, threats of suicide or parasuicide, suicide ideation, and urges to engage in parasuicide. This protocol may be implemented within or following a treatment session, on the telephone, in a hospital setting, or (less frequently) the therapist's or patient's ordinary environment. Information about suicidal behavior may be spontaneously communicated to the therapist, may be elicited from the patient by questioning, or may be obtained via phone calls to the therapist from other professionals or from concerned individuals in the patient's environment.

The Therapeutic Task

The task of the therapist in responding to suicidal behavior is twofold: (1) responding actively enough to block the patient from actually killing or seriously harming herself; and (2) responding in a fashion that reduces the probability of subsequent suicidal behavior. The requirements of these two tasks often conflict. A dialectical tension arises between the demands of keeping a patient safe and the demands of teaching the patient behavioral patterns that will make staying alive worthwhile. Complicating all of this are the fears almost all therapists have of being held responsible for a patient's death if a false step is taken or a mistake made. The strategies described below are designed to address both the therapeutic needs of the patient and the limits of the therapist.

How a therapist responds to any single instance of suicidal behavior or threat will always be mitigated by characteristics of the individual patient, her situation, and the therapeutic relationship. There are only three arbitrary rules in DBT concerning suicidal behavior (which, of course, must be communicated to the patient during treatment orientation). First, parasuicidal acts and suicide crisis behaviors are always analyzed in depth; they are never ignored. Second, a patient who engages in parasuicidal acts cannot call her therapist for 24 hours following the act, except in a medical emergency where she needs the therapist to save her life. Even then, the patient should call emergency services and not the therapist. Third, potentialy lethal patients are not given lethal drugs. (This last point is discussed further under ancillary treatment strategies, below.)

Suicidal behavior strategies should be implemented in at least four situations: (1) The patient reports previous suicidal behavior to her individual or primary therapist during an individual therapy session (and is not now at any medical risk); (2) the patient threatens imminent suicide or parasuicide to her primary therapist; (3) the patient engages in parasuicide while in contact with her primary therapist, or contacts him or her immediately following a parasuicidal act; (4) the patient reports or threatens suicidal behavior to a collateral therapist. When the patient is in crisis and also suicidal, the crisis strategies just described should be integrated with the steps outlined in this section and summarized in Table 15.2.

PREVIOUS SUICIDAL BEHAVIORS: PROTOCOL FOR THE PRIMARY THERAPIST

A patient may spontaneously volunteer information on previous suicidal behavior during any therapy interaction, including phone conversations, skills training or process group therapy sessions, or individual therapy sessions. DBT

TABLE 15.2. Suicidal Behavior Strategies Checklist

FOR PRIMARY THERAPIST, WHEN SUICIDE CRISIS/PARASUICIDAL BEHAVIOR HAS OCCURRED:

____ T has no phone contact with P for 24 hours after an incident (except in a medical emergency); behavior is discussed at the next individual therapy session.)

____ T ASSESSES the frequency, intensity, and severity of suicidal behavior.

____ T does a CHAIN ANALYSIS of the behavior.

____ T discusses ALTERNATIVE SOLUTIONS VERSUS TOLERANCE.

____ T focuses attention on NEGATIVE EFFECTS of suicidal behavior.

____ T REINFORCES nonsuicidal responses.

____ T helps P COMMIT to nonsuicidal behavioral plan.

____ T VALIDATES P's pain.

____ T CONNECTS current behavior to overall pattern.

FOR PRIMARY THERAPIST, WHEN THREATS OF IMMINENT SUICIDE OR PARASUICIDE ARE OCCURRING:

____ T ASSESSES the risk of suicide or parasuicide.

    ____ T uses known factors related to suicide behavior to predict long-term risk.

    ____ T uses known factors related to imminent suicidal behavior to predict imminent risk.

    ____ T makes, keeps available, and uses a crisis planning sheet.

    ____ T knows the likely lethality of various suicide/parasuicide methods.

    ____ T consults with emergency services or medical consultant about medical risk of planned and/or available method(s).

____ T REMOVES or gets P to remove lethal items.

____ T EMPHATICALLY INSTRUCTS P not to commit suicide or engage in parasuicide.

____ T maintains position that suicide is NOT A GOOD SOLUTION.

____ T generates HOPEFUL statements and solutions.

____ T keeps CONTACT and keeps to TREATMENT PLAN when suicide risk is imminent and high.

    ____ T is more active when suicide risk is high.

    ____ T generally does not actively intervene to prevent parasuicide unless medical risk is high.

    ____ T is more conservative with new P.

    ____ T assesses whether suicidal behavior is respondent behavior.

        ____ T attempts to stop the eliciting events.

        ____ T teaches P how to prevent them in the future.

    ____ T assess whether suicidal behavior is operant behavior.

        ____ T searches for response that both meets the requirements of the treatment plan and is also a natural contingency.

        ____ T provides a somewhat aversive contingency—a therapeutic response that is not a reinforcing response.

    ____ T searches for an optimal response that is natural, reduces eliciting factors (behavior as respondent), and minimally reinforces (behavior as operant).

(cont.)

Table 15.2. (cont.)

_____ T tries to pull some improved behavior from P before actively intervening.

_____ T is flexible in response options considered.

_____ If T considers involuntary intervention, T is honest about reasons for doing so.

_____ T ANTICIPATES a recurrence.

_____ T COMMUNICATES P's suicide risk to others in her network.

FOR PRIMARY THERAPISTS, WHEN PARASUICIDAL ACT IS TAKING PLACE DURING CONTACT OR HAS JUST TAKEN PLACE:

_____ T ASSESSES POTENTIAL MEDICAL RISK of behavior, consulting with local emergency services or other medial resources to determine risk when necessary.

_____ T assesses P's ability to obtain medical treatment on her own.

_____ T determines presence of other people nearby.

_____ If a medical emergency exists, T ALERTS individuals near P, and CALLS EMERGENCY SERVICES.

_____ T calls P back and remains in contact until aid arrives.

_____ If nonemergency medical treatment is required, and P is willing, T COACHES P in obtaining medical treatment.

_____ T instructs P to call and check in from site of medical treatment, limiting call to summarizing treatment and medical status.

_____ If nonemergency medical treatment is required, and P is unwilling to get it, T uses PROBLEM-SOLVING STRATEGIES.

_____ T does not take no for an answer.

_____ T troubleshoots P's fears of involuntary hospitalization.

_____ T coaches P in how to interact with medical professionals.

_____ T tells ancillary professionals to follow their normal procedures.

_____ T intervenes, if necessary, to prevent involuntary hospitalization.

_____ If it is clear that medical attention is not needed, T KEEPS TO THE 24-HOUR RULE.

FOR COLLATERAL THERAPISTS:

_____ T keeps P SAFE.

_____ Skills trainer T helps P apply behavior skills until individual T can be contacted.

_____ Pharmacotherapy T consults P about medication adjustments that might help until individual T can be contacted.

_____ Inpatient staff T uses crisis intervention, problem-solving, and/or skills training strategies until P's next appointment with individual T.

_____ T REFERS P to individual or primary T.

diary cards collected at the beginning of each individual therapy session ask for information on daily suicide ideation and urges to engage in parasuicide, and also ask whether or not the patient actually engaged in a parasuicidal act since the previous individual therapy session. Without fail, this information should be reviewed by the therapist at the beginning of each individual therapy session. How the therapist responds to reports of previous suicidal behaviors will influence the probability of subsequent suicidal behaviors. Great care is needed.

If either suicide crisis behaviors (e.g., suicide threats) or parasuicidal acts have occurred since the last individual therapy session, problem-solving strategies are implemented. Detailed analyses of previous suicidal behaviors, however, are only conducted during individual sessions. If the primary therapist hears between sessions (from the patient or another source) about previous parasuicide or suicide crisis behaviors, including threats made to others, intervention directed at that behavior should be postponed until the next session, unless the patient is in danger of further behavior or is at medical risk.

The first step in responding to prior parasuicidal behavior is to conduct a detailed and thorough behavioral assessment. This assessment is *always* conducted during the next individual therapy session (although its timing within the session is optional). At times, the behavioral analysis can take an entire session; it will generally take at least 15 to 20 minutes. (If it is any shorter, either the therapist or the patient is probably avoiding the topic.) A solution analysis follows, or is interwoven. The therapist and patient examine what other behaviors could have been employed or could be used the next time. Often a number of points can be identified where a different response might have led to a different outcome. The behavioral and solution analyses lead, optimally, to relapse prevention planning—an approach developed by Alan Marlatt (Marlatt & Gordon, 1985) for treating alcoholics.

There simply are no exceptions to the implementation of these strategies. Their use does not depend on whether a behavior is medically severe or high in risk versus less severe or lower in risk; on the mood or cooperation of the patient (or the mood of the therapist); or on whether other, more immediate crises have come up since the suicidal behavior. The strategies are also not short-circuited if the patient says she does not remember or does not know the answer to a question. In such instances, the therapist simply analyzes what led up to the point where the patient's memory has failed, and picks up at the next point in time. If *no* cooperative behavior occurs, then the therapist moves back to the commitment strategies (see Chapter 9) or to the therapy-interfering behavior strategies (described below). If time is short, the therapist should shorten the solution analysis in favor of the behavior analysis. If there is current suicide crisis behavior that must be attended to immediately, previous suicide crisis behavior or parasuicide is next on the priority list, even if it must await the next session.

Over time, behavior analyses will go faster as the typical precipitants of suicidal behaviors become clarified. However, therapists of patients in long-term therapy should be cautious about assuming that they understand current suicidal behaviors on the basis of their information about past behavior. The determinants of suicidal behaviors can and do change over time.

As I have discussed in Chapters 9 and 10, behavioral analysis (and, to a lesser extent, solution analysis) can be considered use of behavioral correction and overcorrection—a contingency management procedure. Discussing past suicide crisis behaviors and parasuicide can be aversive for a number of reasons. It requires effort; the patient has to focus her attention, rather than speaking of what comes to mind without effort. Often shame is associated with thinking and talking about suicidal actions. Talking about suicidal behaviors also means that other topics important to the patient may not be discussed because of time constraints.

If parasuicide and suicide crisis behaviors have not occurred since the last session, the therapist should focus on any suicide ideation or urges to engage in parasuicide that have occurred, as well as the cognitive and affective components of suicidal behavior. The amount of time and attention devoted to discussion of ideation and urges is rarely as extensive as that afforded to suicide crisis behaviors and parasuicide. At times only a question or two, or a highlighting comment, is needed. Low levels of these behaviors are not addressed in every instance; otherwise, there would be little time for attention to other targets.

Reinforcement of nonsuicidal responses to events that previously elicited a suicidal response is crucial until changes are stabilized. Sometimes, however, the only evidence of these nonsuicidal responses is an absence of or decrease in suicidal behaviors. In my experience, many therapists have great difficulty spending time on suicidal behaviors that do not occur. Since the entire topic is so aversive to both a patient and a therapist, it often seems easier just to ignore it. However, an analysis of how the patient actually avoids suicidal behaviors, especially in the presence of high suicide ideation, parasuicidal urges, and/or general misery, can be extremely useful in affording opportunities for the therapist to reinforce alternative problem-solving behaviors. Attention should be faded over time to insure that resistance to suicidal behaviors comes under the control of natural reinforcers.

Within the individual session, the following steps should be taken.

1. ASSESSING FREQUENCY, INTENSITY, AND SEVERITY OF SUICIDAL BEHAVIOR

The first step in responding to a patient's previous suicidal behavior is to obtain detailed, descriptive information. When suicide crisis behaviors have occurred in an interaction with the therapist, these behaviors are reviewed to be sure there is agreement on just what the behaviors were, including what was said, how it was said, and any other activities engaged in (writing a suicide note, obtaining lethal means, etc.). If the suicide threat was made to other mental health professionals, a description of exactly what was said and done, how it was said and done, and under what circumstances is obtained. Descriptive case notes should be written following the session.

With respect to parasuicidal acts, the therapist assesses the exact nature of the self-injurious behavior (e.g., where and how deep was the cut, exactly what chemicals or drugs were ingested and how much), the environmental context (alone vs. with others), the physical effects, any medical attention that was needed, the presence of accompanying suicide ideation, and conscious intentions the patient can recall. The therapist should carefully assess the actual lethality or medical risk of the parasuicide episode. The scale points listed in Appendix 15.1 can be used. This scale, developed by Smith, Conroy, and Ehler (1984) and then updated by Bongar (1991), can be reliably used by nonmedical clinicians and does not depend on a patient's willingness to accrurately discuss her "intent" at the time of the parasuicide episode. Instructions for use of the scale were provided by Smith et al. and have also been updated by Bongar.

The frequency and emotional intensity of suicidal ideation since the last contact should be explored. As noted above, continued suicide ideation and parasuicidal urges do not always need to be discussed; however, significant changes (either increases or decreases) should be explored, even if only briefly. Periodically, the therapist should assess whether the patient has made plans to attempt suicide and has the means needed to carry out a suicide attempt; similar information should be elicited regarding parasuicidal urges. It is particularly important to keep up on whether or not the patient is obtaining and keeping parasuicide implements (hoarding drugs, carrying razors around, etc.). A healthy suspicion is useful at times.

2. CONDUCTING A CHAIN ANALYIS

A chain analysis should be carried out in excruciating, moment-to-moment detail. The therapist should elicit enough detail to clarify the environmental events, emotional and cognitive responses, and overt actions that led up to the critical behavior, as well as the behavior's consequences (and thus the functions it served). The starting point of the analysis is the moment the patient identifies as the beginning of the suicidal crisis, or the moment of the first thought or urge to commit suicide, threaten suicide, or engage in parasuicide. One indirect (but intended) consequence of such a detailed and specific assessment is that the questions—for example, "And did the thought of suicide cross your mind then or before then?", "At that moment, were you feeling like you wanted to kill yourself, or did that feeling come up later?", or "You said you feel suicidal because he is leaving you for another woman. Did that feeling (wanting to kill yourself or be dead) start the second he said he was leaving, or did you first start thinking about it or thinking about what it means for you and then start feeling suicidal?"—highlight that (contrary to the patient's beliefs) suicidal responses are not *necessary* responses to the moment under discussion. The assessment model set forth in Chapter 9 should be followed.

3. DISCUSSING ALTERNATIVE SOLUTIONS VERSUS TOLERANCE

Once the problematic situation has been identified, therapist and patient should discuss alternative solutions to the problematic situation that the patient could have used. The therapist should always suggest that one solution to the problem could have been simply to tolerate the painful consequences, including negative affect, that the situation has generated. Furthermore, it should be emphasized that there is *always* more than one possible solution to even the toughest problem. The model for solution analysis set forth in Chapter 9 should be followed.

4. FOCUSING ON NEGATIVE EFFECTS OF SUICIDAL BEHAVIOR

The therapist should enumerate or elicit from the patient the actual or potential negative effects of the suicidal behavior. The strategies and procedures used here are those of solution analysis, contingency clarification, and at times reciprocal communication. It is important for the patient to begin to see the negative interpersonal consequences of both suicide crisis behaviors and parasuicidal acts. The patient may need considerable help in understanding the emotional impact of her behavior on others, as well as the seriousness with which suicidal behavior is viewed by others. The reciprocal communication strategies can be used to give the patient feedback on any negative impact of the suicidal behaviors on the therapeutic relationship or on the therapist's feelings and attitudes toward the patient.

Even if the behavior was conducted in private and negative environmental effects are not immediately obvious, the therapist should point out that over the long run suicidal behavior is not going to work as a means of resolving problems, even if it does temporarily alleviate painful affective states or obtain needed help from the environment. The negative effects of the suicidal behavior on the patient's self-esteem should be discussed. In the case of suicide ideation, the therapist should address the fact that thinking about suicide in response to problems in living serves only to divert attention from ways of solving the problem to ways of escaping the problem. Threatening suicide or preparing for suicide can also divert the patient from finding more effective solutions, as well as create further negatiave consequences of their own.

5. REINFORCING NONSUICIDAL RESPONSES

It is important to reinforce the patient for coping with problematic situations in ways other than suicide crisis behaviors or parasuicide. The procedures described in Chapter 10 should be applied. Reinforcers may include increased therapist warmth, a more ambient therapeutic session, and control over the use of session time. Attention and positive feedback are generally effective here, but the therapist must be very careful that praise is not interpreted as lack of concern about the patient's continued emotional distress. The patient's reports of high misery, but low suicide ideation or parasuicidal urges, should be met with as much care and concern as high suicide ideation. If the patient has to continue suicidal behavior to elicit concern and active therapeutic help, suicidal behaviors will undoubtedly continue. Also, the patient may well need reassurance that therapy is not going to end just because her suicidal behavior is improving.

6. OBTAINING COMMITMENT TO A NONSUICIDAL BEHAVIORAL PLAN

The therapist should help the patient make behavioral plans for avoiding suicidal behavior in the future when encountering similar problematic situations. Again, the solution analysis strategies outlined in Chapter 9 should be used. Frequently, the patient will maintain that there is no solution to the problem except suicidal behavior. Two responses are possible. First, the therapist can review with the patient her commitment to try her best to avoid suicidal behavior. Second, the therapist can generate other alternative behaviors and elicit a commitment from the patient to try such behaviors on an experimental basis. One alternative behavior is for the patient to call for help *before* engaging in suicidal behaviors.

7. VALIDATING THE PATIENT'S PAIN

No matter how unreasonable the suicidal behavior may appear to be, the therapist must always be careful to express understanding of the feelings of unbearable psychological pain that led the patient to engage in parasuicide or consider suicide. It is quite easy to get carried away with invalidating suicidal behavior as a solution to problems and to neglect to validate the feelings that led up to the behavior. Shneidman (1992) puts this perspective most eloquently:

> Suicide is best understood as a combined movement toward cessation *and* a movement away from intolerable, unendurable, unacceptable anguish. It is psychological pain of which I am speaking; "metapain," the pain of feeling pain. From a traditional psychodynamic view, hostility, shame, guilt, fear, protest, longing to join a deceased loved one, and the like have singly and in combination been identified as the root factor(s) in suicide. It is none of these; rather, it is the pain involved in any or all of them. (p. 54)

Parasuicide differs from suicide only insofar as the movement toward cessation (i.e., death) may or may not be present.

8. RELATING CURRENT BEHAVIOR TO OVERALL PATTERNS

The therapist should help the patient see patterns of suicidal behavior that are occurring. The insight (interpretation) strategies, outlined in Chapter 9, constitute the model here. Once such patterns become clear, the therapist and patient can focus more attention on learning how to generate desired outcomes in nonsuicidal ways or how to handle problematic situations more effectively.

THREATS OF IMMINENT SUICIDE OR PARASUICIDE: PROTOCOL FOR THE PRIMARY THERAPIST

An active response is called for when a patient directly or indirectly communicates an intent to commit suicide or to engage in a nonlethal parasuicidal act. Such communications can occur under crisis conditions, and the therapist is faced with determining the immediate risk, possibly at an inconvenient time and over the telephone. In other instances, the patient's intent to engage in parasuicide or commit suicide may be communicated during a scheduled treatment session, with the suicidal behavior threatened to take place either very soon (e.g., that day) or only if some future event occurs (e.g., an anticipated rejection or failure of the therapy). In the event of any threat, the following steps should be carried out.

I. ASSESSING THE RISK OF SUICIDE OR PARASUICIDE

Two types of risk assessment are crucial: short-term or imminent risk and long-term risk. The question in the assessment of long-term risk is whether the person falls into a group at high risk for suicide or parasuicide. Meeting criteria for BPD, for example, increases long-term risk for both. Being female increases risk for parasuicide and decreases risk for suicide. Age is positively correlated with suicide and negatively correlated with parasuicide. Factors related to long-term risk for both suicide and parasuicide are listed in Table 15.3; these risk factors are discussed more extensively in Linehan (1981) and Linehan and Shearin (1988). Factors that are useful in assessing risk for imminent suicide and parasuicide are listed in Table 15.4 and are also discussed extensively in Linehan (1981).[1] Bongar (1991) and Maris, Berman, Maltsberger, and Yufit (1992) also provide excellent reviews of risk assessment strategies. Therapists must have the risk factors so firmly committed to memory they are available to recall at a moment's notice. It is not possible to look these up in the middle of a crisis.

Both persons who commit suicide and those who engage in nonlethal parasuicide acts frequently communicate their intent ahead of time. Borderline patients who habitually engage in parasuicide, for example, may report urges or intentions to mutilate themselves, put themselves to sleep for a week, or the like. These individuals may make it very clear that they have no intent to commit suicide; a person planning to cut her wrists or arm, for instance, may communicate that she plans to cut herself to relieve unbearable tension. An individual planning suicide may similarly be very direct about her plan to die.

Patients also often think about or plan suicidal behavior without directly informing their therapists. A question, then, is whether a therapist ought to ask about suicidal ideation if a patient has not brought up the topic. Several events may suggest probing for suicidal ideation. The occurrence of any event known to have been a precipitant of prior parasuicide or suicide ideation should prompt such questioning. In addition, statements by the individual that she can't stand it any longer, wishes she were dead, believes others would be better off without her, or the like should alert the therapist to probe further.

Once it is clear that the patient is considering suicide or parasuicide, the therapist should move to an assessment of the immediate risk factors outlined in Table 15.4. It is extremely important that the therapist question the

TABLE 15.3. Factors Associated with Long-Term Risk for Suicide or Parasuicide

Factor	Parasuicide	Suicide
I. Environmental characteristics		
A. Life changes	Losses	Losses; bereavement
	Disrupted relationships	—
	Separations	—
	More change events	—
		Discharge from psychiatric hospital (within 6–12 months)
		Adverse events after discharge
B. Social support		
1. Work	Absent	Absent
2. Marital rates	Unmarried > married	Unmarried > married
3. Family	Hostile	Less available
4. Interpersonal contact	Low/lack of confidant	Low/lives alone
C. Models	Socially linked to other parasuicides	Family suicide rate higher
	Higher after widespread suicide publicity	Higher after widespread suicide publicity
D. Method availablity	Available	Available
II. Demographic characteristics		
A. Sex	Female > male	Male > female (almost equal among psychiatric patients)
B Age	Decrease with age	Increases with age (decreases with age for blacks, Hispanics, Native Americans)
C Race	Nonwhites overrepresented	White > nonwhite
III. Behavioral characteristics		
A. Cognitive		
1. Style	Rigid	—
	Possibly impulsive	—
	Poor problem solving	—
	Passive in problem solving	
2. Content	Possibly hopeless	Hopeless
	Powerless	—
	Negative self-concept	—
B. Physiological/ affective		
1. Affective	Angry, hostile	Apathetic, anhedonic
	Depressed	Depressed
	Dissatisfied with treatment	Indifferent to treatment
	High preference for affiliation and affection	Possibly dependent, dissatisfied

(cont.)

TABLE 15.3. (cont,)

Factor	Parasuicide	Suicide
	Uncomfortable with people	Psychic anxiety, panic attacks
2. Somatic	Possibly poor health	Poor health (increases with age)
	—	Insomnia
	Low frustration tolerance	Low pain tolerance
	—	Suicide in biological relative
C. Overt motor		
1. Interpersonal	Low social involvement	Low social involvement
	Less likely to ask for help	Less likely to ask for support or attention
	High friction and conflict	Data mixed on friction and conflict
2. General behavioral	20–55% previous parasuicide	20–55% previous parasuicide
	Alcohol and drug abuse	Alcohol and drug abuse
	—	Criminal behavior (young men)
	Unemployed	Unemployed/retired

Note. Adapted from "A Social–Behavioral Analysis of Suicide and Parasuicide: Implications for Clinical Assessment and Treatment" by M. M. Linehan, 1981, in H. Glaezer and J. F. Clarkin (Eds.), *Depression: Behavioral and Directive Intervention Strategies.* New York: Garland. Copyright 1981 by Garland Publishing. Adapted by permission.

patient about the method she intends to use (and whether the implements for such a method are currently available or easily obtained). In the case of a proposed drug overdose, the therapist should ask for the name of every drug that is in the patient's possession now (or easily accessible), together with the number of pills left and their dosage leve. In addition, the therapist should determine whether the patient has written a suicide note, has any plans for isolating herself, or has taken any precautions against discovery or intervention. It is important also to assess how available other people are to her now and how available they will be over the next several days. If the patient refuses to divulge this information, the risk is, of course, higher. The therapist should be alert to signs of severe or deepening depressive affect and of emerging panic attacks. If the risk assessment is taking place over the phone, it is important to determine whether the patient has been drinking or taking nonprescribed drugs recently, where she is at the moment of the call, and where other people are in relationship to the patient.

Lethal Drugs: Use of the Crisis Planning Sheets. Patients threatening to overdose have frequently stolen drugs from a friend or family member. They may have a vague idea of what they have, or may be able to describe it, but often will not know the exact name or dosage. The *Physicians' Desk Reference*

TABLE 15.4. Factors Associated with Imminent Risk for Suicide or Parasuicide

I. Direct indices of imminent risk for suicide or parasuicide

1. Suicide ideation
2. Suicide threats
3. Suicide planning and/or preparation
4. Parasuicide in the last year

II. Indirect indices of imminent risk for suicide or parasuicide

5. Patient falls into suicide or parasuicide risk populations
6. Recent disruption or loss of interpersonal relationship; negative environmental changes in past month; recent psychiatric hospital discharge
7. Indifference to or dissatisfaction with therapy; elopements and early pass returns by a hospitalized patient
8. Current hopelessness, anger, or both
9. Recent medical care
10. Indirect references to own death, arrangements for death
11. Abrupt clinical change, either negative or positive

III. Circumstances associated with suicide and/or parasuicide in the next several hours/days

12. Depressive turmoil, severe anxiety, panic attacks, severe mood cycling
13. Alcohol consumption
14. Suicide note written or in progress
15. Methods available or easily obtained
16. Isolation
17. Precautions against discovery or intervention; deception or concealment about timing, place, etc.

Note. Adapted from "A Social–Behavioral Analysis of Suicide and Parasuicide: Implications for Clinical Assessment and Treatment" by M. M. Linehan, 1981, in H. Glaezer and J. F. Clarkin (Eds.), *Depression: Behavioral and Directive Intervention Strategies.* New York: Garland. Copyright 1981 by Garland Publishing. Adapted by permission.

(PDR) can be very useful in determining the specific drugs and dosage levels the patient has on hand or has ingested. Individuals who are not medically trained should not under ordinary circumstances make decisions about the lethality or medical risk of what a patient has ingested or is threatening to ingest. The effects of combining drugs with one another or with alcohol, specific medical conditions, the patient's weight, and other factors make such decisions complicated.

The response to a patient threatening suicide, however, will depend on the therapist's estimate of the actual risk of death or substantial harm. Therefore, it is important to make some attempt to ascertain the lethality of the drugs the patient has on hand or has ingested. There are a number of aids and procedures. First, the therapist should have a crisis planning sheet formulated and kept up to date for the patient (see Figure 15.1). The crisis planning sheet should contain information about all of the prescription and nonprescription drugs the patient is known to possess or take, together with dosage levels, prescribing physician, and the patient's weight in kilograms. The crisis planning sheet should also indicate the average daily dose for each drug regularly taken or in the possession of the patient. It is important to remember that a dose that is not potentially lethal can still be medically dangerous. Thus, knowing the lethality of a drug is insufficient for a skillful response.

Second, a therapist who is not medically trained should always check an assessment of drug lethality immediately with a medically qualified person. Sometimes, the problem here is getting anyone to provide the needed information, others are often afraid of liability. In my experience, the best place to call is the local public emergency room (preferably the busiest one). This is the place least likely to want unnecessary hospitalizations, and thus most likely to want to help. A therapist who knows the exact dose taken or threatened, the patient's weight in kilograms, whether alcohol or illicit drugs are involved, and any medical problems the patient has can usually get a very good consultation. If the therapist cannot get a medical consultation, there is little choice but to err on the side of caution.

Unless the therapist is medically trained, he or she should follow medical advice as to whether the patient must get medical attention. (If the therapist is in doubt about the advice, a second consultation call can be placed to discuss the problem again.) This point cannot be made too strongly. It is very easy for a tired or overburdened therapist, who is in a rush to do something else, to underestimate the medical consequences of a drug overdose. Medical reactions can be delayed, and the fact that a patient is not groggy or looks OK is not sufficient reason for inaction. Often a therapist justifies inaction by deciding that requiring medical attention would reinforce the behavior, but this line of reasoning can sometimes have life-threatening consequences.

Other Lethal Means. Patients may threaten suicide by other means than a drug overdose. Thus, a therapist must know the likely lethality of various methods of suicide. Obviously, the threat to jump from 3 feet is lower than the threat to jump from 50 feet. Common methods, in decreasing order of lethality, are (1) firearms and explosives, (2) jumping from high places, (3) cutting and piercing vital organs, (4) hanging, (5) drowning (cannot swim), (6) poisoning (solids and liquids), (7) cutting and piercing nonvital organs, (8) drowning (can swim), (9) poisoning (gases), and (10) analgesic and soporific substances. (Schutz, 1982).

2. REMOVING OR CONVINCING THE PATIENT TO REMOVE LETHAL ITEMS

Once the therapist has determined that the patient is suicidal and possesses lethal means, attention should be focused on convincing the patient to remove or dispose of the lethal items. During telephone conversations, this can

FIGURE 15.1. DBT crisis planning sheet.

Date _____

Patient's
name _____ Clinic No. _____ DOB _____ Weight (kg)_____

Home address _____

Work address _____

Phone (Home) _____ (Work) _____
Significant others:
Name _____ Phone _____ City _____

Relationship _____
Relative:
Name _____ Phone _____ City _____

Relationship _____
Referring therapist:
Name _____ Phone _____ City _____
Current individual therapist:
Name _____ Phone (Day) _____

                                         Phone (Eve) _____
Primary skills training therapist:
Name _____ Phone (Day) _____

                                         Phone (Eve) _____
Skills training cotherapists:
Name _____ Phone (Day) _____

                                         Phone (Eve) _____
Pharmacotherapist:
Name _____ Phone (Day) _____

                                         Phone (Eve) _____

CRISIS PLAN

Reference notes (brief parasuicide history, treatment plan)

_____
_____
_____
_____
_____
_____
_____
_____
_____
_____

(cont.)

Figure 15.1. (cont.)

MEDICATIONS

#1 Rx _____ Generic name _____ Date _____

M.D. _____ Phone _____

Pharmacist _____ Phone _____

   Daily dose ____mg/g No. tabs/caps per day ____ Dose per tab/Cap ____mg/g

   Usual no. prescribed _____ Cautions_____

   Notes _____

Date stopped taking _____ Number tabs/caps remaining _____

#2 Rx _____ Generic name _____ Date _____

M.D. _____ Phone _____

Pharmacist _____ Phone _____

   Daily dose ____mg/g No. tabs/caps per day ____ Dose per tab/Cap ____mg/g

   Usual no. prescribed _____ Cautions _____

   Notes _____

Date stopped taking _____ Number tabs/caps remaining _____

#3 Rx _____ Generic name _____ Date _____

M.D. _____ Phone _____

Pharmacist _____ Phone _____

   Daily dose ____mg/g No. tabs/caps per day ____ Dose per tab/Cap ____mg/g

   Usual no. prescribed _____ Cautions _____

   Notes _____

Date stopped taking _____ Number tabs/caps remaining _____

be done by instructing the patient to throw potentially lethal drugs down the toilet or give them to another individual in the house. If the patient is both drinking alcohol and planning to take drugs, she should also be asked to dispose of any available alcohol. Razor blades and other cutting instruments, matches, poisons, and so forth should be thrown in a trash bin outside the home. A gun or its ammunition can be locked in the trunk of a car or in a locker, and the key can be given to someone else. The general idea is to put distance and effort between the patient and the means; the therapist may need to be creative here. During a session, the patient should be asked to hand over whatever she has with her for safekeeping.

    The therapist should give these instructions to the patient in a matter-of-fact way, and communicate a positive expectancy that the patient will in fact carry them out. On the phone, the therapist should simply tell the patient what she is to do and wait while she disposes of the lethal items. If the suicidal threat occurs during a regular session, the patient should be instructed to bring the lethal items to the next session, or even to go home and bring the items in immediately. Keeping lethal means around can be considered a therapy-interfering behavior and treated as such. This is the time for using reciprocal communication paired with observing limits.

It is important that the therapist not be diverted from the task of removing lethal items. Possession of lethal means is often perceived by the patient as a safety factor; she may become very anxious at the prospect of removing any possibility of killing herself. A useful rationale for removing lethal items is that the presence of such items may lead to an accidental suicide, even if in retrospective analysis of the situation she would probably not have decided to kill herself. The therapist can also emphasize that the patient can always stock up on lethal items again at a future point. The removal of lethal items should be presented as a technique to give the patient more time to think, rather than an absolute ruling out of any suicidal behavior in the future.

It is also important not to overfocus on the task when it becomes clear that the patient is simply not going to comply. The power struggle that ensues may be very hard to win. If the patient refuses, the therapist should simply back off and bring it up another day; persistence in bringing it up at opportune times should eventually result in success. However, the therapist should not underestimate the importance of the patient's bringing in lethal items or throwing them away. A patient of mine hoarded a stock of various medications that would have killed her many times over. For 2 years she refused to give them up, because they were her safety valve. She finally brought them in a box wrapped in black electrical tape, with a cross and flower taped to the top of the box. She had brought me her coffin, and this marked a significant turning point in therapy.

3. EMPHATICALLY INSTRUCTING THE PATIENT NOT TO COMMIT SUICIDE OR PARASUICIDE

Often, it is helpful simply to tell the patient emphatically that she should not kill or harm herself. Once again, the therapist can tell the patient that refraining from suicidal behavior now does not prevent her from doing it *in the future.*

4. MAINTAINING THAT SUICIDE IS NOT A GOOD SOLUTION

Suicidal patients often try to get their therapists to agree that suicide is a good solution, so that they can have "permission" to go ahead and kill themselves. It is essential not to give such permission. Thus, a DBT therapist should *never* instruct a patient to go ahead and do something, under a mistaken assumption that such statements may arouse in the patient sufficient anger and inhibit any suicidal behavior (i.e., the therapist should not use paradoxical instruction). Nor should the patient be "baited" with statements implying that she will never carry out her threats. Such statements may force the patient to prove that she *is* actually serious. Rather, the therapist should validate the emotional pain that has led to suicidal behavior, while at the same time refusing to validate such behavior as an appropriate solution. (See Chapter 5 for further arguments against suicidal behaviors.)

5. GENERATING HOPEFUL STATEMENTS AND SOLUTIONS

In some crises, the best thing the therapist can do is to generate as many hopeful statements and solutions as possible and hope that one of these will help the patient acknowledge that other solutions to the problem may exist. If one doesn't "catch," another should be proposed. I was once making an emergency home visit to a woman who was threatening suicide because her husband and children were treating her very cruelly. She felt completely hopeless. I spent over an hour talking with her while my teammate spoke with the family. It was late and I wanted to resolve the crisis so I could go home. But nothing seemed to help, and she rejected every idea and solution I could think of. Finally, I said, "Well, just because your marriage and family may be a catastrophe doesn't mean that your whole life and future has to be a catastrophe." She looked at me in complete surprise and said, "I never thought of it that way but you are right." We talked another few minutes, and the crisis was resolved for the moment. I had expanded the boundaries of her frame, which led to a new interpretation of her life and allowed affective change.

Focusing on the problem situation rather than on the planned suicidal behavior is useful, because undue emphasis on the latter will divert attention from finding alternative solutions. Some problems may be so complex that even the therapist is unable to arrive at alternatives likely to reduce the scope of the problem. In these instances, the therapist should simply state that although neither can think of a nonsuicidal solution at the moment, this does not *prove* there is no recourse but suicide. The finality of suicide as a solution can then be discussed, and the possibility of holding off on suicide can be presented.

6. WHEN SUICIDE RISK IS IMMINENT AND HIGH: KEEPING CONTACT AND KEEPING TO THE TREATMENT PLAN

Perhaps the most difficult treatment situation encountered by a therapist is that of the patient who convincingly threatens suicide, is alone, and refuses to be dissuaded from her purpose. The general rule is to stay in contact with the patient, either in person or by phone, until the therapist is convinced that the patient will be safe (from suicide or serious harm) once contact is broken off. If possible, a therapy session or phone call should be extended until the therapist is able to develop a satisfactory plan with the patient. A home visit may be called for if such a visit will not inadvertently reinforce the suicide communication. Home visits in DBT must be carried out with another team member (never alone), and a male therapist should always be accompanied by a female therapist. Home visits are extremely rare in DBT.

A therapist who is unable to stay in contact should elicit help from significant others, family members, or other treatment personnel (such as case managers or house counselors if the patient lives in a group home), or should suggest temporary hospitalization. The threat of imminent suicide is not the time for confidentiality. If the patient is willing, she can be referred to area emergency services, such as emergency rooms. The rule of thumb is to select the least intrusive intervention necessary.

Risk Factors and Operant versus Respondent Behavior. Two factors are important to keep in mind when planning treatment and deciding on how active to be in response to a suicidal crisis. The first factor is the short-term risk of suicide if the therapist does not actively intervene. The second factor is the long-term risk of suicide, or a life not worth living, if the therapist does actively intervene. The response to the patient in any given case requires a good knowledge of current risk factors and of the functions of suicidal behavior for this patient. Therapist will know much less clear about risk factors and the functions of suicidal behavior for new patients; thus, in the early stages of therapy, treatment should be much more conservative and active.

Risk factors have been described above. The general rule is that the higher the risk, the more active the response should be; mitigating this, however, are the functions of the behavior and the likely long-term consequences of various courses of action. Although in the short run a certain response may decrease the probability of suicide, the same response may actually increase the likelihood of future suicide. The key analysis that must be made is whether in the specific instance, the patient's suicide ideation, preparations, and communications are operant or respondent behaviors. A behavior is respondent when it is automatically elicited by a situation or specific stimulus event; the behavior is under the control of the preceding events, not of the consequences. Suicide ideation and threats elicited by extreme hopelessness and a wish to die, by "voices" telling her to kill herself, or by severe depression, are examples here. When suicidal behavior is respondent, therapists do not have to be as wary that they will accidentally reinforce it by intervening.

When the behavior is operant, it is under the control of the consequences. Operant behaviors function to affect the environment. When suicide ideation and threats function to get others actively involved (e.g., to get help, to command attention or concern, to get others to solve problems, to obtain admission to a hospital, etc.), they are functionally operant. In these cases therapists have to be very wary of inadvertently reinforcing the very behaviors—high-risk suicidal behaviors—they are trying to stop. The difficulty is that if a therapist withholds active involvement, a patient can always escalate her behavior to a point where the therapist does intervene. This can reinforce more lethal behavior than was happening previously. As such escalation continues, suicidal behavior can become lethal.

Much of the time, suicidal behaviors among borderline patients are simultaneously respondent and operant. Hopelessness, despair, and the unbearableness of life elicit the behavior. The community's responses—giving help, taking the person seriously, taking the person out of difficult situations, and so on—reinforce the behavior. The best response is one that both reduces the eliciting factors and minimally reinforces the behavior. Unless there is a medical emergency, an active intervention that is potentially reinforcing should both require some improved patient behavior first and keep the patient safe.

Flexibility of response options is essential. The therapist must figure out the function of the behavior and then be active, but not in a manner that keeps the behavior functional. There are many ways to keep a patient safe. For example, if the behavior functions to get the therapist's time and attention, and if going into the hospital is aversive for that patient, insisting that the problem is obviously so serious that she must get to the hospital right away maintains safety without reinforcement. Of course, the therapist should not give her extra time once she is in the hospital. When the functional value of the behavior is to get the patient into a hospital, then the response should, of course, be different. Here the therapist may need to give the patient far more attention and active support outside of the hospital, or line up sufficient community resources to keep her safe outside of a hospital. Or perhaps involuntary hospitalization should be considered (assuming that this is not a reinforcing option). It is always a good idea to have area hospitals ordered in terms of the patient's preference. A patient who becomes suicidal to gain admission should be admitted to her *least* preferred place, if possible.

Complicating matters further, however, is the fact the therapist must remember that the object is to remove consequences that actually reinforce suicidal behavior for the particular patient. As the reader may remember from Chapter 10, what is and is not reinforcing or punishing for a particular patient can only be determined by close empirical observation. The fact that a patient doesn't like a consequence, or even that she complains bitterly about it, does not necessarily mean that the consequence is not a reinforcer nonetheless. The necessity of having some idea of what consequences are maintaining the patient's suicidal behaviors is the principal reason behind the emphasis in DBT on minute behavioral assessment of every episode of parasuicide and suicide crisis behavior.

In summary, for operant suicidal behavior, the plan is to design a response that is natural instead of arbitrary, somewhat aversive (but not so aversive that it only temporarily suppresses the behavior or drives it into secrecy), and is not a reinforcer for that particular patient. Usually, but not always, this means selecting something other than the patient's preferred therapeutic response. For respondent suicidal behavior, the plan is to design a therapeutic response that stops (or at least reduces) the eliciting events, teaches the patient how to prevent them in the future, and reinforces alternative problem-solving behaviors. For combined operant and respondent suicidal behaviors, the strategies should be combined.

Two points are important here. First, the decision as to whether suicidal behavior is operant or respondent should be based on careful assessment. Theory cannot answer this question; only close observation can. Second, in working with chronically suicidal individuals, there will be times when reasonably high short-term risks must be taken to produce long-term benefits. It is very difficult to feel secure when a patient is directly or indirectly threatening suicide. Difficulty in finding the best response is most likely when suicidal behavior is both respondent and operant and has previously been on an intermittent reinforcement schedule. The risks required in these cases are what make DBT somewhat like playing the car game of "chicken." In that game, two car drivers speed toward an obstacle; the object is to be the last to swerve the car to safety.

Generally, active intervention is taken to prevent suicide but not to prevent parasuicide, unless there is reason to believe that the parasuicidal act will result in serious medical harm. Ordinarily, burning, cutting, ingesting a few more drugs than recommended, or similar acts are not cause for environmental intervention by the therapist. The choice here is between a consultation-to-the-patient approach and an environmental intervention approach; the therapist ordinarily chooses the former. With a chronically parasuicidal patient, the therapist can expect a number of repeated parasuicides before the behavior comes under control. However, it is ultimately essential that the behavior come under the patient's control, not the therapist's or the community's.

Involuntary Intervention. Guidelines on when and how to hospitalize patients, including suicidal patients, are given in connection with ancillary treatment strategies (see below). DBT does not have a specific policy regarding involuntary commitment of individuals at risk for suicide. Some therapists are more willing than others to use this option; opinions differ as to its ethics and efficacy. The important point in DBT is that therapists absolutely must know where they stand on this issue *before* patients become suicidal. The middle of a suicide crisis is no time to be figuring this out. Also, therapists must know the applicable legal guidelines, procedures, and legal precedents in their own state for involuntary commitment.

It is important to be direct and clear about the reasons for interventions against the wishes of the patient. Often a therapist is acting in his or her own best interest (because of fear or exhaustion), and not necessarily the interest of the patient. In any case, when intervention is involuntary the therapist's and the patient's view of her interests conflict. Fortunately or unfortunately, when a person threatens suicide in a credible manner, in our legal system he or she gives up power to mental health professionals and loses individual rights of freedom. This is in spite of the fact that there is no empirical evidence whatsoever that involuntary intervention or psychiatric hospitalization actually decreases suicide risk in any way.

In cases when the therapist's self-interest is at issue, observing limits and reciprocal communication can be used to indicate this to the patient. For example, a therapist may involuntarily commit a suicidal patient to avoid the threat of being sued or held liable if the patient commits suicide. The therapist may be aware that hospitalizing reinforces the behavior, but may be afraid to take the risk of suicide if the patient is not hospitalized. Some therapists are willing to take many fewer personal risks than others. Not all active interventions must be justified as designed to protect the welfare of the patient, independent of the therapist's own welfare. If the patient has frightened the therapist, this should be made clear, and the therapist's right to maintain a comfortable existence should be explained. When the therapist's self-interest is not at issue—usually, when suicide risk appears very high and the individual does not seem capable of acting in her own best interest—this should be made clear also. For example, although I am generally opposed to involuntary commitment as a method of suicide prevention, I would not hesitate to commit an actively suicidal individual in the middle of a psychotic episode. An important focus in working a with suicidal patient is on helping the patient appreciate the motivations of individuals in the community who must respond to her suicidal behavior.

The therapist's position on involuntary commitment and probable response to threats of imminent suicide should be made very clear to the patient at the beginning of therapy. I tell my patients that if they ever convince me that they are going to commit suicide, I will probably actively intervene to stop them. Although I believe in the individual's right of self-determination (including the rights of a borderline patient in therapy), I have no intention of having my professional life and treatment program threatened by a lawsuit because of a patient's committing suicide when I could have stopped it. I go on to express my personal philosophy against involuntary commitment, but make it clear that I may violate that if necessary. I explain that in the final analysis, if there is an irresolvable conflict between a patient's rights to engage in a certain behavior (suicide) and to remain free from involuntary confinement versus my rights to maintain a professional practice and a treatment program for other persons struggling with issues of life and death, I will most likely put my rights first. Although the communication style is irreverent, the therapeutic point is important. Suicide cannot be divorced from its interpersonal context; by entering therapy, the patient is entering into an interpersonal relationship where her behavior will have consequences within the relationship. The same is true, of course, for the therapist's behavior, and the patient's view on voluntary commitment and right to choose suicide should also be explored.

7. ANTICIPATING A RECURRENCE OF THE SUICIDAL URGES

Once the patient is no longer threatening imminent suicide, the therapist should anticipate and plan for a recurrence of suicidal urges or urges to inflict self-injury.

8. LIMITING CONFIDENTIALITY

The patient who threatens suicide or engages in potentially lethal suicidal behaviors often requests that the therapist keep such behavior confidential. The therapist should not agree to this. This point should be made very clearly to the patient and her family during the therapy orientation phase.

ONGOING PARASUICIDAL ACT: PROTOCOL FOR THE PRIMARY THERAPIST

I. ASSESSING AND RESPONDING TO EMERGENCIES

If a patient phones her therapist after initiating self-injurious behavior, or if such behavior is initiated on the phone, the therapist should immediately focus the conversation on assessing the potential lethality of the behavior and obtaining the patient's current address and phone number. In the case of a drug overdose, the crisis planning sheet should be used to determine the potential lethality of the behavior for that particular patient. If the patient is cutting herself, the therapist should ascertain the amount of blood and whether the cut appears to need medical attention. If the patient has turned on the gas in her house, the degree of ventilation and time that the gas was turned on should be ascertained. If the patient is ingesting chemical substances (e.g., drano, bleach), the type and amount should be determined.

   If the self-injurious behavior is possibly life-threatening, the immediacy of the medical danger should be assessed, along with the patient's ability to obtain medical treatment on her own and the presence of other people with her. If the risk constitutes a medical emergency, the therapist should both attempt to alert any individuals currently near the patient and immediately call the appropriate community emergency services, giving them the location of the patient and information about the patient's parasuicidal behavior. (This potential necessity requires that all therapists have patient's phone numbers and addresses always available.) The therapist should then call the patient back and stay in contact until aid arrives. If medical attention is required, but time is not of the essence, the therapist should first assess whether the patient is willing to get the required attention voluntarily; if so, he or she should help the patient figure out how to get to the physician, medical clinic, or emergency room. Depending on the patient's condition and her circumstances, people in her environment should be recruited for transportation or the patient should be sent on her own or in a cab. Depending on the therapist's trust in the patient, it may also be wise to instruct the patient to call and check in from the emergency room. This conversation, however, should be limited to checking on treatment and medical status.

   Patients are often unwilling to get medical attention for a parasuicide, fearing (often reasonably) that it will result in involuntary psychiatric hospitalization. The therapist should apply problem-solving strategies here. If it is medically indicated (or sometimes if the therapist simply fears that it might be), not getting at least a medical examination should simply not be one of the options. The therapeutic relationship is the therapist's chief ally at this point. Unless the patient is at high risk of killing herself if she is not hospitalized (or, of course, needs continuing medical attention), the DBT therapist does not recommend hospitalization following a parasuicide episode. In our clinic, patients are instructed to tell the emergency room staff that they are in our treatment program and that hospitalization is not part of the treatment plan. The idea is for a patient to use all of her interpersonal skills. If the physician or mental health professionals are not persuaded, they can be asked to call the therapist. The therapist can then verify the patient's description of the treatment program. At times, members of the emergency room staff will be quite fearful themselves of liability if the patient is not hospitalized. I have been asked more than once to agree to take clinical responsibility for a patient if she is released. This can be a difficult situation for any therapist, since it generally occurs by phone rather than in the patient's presence. How the therapist responds should depend on his or her knowledge of the patient and the patient's current risk status. How the therapist responds, however, can also be very important to the therapeutic relationship.

For example, one of my patients who was new in therapy took a moderately serious overdose of several medications. Her mother called me, and I sent both to the emergency room. From there the patient called me, begging me to talk to the physician, who was threatening to arrange involuntary commitment to the psychiatric unit. Although the patient was clearly out of medical danger, the physician believed that anyone who overdosed should be hospitalized for the night. He insisted that I agree to take all clinical responsibility for the patient if he discharged her. In talking to the patient, I pointed out to her that I was putting myself on the line for her, and quizzed her on her commitment to avoid further suicidal behavior and her willingness and ability to carry through on such a commitment. After coaching her on appropriate emergency room behavior and verifying our next appointment, I told the physician that I would accept responsibility for her continued care if he discharged her. It was a very difficult act of trust on my part, but one that I thought the patient needed. Most of the time, however, the patient's interpersonal skills (perhaps with a lot of coaching) will be sufficient; the therapist's best strategy is then to recommend that emergency room personnel, paramedics, or police officers on the scene carry out normal procedures.

Although the overriding concern in such a medical crisis is to keep the patient alive, two secondary issues are important in the long-range management of suicidal individual. First, therapists should work with community agents in developing *general* crisis response strategies that are minimally reinforcing of suicidal behavior. Second, the social consequences of serious suicidal behavior should not be interfered with. The therapist should constantly reiterate to the patient that he or she has no control over community agencies. Thus, the patient can develop realistic expectations about likely community responses to her suicidal behavior.

The suicidal patient will quickly appreciate the differences between the DBT therapist's and the community's responses to suicidal behavior. Generally, community agencies will respond far more actively than the DBT therapist. In these instances, the therapist should discuss matter-of-factly with the patient the effect of her engaging in behavior that frightens other individuals.

2. KEEPING THE 24-HOUR RULE

If the self-injurious behavior is *clearly* not now or potentially life-threatening or dangerous, the therapist should revert to the 24-hour rule, which is described more fully later in connection with the telephone strategies. The therapist should remind the patient that calling after engaging in self-injurious behavior is not appropriate, and should instruct her to contact other resources (family, friends, emergency services). Except in very unusual circumstances, the conversation should then be terminated. The inappropriate call as well as the parasuicideal behavior should be discussed in the next therapy session.

SUICIDAL BEHAVIORS: PROTOCOL FOR COLLATERAL THERAPISTS

I. KEEPING THE PATIENT SAFE

If the patient engages in behaviors that suggest high imminent risk for suicide, all therapists attend to the behavior. All therapists other than the primary therapist should do what is necessary to keep the patient safe (see above) until contact can be made with the primary therapist.

2. REFERRING TO THE PRIMARY THERAPIST

Once safety is assured, contacting the primary therapist is the first response. All therapists make it clear to the patient that help with the suicidal crisis, even if the patient feels that a collateral therapist is the source of the crisis, must be obtained from the primary therapist. Skills trainers may help the patient use distress tolerance skills until such contact can be made; pharmacotherapists may adjust medications (e.g., give a hypnotic to a patient with insomnia) to increase her tolerance; and so on. But, other than attending to safety issues and observing their own limits with respect to the amount of suicide risk they are willing to tolerate, all therapists except the primary therapist respond to suicide crisis behaviors by referral. The primary therapist responds with relevant problem-solving strategies discussed above.

Exceptions: Skills Training and Supportive Process Groups. One rule in skills training and supportive process groups is that parasuicidal acts cannot be discussed with other patients outside of group meetings. If the topic is brought up in a group session, attention is immediately focused on how the behavior could have been avoided or could be avoided in the future (i.e., to other solutions). In a group, the therapist directs attention in a very matter-of-fact manner to how DBT or other behavioral skills could be applied in such instances. A similar approach is used when suicide ideation and urges are discussed. Displays of parasuicidal sequelae, (e.g., bandaged arms, uncovered cuts) or discussions of outcomes (e.g., being hospitalized) are generally ignored. The only behavior directly attended to is an attempt to engage in parasuicide during a therapy session; the individual is told to stop and, if necessary, the behavior is prevented. If the behavior persists, the primary therapist is called for instructions or the patient is asked to leave. (Of course, if there is high medical or suicide risk, safety is the first concern.)

Exceptions: Inpatient and Day Treatment. Inpatient and day treatment environments offer unique possibilities for enhancing the application of problem-solving strategies to suicidal behaviors, because of the increased number of individuals who can respond to such behaviors in a focused, problem-solving manner.

For example, in one inpatient setting, the nursing staff and/or mental health technicians conduct immediate, in-depth behavioral and solution analyses of all parasuicidal or suicide crisis behaviors. The analyses are then repeated during the weekly community meeting where patient and staff interactions are reviewed. The key to the success of this public procedure is conducting of the analyses in a nonjudgmental, matter-of-fact, and validating manner. Staff members must provide an exposure atmosphere that does not further reinforce the shame, guilt, and fear patient's feel about admitting and discussing the behavior. Thus, not only are behavioral and solution analyses modeled for the patients, but they have a chance to participate in the conduct of these analyses (presumably increasing their skill), and also may benefit from the vicarious exposure and contengencies applied. Finally, the behavioral and solution analyses, together with other problem-solving strategies, are also applied by the individual therapist.

In another setting, patients were formerly put on public, constant observation following parasuicidal or suicide crisis behaviors. With minor exceptions, a patient was not allowed to talk to anyone during the 24 hours following such a behavior. The procedure was modified in accord with DBT principles to drop the enforced silence. The new rule was that for the 24 hours following a parasuicidal or suicide crisis behavior, the *only* topics of conversation allowed with staff or other patients would be formal behavioral and solution analyses of the behavior. In each of these protocols, suicidal behaviors and their attendant pain are taken very seriously.

Principles of Risk Management with Suicidal Patients

DBT as a whole was developed for the chronically suicidal, borderline patient. Thus, most modifications of "ordinary" psychotherapy to handle suicidal behaviors have been included within the fabric of the therapy. However, not all borderline patients present as being at high risk for suicide. For patients who do, or who become high-risk patients during the course of treatment, the therapist should of course be particularly careful to employ strategies that minimize the risk of such patients' suicide. The therapist should also, however, take steps to minimize the risk of his or her own legal liability if a patient does commit suicide. As Bongar (1991) and others have suggested, it is naive for the clinician not to consider appropriate clinical and legal issues when treating high-risk populations. Bongar suggests a number of clinical and legal risk management strategies that are or can be easily incorporated into DBT. These include the following:

1. *Self-assessment of technical and personal competence* to treat suicidal behaviors is essential. Such competence should include knowledge of the specific clinical and research literature on recommended interventions for suicidal behaviors, as well as for other disorders the patient presents with. Not all clinicians are cut out to work with suicidal patients, and certainly many are not equipped by temperament or by training to work with suicidal borderline patients. A therapist should refer a patient or obtain supervision and additional training if his or her competence is not sufficient.

2. *Meticulous and timely documentation* is required. The therapist should keep thorough records of suicide risk assessments; analyses of the risks and benefits of various treatment plans; treatment decisions and their rationales (including decisions not to hospitalize a patient or not to take other precautions); consultations obtained and advice received; communications with the patient and with others about treatment plans and associated risks; and informed consents obtained. The general rule of thumb here is "What isn't written didn't happen."

3. *Previous medical and psychotherapy records* should be obtained for each patient, especially as these relate to treatment for suicidal behaviors. In DBT, the optimal procedure here would be to make the patient responsible for obtaining these records and bringing them into therapy.

4. *Involving the family,* and if necessary the patient's support system (with the permission of the patient), in management and treatment of suicidal risk; informing family members of risks and benefits of proposed treatment versus alternative treatments; and actively seeking the family's support for keeping the patient engaged in treatment can be very useful. This is all compatible with DBT when the patient is seen jointly with the family or support network, and it is often recommended by suicide experts.

5. *Consultation with other professionals* about general management and risk assessment is a definitional part of DBT and is also a part of standard treatment of suicidal behaviors. The nonmedical clinician should consult specifically with medical colleagues about the advisability of using medication or the need for additional medical evaluation. Ancillary pharmacotherapy is compatible with DBT and may be useful in the individual case.

6. *Postvention* following a patient's suicide—including addressing per-

sonal and legal issues, counseling with other staff members involved in the patient's care, and meeting and working with family and friends — can be extremely difficult, but is nonetheless essential. Consultation with a knowledgeable colleague about postvention steps, including legal consultations, is strongly recommended by many.

THERAPY-INTERFERING BEHAVIOR STRATEGIES

As I have emphasized throughout this volume, DBT requires active, collaborative participation on the part of the patient. There are three main types of patient therapy-interfering behaviors: (1) behaviors that interfere with receiving therapy (nonattentive, noncollaborative, noncompliant behaviors); (2) patient-to-patient interfering behaviors; and (3) behaviors that burn out the therapist (i.e., behaviors that push the therapist's personal limits or decrease his or her motivation). Specific instances of these behaviors are discussed in Chapter 5. The overall strategy for dealing with patient therapy-interfering behavior is to approach it as a problem to be solved and to assume that the patient is motivated to solve her problems. (Special methods for dealing with therapist therapy-interfering behaviors are discussed below in connection with the relationship strategies.)

As noted in Chapter 3, a borderline patient oscillates between two distinct types of self-invalidation. On the one hand, she believes that all of her behavioral failures, including failures within therapy, are at root motivational problems and demonstrate that she is not trying hard enough, is lazy, or simply does not want to improve. On the other hand, she believes that all of these failures result from irremediable character deficits. In contrast, the therapist assumes that the patient is trying, is doing her best, and is not fatally flawed, and makes clear statements to this effect when discussing problematic behavior. Such an orientation prompts both therapist and patient to view interfering behavior as evidence of a problem in the treatment itself, rather than as evidence in support of negative conclusions about certain traits of the patient. The therapy-interfering behavior strategies are discussed below and outlined in Table 15.5.

I. DEFINING THE INTERFERING BEHAVIOR

The first step is to specify interfering behaviors as accurately and precisely as possible. The nature of the interfering behavior should be discussed with the patient and discrepancies in the patient's and therapist's perceptions should be resolved.

2. CONDUCTING A CHAIN ANALYSIS OF THE BEHAVIOR

The therapist should not begin an analysis by asking the patient *why* she did or did not engage in some specified behavior. Instead, as for suicidal behaviors,

TABLE 15.5. Therapy-Interfering Behavior Strategies Checklist

___ T behaviorally DEFINES what P is doing to interfere with therapy.

___ T conducts a CHAIN ANALYSIS of the interfering behaviors; T offers hypothese about function of behavior and does not assume function.

___ T adopts a problem-solving PLAN.

___ When P refuses to modify behavior:
    ___ T discusses goals of therapy with P.
    ___ T avoids unnecessary power struggles.
    ___ T considers vacation from therapy or referral to another T.

Anti-DBT tactics

___ T blames the patient.

___ T infers, without assessment, that P does not want to change or progress.

___ T is rigid in interpretaion of P's behavior.

___ T places all responsibility for change on P.

___ T stakes out a position and refuses to change.

___ T is defensive.

___ T fails to see own contribution to P's behavior.

a chain analysis should specify the antecedents that produce the response, the response itself, and the consequences that follow the response, all in exhaustive detail. When the patient has difficulty identifying or communicating variables influencing her interfering behavior, the therapist should generate hypotheses for discussion; these should be based on knowledge of the specific individual and of suicidal patients in general. A large variety of situations can produce interfering behavior, and each instance of such behavior must be approached ideographically. For example, one patient may miss therapy sessions because she does not believe that they are helpful or feels hopeless about her chances of improvement. Another patient may miss sessions because of anticipatory anxiety, depression, or other negative feelings. A third patient may miss sessions because of the inability to produce the behaviors needed for session attendance (e.g., leaving work on time, arranging for babysitting, telling friends that she has to leave for an appointment). A fourth patient may miss sessions because of pressure in her environment. For example, people in her family or those she lives with may pressure her to stop therapy, may ridicule her for going to therapy, or may otherwise punish session attendance.

3. ADOPTING A PROBLEM-SOLVING PLAN

Once the problem is defined and the determinants identified, patient and therapist must agree on a program for reducing the interfering behavior. Such a program should be based on the results of the analysis of the interfering behavior. A program may focus on motivational issues and changing contingencies, teaching skills necessary for performing the requisite behaviors, reducing inhibiting emotions, changing beliefs and expectancies, or manipulating environmental determinants. As with all problems in therapy, the therapist should verbally emphasize and model a problem-solving approach.

4. RESPONDING TO THE PATIENT WHO REFUSES TO MODIFY INTERFERING BEHAVIOR

At times, a borderline patient will simply refuse to comply with requirements of therapy. The patient may say that she does not need to attend so many sessions; may refuse to role-play or carry out homework assignments; may simply refuse to abide by other therapeutic agreements; may demand that the therapist cure her; or may say that it is the therapist's responsibility to be helpful, which he or she is not. In these instances, the therapist should engage the patient in a discussion of the overall goals of the treatment, as well as of the initial agreements that the patient endorsed upon entering therapy and that were conditions for her acceptance into the treatment program. As with many targets in DBT, the strategy is to talk the problem behavior to death.

The therapist should be very careful to avoid unnecessary power struggles. If an issue does not seem important, it should not be pursued. Learning how to retreat is very important in DBT, as is choosing battles wisely. The therapist should be prepared, though, to fight and win *some* battles in order to help the patient. The patient should not be described as not caring or as being lazy, accused of intentionally sabotaging therapy or described the in any other pejorative language.

If the patient simply refuses to go along with the therapy, the possibility of a vacation from therapy, or of a referral to another therapist, should be brought up for discussion. Such discussions should always stress that it is the patient who would be choosing to go on vacation or to terminate, not the therapist. Indeed, the therapist emphasizes firmly that he or she cares about the patient and hopes that they can work together to solve the current impasse. Such discussions should be carried out only when the patient refuses to work on resolving the problem and other less drastic options have been explored with both the patient and the supervision/consultation team.

TELEPHONE STRATEGIES

The DBT telephone strategies are designed with several points in mind. First, the overriding principle is that a patient should not be required to be suicidal in order to obtain extra time and attention from her primary therapist. Thus, the strategies are designed to minimize the therapist's phone contact as a reinforcer for parasuicide and suicide ideation. Second, the strategies are designed to teach the patient how to apply the skills she is learning in therapy to the problem situations of her everyday life—in other words, to encourage skills generalization.

Third, the phone strategies provide additional therapy time to the patient between sessions when crises arise or the patient is otherwise unable to cope with problems in living. Suicidal and borderline patients frequently need more therapeutic contact than can be provided in one individual session per week, especially since individual patients' concerns can rarely be discussed in skills training sessions. Although extra therapy sessions may occasionally be scheduled, the need for more therapy time is usually addressed via the therapist's availability to phone calls from the patient.

Fourth, the phone strategies are designed to provide training for the patient in how to request help from others appropriately. In DBT, the patient may call her primary therapist for assistance when necessary. Phone calls to collateral therapists, including group therapists, are severely limited; calls can be made to obtain information about meeting times, to make appointments, or to resolve a problem that would lead to therapy termination otherwise. These conditions are discussed in the companion manual to this volume.

Although patients' phone calls to their therapists occur on a continuum from "few or none" to "excessive," the calls of borderline patients often either fall at one end of the continuum or vacillate at different periods between one end and the other. Some patients call their therapists at the least sign of trouble, often calling at inappropriate times and interacting with the therapists in a demanding and hostile manner. Other patients refuse to call their therapists under any circumstances, with the possible exception of already initiated or completed parasuicidal behavior. It is often useful to make calling the therapist between sessions a homework assignment for this type of patient. Or a patient may, at different times in therapy, call either not often enough or too often.

The application of the phone strategies will be somewhat different for the noncalling patient versus the patient who calls excessively. Often the noncalling patient must learn to ask for help earlier in the crisis sequence, so that suicidal behavior does not function to get attention. The excessive phone caller often needs to improve her distress tolerance skills. There are three main types of telephone contact with the patient: (1) phone calls from the patient to the therapist because of a crisis or inability to solve a current problem in living, or because of a rupture in the therapeutic relationship; (2) preplanned regular phone calls from the patient to the therapist; and (3) phone calls to the patient from the therapist. Strategies for each are discussed below and summarized in Table 15.6.

I. ACCEPTING PATIENT-INITIATED PHONE CALLS UNDER CERTAIN CONDITIONS

Phone Calls and Suicidal Behavior: The 24-Hour Rule

Patients are told as part of orientation that they are expected to call their individual therapists *before* they engage in parasuicidal behavior rather than

TABLE 15.6. Telephone Strategies Checklist

_____ T ACCEPTS phone calls from P as appropriate in various situations.

    _____ T informs P of the 24-hour rule on phone calls after parasuicidal behavior, and sticks to it.

    _____ During problem-solving phone calls, T coaches P on using crisis survival and other skills to tider her over until the next session.

    _____ T is willing to repair P's alienation during phone calls.

_____ T considers SCHEDULING P-initiated phone calls for regular times.

_____ T INITIATES phone contacts:

    _____ To extinguish functional connection between T's attention and suicidal behavior.

    _____ To interfere with P's avoidance.

_____ T gives P FEEDBACK about phone call behavior during therapy sessions.

Anti-DBT tactics

_____ T does psychotherapy on the phone.

_____ T is mean-spirited about accepting phone calls.

_____ T gives pejorative interpretations of P's phone calls to T.

_____ T is not available during crisis periods.

---

after; indeed, they do not have to be suicidal in order to call. As noted earlier in this chapter, once parasuicideal behavior has occurred, a patient is not allowed to call her therapist for 24 hours afterward (unless her injuries are life-threatening). The idea here is that a therapist can be more helpful before than after an attempt to solve problems via a parasuicidal act. The rationale given is that a phone call is no longer useful after a patient has engaged in self-injurious behavior, because the patient has already solved the problem (albeit maladaptively) and now has little need for the therapist's attention. The role of therapist reinforcement in precipitating suicidal ideation should be clearly described to the patient. In addition, the therapist should clearly indicate to the patient that it is extraordinarily difficult for anyone to be very helpful to a person who waits until a crisis is full-blown before asking for help.

Typically, a patient's existing behavior is to call after a parasuicidal act. These calls should be handled in the manner described earlier in this chapter. The goal is to shape the patient into calling the therapist at earlier stages of crisis. An intermediate step in this shaping might be calling before the parasuicide but after the suicide ideation is initiated; the final goal, of course, is calling before engaging in suicidal ideation.

This strategy achieves different effects, depending on the patient's willingness to call the therapist. For a patient who finds calling the therapist aversive, the strategy offers an opportunity for learning to replace destructive behavior with asking for help appropriately. Parasuicidal behavior not preceded by an attempt to call the therapist is viewed as a therapy-interfering behavior, and thus becomes a focus of therapy time. For the patient who finds talking to the therapist comforting, by contrast, any behaviors associated with a phone call will be reinforced. Thus the therapist has a choice of reinforcing adaptive behavior or suicidal behavior. A call to the therapist is permitted following 24 hours of nonparasuicidal behavior; if the patient engages in parasuicide again in the first 24 hours, the clock starts again. Very occasionally, this time frame can be reduced to 12 hours. The therapist must be careful to provide the same sort of time and attention for less crisis-oriented moments as for peak suicidal periods. It is essential to instruct the patient that she does not have to feel suicidal in order to call the therapist.

Types of Calls

Calls to the therapist are encouraged under two conditions, and those conditions determine the conduct of a call. The first condition is when the patient is in a crisis or is facing a problem she cannot solve on her own. The second condition is when the therapy relationship is in disrepair and mending is needed. Generally, phone calls will last for no longer than 10 to 20 minutes, although exceptions can be made in crisis situations. If a longer amount of time is needed, it may be useful for the therapist to schedule an extra session with the patient or suggest that the patient call the therapist again in a day or so.

Focusing on Skills. The rationale of these calls (at least from the therapist's viewpoint) is that the patient often needs help in applying the behavioral skills she has learned to date, or is learning, to problems or crises in daily living. The focus of these calls should be applying skills—*not* on analyzing the entire problem, analyzing the patient's response to the problem, or providing catharsis. The crises strategies described earlier should be implemented. With a relatively easy problem, the focus may be on skills for actually resolving the problem. For more intransigent or complex problems, the focus may be on responding in a way that will enable the patient to get to the next session without engaging in maladaptive behavior. That is, dysfunctional behavior is averted, but the problem is not necessarily solved. It is essential to keep this in mind and to remind the patient of it. Problems often need to be tolerated for some time. Distress tolerance skills should be recommended.

All patients and therapists should have readily available near the phone the crisis survival strategies (see the companion manual to this volume). After getting a brief description of a patient's problem or crisis, the therapist should ask which skills the person has already tried (either ones she is learning in DBT or other skills she has developed independently). Then the therapist should review other DBT skills that might help or other ideas the patient has. I may ask the patient to try one or two more skillful responses and then call me back to check in; at that point, we can figure out a new response if that is needed.

The trap to avoid is conducting DBT individual psychotherapy over the phone. This can be difficult because the patient often presents a crisis as irreparable or may be so emotionally aroused that her problem-solving skills are compromised. Rigid thinking and inability to see new solutions are common. The therapist should respond to this in three ways. First, the crisis strategies described earlier in this chapter should be used as appropriate. Second, the focus should be kept on what skills the person can use; the therapist is responsible for keeping the call on track. Third, all problem-solving efforts should be interwoven with validation of the patient's misery and difficulty. Persistent "Yes, but. . ." behavior is therapy-interfering and should be analyzed (at the next session) if common. Within a phone call, the therapist should respond to such behavior with reciprocal communication, disclosing the effect of that behavior on his or her willingness to continue.

Over time, if the therapist persists with this strategy, both the patient's skills in everyday life and her skills in obtaining help on the phone should improve. The frequency and duration of calls will decrease. As several of our clinic patients have said after some time and a large reduction in phone calls, after a while they know exactly what we are going to do and say, and they can just as well do and say it themselves. Or, as one patient said, "Talking about skills all the time is not much fun."

Repairing the Relationship. If there is a rupture in the therapeutic relationship, I have not thought it reasonable to require the patient to wait up to a whole week before it can be repaired. Such a rule is arbitrary and seems to me lacking in compassion. Thus, when the relationship is in disrepair and the patient feels alienated, it is appropriate for her to call for a brief "heart-to-heart"—that is, to process her feelings about the therapist and the therapist's treatment of her. Usually these calls will be precipitated by intense anger, fears of abandonment, or feelings of rejection. It is also appropriate for the patient to call just to "check in." The therapist's role in these calls is to soothe and reassure (except in the final phase of treatment, when the focus is on the patient's learning to soothe herself). In-depth analysis should wait until the next session; however, without the phone call, there might not be a next session.

Some therapists are afraid that if they allow patients to call them when the relationship is ruptured, this will inadvertently reinforce ruptures, and the therapy relationship will gradually worsen. This is a likely outcome if two conditions are met: (1) Talking to a therapist on the phone is more reinforcing than avoiding ruptures and alienation, and (2) phone calls become paired with relationship-rupturing responses. The solution here is twofold. First, the therapist should break the rupture–reinforcement link by making sure that the patient is free to call for brief "check-ins" when there is no relationship rupture. For example, the phone scheduling described in the next section can be used; this can be particularly important for a patient who finds it difficult to go an entire week with no contact. Second, the therapist should try to make a relationship with no ruptures and no relationship calls more reinforcing than a relationship with ruptures plus calls. Steps in this direction include systematic behavioral analysis and problem solving in subsequent therapy sessions of events that lead to excessive phone calls. In addition, the therapist should not give the patient more control over therapy or more validation, praise, or other social reinforcement only when the relationship is not going well. The therapist must pay attention to the contingencies provided when the relationship *is* going well. Social reinforcement should not be faded too quickly.

2. SCHEDULING PATIENT-INITIATED PHONE CALLS

At times, the patient may need more time and attention on a regular basis than the therapist can provide in the weekly individual session. For example, the patient may be calling three or more times per week on a continuing basis. In such instances, the therapist should consider scheduling calls for preset, regular intervals. Such a policy recognizes the patient's need for greater assistance; minimizes the positive consequences for being in a crisis; and, by inserting a waiting period between calls, requires the patient to develop greater distress tolerance skills. Although the patient receives more therapist time, the extra time is not temporally contingent on the patient's feeling panicked or in a state of crisis. In essence, this strategy is similar to giving medical patients regular pain cocktails noncontingently rather than making them contingent upon the presence of pain. If regular phone sessions are scheduled, the therapist should resist the temptation to talk with the patient at an unscheduled time, even if a crisis is present.

3. INITIATING THERAPIST PHONE CONTACTS

Therapist-initiated phone calls are designed to further extinguish any functional connection between the therapist's attention and the patient's suicidal behavior and intense negative affect. Such calls should be independent of patient-initiated calls to the therapist, although generally they will only be planned when it is known that the patient is having an unusually difficult time or is facing a very stressful event. These phone calls can be quite brief and should focus on how the patient is doing in applying therapeutic principles to her current daily problems.

A second time for therapist-initiated phone contact is when the patient is trying to avoid therapy or work on a problem; in these cases, the phone call breaks up the avoidance. For example, if a patient is afraid of coming to therapy and does not show up, I may call right away and be rather directive about figuring out a way for her to get to the session while time still remains or scheduling her for later in the day. Once again, the therapist must analyze the function of the patient's maladaptive behaviors and respond accordingly.

4. GIVING FEEDBACK ABOUT PHONE CALL BEHAVIOR DURING SESSIONS

As noted previously, one goal of the telephone strategies is to help the patient learn how to ask other individuals for help appropriately. Help-seeking behavior requires the individual to be socially sensitive, so that she does not ask for help excessively or at inappropriate times. In addition, the request must be neither made in a demanding manner nor presented in such a fashion that the recipient is not actually able to help. Thus it is essential to give the patient feedback about both her behavior in asking for help and, when appropriate, the responses these requests have elicited in the therapist.

A major treatment goal in DBT is to help the patient find other individuals in her environment to turn to for help. However, it must be recognized that if the patient's skills are not at a reasonable level, asking others for help may lead to increased isolation rather than increased social networking. On the other hand, the therapist must be alert to fostering too much dependency on the part of the patient.

This is a special problem when treatment is time-limited. No matter how inept the patient is at asking for help, at the end of the time limit she will be required to ask others rather than the therapist for needed assistance. By at least the midpoint of therapy, the therapist should be actively working with the patient on finding other individuals in her environment for her to call when she is having problems in living. If these calls do not produce positive results, they should be discussed and analyzed within the therapy sessions. Strategies for improving the results should be planned and practiced by the patient.

Therapist Availability and Management of Suicidal Risk

When I conduct workshops with therapists, one of the most persistent fears raised is that of being called too frequently after work hours by borderline patients. Many therapists feel overwhelmed and unable to limit what feel to them like intrusions in their everyday lives. Some therapists cope with this by developing arbitrary rules limiting phone calls at home. Others cope by using an answering service or machine as a go-between, instructing the service to tell patients that they are unavailable or having the machine do so when they do not wish to be disturbed. Others cope by getting so angry at their patients that they quickly learn not to call. Still others simply refuse to see suicidal and/or borderline patients. The DBT observing-limits procedures, together with the therapy-interfering behavior strategies, are designed to give therapists some control over the potentially unmanageable phone calls of their patients.

The tension between a therapist's wishes and needs and a patient's wishes and needs, however, can be very real and potentially very serious. There will be times when a therapist must extend his or her limits, sometimes for fairly long periods of time, and be available to a patient by phone and during the evening hours. I believe strongly, as do a number of experts (see Bongar, 1991) in the treatment of suicidal patients (including those who meet criteria for BPD) must be told that they can call their therapists at any time—night or day, work days or holidays if necessary. A high risk suicidal patient must be given a phone number where she can reach her therapist at home. If an answering service is used, it must be instructed to contact the therapist for calls from suicidal patients unless very special circumstances require therapists to limit access. If access is limited, a therapist must provide access to other backup professional care.

With my own patients, for example, I tell them that whenever they call me and I am unavailable, they can be assured that, at the latest, I will call them back before I go to bed that night. If they cannot wait, they have back-up phone numbers they can call. (I have also spent countless hours with actively parasuicidal patients discussing alternate solutions they could have employed to cope with their crises and/or rage at not getting me on the phone immediately.) When a patient is in a suicidal crisis, I may give her my daily schedule, letting her know when she can most easily get me by phone. I may plan periodic calls to be sure we connect. When I am out of town, I either give patients my phone numbers or am available for emergency contact through my phone service; the skills training leaders also provide backup coverage. Thus, continuity of care is assured. I have never had access to me abused when I am out of town, but knowing that I can be reached is very soothing for many patients.

In my experience, very few DBT patients actually abuse their ability to telephone their therapists when DBT strategies are used consistently. For those who do, inappropriate calling simply becomes a therapy-interfering behavior to work on in sessions. If it is discussed every single time a patient abuses the phone, the behavior will not continue long. It is essential, of course, that the therapist not view all (or most) calls during a crisis or calls for help in averting a crisis as abusive or manipulative.

ANCILLARY TREATMENT STRATEGIES

I. RECOMMENDING ANCILLARY TREATMENT WHEN NEEDED

There is nothing in DBT that proscribes ancillary mental health treatments, as long as these programs are clearly ancillary to DBT and not the primary treatments. Outpatients may be admitted for brief psychiatric inpatient visits or residential substance abuse programs (as long as they do not miss more than 4 scheduled weeks of DBT); take psychotropic medications and see a physician, nurse, or other pharmacotherapist for monitoring; participate in behavioral skills classes offered in the community; attend group meetings and meet with their counselors in residential treatment communities; see case managers associated with ancillary treatment; go to marriage counseling, vocational counseling, or movement therapy; and attend day treatment. Patients are likely to make occasional contact with other mental health care providers (e.g., crisis clinics and emergency rooms). In my experience, any attempt at proscribing ancillary treatment for borderline patients would lead to either dishonesty by the patients or open rebellion. Thus, in the usual treatment situation with a borderline patient, the mental health network is often large

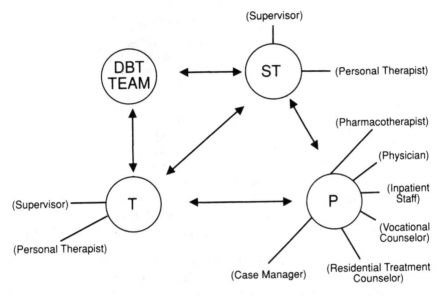

NOTE: T = Individual (Primary) Therapist   Possible ancillary relationships are in ( )
      P = Patient
      ST = Skills Training Therapist

FIGURE 15.2. A possible ancillary treatment scenario in DBT.

and complex. A possible scenario is illustrated in Figure 15.2. Circles enclose units required by DBT; those in parentheses are optional ancillary consultants. The ancillary treatment strategies are outlined in Table 15.7.

The chances that the patient will be admitted to an inpatient psychiatric unit and take psychotropic medications are so great that special DBT hospital and medication protocols have been developed and are discussed below. With all ancillary treatments, the case management strategies, especially the consultation-to-the-patient strategies discussed in Chapter 13, should be applied. When interacting with ancillary treatment professionals and with the patient in regard to these professionals, the therapist must remember that his or her role is that of consultant to the patient, not consultant to the ancillary treatment unit. It is useful to remember the DBT dialectical strategies, especially the emphasis on truth as constructed rather than absolute and the principle that consistency need not be maintained. If the patient receives conflicting advice, opinions, or interpretations, the primary therapist can assist the patient in thinking through how she herself wants to consider herself and her own life and problems.

2. RECOMMENDING OUTSIDE CONSULTATION FOR THE PATIENT

The primary therapist should be very free in recommending that the patient obtain outside consultation when she is unhappy with the individual therapy

TABLE 15.7. Ancillary Treatment Strategies Checklist

_____ T RECOMMENDS ancillary treatment when needed.
  _____ T recommends appropriate pharmacotherapy.
  _____ T recommends inpatient hospitalization when appropriate.
_____ T helps P find a THERAPY CONSULTANT when P is dissatisfied with T's therapy.

MEDICATION PROTOCOL
WHEN PHARMACOTHERAPISTS ARE ANCILLARY PROFESSIONALS:
_____ T SEPARATES psychotherapy from pharmocotherapy.
_____ T acts as CONSULTANT TO P on pharmocotherapy consumer issues.
_____ T TREATS PRESCRIPTION ABUSE by P as appropriate (as suicidal behavior, therapy-interfering behavior, or quality-of-life-interfering behavior.

WHEN T IS ALSO THE PHARMACOTHERAPIST:
_____ T knows the CURRENT RESEARCH LITERATURE on pharmocotherapy of BPD.
_____ T addresses P's HISTORY AND SUBSTANCE ABUSE RISK.
_____ T does not give LETHAL DRUGS TO LETHAL P.
_____ T DIFFUSES power struggles by referral.

HOSPITAL PROTOCOL
_____ T AVOIDS inpatient psychiatric hospitalization whenever possible.
_____ T RECOMMENDS brief hospitalization under certain conditions (see Table 15.8)
_____ T DOES NOT ACT as P's inpatient attending physician.
_____ T acts as CONSULTANT TO P on inpatient treatment issues.
_____ T teaches P how to get herself hospitalized on her own when T does not believe it necessary.
  _____ T maintains own position and opinion.
  _____ T validates P's right to maintain her own position.
  _____ T insists that P take care of herself.
    _____ T teaches P to take responsibility for her own welfare.
    _____ T teaches P to trust her own "wise mind" even when respected others disagree.
  _____ T teaches P how to get herself admitted.
  _____ T reinforces self-validation by not punishing P for admitting herself.

Anti-DBT tactics

_____ T interprets P's wish for outside consultation in a pejorative manner.
_____ T has a position of too much power relative to P.
_____ T punishes P for following her own "wise mind" and going against T's recommendations.

or with her relationship with the primary therapist or the treatment team. One of the inequities in DBT is that the therapist has a helper team in his or her relationship with the patient, but the patient may not have a similarly competent team to help her in relating to the therapist. The inequity is mitigated somewhat by group therapy, where group members and leaders assist patients in their episodic traumas with individual therapists. Not only is finding other consultation viewed as desirable, but the therapist should be willing to assist the patient in finding such help. As I discuss below, psychiatric inpatient staff members can often be extremely useful here.

A patient should not participate in more than one individually oriented psychotherapy relationship at a time. That is, there can only be one primary therapist at a time. Within DBT, all therapists other than the individual psychotherapist are clearly complementary to the individual psychotherapist; the same relationship must obtain with outside professionals. Within the context of DBT, seeing an outside individual consultant is allowed for up to three sessions in close succession. More than that should be considered being in dual therapy. This is considered a form of therapy-interfering behavior and is thus high in priority for session focus.

MEDICATION PROTOCOL

PROTOCOL WHEN PHARMACOTHERAPISTS ARE ANCILLARY PROFESSIONALS

1. SEPARATING PHARMACOTHERAPY FROM PSYCHOTHERAPY. In standard DBT, the primary therapist does not supervise, manage, or prescribe psychotropic medications. With the exceptions discussed below, this strategy holds even when the primary therapist is a physician or nurse-practitioner. The approach was derived both from our clinical experiences in trying to combine pharmacotherapy and psychotherapy, and from behavioral principles underlying the teaching of patients to be responsible and competent medical consumers. My clinical experiences suggested that patients were often dishonest about their use of medications. As one patient told me, if I proscribed certain medications she wanted, she would just get them somewhere else and not tell me about it. It became clear that if a patient's primary therapist has the role of medication manager, the patient has an incentive to lie about medication abuse as a means of obtaining more drugs from the therapist. From a behavioral point of view, this renders the therapist almost totally ineffective in the role of teacher of proper use of medications and medical consultation. Essentially, the therapist is in the power position of drug prescriber, and such a role interferes with his or her ability to work collaboratively with the patient regarding the proper use of medications.

In the years since I instituted the policy of separating psychotherapy from pharmacotherapy in my treatment program, we have discovered a troubling tendency on the part of patients to overuse, underuse, and generally misuse prescribed medications; combine medications in idiosyncratic ways; hoard medications for a possible future suicide attempt or in case medical benefits are cut off; and interact with the prescribing psychiatrist or nurse in an ineffective manner at times and a dissembling manner at other times. I am not sure whether this tendency is any greater in suicidal and borderline patients than it is in any other patient population. However, it was clear in our clinic that we learned a lot more about these practices as soon as we separated the two types of therapy.

2. CONSULTING TO THE PATIENT ON PHARMACOTHERAPY CON-SUMER ISSUES. Once the two roles are separated, the psychotherapist becomes the consultant to the patient about how to interact effectively with medical personnel; how to communicate what her needs are in a way that can be heard and responded to; how to obtain the information she needs about risks and benefits of various pharmacotherapy regimens; how to evaluate the advice and medical treatment plan she is given; how to comply with prescriptions; how to get prescriptions changed when needed; and so on. Because some borderline patients are hospitalized frequently, the therapist also must teach the patient how to insist that new medical treatment teams consult with ongoing medical treatment teams before changing all of her medications. In DBT, it is ultimately the responsibility of the patient to make sure that she does not remain in iatrogenic treatments. Thus, the psychotherapist also teaches the patient how to get second opinions and how to find pharmacotherapists she can work well with. The long-term goal of DBT, of course, is to replace medical management of behavior, including mood and cognitive processes, with behavioral management or self-management. For some patients, however, this is not a short-term goal.

3. TREATING PRESCRIPTION ABUSE. When a patient is abusing prescription medications, this behavior is treated as suicidal behavior if the abuse is potentially life-threatening or is instrumental to parasuicidal behaviors; as therapy-interfering behavior if medication is formally a part of the treatment plan; and as quality-of-life-interfering behaviors if it is not. The DBT diary card elicits information on medications (both licit and illicit), as well as the patient's daily intake of each. The primary therapist should regularly review this information. A patient will often decide on her own to stop recording medication use, saying usually that it is the same each day, and therefore doesn't need to be written down. The therapist should not go along with this. Instead, patient and therapist should work out some sort of shorthand notation so that the patient can record the information more easily. In this manner, the patient can keep the therapist from knowing about medication use only by lying.

Whether the patient lies to the psychotherapist about misuse of medications will depend largely on the therapist's response both to the misuse and to lying. Generally the therapist should respond more negatively to lying and/or withholding information than to misuse. Problem-solving strategies, contingency procedures, and skills training procedures will be the most important approaches to changing a patient's inappropriated use of medications and medical consultation. Consultation to the patient rather than environmental intervention (i.e., calling the pharmacotherapist) is the usual response to medication misuse in DBT. It is crucial, however, that the psychotherapist insure that every pharmacotherpist working with the patient knows about the DBT consultation and case management strategies. This is especially important because the DBT approach is not the expected one in many communities. In a sense, then, a pharmacotherapist should be alerted to treat the patient as carefully as if the patient were not in collateral-to-pharmacotherapy psychotherapy.

A patient at risk for suicidal behavior needs help in limiting access to lethal amounts of medication. The general rule in DBT is that lethal drugs are not given to lethal people. Once patients know this rule, they are usually quite good about conveying it to their physicians and/or nurse-practitioners. The patient and therapist should discuss and devise methods of controlling the amount of medication available and of insuring prescription compliance. These methods can include the use of a public health nurse, the cooperation of family members, the use of small prescriptions, and the use of blood or urine level monitoring (e.g., lithium levels) to track whether medication is being taken or is being hoarded. A fair amount of caution is useful here. It should be the prescribing physician's responsibility to setup and monitor such a formal program, but often the psychotherapist and patient will need to reach a working agreement within the context of managing suicidal behavior.

PROTOCOL WHEN THE PRIMARY THERAPIST IS ALSO THE PHARMACOTHERAPIST

Although DBT favors separating psychotherapy from pharmacotherapy, there are times when this is not practical. The patient may not be able to see someone else; especially in rural areas, there may not be anyone else available. Or, if a therapist is also a physician or nurse-practitioner, such a separation may violate his or her own principles of practice. For therapists who manage both psychotherapy and pharmacotherapy, DBT guidelines are as follows:

1. KNOWING THE CURRENT RESEARCH LITERATURE. The research literature on pharmacotherapy of BPD is growing at a steady clip, and keeping up with it is essential. It is important to remember that responses to specific medications may be quite different for borderline individuals than for others, even when they meet the same criteria for Axis I disorders. For example, a depressed borderline patient and a depressed nonborderline patient may need different medication regimens; some medications increase behavioral dyscontrol, a special problem when treating the borderline individual (Gardner & Cowdry, 1986; Soloff, George, Nathan, Shulz, & Perel, 1985).

2. ADDRESSING THE PATIENT'S HISTORY AND RISK OF SUBSTANCE ABUSE. Substance abuse is a special problem with borderline individuals. Thus, a patient may well abuse the medications she is prescribed. This is a special problem with benzodiazepines, and for this reason they should be used rarely, if ever. Abuse can be very difficult to detect (or, once detected, to control). It is one of the major reasons for separating pharmacotherapy and psychotherapy in standard DBT. The prescribing therapist should intermittently address this issue matter-of-factly, analyzing with the patient the factors that

promote deception and those that favor honesty. That is, the therapist should help the patient analyze the pros and cons of lying or withholding information about substance use. The therapist should periodically highlight the consequences for the therapeutic relationship if the patient is not fully honest with the therapist.

3. NOT GIVING LETHAL DRUGS TO LETHAL PEOPLE.

Therapists must be very careful about prescribing drugs that patients can then use to overdose or commit suicide. The general principle here is that when patients have a history of misusing or overdosing on drugs, they should not be given amounts of those drugs that, if taken all at once, are harmful. For some patients, this will mean sharply curtailing pharmacotherapy; for others, it may mean having their medications managed by other people in their social environment; for all, it should mean prescribing small quantities and making prescriptions refillable. When for financial reasons patients must buy larger quantities at once, a method for dispensing them in small amounts should be developed.

4. DIFFUSING POWER STRUGGLES BY REFERRAL.

A patients will sometimes want a medication regimen different from the one the therapist is willing to prescribe. If therapist and patient cannot reach an agreement on this issue, the therapist should consider referring the patient to another professional for a consultation or for medication management. The rationale here is twofold. First, the therapist should accept that he or she may be wrong, or that there may be more than one "right" way to handle medications. Second, the therapist and the patient do not have to agree on this issue immediately. In the long run, teaching the patient to utilize medical resources effectively is more important than getting the medications exactly correct at this very moment.

HOSPITAL PROTOCOL

I. STRIKING WHILE THE IRON IS HOT: AVOIDING PSYCHIATRIC INPATIENT ADMISSIONS

In DBT, inpatient hospitalization is avoided whenever possible. To date there are no empirical data to suggest that acute, inpatient hospitalization is effective in reducing suicide risk, even when the individual is considered high in such risk. Nor does available evidence suggest that hospitalization is the treatment of choice for borderline behaviors. The DBT treatment model in this respect is most similar to a rehabilitation medicine model: Therapists keep individuals in their stressful enviornments and go in themselves and help the individuals learn to cope with life as it is. The patients are strengthened in the situation, not out of it. In a crisis, DBT says, "Now is the time to learn new behavior." The notion is to "strike while the iron is hot." Taking patients out of stressful environments puts therapy on hold temporarily, and sometimes it actually sets back therapy. Thus, it is rarely the treatment of choice.

2. RECOMMENDING BRIEF HOSPITALIZATION . . . UNDER CERTAIN CONDITIONS

This bias notwithstanding, there are some situations in which the DBT therapist will recommend or consider brief inpatient hospitalizations. These situations are listed in Table 15.8. When hospitalization is recommended, the therapist does most of the work involved in arranging for it; that is, he or she ordinarily uses the environmental intervention strategies and arranges the admission. The therapist should be knowledgeable about the acute psychiatric and emergency services in the local area, as well as thoroughly familiar with how to arrange for the admission of an individual patient. Each hospital will have its own policies and preferences. In additions, hospitals should be prioritized in terms of patients' preferences.

The therapist should discuss his or her policy on hospitalization with the patient during orientation to therapy. A patient may in the therapist's opinion require emergency hospitalization, but may refuse to be hospitalized. This situation is covered by state laws regarding conditions and means of involuntary treatment. Therapists should be thoroughly familiar with their locality's and state's procedures; a crisis is no time to learn these. As I have said earlier, therapists should also know where they stand on involuntary commitment, and should make this clear to their patients. Finally, therapists should have readily available, at work and at home, relevant phone numbers for emergency admissions.

3. SEPARATING THE PRIMARY THERAPIST'S ROLE FROM THE INPATIENT ATTENDING PHYSICIAN'S ROLE

In standard DBT, the primary therapist does not function also as the inpatient attending physician for a patient; nor does the primary therapist admit a patient. A therapist who wants a patient admitted to a hospital where the therapist has admitting privileges should find another person to admit the patient. The rationale here is the same as that given above for the primary therapist's not being the pharmacotherapist. In this case, the therapist's role is to consult with the patient about how to interact appropriately with inpatient staff. A recurrent task will usually be to teach the patient how to communicate about suicidal behavior in a manner that does not unduly scare the staff and create negative consequences for the patient. Going around threatening suicide on an inpatient unit, for example, is usually not a very effective strategy. Teaching the patient how to blend assertiveness with appropriate cooperation, and advising her how to function in a sometimes arbitrary system with very high power, are also common issues of consultation. A primary therapist who has the power either to keep the patient in the hospital or let her out, or to give or take away privileges, cannot be a good consultant.

TABLE 15.8. Situations in Which Brief Inpatient Psychiatric Hospitalization Should Be Recommended or Considered

Recommend:

1. The patient is in a psychotic state and is threatening suicide, unless there is convincing evidence to suggest that the patient is not at high risk.

2. The risk of suicide outweighs the risk of inappropriate hospitalization. (See suicidal behavior strategies for further discussion.)

3. Operant suicide threats are escalating and the patient does not want hospitalization. The patient should not be hospitalized for escalating parasuicide unless the behavior represents a clear danger to health or life. (See suicidal behavior strategies for further discussion.)

4. The relationship between the patient and therapist is seriously strained, the strain is creating a suicide risk or unmanageable crisis for the patient, and outside consultation seems necessary. Inpatient staff can be very helpful in counseling both parties and in assisting in repairing the relationship. A joint meeting with the therapist, the patient, and an inpatient therapist should be considered.

5. The patient is on psychotropic medications, has a history of serious medication abuse or overdose, and is having problems that necessitate close monitoring of medication and/or dose.

6. The patient needs protection during the early stages of exposure treatment of posttraumatic stress, or during later stages that are particularly taxing. This should be arranged at a full conference of the inpatient staff. (Many inpatient staff members are afraid of patient "regression" and do not want to or are unable to treat patients going through exposure treatment.)

7. The therapist needs a vacation. Although DBT is biased against hospitalization, it does not advocate that the therapist become the hospital. Sometimes the patient needs so much assistance during a crisis period that the therpaist approaches burnout and simply needs a few days off from the patient. DBT recommends this as long as the therapist is honest with everyone about the reason for it. (In my experience, inpatient units are very willing to accommodate outpatient therapists on this point.)

Consider:

1. The patient is not responding to outpatient DBT and there is severe depression or disabling anxiety.

2. The patient is in an overwhelming crisis and cannot cope with it alone without significant risk of harm to herself, and no other safe environment can be found. The risk to a life worth living outweighs the risk of inappropriate hospitalization. (This reason should be used *very* sparingly.)

3. There is emergent psychosis for the first time; there is emergent psychosis thereafter, the patient cannot easily cope with such a state, and the patient has little or no social support.

4. CONSULTING TO THE PATIENT ON INPATIENT TREATMENT ISSUES

When a patient is admitted to an inpatient unit, the therapist should remain in the consultant-to-the-patient role unless the exceptions described in Chapter 13 hold. The therapist should expect the patient to get passes to go to individual and skills training sessions, and to arrange for transportation and a travel companion if these are necessary. In our experience, once staff members on an inpatient unit know that missing 4 weeks of scheduled treatment, *for any reason,* will result in termination of outpatient therapy, they are quite eager to see to it that the patient attends. If absolutely essential, the therapist can see the patient for individual sessions on the inpatient unit.

When requested, the individual therapist should attend case conferences with the patient and inpatient staff. An inpatient treatment milieu can also be a good place for other large meetings with the patient, such as meetings with family members, all ancillary therapists, and/or collateral DBT therapists. If a case conference is not requested but the therapist thinks one is advisable, the first approach should be to help the patient set up and coordinate a meeting. (As I have noted in Chapter 13, this policy can backfire and create anger directed at the patient if the inpatient unit has not been oriented to the DBT consultation-to-the-patient strategies.) It is usually a good idea to stay in close contact with the patient by telephone to monitor progress. I generally call inpatients regularly.

Guidelines When the Patient Wants Hospitalization and the Therapist Disagrees

A borderline patient often wants to be hospitalized when the therapist thinks it is not in her best interest. She may be in the midst of a crisis, report feeling suicidal, and may ask to be admitted. It can be extremely difficult in some situations to assess such a person's actual risk and need for hospitalization. In these situations, DBT guidelines are as follows:

1. *Maintaining one's own position.* The fact that a patient feels she cannot cope outside of a hospital without killing herself does not mean that the therapist has to agree with her. The therapist can believe (following an appropriate risk assessment) that she is capable of coping and surviving, at least with help.

2. *Validating the patient's right to maintain her position.* Conversely, the fact that a therapist thinks a patient can cope does not mean she can; the therapist may be wrong. Honesty, humility, and a spirit of willingness are needed here. The therapist should encourage the patient to use "wise mind" to evaluate the two positions, and should support her right to maintain a position independent of the therapist's. Pretending to agree with her robs her of the opportunity to learn this.

3. *Insisting that the patient take care for herself.* The therapist should tell the patient that in this situation, she has to do for herself what she thinks is best for herself, even if the therapist disagrees. If she herself believes hospitalization is important, she should pursue it. She must follow "wise mind." She is ultimately responsible for her own life, and she must take care for it.

4. *Helping the patient get herself admitted.* The therapist should teach

the patient how to get herself admitted to an inpatient, acute care hospital unit. This is almost always possible, of course, if the patient goes to an emergency room and says she is going to kill herself. However, there are a number of less drastic options, and the therapist should consult with the patient on these. The therapist should be as skillful in teaching here as he or she would be in teaching a therapist-preferred option.

5. *Not punishing the patient for going against advice.* It is absolutely essential not to punish the patient if she gets herself admitted to a hospital against the therapist's advice. The only important thing to consider is whether the patient is acting in accord with her own "wise mind," rather than according to "emotion mind" or (much more rarely) "reasonable mind."

RELATIONSHIP STRATEGIES

A strong, positive relationship with a suicidal patient is absolutely essential. Although some therapies may be effective with certain individuals or target complaints in the absence of such a relationship, or with a considerably diluted one, this is not true of work with borderline suicidal patients. Indeed, the strength of the relationship is what keeps such a patient (and often the therapist as well) in the therapy. At times, if all else fails, the strength of the relationship will keep a patient alive during a crisis. The effectiveness of many DBT strategies and procedures, such as cheerleading, emotional validation, contingency management, and both reciprocal and irreverent communication, depend upon the presence of a positive relationship between patient and therapist. There are also times when the positive relationship will help the therapist maintain a working alliance with the patient or prevent him or her from responding with hostility, frustration, or other countertherapeutic behaviors. Although DBT was designed to enhance the therapeutic relationship, the strength of the relationship will reciprocally enhance the effectiveness of DBT.

The relationship in DBT has a dual role. The relationship is the vehicle through which the therapist can effect the therapy; it *is* also the therapy. There is a dialectical tension between these two views. The latter implies that the therapy will be successful if the therapist can be a certain way—in this case, compassionate, sensitive, flexible, nonjudgmental, accepting, and patient. With the provision of a relationship having these qualities, the wounds of the patient's past experiences will heal; her developmental deficiencies will be rectified; and her innate potential and capability for growth will be stimulated. Control over behavior and the course of therapy in general resides primarily with the patient. In contrast, when the relationship is used as the vehicle to bring about therapy, the therapist controls therapy with the consent of the patient. The relationship is then a means to an end—a way of having sufficient contact and leverage with the patient to cause change and growth. In this view, wounds heal only because of active exposure of the patient to similar but benign situations; deficiencies are rectified by the acquisition of coping strategies; and growth occurs because it is made more reward-ing than other alternatives.

In DBT, a dialectic is thus intrinsic in the therapeutic relationship; the therapist must choose an appropriate balance between these two approaches at each moment. "The relationship as therapy" facilitates both acceptance of the client as she is and development. "Therapy through the relationship" facili-tates the therapist's control of behavior the patient cannot control, as well as the patient's acquisition of skills previously unknown or insufficiently gener-alized.

Before either approach can proceed, however, there must be a therapist–patient relationship. Therefore, one of the goals of the initial phase of thera-py is to develop the patient–therapist attachment quickly. Means of achiev-ing this include the emphasis upon validation of the patient's affective, cognitive, and behavioral experiences; the clarity of the contract (ending sui-cidal behaviors and building a life worth living); the focus upon therapy-interfering behavior; outreach and availability through telephone calls; the therapist's reciprocal communication style; and problem solving of feelings re-garding the relationship. Through these, the therapist nurtures the patient's feelings of attachment and trust. Equally important, however, is the therapist's attachment to the patient. If the therapist feels ambivalence or dislike for the patient, this will be communicated through omissions if not direct actions, and the relationship will suffer. Resolution is facilitated by the focus upon suici-dal behaviors (which will reduce therapist stress), therapy-interfering be-haviors, and feelings about the relationship, as well as by supervision and consultation.

The therapeutic relationship is usually not as intense in other modes of DBT, such as skills training or supportive process group therapy. Nevertheless, the patient–therapist attachment is still quite important and must receive the same kinds of attention described above. As in individual therapy, the relation-ship may be the only therapeutic ingredient that keeps the patient alive at times.

Although most DBT strategies attend to and enhance the therapeutic rela-tionship, a specific focus on the relationship is sometimes called for. There are three particularly important issues, each marked by a relationship strate-gy. Once again, these strategies do not require new learning, but do require a different integration of strategies I have already discussed. The strategies are (1) relationship acceptance, (2) relationship problem solving, and (3) rela-tionship generalization. Unless a dialectical approach is kept clearly in mind, the presence of such opposite techniques as relationship acceptance and rela-tionship problem solving in the same set of strategies will seem paradoxical indeed. Relationship strategies are summarized in Table 15.9.

I. RELATIONSHIP ACCEPTANCE

In relationship acceptance the therapist recognizes, accepts, and validates both the patient and himself or herself as a therapist with this patient as well as

TABLE 15.9. Relationship Strategies Checklist

_____ T attaches to P.

_____ T uses relationship to keep P alive.

_____ T balances "the relationship as therapy" and "therapy through the relationship."

_____ T ACCEPTs the therapeutic relationship as it is in the current moment.
     _____ T accepts and validates P as she is right now.
     _____ T accepts himself or herself as he or she is right now.
     _____ T accepts the level of progress as it is right now.
     _____ T is willing to suffer with P.
     _____ T accepts that therapeutic mistakes will be made; T emphasizes repairing mistakes well.

_____ T focuses PROBLEM SOLVING on the relationship when problem arise.
     _____ T assumes that both T and P are motivated to solve relationship problems.
     _____ T assumes a dialectical approach, believing that problems are a result of transactions in therapy.
     _____ T consults with the supervision/consultation team about how to repair therapy mistakes.

_____ T attends directly to GENERALIZATION of behaviors learned in the therapy relationship to other relationships.

Anti-DBT tactics

_____ T manipulates the moment to stop the pain.

_____ T is defensive.

_____ T assumes that learning in therapy will generalize to outside therapy.

---

the quality of the patient–therapist relationship. Each is accepted _as it is_ in the current moment; this includes an explicit acceptance of the stage of therapeutic progress or lack thereof. Relationship acceptance, like all other acceptance strategies, cannot be approached as a technique for change—acceptance in order to get past a particular point. Relationship acceptance requires many things, but most importantly it requires a willingness to enter into a situation and a life filled with pain, to suffer along with the patient, and to refrain from manipulating the moment to stop the pain. Many therapists are not prepared for the pain they will encounter in treating borderline patients, or for the professional risks, personal doubts, and traumatic moments they will encounter. The old saying "If you cannot stand the heat, don't go into kitchen" is nowhere more true than in working with suicidal and borderline patients. In addition, a high tolerance for criticism and hostile affect, and the ability to maintain a nonjudgmental, behavioral approach, are extremely important for relationship acceptance.

To put it another way, relationship acceptance means that the therapist must radically enter into the therapeutic relationship, meeting the patient where she is just at this one moment. "Meeting the patient where she is" may be a trite saying, but in my consulting experience it is a stance that therapists of borderline patients often find almost impossible. Relationship acceptance is "radical" because it cannot be used in a discriminative way. Radical acceptance does not choose what to accept and what not to accept. Thus, it requires an acceptance of the patient, of oneself, of the therapeutic endeavor, and of the "state of art" without distortion, without adding judgment of good or bad, and without trying to keep or get rid of the experience (in the moment). Another way to think of acceptance, including relationship acceptance, is that it is radical truth. It is seeing the therapeutic relationship clearly, without the haze of what one wants it or doesn't want it to be. From an analytic point of view, it is the ability to respond, both privately and publicly, without defense.

One of the most important things a therapist with a borderline patient has to accept is that therapeutic mistakes will be made. Mistakes may be serious and may cause both patient and therapist great pain. DBT does not put its major emphasis on avoiding mistakes; instead, the major emphasis is on repairing mistakes skillfully and well. A mistake may be thought of as a tear or rip in a piece of fabric. A good DBT therapist is not one who never tears the fabric, but one who can sew well and makes good repairs. Learning that relationships can be repaired is possibly much more important to a borderline patient than learning that repairs are not needed in this particular relationship (see Kohut, 1984, for a similar view).

2. RELATIONSHIP PROBLEM SOLVING

Relationship problem solving is needed whenever the relationship is a source of problems for either member. Unhappiness, dissatisfaction, or anger by either patient or therapist at the other is treated as a signal that the relationship needs problem-solving attention. All of the problem-solving strategies discussed in Chapter 9 are appropriate here. Relationship problem solving in DBT is based on the view of the therapeutic relationship as a "real" relationship in which either or both parties may be the source of the problem.

Common elements of case conferences when borderline patients are discussed are comments having to do with how a certain patient is "playing games," is trying to manipulate the therapist, is engaging in "staff splitting," or is otherwise out to get the therapist and destroy the therapy. The assumption is that if a patient is hurting, humiliating, or enraging her therapist, or otherwise causing problems, she must intend such outcomes (either consciously or unconsciously). As I have stressed over and over, such reasoning is based on faulty logic. Therapists often feel that borderline patient have an uncanny ability to figure out their weak spots and attack there; I doubt it. Instead, I think that borderline patients often engage in so many troublesome interpersonal behaviors that by the law of averages they are bound to hit a weak spot in almost any therapist.

Patients, of course, have a number of complaints about their therapists. I have discussed these extensively in Chapter 5 and will not go into them again here. Most problems have to do with patient's wanting more respect, more emotional reciprocity, less arbitrariness, and more help. Above all, border-line patients want to be heard. (More than one clinic patient has told us that our willingness to admit mistakes is one of their favorite parts of DBT.)

The general approach to treating both therapist and patient relationship-interfering behaviors is to approach them as problems to be solved, to as-sume that the individuals are motivated to solve problems in the therapy rela-tionship, and to believe that such problems can be solved. It is not *assumed* that one party or the other is primarily responsible for problems that arise. Such an approach will often provide a distinct change in orientation to the patient. The idea that the patient is trying to cause problems, rather than doing her best to help herself, repeats a common communication she has received all her life. When self-invalidating, the patient views all relationship problems as her own fault; at the other extreme, aware that she is doing her best, she may attribute all relationship problems to flaws in the therapist. Ther-apists sometimes show a not dissimilar tendency to blame all relationship problems on patient pathology. They less often attribute all problems to per-sonal deficiencies and "countertransference." The "truth," of course, is some-where in the middle of the dialectical contrast.

Where and how relationship problems are discussed and solved depends to some extent on where the problem is taking place (group therapy or indi-vidual therapy), what the problem is, and who is unhappy (a patient or a ther-apist). Relationship problems in group therapy may be taken up within the group setting or individually. (A number of factors enter into the decision here, such as time constraints of the group sessions and the patient's ability to handle working on her own behavior within the group.) Some problems, such as fear or anger so extreme that the patient can not return or serious rela-tionship mistakes by the therapist not admitted during a session (group or individual), are often handled in phone calls. Often, the impact of an inter-action is not fully appreciated until after the session; phone calls to alleviate a sense of alienation or to resolve intolerable rage are acceptable in DBT. This point has been discussed more fully above in connection with telephone strategies.

Therapist behaviors that cause relationship problems are dealt with either in consultation team meetings, in individual supervision, or with the patient in the therapy session. Complaints of the patient to the therapist about his or her behavior are always discussed in therapy. Usually, the key to resolu-tion is the therapist's openness to the fact that a mistake has been made (when this is, indeed, the case). Although the influence of the patient's behavior on the therapist's behavior (and vice versa) is an important topic for the discus-sion, the therapist must be careful not to turn the discussion into blaming the patient for the therapist's own inappropriate behavior. Relationship-interfering problems not brought up by the patient are usually solved within the consultation or individual supervision meetings. In these situations, the therapist's colleagues apply DBT strategies to the therapist.

3. RELATIONSHIP GENERALIZATION

Generalization from the therapy relationship to other relationships is not assumed in DBT. Although there are many differences between a therapeutic relationship and a "real" one, the therapist should use times of relationship difficulties and relationship problem solving to explore the similarities with relationships in the patient's life and to suggest how analogous approaches in those might be productive. When the relationship is going well, this fact should also be acknowledged, and the relationship with the therapist should be compared to other relationships the patient is engaged in. Such a comparison can highlight what the patient wants from a relationship and what is missing from her day-to-day relationships. All of the skill generalization strategies, discussed in Chapter 11, should be employed here.

Concluding Comments

The one protocol that is not included in this book is the protocol for conducting the actual behavioral skills training with borderline patients. The content and process of skill training are covered in detail in the companion manual to this volume. The actual skills are described in Chapter 5, and skills training procedures for individual therapy are described in Chapter 11. By putting the two together, you can create your own skills training approach. The important point to remember is that whether you follow the companion manual or not, a borderline patient must be taught how to respond and act differently than she does. It is your task as a therapist to teach, coach, cajole, and gently lead her into a new way of being and behaving in this world. The strategies described in this chapter are vehicles to keep the treatment frame in existence while you accomplish the necessary teaching and the patient learns how to be different.

APPENDIX 15.1
Scale Points for Lethality Assessment*

0.0   Death is an impossible result of the "suicidal" behavior.
Cutting. Light scratches that do not break the skin; usually done with pop can "pull tabs," broken plastic, pins, paper clips; reopening old wounds also is included at this level. Wounds requiring sutures must be rated at a higher level.

*From *The Suicidal Patient: Clinical and Legal Standards of Care* (pp. 277–283) by B. Bongar, 1991, Washington, DC: American Psychological Association. Copyright 1991 by the American Psychological Association. Reprinted by permission. Updated and revised by Bongar from "Lethality of Suicide Attempt Rating Scale" by K. Smith, R. W. Conroy, and B. D. Ehler, 1984. *Suicide and Life-Threatening Behavior, 14*(4), 215–242. Copyright 1984 by Guilford Publications, Inc. Adapted by permission. The scale points were originally suggested by T. L. MacEvoy (1974).

Ingestion: This includes mild overdoses and the swallowing of objects such as money, paper clips, and disposible thermometers. Ten or fewer ASA, Tylenol® , "cold pills," laxatives, or other over-the-counter drugs; mild doses of tranquilizers or prescribed medications (usually fewer than 10 pills). Putting broken glass into one's mouth but not swallowing would be rated in this category.

Other: Clearly ineffective acts which are usually shown by the patient to staff or others (e.g., going outside in cold weather with only a nightgown on after telling parents she was going to commit suicide by "freezing myself to death").

1.0   Death is very highly improbable. If it occurs it would be a result of secondary complication, an accident, or highly unusual circumstances.

Cutting: Shallow cuts without tendon, nerve, or vessel damage. These wounds may require some very minor suturing. Cutting is often done with something sharp such as a razor. Very little blood loss. Scratches (as opposed to cuts) to the neck are first rated here.

Ingestion: Relatively mild overdoses or swallowing of nonsharp glass or ceramics, events usually brought by the patient to staff attention. Twenty or fewer ASA, laxatives, and/or over-the-counter meds (e.g., Sominex, Nytol® , 15 or fewer Tylenol). Small doses of potentially lethal medications (e.g., six Tuinal, four Seconal) are also common; fewer than 20 (10-mg) Thorazine tablets.

Other: Tying a thread, string, or yarn around neck and then showing to staff.

2.0   Death is improbable as an outcome of the act. If it occurs it is probably due to unforeseen secondary effects. Frequently the act is done in a public setting or is reported by the person or by others. While medical aid may be warranted, it is not required for survival.

Cutting: May receive but does not usually *require* medical intervention to survive.

> *Examples:* Relatively superficial cuts with a sharp instrument that may involve slight tendon damage. Cuts to the arms, legs, and wrists will require suturing. Cuts to the side of the neck are first rated in this category and should not require suturing.

Ingestion: May receive but does not usually *require* medical intervention to survive.

> *Examples:* Thirty or fewer ASA and/or other over-the-counter pills; fewer than 100 laxatives; 25 or fewer Regular Strength Tylenol; drinking of toxic liquids (12 ounces of less), shampoo or astringent (e.g., Ten-O-Six® Lotion), lighter fluid or other petroleum-based products (less than two ounces). Small doses of potenially lethal medications (e.g., 21 65-mg Darvon, 12 tablets of Fiorinal, "overdosed on phenobarbital but only enough to make him very drowsy," 10–15 50-mg Thorazine tablets), greater quantities of aspirin might be taken when staff is notified within minutes by the patient. Fourteen or fewer lithium carbonate tablets. The patient may swallow small quantities of cleaning compounds or fluids such as Comet® cleanser (less than four tablespoons).

Other: Nonlethal, usually impulsive and ineffective methods.

> *Examples:* Inhaling deodorant without respiratory distress occuring, swallowing several pieces of sharp glass, evidence of failed attempt to choke self with a piece of pillowcase (e.g., rash-type abrasions).

3.5   Death is improbable so long as first aid is administered by victim or other agent. Victim usually makes a communication or commits the act in a public way or takes no measures to hide self or injury.

Cutting: Deep cuts involving tendon damage (or severing) and possible nerve, vessel, and artery damage; cuts to the neck will require sutures but not major vessels were severed. Blood loss is generally less than 100 cc. Cuts to neck go beyond scratching but do not actually sever main veins or arteries.

Ingestion: This is a significant overdose and may correspond to the lower part of the LD_{50} range.

> *Examples:* Fewer than 60 ASA or other over-the-counter pills. Higher doses may be taken but patient insures intervention (e.g., 64 Sominex). Over 100 laxatives; 50 or fewer Tylenol. Potentially lethal overdoses (e.g., 60 Dilantin capsules plus half a fifth of rum) but done in such a way as to insure intervention (e.g., in front of nursing staff, telling someone within 1 hour). Signs of physiological distress may be present such as nausea, elevated blood pressure, respiratory changes, convulsions, and altered consciousness stopping short of coma. Lighter fluid (3 or more ounces); 15–20 lithium carbonate tablets.

Other: Possibly serious actions that are quickly brought by the patient to staff's attention (e.g., tied a shoelace tightly around neck but came to staff immediately).

5.0   Death is a 50-50 probability directly or indirectly, or in the opinion of the average person, the chosen method has an equivocal outcome. Use this rating only when (a) details are vague; (b) a case cannot be made for rating either a 3.5 or 7.0.

Cutting: Severe cutting resulting in sizable blood loss (more than 100 cc) with some chance of death. Cutting may be accompanied by alcohol or drugs, which may cloud the issue.

Ingestion: Reports of vague but possibly significant quantities of lethal medications. Unknown quantities of drugs that are lethal in small dosages. . . also belong here.

> *Examples:* "Take a large number of chloral hydrate and Doriden"; "took 60 ASA and an undetermined amount of other medications."

Other: Potentially lethal acts.

> *Examples:* Trying to put two bare wires into an electrical outlet with a nurse present in the room; jumping headfirst from a car driven by staff going 30 miles an hour; unscrewing a light bulb in the lounge and putting finger in socket with patients around.

7.0   Death is the probable outcome unless there is "immediate" and "vigorous" first aid or medical attention by victim or other agent. One or both of the following are also true: (a) makes communication (directly or indirectly); (b) performs act in public where he [or she] is likely to be helped or discovered.

Cutting: Cuts are severe.

> *Examples:* Eloping and "slashing neck with razor" (including severing jugular) but returning to hospital on own and asking for help; while alone cut head with shard of glass and "almost bled to death"–called doctor after cutting. Eloping and very severely cutting self in a public restroom or motel – cuts led to hemorrhage shock with vascular collapse – patient makes direct request for help after cutting.

Ingestion: Potentially lethal medications and quantities. This would involve a dose which, without medical intervention, would kill most people (usually at the upper end of the LD_{50} range or beyond).

> *Examples:* Eloping and ingesting approximately two bottles of ASA and then return-ing to the hospital; 50 Extra-Strength Tylenol, eloping to motel and ingesting large quantities of Inderal, Dalmane, Mellaril, and three-quarters of a fifth of bourbon, then making indirect communication of distress; took 23 100-mg tablets of phenobar-bital but told roommate immediately who told staff; 16–18 capsules of Nembutal—left note with a friend who missed the note resulting in the patient almost dying.

Other: Lethal actions performed in a way that maximizes chances of intervention.

> *Examples:* Tied towel tightly around neck—airway cut off—tried to untie it but passed out on floor—found cyanotic and in respiratory arrest—had seen staff making rounds before attempt; string wrapped several times around neck and tied to bed—face flushed when found.

8.0   Death would ordinarily be considered the outcome to the suicidal act, unless saved by another agent in a "calculated" risk (e.g., nursing rounds of expecting a room-mate or spouse at a certain time). One or both of the following are true: (a) makes no direct communications; (b) takes action in private.

Cutting: Severe gashes with major and quick blood loss. May be partially hidden from staff, spouse, or friends.

> *Examples:* Patient went into bathroom of his room, left the door open and severely cut one wrist resulting in major blood loss; death would have occurred had he not been found 30 minutes later by nursing staff on rounds.

Ingestion: Clearly lethal doses and no communication is made.

> *Examples:* Taking a lethal overdose of barbituates but vomiting before going into a coma; overdosed on 900 mg Stelazine in apartment alone; overdoses on phenobarbi-tal plus alcohol, found comatose in her bed. Took 20 Tuinal and became very sleepy while visiting friends—the friends became suspicious and took her to emergency room—in coma for 36 hours; took 15 Tuinal—found unconscious at home in tub of warm water.

Other: Most common here are hangings and suffocations which may or may not suc-ceed but are performed so that a calculated chance of intervention could interrupt.

> *Example:* Tying belt very tightly around neck and strangling self in shower; tied shoe-lace lightly around neck and going to bed—found at rounds to be cyanotic; blocked airways with plastic and had tied a stocking tightly around neck—found on top of her bed gurgling and pale but not cyanotic; elopes and attempts to drown self in near-by pond but in broad daylight; jumps in front of fast-moving car (over 30 mph); plas-tic bag over head—found deeply cyanotic; played Russian roulette and drew a "pass."

9.0   Death is a highly probable outcome: "Chance" intervention and/or unforeseen circumstance may save victim. Two of the following conditions also exist: (a) no com-munication is made; (b) effort is put forth to obscure act from helpers' attention; (c) precautions against being found are instituted (e.g., eloping).

Cutting: Severe, usually multiple cuts involving severe blood loss.

Examples: Severly cutting arm with razor and bleeding into wastebasket then got into bed (it was bedtime so being in bed did not arouse suspicion)—found unconscious and in shock; savagely biting a 2-cm piece of skin out of wrist, losing 4 pints of blood, and found in shock under bed covers; cut neck in arts and crafts bathroom (when shop was closed) with 3-inch blade, found unconscious; severely cut throat with a broken pop bottle in unit shower—this was done when most patients were away from the unit—difficulty breathing when found; cut neck and wrist in bathtub at home—died by drowning—had "hoped" husband would happen to discover.

Ingestion: Clearly lethal doses.

> *Examples:* Drinking several ounces of nail polish remover—found covered in bed gagging, pale with large amount of foaming exudate coming from mouth—mildly comatose; took 30 500-mg Doriden tablets right before bedtime—in bed, appeared to be asleep but was actually unconscious in a deep coma.

Other: Highly lethal means employed.

> Example: Plastic bag over head tied with a scarf—found unconscious with head in toilet; drove head on into a gasoline truck but survived with minor scratches and bruises; stuffed plastic in both nostrils and oral pharynx, completely closing airways—she appeared to be sleeping in bed under covers; eloped to another city in car, tied plastic hose to exhaust and suffocated in parking lot; hanged self in closet with door closed— not breathing when cut down; jumped from 90-foot bridge into water—was unconscious when found. Gunshot to chest area (if shotgun used, rate 10.0); jumped headfirst from three-story building.

10.0   Death is almost a certainty regardless of the circumstances or interventions by an outside agent. Most of the people at this level die quickly after the attempt. A very few survive through no fault of their own.

Cutting: Just cuts as severe as in 9.0, except that the likelihood for intervention is even more remote. Blood loss is severe and quick.

> *Examples:* Eloping to an empty house and severely cutting wrists and neck with razor— when a policeman happened by the patient was sitting in a large pool of blood, warded off the policeman with the razor.

Ingestion: Because of the time usually involved before a toxin can take effect, there are very few instances of overdosing that can be considered this serious.

> *Example:* Some that have been serious are [as follows]: ingesting furniture polish, paint thinner, and many prescription medications while alone in the house with no one expected by; overdose on large quantities of Dalmane and barbiturates with husband out of town and no children or other live-in companions in the household; ingested 60 Nembutal, went into secluded, wooded area in midwinter, covered self with leaves which caused him not to be found for several days.

Other: These are the most common type of attempts at this level.

> *Examples:* Jumping off a tall building (four or more floors); jumping in front of cars on a freeway and being hit; eloping and hanging self in gym locker building at night; secretly eloping and drowning self in lake at a time when there was no activity in the lake area and when he would not be expected to be on the unit; gunshot to the head and any effort involving a shotgun.

Note

1. These risk factors are for adult patients. Risk factors for children and adolescents, though similar, differ in some important respects. See Berman and Jobes (1992) and Pfeffer (1986) for reviews of risk factors for children and adolescents.

Appendix: Suggested Reading

* Strongly recommended

** Strongly recommended (one or more) for readers with no behavior therapy background

Barker, P. (1985). *Using metaphors in psychotherapy.* New York: Brunner/Mazel.

Metaphors are crucial to DBT and form an important set of dialectical strategies. This book is an interesting discussion of metaphor and psychotherapy, and also gives examples of many metaphors potentially useful in DBT.

* Barlow, D. H. (1988). *Anxiety and its disorders: The nature and treatment of anxiety and panic.* New York: Guilford Press.

Barlow's book is one of the best resource books to date for the treatment of anxiety-based disorders. Barlow provides a good description of theory and research on the role of "emotional processing" and exposure-based strategies in therapy. The theory and treatment are also applicable to shame and guilt—key emotions addressed in DBT. An understanding of the points made here is important for application of exposure-based strategies in DBT, given that many (or most) borderline individuals are emotion-phobic.

* Basseches, M. (1984). *Dialectical thinking and adult development.* Norwood, NJ: Ablex.

This book provides an excellent overview of what is meant by a "dialectical thinking style." It also gives a brief review of dialectical philosophy. Understanding the points made here is essential for the conduct of DBT.

* Berg, J. H. Responsiveness and self-disclosure. In V. J. Derlega & J. H. Berg (Eds.), *Self-disclosure: Theory, research, and therapy.* New York: Plenum Press.

Responsiveness and self-disclosure form the backbone of the reciprocal communication strategies. This is a nice summary of the principles.

* Bongar, B. (1991). *The suicidal patient: Clinical and legal standards of care.* Washington, DC: American Psychological Association.

This book provides an excellent overview of clinical and legal issues surrounding the treatment of suicidal behaviors. It is one of the best clinical guides published to date. Bongar reviews the theoretical and empirical literature on high-risk suicidal behaviors, and summarizes case law as it pertains to treatment of suicidal patients. The book provides sophisticated risk management strategies in the context of clinically sensitive treatment recommendations. Numerous risk assessment scales are reprinted in the back of the book.

Egan, G. (1982). *The skilled helper: Model, skills, and methods for effective helping* (2nd ed.). Monterey, CA: Brooks/Cole. (See especially Chapters 3, 4, and 5.)

The first two steps in validation—observing and describing (active listening, accurate empathy)—are very well described and discussed here. The discussions of respect, genuineness, and social influence are relevant to the reciprocal communication strategies.

* Hanh, T. N. (1976). *The miracle of mindfulness: A manual on meditation.* Boston: Beacon Press.

This book presents the rationale and methods of mindfulness practice. Although it is essentially spiritual in orientation, the approach is not religious. Mindfulness is the quality of being awake. Understanding it is crucial for teaching the core mindfulness skills. The importance of "acceptance" is highlighted in the practice of mindfulness. Thus it is not possible to conduct DBT without an inner understanding of this practice.

Hollandsworth, J. G. (1990). *The physiology of psychological disorders: Schizophrenia, depression, anxiety, and substance abuse.* New York: Plenum Press.

DBT is based on a biosocial theory of behavior and behavior disorder. Thus, it is very important to have a reasonable understanding of how biology, environment, and experience interact to influence functioning. The systemic model of functioning presented by Hollandsworth is compatible with a biosocial dialectical view. The book provides a nice introduction to behavioral genetics and to the research literature on physical, biochemical, and psychophysiological factors in schizophrenia, depression, anxiety, and substance abuse.

* Kabat-Zinn, J. (1990). *Full catastrophe living: Using the wisdom of your body and mind to face stress, pain, and illness.* New York: Dell.

This book describes the program of the stress reduction clinic at the University of Massachusetts Medical Center. Although designed within the context of a behavioral medicine program, the program teaches a full array of mindfulness practices. As the author says, it is an intensive, self-directed training program in the art of conscious living. This is an invaluable resource for the therapist who wants to expand mindfulness skills training.

Kanter, J. (1989). Clinical case management: Definition, principles, components. *Hospital and Community Psychiatry, 40.* 361–368.

This is a brief summary of principles of case management. It emphasizes environmental intervention more than DBT does, but otherwise addresses the issues and the integration of consultation to the patient and environmental intervention quite well.

Kohlenberg, R. J., & Tsai, M. (1991). *Functional analytic psychotherapy: Creating intense and curative therapeutic relationships.* New York: Plenum Press.

This book describes in very good detail how to apply principles of operant learning within the framework of intensive, interpersonally oriented psychotherapy. These are the same principles that underlie the contingency procedures in DBT. In the third (and last) stage of treatment, DBT is quite similar in many ways to this treatment.

Kopp, S. B. (1971). *Metaphors from a psychotherapist guru.* Palo Alto, CA: Science & Behavior Books.

Kopp provides many metaphors from primitive religion, Judaism, Christianity, the Orient, ancient Greece and Rome, the Renaissance, children's tales, and science fiction. There is a nice reading list at the end.

Maris, R. W., Berman, A. L., Maltsberger, J. T., & Yufit, R. I. (Eds.). (1992). *Assessment and prediction of suicide.* New York: Guilford Press.

This is a handbook summarizing the literature to date on assessment and prediction of suicide. It reviews and discusses most methods of suicide assessment, including suicide prediction scales, psychological tests, clinical interviews, and so forth.

** Martin, G., & Pear, J. (1992). *Behavior modification: What it is and how to do it* (4th ed.). *Part II: Basic behavioral principles and procedures.* Englewood Cliffs, NJ: Prentice-Hall.

This is a very good, very basic review of principles of behavior modification, including operant and classical conditioning, shaping, chaining, etc. It is especially relevant to the skills training and contingency procedures.

** Masters, J. C., Burish, T. G., Hollon, S. T., & Rimm, D. C. (1987). *Behavior therapy: Techniques and empirical findings* (3rd. ed.). New York: Harcourt Brace Jovanovich.

This is a good basic overview of behavior therapy techniques. The chapters are organized by techniques rather than disorder. There is a good appendix covering basic principles of learning.

* Whitaker, C. A., Felder, R. E., Malone, T. P., & Warkentin, J. (1982). First-stage techniques in the experimental psychotherapy of chronic schizophrenic patients. In J. R. Neill & D. P. Kniskern (Eds.), *From psyche to system: The evolving therapy of Carl Whitaker.* New York: Guildford Press. (Original work published in 1962)

First-stage techniques for working with schizophrenic patients are very similar to the irreverent communication strategies used in DBT. This chapter is a good summary with lots of examples. Some of the techniques suggested by Whitaker and colleagues would not be used in DBT because they are too susceptible to abuse or insensitive use. Also, personal style is important here, and many simply do not fit my own style.

Wilber, K. (1981). *No boundary: Eastern and Western approaches to personal growth.* Boulder, CO: New Science Library.

Wilber presents a compelling discription of how we create polarities, boundaries, and parts out of the whole. Understanding of the essential unity of polarities and of the artificial nature of these boundaries is essential to a dialectical view.

References

Abel, E. L. (1981) Behavioral teratology of alcohol. *Psychological Bulletin, 90,* 564–581.

Abel, E. L. (1982). Consumption of alcohol during pregnancy: A review of effects on growth and development of offspring. *Human Biology, 54,* 421–453.

Adam, K. S., Bouckoms, A., & Scarr, G. (1980). Attempted suicide in Christchurch: A controlled study. *Australian and New Zealand Journal of Psychiatry, 14,* 305–314.

Adler G. (1985). *Borderline psychopathology and its treatment.* New York: Aronson.

Adler, G. (1989). Psychodynamic therapies in borderline personality disorder. In A. Tasman, R. E. Hales, & A. J. Frances (Eds.), *Review of psychiatry* (vol. 8, pp. 49–64) Washington, DC: American Psychiatric Press.

Aitken, R. (1987). The middle way. *Parabola, 12* (9), 40–43.

Akhtar, S., Byrne, J. P., & Doghramji, K. (1986). The demographic profile of borderline personality disorder. *Journal of Clinical Psychiatry, 47,* 196–198.

Akiskal, H. S. (1981). Subaffective disorders: Dysthymic, cyclothymic and bipolar II disorders in the "borderline" realm. *Psychiatric Clinics of North America, 4,* 25–46.

Akiskal, H. S. (1983). Dysthymic disorder: Psychopathology and proposed chronic depressive subtypes. *American Journal of Psychiatry, 140,* 11–20.

Akiskal, H. S., Chen, S. E., Davis, G. C., Pusantian, V. R., Kashgariam, M., & Bolinger, J. M. (1985a). Borderline: An adjective in search of a noun. *Journal of Clinical Psychiatry, 46,* 41–48.

Akiskal, H. S., Yerevanian, B. I., Davis, G. C., King, D. & Lemmi, H. (1985b). The nosologic status of borderline personality: Clinical and polysomnograph study. *American Journal of Psychiatry, 142,* 192–198.

American Psychiatric Association. (1987). *Diagnostic and statistical manual of mental disorders* (3rd ed., rev.). Washington, DC: Author.

American Psychiatric Association. (1991). *DSM-IV options book: Work in progress.* Washington, DC: Author.

Andrulonis, P. A., Glueck, B. C., Stroebel, C. F., Vogel, N. G., Shapiro, A. L., & Aldridge, D. M. (1987). Organic brain dysfunction and the borderline syndrome. *Psychiatric Clinics of North America, 4,* 47–66.

Arnkoff, D. B. (1983). Common and specific factors in cognitive therapy. In M.J. Lambert (Ed.), *Psychotherapy and patient relationships* (pp. 85–125). Homewood, IL: Dorsey Press.

Arnold, M. B. (1960). *Emotion and personality* (2 vols.). New York: Columbia University Press.

Arnold, M. B. (1970). Brain function in emotion: A phenomenological analysis. In P. Black (Ed.), *Physiological coorelates of emotion* (pp. 261–285). New York: Academic Press.

Averill, J. R. (1968). Grief: Its nature and significance. *Psychological Bulletin, 70,* 721–748.

Bahrick, H. P., Fitts, P. M., & Rankin, R. E. (1952). Effect of incentives upon reactions to peripheral stimuli. *Journal of Experimental Psychology, 44,* 400–406.

Bancroft, J., & Marsack, P. (1977). The repetitiveness of self-poisoning and self-injury. *British Journal of Psychiatry, 131,* 394–399.

Bandura, A. (1973). *Aggression: A social learning analysis.* Englewood Cliffs, NJ: Prentice-Hall.

Barker, P. (1985). *Using metaphors in psychotherapy.* New York: Brunner/Mazel.

Barley, W. D., Buie, S. E., Peterson, E. W., Hollingsworth, A. S., Griva, M., Hickerson, S. C., Lawson, J. E., & Bailey, B. J. (in press). The development of an inpatient cognitive–behavioral treatment program for borderline personality disorder. *Journal of Personality Disorders.*

Barlow, D. H. (1988). *Anxiety and its disorders: The nature and treatment of anxiety and panic.* New York: Guilford Press.

Baron, M., Gruen, R. Asnis, & Lord, S. (1985). Familial transmission of schizotypal and borderline personality disorders. *American Journal of Psychiatry, 142,* 927–933.

Basseches, M. (1984). *Dialectical thinking and adult development.* Norwood, NJ: Ablex.

Baumeister, R. F. (1987). How the self became a problem: A psychological review of historical research. *Journal of Personality and Social Psychology, 52,* 163–176.

Beck, A. T. (1976). *Cognitive therapy and the emotional disorders.* New York: International Universities Press.

Beck, A. T., Brown, G., & Steer, R. A. (1989). Prediction of eventual suicide in psychiatric inpatients by clinical ratings of hopelessness. *Journal of Consulting and Clinical Psychology, 57,* 309–310.

Beck, A. T., Brown, G., Steer, R. A., Eidelson, J. I., & Riskind, J. H. (1987). Differentiating anxiety and depression: A test of the cognitive content-specificity hypothesis. *Journal of Abnormal Psychology, 96,* 179–183.

Beck, A. T., Davis, J. H., Frederick, C. J., Perlin, S., Pokorny, A. D., Schulman, R. E., Seiden, R. H., & Wittlin, B. J. (1973). Classification and nomenclature. In H. L. P. Resnick & B. C. Hawthorne (Eds.), *Suicide prevention in the 70's* (pp. 7–12). Rockville, MD: Center for Studies of Suicide Prevention, National Institute of Mental Health.

Beck, A. T., Freeman, A., & Associates. (1990). *Cognitive therapy of personality disorders.* New York: Guilford Press.

Beck, A. T., Rush, A. J., Shaw, B. F., & Emery, G. (1979). *Cognitive therapy of depression.* New York: Guilford Press.

Beck, A. T., Steer, R. A., Kovacs, M., & Garrison, B. (1985). Hopelessness and eventual suicide: A ten year prospective study of patients hospitalized with suicidal ideation. *Journal of Personality and Social Psychology, 142,* 559–563.

Benjamin, L. S. (in press). *Interpersonal diagnosis and treatment of the DSM personality disorders.* New York: Guilford Press.

Berent, I. (1981). *The algebra of suicide.* New York: Human Sciences Press.

Berg, A. B., & Sternberg, R. J. (1985). A triarchic theory of intellectual development during adulthood. *Developmental Review, 5,* 334–370.

Berkowitz, L. (1983). Aversively stimulated aggression: Some parallels and differences in research with animals and humans. *American Psychologist, 38*, 1135–1144.

Berkowitz, L. (1989). Frustration–aggression hypothesis: Examination and reformation. *Psychological Bulletin, 106, 59–73.*

Berkowitz, L. (1990). On the formation and regulation of anger and aggression: A cognitive–neoassociationistic analysis. *American Psychologist, 45*, 494–503.

Berman, A. L., & Jobes, D. A. (1992). *Adolescent suicide: Assessment and intervention.* Washington, DC: American Psychological Association.

Beutler, L. E., Engle, D., Oro'-Beutler, M. E., Daldrup, R., & Meredith, K. (1986). Inability to express intense affect: A common link between depression and pain? *Journal of Consulting and Clinical Psychology, 54, 752–759.*

Bogard, H. M. (1970). Follow-up study of suicidal patients seen on emergency room consultation. *American Journal of Psychiatry, 126*, 1017–1020.

Bongar, B. (1991). *The suicidal patient: Clinical and legal standards of care.* Washington, DC: American Psychological Association.

Bower, G. H. (1981). Mood and memory. *American Psychologist, 36*, 129–148.

Brasted, W. S., & Callahan, E. J. (1984). A behavioral analysis of the grief process. *Behavior Therapy, 15, 529–543.*

Briere, J. (1988). The long-term clinical correlates of childhood sexual victimization. In R.A. Prentky & V.L. Quinsey (Eds.), *Human sexual aggression: Current perspectives* (pp. 327–334). New York: New York Academy of Sciences.

Briere, J. (1989). *Therapy for adults molested as children.* New York. Springer.

Briere, J., & Runtz, M. (1986). Suicidal thoughts and behaviours in former sexual abuse victims. *Canadian Journal of Behavioural Science, 18*, 413–423.

Bryer, J. B., Nelson, B. A., Miller, J. B., & Krol, P. A. (1987). Childhood sexual and physical abuse as factors in adult psychiatric illness. *American Journal of Psychiatry, 144*, 1426–1430.

Buck, R. (1984). The evolution of emotion communication. In R. A. Baron & J. Rodin (Eds.), *The communication of emotion* (pp. 29–67). New York: Guilford Press.

Bursill, A. E. (1958). The restriction of peripheral vision during exposure to hot and humid conditions. *Quarterly Journal of Experimental Psychology, 10*, 123–129.

Callahan, E. J., Brasted, W. S., & Granados, J. L. (1983). Fetal loss and sudden infant death: Grieving and adjustment for families. In E. J. Callahan & K. A. McCluskey (Eds.), *Life-span developmental psychology: Nonnormative life events* (pp. 145–166). New York: Academic Press.

Callahan, E. J., & Burnette, M. M. (1989). Intervention for pathological grieving. *The Behavior Therapist, 12*, 153–157.

Callaway, E., III, & Stone, G. (1960). Re-evaluating focus of attention. In L. Uhr & J. G. Miller (Eds.), *Drugs and behavior* (pp. 393–398). New York: Wiley.

Cannon, S. B. (1983). A clarification of the components and the procedural characteristics of overcorrection. *Educational and Psychological Research, 3*, 11–18.

Carpenter, W. T. Gunderson, J. G., & Strauss, J. S. (1977). Considerations of the borderline syndrome: A longitudinal comparative study of borderline and schizophrenic patients. In P. Hartcollis (Ed.), *Borderline personality disorder: The concept, the syndrome, the patient* (pp. 231–253). New York: International Universities Press.

Carrol, J. F. X., & White, W. L. (1981). Theory building: Integrating individual and environmental factors within an ecological framework. In W.S. Paine (Ed.), *Job stress and burnout.* Beverly Hills, CA: Sage.

Chamberlain, P., Patterson, G., Reid, J., Kavanagh, K., & Forgatch, M. (1984). Observation of client resistance. *Behavior Therapy, 15*, 144–155.

Chatham, P. M. (1985). *Treatment of the borderline personality.* New York: Jason Aronson.

Cherniss, C. (1980). *Staff burnout: Job stress in the human services.* Beverly Hills, CA: Sage.

Chess, S., & Thomas, A. (1986). *Temperament in clinical practice.* New York: Guilford Press.

Cialdini, R. B., Vincent, J. E., Lewis, S. K., Catalan, J., Wheeler, D., & Darby, B. L. (1975). Reciprocal concessions procedure for inducing compliance: The door-in-the-face technique. *Journal of Personality and Social Psychology, 31*, 206–215.

Clarkin, J. F., Hurt, S. W., & Hull, J. W. (1991). Subclassification of borderline personality disorder: A cluster solution. Unpublished manuscript. New York Hospital-Cornell Medical Center. Westchester, NY.

Clarkin, J. F., Marziali, E., & Munroe-Blum, H. (1991). Group and family treatments for borderline personality disorder. *Hospital and Community Psychiatry, 42*, 1038–1043.

Clarkin, J. F., Widiger, T. A., Frances, A., Hurt, S. W., & Gilmore, M. (1983). Prototypic typology and the borderline personality disorder. *Journal of Abnormal Psychology, 92*, 263–275.

Cornelius, J. R., Soloff, P. H., George, A. W. A., Schulz, S. C., Tarter, R., Brenner, R. P., & Schulz, P. M. (1989). An evaluation of the significance of selected neuropsychiatric abnormalities in the etiology of borderline personality disorder. *Journal of Personality Disorders, 3*, 19–25.

Cornsweet, D. J. (1969). Use of cues in the visual periphery under conditions of arousal. *Journal of Experimental Psychology, 80*, 14–18.

Costa, P. T., Jr., & McCrea, R. R. (1986). Personality stability and its implications for clinical psychology. *Clinical Psychology Review, 6*, 407–423.

Cowdry, R. W., & Gardner, D. L. (1988). Pharmacotherapy of borderline personality disorder: Alprazolam, carbamazepine, trifluoperazine, and tranylcypromine. *Archives of General Psychiatry, 45*, 111–119.

Cowdry, R. W., Pickar, D., & Davies, R. (1985). Symptoms and EEG findings in the borderline syndrome. *International Journal of Psychiatry in Medicine, 15*, 201–211.

Crook, T., Raskin, A., & Davis, D. (1975). Factors associated with attempted suicide among hospitalized depressed patients. *Psychological Medicine, 5*, 381–388.

Dahl, A. A. (1990, November). *The personality disorders: A critical review of family, twin, and adoption studies.* Paper presented at the NIMH Personality Disorders Conference, Williamsburg, VA.

Davids, A., & Devault, S. (1962). Maternal anxiety during pregnancy and childbirth abnormalities. *Psychosomatic Medicine, 24*, 464–470.

Deikamn, A. J. (1982). *The observing self: Mysticism and psychotherapy.* Boston: Beacon Press.

Dennenburg, V. H. (1981). Hemispheric laterality in animals and the effects of early experience. *Behavioral and Brain Sciences, 4*, 1–49.

Derlega, V. J., & Berg, J. H. (1987). *Self-disclosure: Theory, research and therapy.* New York: Plenum Press.

Derryberry, D. (1987). Incentive and feedback effects on target detection: A chronometric analysis of Gray's model of temperament. *Personality and Individual Differences, 6*, 855–866.

Derryberry, D., & Rothbart, M. K. (1984). Emotion, attention, and temperament. In C. E. Izard, J. Kagan, & R. B. Zajonc (Eds.), *Emotions, cognition, and behavior* (pp. 132–166). Cambridge, England: Cambridge University Press.

Derryberry, D., & Rothbart, M. K. (1988). Arousal, affect, and attention as components of temperament. *Journal of personality and Social Psychology, 55,* 958–966.

Deutsch, H. (1942). Some forms of emotional disturbance and their relationship to schizophrenia. *Psychoanalytic Quarterly, 11,* 301–321.

Diener, C. I., & Dweck, C. S. (1978). Analysis of learned helplessness: Continuous changes in performance, strategy, and achievement cognitions following failure. *Journal of Personality and Social Psychology, 36,* 451–462.

Duclos, S. E., Laird, J. D., Schneider, E., Sexter, M., Stern, L., & Van Lighten, O. (1989). Emotion-specific effects of facial expressions and postures on emotional experience. *Journal of Personality and Social Psychology, 57,* 100–108.

Duncan, J., & Laird, J. D. (1977). Cross-modality consistencies in individual differences in self-attribution. *Journal of Personality, 45,* 191–196.

Dweck, C. S., & Bush, E. S. (1976). Sex differences in learned helplessness: I. Differential deliberation with peer and adult evaluations. *Developmental Psychology, 12,* 147–156.

Dweck, C. S., Davidson W., Nelson, S., & Emde, B. (1978). Sex differences in learned helplessness: II. The contingencies of evaluative feedback in the classroom and III. An experimental analysis. *Developmental Psychology, 14,* 268–276.

Easser, R., & Less, S. (1965). Hysterical personality: A reevaluation. *Psychoanalytic Quarterly, 34,* 390–402.

Easterbrook, J. A. (1959). The effect of emotion on cue utilization and the organization of behavior. *Psychological Review, 66,* 183–201.

Edwall, G. E., Hoffman, N. G., & Harrison, P. A. (1989). Psychological correlates of sexual abuse in adolescent girls in chemical dependency treatment. *Adolescence, 24,* 279–288.

Efran, J., Chorney, R. L., Ascher, L. M., & Lukens, M. D. (1981), April. *The performance of monitors and blunters during painful stimulation.* Paper presented at the meeting of the Eastern Psychological Association, New York.

Ekman, P., Friesen, W. V., & Ellsworth, P. (1972). *Emotion in the human face: Guidelines for research and an integration of findings.* New York: Pergamon Press.

Ekman, P., Friesen, W. V., O'Sullivan, M., Chan, A., Diacoyanni-Tarlatzis, I., Heider, K., Krause, R., LeCompte, W. A., Pitcairn, T., Ricci-Bitti, P. E., Scherer, K., Tomita, M., & Tzavaras, A. (1987). Personality processes and individual differences: Universals and cultural differences in the judgments of facial expressions of emotion. *Journal of Personality and Social Psychology, 53,* 712–717.

Ekman, P., Levenson, R., & Friesen, W. V. (1983). Autonomic nervous system activity distinguishes among emotions. *Science, 221,* 1208–1210.

Ekstein, R. (1955). Vicissitudes of the "internal image" in the recovery of a borderline schizophrenic adolescent. *Bulletin of the Menninger Clinic, 19,* 86–92.

Ellis, A. (1962). *Reason and emotion in psychotherapy.* New York: Lyle Stuart.

Evenson, R. C., Wook, J. B., Nuttall, E. A., & Cho, D. W. (1982). Suicide rates among public mental health patients. *Acta Psychiatrica Scandinavica, 66,* 254–264.

Eysenck, H. J. (1967). *The biological basis of personality.* Springfield, IL: Charles C. Thomas.

Eysenck, H. J. (1968). A theory of the incubation of anxiety/fear responses. *Behaviour Research and Therapy, 6,* 309–321.

Fiedler, K. (1988). Emotional mood, cognitive style, and behavior regulation. In D. Fiedler & J. Forgas (Eds.), *Affect, cognition, and social behavior* (pp. 100–119). Toronto: Hogrefe.

Finkelhor, D. (1979). *Sexually victimized children*. New York. Free Press.

Firestone, S. (1970). *The dialectic of sex: The case for feminist revolution*. New York: Bantam Books.

Firth, S. T., Blouin, J., Natarajan, C., & Blouin, A. (1986). A comparison of the manifest content in dreams of suicidal, depressed and violent patients. *Canadian Journal of Psychiatry, 31,* 48–53.

Flaherty, J., & Richman, J. (1989). Gender differences in the perception and utilization of social support: Theoretical perspectives and an empirical test. *Social Science and Medicine, 28,* 1221–1228.

Foa, E. B., & Kozak, M. J. (1986). Emotional processing of fear: Exposure to corrective information. *Psychological Bulletin, 99,* 20–35.

Foa, E. B., Steketee, G., & Grayson, J. B. (1985). Imaginal and *in vivo* exposure: A comparison with obsessive-compulsive checkers. *Behavior Therapy, 16,* 292–302.

Frances, A. (1988). In (Chair), *Alternative models and treatments of patients with borderline personality disorder*. Symposium conducted at the meeting of the Society for the Exploration for Psychotherapy Integration, Boston.

Frank, J. D. (1973). *Persuasion and healing: A comparative study of psychotherapy*. Baltimore: Johns Hopkins University Press.

Freedman, J. L., & Fraser, S. C. (1966). Compliance without pressure: The foot-in-the-door technique. *Journal of Personality and Social Psychology, 4,* 195–202.

Frijda, N. H., Kuipers, P., & Schure, E. (1989). Relations among emotion, appraisal, and emotional action readiness. *Journal of Personality and Social Psychology, 57,* 212–228.

Garber, J., & Dodge, K. A. (1991). *The development of emotion regulation and dysregulation*. Cambridge, England: Cambridge University Press.

Gardner, D. L., & Cowdry, R. W. (1986). Alprazolam-induced dyscontrol in borderline personality disorder. *American Journal of Psychiatry, 143,* 519–522.

Gardner, D. L., & Cowdry, R. W. (1988). *Anticonvulsants in personality disorders*. Clifton, NJ: Oxford Health Care.

Gauthier, J., & Marshall, W. (1977). Grief: A cognitive–behavioral analysis. *Cognitive Therapy and Research, 1,* 39–44.

Gilligan, C. (1982). *In a different voice: Psychological theory and women's development*. Cambridge, MA: Harvard University Press.

Gilligan, S. G., & Bower, G. H. (1984). Cognitive consequences of emotional arousal. In C. E. Izard, J. Kagan, & R. B. Zajonc (Eds.), *Emotions, cognition, and behavior* (pp. 547–588). Cambridge, England: Cambridge University Press.

Goldberg, C. (1980). The utilization and limitations of paradoxical intervention in group psychotherapy. *International Journal of Group Psychotherapy, 30,* 287–297.

Goldfried, M. R.. & Davidson, G. C. (1976). *Clinical behavior therapy*. New York: Holt, Rineholt & Winston.

Goldfried, M. R., Linehan, M. M., & Smith, J. L. (1978). The reduction of test anxiety through cognitive restructuring. *Journal of Consulting and Clinical Psychology, 46,* 32–39.

Goldman, M. (1986). Compliance employing a combined foot-in-the-door and door-in-the-face procedure. *Journal of Social Psychology, 126,* 111–116.

Goodstein, J. (1982). *Cognitive characteristics of suicide attempters.* Unpublished doctoral dissertation, The Catholic University of America.

Goodyer, I. M.. Kolvin, I., & Gatzanis, S. (1986). Do age and sex influence the association between recent life events and psychiatric disorders in children and adolescents? A controlled enquiry. *Journal of Child Psychology and Psychiatry, 27,* 681–687.

Gottman, J. M., & Katz, L. F. (1990). Effects of marital discord on young children's peer interaction and health. *Developmental Psychology, 25,* 373–381.

Gottman, J. M., & Levenson, R. W. (1986). Assessing the role of emotion in marriage. *Behavioral Assessment, 8,* 31–48.

Green, S. A., Goldberg, R. L., Goldstein, D. M., & Liebenluft, E. (1988). *Limit setting in clinical practice.* Washington, DC: American Psychiatric Press.

Greenberg, L. S. (1983). Psychotherapy process research. In C.E. Walker (Ed.), *Handbook of clinical psychology.* Homewood, IL: Dow Jones-Irwin.

Greenberg, L. S., & Safran, J. D. (1987). Emotion in psychotherapy. New York: Guilford Press.

Greenberg, L. S., & Safran, J. D. (1989). Emotion in psychotherapy. *American Psychologist, 44,* 19–29.

Greenough, W. T. (1977). Experimental modification of the developing brain. In I.L. Janis (Ed.), *Current trends in psychology* (pp. 82–90). Los Altos, CA: William Kaufmann.

Greenwald, A. G. (1992). New Look 3: Unconscious cognition reclaimed. *American Psychologist, 92,* 766–779.

Greer, S., & Gunn, J. C. & Koller, K. M. (1966) A etiological factors in attempted suicide. *British Medical Journal, ii,* 1352–1355.

Greer, S., & Lee, H.A. (1967). Subsequent progress of potentially lethal attempted suicides. *Acta Psychiatrica Scandinavica, 40,* 361–371.

Grinker, R. R., Werble, B., & Drye, R. (1968). *The borderline syndrome: A behavioral study of ego functions.* New York: Basic Books.

Grotstein, J. S. (1987). The borderline as a disorder of self-regulation. In J. S. Grotstein, M. F. Solomon, & J. A. Lang (Eds.), *The borderline patient: Emerging concepts in diagnosis, psychodynamics, and treatment* (pp. 347–384). Hillsdale, NJ: The Analytic Press.

Gunderson, J. G. (1984). *Borderline personality disorder.* Washington DC: American Psychiatric Press.

Gunderson, J. G., & Elliott, G. R. (1985). The interface between borderline personality disorder and affective disorder. *American Journal of Psychiatry, 142,* 277–288.

Gunderson, J. G., & Kolb, J. E. (1978). Discriminating features of borderline patients. *American Journal of Psychiatry, 135,* 792–796.

Gunderson, J. G., Kolb, J. E., & Austin, Y. (1981). The Diagnostic Interview for Borderline Patients. *Journal of Personality and Social Psychology, 138,* 896–903.

Gunderson, J. G., & Zanarini, M. C. (1989). Pathogenesis of borderline personality. In A. Tasman, R. E. Hales, & A. J. Frances (Eds.). *Review of psychiatry* (Vol. 8, pp. 25–48) Washington, DC: American Psychiatric Press.

Guralnik, D. B. (Ed.). (1980). *Webster's new world dictionary of the American language* (2nd college ed.). Cleveland, OH: William Collins.

Hall, S. M., Havassy, B. E., & Wasserman, D. A. (1990). Commitment to abstinence and acute stress in relapse to alcohol, opiates, and nicotine. *Journal of Consulting and Clinical Psychology, 58,* 175–181.

Hankoff, L. D. (1979). Situational categories. In L. D. Hankoff & B. Einsidler (Eds.), *Suicide: Theory and clinical aspects* (pp. 235–249). Littleton, MA: PSG.

Hayes, S. C. (1987). A contextual approach to therapeutic change. In N.S. Jacobson (Ed.), *Psychotherapists in clinical practice: Cognitive and behavioral perspectives*. New York: Guilford Press.

Hayes, S. C., Kohlenberg, B. S., & Melancon, S. M. (1989). Avoiding and altering rule-control as a strategy of clinical intervention. In S. C. Hayes (Ed.), *Rule-governed behavior: Cognition, contingencies, and instructional control* (pp.359–385). New York: Plenum Press.

Heard, H. L., & Linehan, M. M. (in press). Problems of self and borderline personality disorder. In Z. V. Segal & S. J. Blatt (Eds.), *Cognitive and psychodynamic perspectives* New York: Guilford Press.

Hellman, I. D., Morrison, T. L., & Abramowitz, S. I. (1986). The stresses of psychotherapeutic work: A replication and extension. *Psychological Medicine, 42,* 197–205.

Herman, J. L. (1986). Histories of violence in an outpatient population. *American Journal of Orthopsychiatry, 56,* 137–141.

Herman, J. L. (1992). *Trauma and recovery: The aftermath of violence—from domestic abuse to political terror.* New York: Basic Books.

Herman, J. L., & Hirschman, L. (1981). Families at risk for father-daughter incest. *American Journal of Psychiatry, 138,* 967–970.

Herman, J. L., Perry, J. C., & van der Kolk, B. A. (1989). Childhood trauma in borderline personality disorder. *American Journal of Psychiatry, 146,* 490–495.

Hoffman, L. W. (1972). Early childhood experiences and women's achievement motives. *Journal of Social Issues, 28,* 129–156.

Hooley, J. M. (1986). Expressed emotion and depression: Interactions between patients and high-versus low-expressed-emotion spouses. *Journal of Abnormal Psychology, 95,* 237–246.

Horowitz, M. J. (1986). Stress-response syndromes: A review of posttraumatic and adjustment disorders. *Hospital and Community Psychiatry, 37,* 241–249.

Howard, J. (1989). Cocaine and its effects on the newborn. *Developmental Medicine and Child Neurology, 31,* 255–257.

Howard, J. A. (1984). Societal influences of attribution: Blaming some victims more than others. *Journal of Personality and Social Psychology, 47,* 494–505.

Howe, E. S., & Loftus, T. C. (1992). Integration of intention and outcome information by students and circuit court judges: Design economy and individual differences. *Journal of Applied Social Psychology, 22,* 102–116.

Hurt, S. W., Clarkin, J. F., Monroe-Blum, H., & Marziali, E. A. (1992). Borderline behavior clusters and different treatment approaches. In J. F. Clarkin, E. A. Marziali, & H. Monroe-Blum (Eds.), *Borderline personality disorder: clinical and empirical perspectives* (pp. 199–219). New York: Guilford Press.

Hurt, S. W., Clarkin, J. F., Widiger, T. A., Fyer, M. R., Sullivan, T., Stone, M. H., & Frances, A. (1990). Evaluation of DSM-III decision rules for case detection using joint conditional probability structures. *Journal of Personality Disorders, 4,* 121–130.

Hyler, S. E., Reider, R. O., Williams, J. B., Spitzer, R. L., Hendler, J., & Lyons, M. (1987). *Personality Diagnostic Questionnaire—Revised (PDQ-R).* New York: New York State Psychiatric Institute.

Ingram, R. E. (1989). Affective confounds in social-cognitive research. *Journal of Personality and Social Psychology, 57,* 715–722.

Isen, A. M., Daubman, K. A., & Nowicki, G. P. (1987). Positive affect facilitates creative problem solving. *Journal of Personality and Social Psychology, 52,* 1122–1131.

Isen, A. M., Johnson, M., Mertz, E., & Robins, G. (1985). Positive affect and the uniqueness of word association. *Journal of Personality and Social Psychology, 48*, 1413–1426.

Izard, C. E. (1977). *Human emotions.* New York: Plenum Press.

Izard, C. E., Kagan, J., & Zajonc, R. B. (Eds.) (1984). *Emotions, cognition, and behavior.* Cambridge, England: Cambridge University Press.

Izard, C. E., & Kobak, R. R. (1991). Emotions systems functioning and emotion regulation. In J. Garber & K. A. Dodge (Eds.), *The development of emotion regulation and dysregulation* (pp. 303–322). Cambridge, England: Cambridge University Press.

Jacobson, A., & Herald, C. (1990). The relevance of childhood sexual abuse to adult psychiatric inpatient care. *Hospital and Community Psychiatry, 41*, 1545–158.

Jacobson, N. S. (1992). Behavioral couple therapy: A new beginning. *Behavior Therapy, 23*, 493–506.

Janoff-Bulman, R. (1985). The aftermath of victimization: Rebuilding shattered assumptions. In C. R. Figley (Ed.), *Trauma and its wake: The study and treatment of post-traumatic stress disorder* (pp. 15–35). New York: Brunner/Mazel.

The Jerusalem Bible. (1966). (A. Jones, Ed.). Garden City, NY: Doubleday.

Johnson, P. (1976). Women and power: Toward a theory of effectiveness. *Journal of Social Issues, 32*, 99–109.

Kanter, J. S. (1988). Clinical issues in the case management relationship. In M. Harris & L. L. Bachrach (Series Eds.) and H. R. Lamb (Vol. Ed.), *Clinical case management: No. 40. New directions for mental health services* (pp. 15–27). San Francisco: Jossey-Bass.

Kastenbaum, R. J. (1969). *Death and bereavement* in later life. In A. H. Kutscher (Ed.), Death and bereavement (pp. 28–54). Springfield, IL: Charles C Thomas.

Keele, S. W., & Hawkins, H. H. (1982). Explorations of individual differences relevant to high level skill. *Journal of Motor Behavior, 14*, 3–23.

Kegan, R. (1982). *The evolving self: Problem and process in human development.* Cambridge, MA: Harvard University Press.

Kernberg, O. F. (1975). *Borderline conditions and pathological narcissism.* New York: Aronson.

Kernberg, O. F. (1976). *Object-relations theory and clinical psychoanalysis.* New York: Aronson.

Kernberg, O. F. (1984). *Severe personality disorders: Psychotherapeutic strategies.* New Haven, CT: Yale University Press.

Klein, D. F. (1977). Psychopharmacological treatment & delineation of borderline disorders. In P. Hartocollis (Ed.), *Borderline personality disorder: the concept, the syndrome, the patient* (pp. 365–383). New York: International Universities Press.

Knight, R. P. (1954). Management and psychotherapy of the borderline schizophrenic patient. In R. P. Knight & C.R. Friedman (Eds.), *Psychoanalytic psychiatry and psychology* (pp. 110–122). New York: International Universities Press.

Knussen, C., & Cunningham, C. C. (1988). Stress, disability and handicap. In S. Fisher & J. Reason (Eds.), *Handbook of life, stress, condition and health* (pp. 335–350). New York: Wiley.

Koenigsberg, H. W., Clarkin, J., Kernberg, O. F., Yeomans, F., & Gutfreund, J. (in press). Some measures of process and outcome in the psychodynamic psychotherapy of borderline patients. In *The Integration of Research and Psychoanalytic Practice: The Proceedings of the IPA First International Conference on Research.*

Kohlenberg, R. J., & Tsai, M. (1991). *Functional analytic psychotherapy: Creating intense and curative therapeutic relationships.* New York: Plenum Press.

Kohut, H. (1977). *The restoration of the self.* New York: International Universities Press.

Kohut, H. (1984). *How does analysis cure?* Chicago: University of Chicago Press.

Kopp, S. B. (1971). *Metaphors from a psychotherapist guru.* Palo Alto, CA: Science & Behavior books.

Kreitman, N. (1977). *Parasuicide.* Chichester, England: Wiley.

Kroll, J. L., Carey, K. S., & Sines, L. K. (1985). Twenty-year follow-up of borderline personality disorder: A pilot study. In C. Stragass (Ed.), *IV World Congress of Biological Psychiatry.* New York: Elsevier.

Kuhn, T. S. (1970). *The structure of scientific revolutions* (2nd ed.). Chicago: University of Chicago Press.

Kyokai, B. D. (1966). *The teachings of Buddha.* Tokyo: Author.

Laird, J. D. (1974). Self-attribution of emotion: The effects of expressive behavior on the quality of emotional experience. *Journal of Personality and Social Psychology, 29,* 475–486.

Laird, J. D., Wagener, J. J., Halal, M., & Szegda, M. (1982). Remembering what you feel: The effects of emotion on memory. *Journal of Personality and Social Psychology, 42,* 646–657.

Lamping, D. L., Molinaro, V., & Stevenson, G. W. (1985, March *The effects of perceived control and coping style on cognitive appraisals during stressful medical procedures: A randomized, controlled trial.* Paper presented at the meeting of the Eastern Psychological Association, Boston.

Lang, P. J. (1984). Cognition in emotion: Concept and action. In C.E. Izard, J. Kagan, & R.B. Zajonc (Eds.), *Emotions, cognition, and behavior* (pp. 192–226). Cambridge, England: University Press.

Lanzetta, J. T., Cartwright-Smith, J., & Kleck, R. E. (1976). Effects on nonverbal dissimulation on emotional experience and automatic arousal. *Journal of Personality and Social Psychology, 39,* 1081–1087.

Lazarus, R. S. (1966). *Psychological stress and the coping process.* New York: McGraw-Hill.

Lazarus, R. S. (1991). Cognition and motivation in emotion. *American Psychologist, 46,* 352–367.

Lazarus, R. S., & Folkman, S. (1984). *Stress, coping and adaptation.* New York: Springer.

Leff, J. P., & Vaughn, C. (1985). *Expressed emotion in families: Its significance for mental illness.* New York: Guilford Press.

Leinbenluft, E., Gardner, D. L., & Cowdry, R. W. (1987). The inner experience of the borderline self-mutilator. *Journal of Personality Disorders, 1,* 317–324.

Levenson, M. (1972). *Cognitive and perceptual factors in suicidal individuals.* Unpublished doctoral dissertation, University of Kansas.

Levenson, M., & Neuringer, C. (1971). Problem-solving behavior in suicidal adolescents. *Journal of Consulting and Clinical Psychology, 37,* 433–436.

Leventhal, H. & Tomarken, A. J. (1986). Emotion: Today's problems. *Annual Review of Psychology, 37,* 565–610.

Levins, R., & Lewontin, R. (1985). *The dialectical biologist.* Cambridge, MA: Harvard University Press.

Levis, D. J. (1980). Implementing the technique of implosive therapy. In A. Goldstein & E. B. Foa (Eds.), *Handbook of behavioral interventions: A clinical guide* (pp.92–151). New York: Wiley.

Lewis, M., Wolan-Sullivan, M., & Michalson, L. (1984). The cognitive–emotional fugue. In C. E. Izard, J. Kagen, & R. B. Zajonc (Eds.), *Emotions, cognitions, and behavior* (pp. 264–288). Cambridge, England: Cambridge University Press.

Linehan, M. M. (1979). A structured cognitive–behavioral treatment of assertion problems. In P. C. Kendall & S. D. Hollon (Eds.), *Cognitive–behavioral interventions: Theory, research and procedures* (pp. 205–240). New York: Academic Press.

Linehan, M. M. (1981). A social–behavioral analysis of suicide and parasuicide: Implications for clinical assessment and treatment. In H. Glaezer & J. F. Clarkin (Eds.), *Depression: Behavioral and directive intervention strategies* (pp. 29–294). New York: Garland.

Linehan, M. M. (1986). Suicidal people: One population or two? In J. J. Mann & M. Stanley (Eds.), *Psychobiology of suicidal behavior* (pp. 16–33). New York: New York Academy of Sciences.

Linehan, M. M. (1988). Perspectives on the interpersonal relationship in behavior therapy. *Journal of Integrative and Eclectic Psychotherapy, 7,* 278–290.

Linehan, M. M. (1989). Cognitive and behavior therapy for borderline personality disorder. In A. Tasman, R. E. Hales, & A. J. Frances (Eds.), *Review of psychiatry* (Vol. 8, pp. 84–102). Washington, DC: American Psychiatric Press.

Linehan, M. M., Armstrong, H. E., Suarez, A., Allmon, D., & Heard, H. L. (1991). Cognitive–behavioral treatment of chronically parasuicidal borderline patients. *Archives of General Psychiatry, 48,* 1060–1064.

Linehan, M. M., Camper, P., Chiles, J. A., Strosahl, K., & Shearin, E. (1987). Interpersonal problem solving and parasuicide. *Cognitive Therapy and Research, 11,* 1–12.

Linehan, M. M., & Egan, K. (1979). Assertion training for women. In A. S. Belleck & M. Hersen (Eds.), *Research and practice in social skills training* (pp. 237–271). New York: Plenum Press.

Linehan, M. M., Goldfried, M. R., & Goldfried, A. P. (1979). Assertation therapy: Skill training or cognitive restructuring. *Behavior Therapy, 10,* 372–388.

Linehan, M. M., & Heard, H. L. (1993). Impact of treatment accessibility on clinical course of parasuicidal patients: In reply to R. E. Hoffman [Letter to the editor]. *Archives of General Psychiatry, 50,* 157–158.

Linehan, M. M., Heard, H. L., & Armstrong, H. E. (1993). Standard dialectical behavior therapy compared to psychotherapy in the community for chronically parasuicidal borderline patients. Unpublished manuscript. University of Washington, Seattle, WA.

Linehan, M. M., Heard, H. E., & Armstrong, H. E. (in press). Naturalistic follow-up of a behavioral treatment for chronically suicidal borderline patients. *Archives of General Psychiatry.*

Linehan, M. M., & Shearin, E. N. (1988). Lethal stress: A social-behavioral model of suicidal behavior. In S. Fisher & J. Reason (Eds.), *Handbook of life stress, cognition and health* (pp.265–285). New York: Wiley.

Linehan, M. M., Tutek, D., & Heard, H. L. (1992, November). Interpersonal and social treatment outcomes for borderline personality disorder. Poster presented at the annual meeting of the Association for the Advancement of Behavior Therapy, Boston, Mass.

Links, P. S., Steiner, M. & Huxley, G. (1988). The occurence of borderline personality disorder in the families of borderline patients. *Journal of Personality Disorders, 2,* 14–20.

Loranger, A. W., Oldham, J. M., & Tulis, E. H. (1982). Familial transmission of DSM-III borderline personality disorder. *Archives of General Psychiatry, 39,* 795–799.

Lumsden, E. (1991). *Possible role of impaired memory in the development and/or maintenance of borderline personality disorder.* Unpublished manuscript, University of North Carolina at Greensboro.

Lykes, M. G. (1985). Gender and individualistic vs. collectivist based for notions about the self. *Journal of Personality, 53,* 356–383.

Maccoby, R., & Jacklin, E. (1978). *The psychology of sex differences.* Stanford, CA: Stanford University Press.

Mackenzie-Keating, S. E., & McDonald, L. (1990). Overcorrection: reviewed, revisited and revised. *The Behavior Analyst, 13,* 39–48.

MacLeod, C., Mathews, A., & Tata, P. (1986). Attentional bias in emotional disorders. *Journal of Abnormal Psychology, 95,* 15–20.

Maddison, D. C., & Viola, A. (1968). The health of widows in one year following bereavement. *Journal of Psychosomatic Research, 12,* 297–306.

Mahoney, M. J. (1991). *Human change processes: The scientific foundations of psychotherapy.* New York: Basic Books.

Main, T. F. (1957). The ailment. *British Journal of Medical Psychology, 30,* 129–145.

Malatesta, C. Z. (1990). The role of emotions in the development and organization of personality. In R. A. Thompson (Ed.), *Socioemotional development: Nebraska symposium on motivation, 1988* (pp. 1–56). Lincoln and London: University of Nebraska Press.

Malatesta, C. Z., & Haviland, J. M. (1982). Learning display rules: The socialization of emotion expression in infancy. *Child Development, 53,* 991–1003.

Malatesta, C. Z., & Izard, C. E. (1984). The ontogenesis of human social signals: From biological imperative to symbol utilization. In N. Fox & R. Davidson (Eds.), *The psychobiology of affective development* (pp. 161–206). Hillsdale, NJ: Erlbaum.

Mandler, G. (1975). *Mind and emotion.* New York: Wiley.

Manicas, P. T., & Secord, P. F. (1983). Implications for psychology of the new philosophy of science. *American Psychologist, 38,* 399–413.

Maris, R. W. (1981). *Pathways to suicide: A survey of self-destructive behaviors.* Baltimore: Johns Hopkins University Press.

Maris, R. W., Berman, A. L., Maltsberger, J. T., & Yufit, R. I. (Eds.), 1992. *Assessment and prediction of suicide.* New York: Guilford Press.

Marlatt, G. A., & Gordon, J. R. (Eds.). (1985). *Relapse prevention: Maintenance strategies in the treatment of addictive behaviors.* New York: Guilford Press.

Martin, G., & Pear, J. (1192). *Behavior modification: What it is and how to do it* (4th ed,). *Part III. Basic behavioral principles and procedures.* Englewood Cliffs, NJ: Prentice-Hall.

Marx, K., & Engels, F. (1970). *Selected works* (Vol.3). New York: International.

Marziali, E. A. (1984). Prediction of outcome of brief psychotherapy from therapist interpretive interventions. *Archives of General Psychiatry, 41,* 301–304.

Marziali, E. A., & Munroe-Blum, H. (1987). A group approach: The management of projective identification in group treatment of self-destructive borderline patients. *Journal of Personality Disorders, 1,* 340–343.

Masters, J. C., Burish, T. G. Hollon, S. D., & Rimm, D. C. (1987). *Behavior therapy: Techniques and empirical findings* (3rd ed.). New York: Harcourt Brace Jovanovich.

Masterson, J. F. (1972). *Treatment of the borderline adolescent.* New York, Wiley.

Masterson, J. F. (1976). *Psychotherapy of the borderline adult: A developmental approach.* New York: Brunner/Mazel.

May, G. (1982). *Will and spirit.* San Francisco: Harper & Row.

McGlashen, T. H. (1983). The borderline syndrome: II. Is it a varient of schizophrenia or affective disorder? *Archives of General Psychiatry, 40,* 1319–1323.

McGlashen, T. H. (1986a). The Chestnut Lodge follow-up study: III. Long-term outcome of borderline personalities. *Archives of General Psychiatry, 43,* 20–30.

McGlashen, T. H. (1986b). Schizotypal personality disorder: Chestnut Lodge follow-up study, VI: Long-term follow-up perspectives. *Archives of General Psychiatry, 43,* 329–334.

McGlashen, T. H. (1987). Borderline personality disorder and unipolar affective disorder. *Journal of Nervous and Mental Disease, 175,* 467–473.

McGuire, W. J., & McGuire, C. V. (1982). Significant others in self-space: Sex differences and developmental trends in the social self. In J. Suls (Ed.), *Psychological perspectives on the self* (pp.71–96). Hillsdale, NJ: Erlbaum.

McNamara, H., & Fisch, R. (1964). Effect of high and low motivation on two aspects of attention. *Perceptual and Motor Skills, 19,* 571–578.

Meichenbaum, D., & Turk, D. (1987). *Facilitating treatment adherence: A practitioner's guidebook.* New York: Plenum Press.

Meissner, W. W. (1984). *The borderline spectrum: Differential diagnosis and developmental issues.* New York: Aronson.

The Merriam-Webster dictionary. 1977. Boston: G.K. Hall.

Metalsky, G. I., Halberstadt, L. J., & Abramson, L. Y. (1987). Vulnerability to depressive mood reactions: Toward a more powerful test of the diathesis-stress and causal mediation components of the reformulated theory of depression. *Journal of Personality and Social Psychology, 52,* 386–393.

Miklowitz, D. J., Strachan, A. M., Goldstein, M. J., Doane, J. A., Snyder, K. S., Hogarty, G. E., & Falloon, I. R. H. (1986). Expressed emotion and communication deviance in the families of schizophrenics. *Journal of Abnormal Psychology, 95,* 60–66.

Milgram, S. (1963). Behavioral study of obedience. *Journal of Abnormal and Social Psychology, 67,* 371–378.

Milgram, S. (1964), Issues in the study of obedience. *American Psychologist, 19,* 848–852.

Millenson, J. R., & Leslie, J. C. (1979). *Principles of behavioral analysis.* New York: Macmillan.

Miller, J. G. (1984). Culture and the development of everyday social explanation. *Journal of Personality and Social Psychology, 46,* 961–978.

Miller, M. (1990). *Developing a scale to measure individual's stress-proneness to behaviors of human service professionals.* Unpublished manuscript. University of Washington.

Miller, M. L., Chiles, J. A., & Barnes, V. E. (1982). Suicide attempters within a delinquent population. *Journal of Consulting and Clinical Psychology, 50,* 491–498.

Miller, S. M. (1979). Controllability and human stress: Method, evidence and theory. *Behaviour Research and Therapy, 17,* 287–304.

Miller, S. M., & Mangan, C. E. (1983). Interacting effects of information and coping style in adapting to gynecologic stress: Should the doctor tell all? *Journal of Personality and Social Psychology, 45,* 223–236.

Millon, T. (1981). *Disorders of personality DSM-III: Axis II.* New York: Wiley.

Millon, T. (1987a). On the genesis and prevalence of the borderline personality disorder: A social learning thesis. *Journal of Personality Disorders, 1,* 354–372.

Millon, T. (1987b). *Manual for the Millon Clinical Multiaxial Inventory II (MCMI-II).* Minnetonka, MN: National Computer Systems.

Mintz, R.S. (1968). Psychotherapy of the suicidal patient. In H.L.P. Resnik (Ed.), *Suicidal behaviors: Diagnosis and management* (pp. 271–296). Boston: Little, Brown.

Mischel, W. (1968). *Personality and assessment.* New York: Wiley.

Mischel, W. (1984). Convergences and challenges in the search for consistency. *American Psychologist, 39,* 351–364.

Morris, R. J., & Magrath, K. H. (1983). The therapeutic relationship in behavior therapy. In M. J. Lambert (Ed.), *Psychotherapy and patient relationships* (pp. 145–189). Homewood, IL: Dorsey Press.

Morris, W. (Ed.) (1979). *The American heritage dictionary of the English language.* Boston: Houghton Mifflin.

Munroe-Blum, H., & Marziali, E. (1987). *Randomized clinical trial of relationship management time-limited group treatment of borderline personality disorder.* Unpublished manuscript. Hamilton, Ontario Mental Health Foundation.

Munroe-Blum, H., & Marziali, E. (1989). *Continuation of a randomized control trial of group treatment for borderline personality disorder.* Unpublished manuscript. Hamilton, Canadian Department of Health and Human Services.

Murray, N., Sujan, H., Hirt, E. R., & Sujan, M. (1990). The influence of mood on categorization: A cognitive flexibility interpretation. *Journal of Personality and Social Psychology, 59,* 411–425.

Napalkov, A. V. (1963). Information process and the brain. In N. Wiener & J. P. Schade (Eds.), *Progress in brain research* (pp. 59–69). V 2 Amsterdam: Elsevier.

Neill, J. R., & Kniskern, D. P. (Eds.). (1982). *From Psyche to System: The evolving therapy of Carl Whitaker.* New York: Guilford Press.

Nelson, V. L., Nielsen, E. C., & Checketts, K. T. (1977). Interpersonal attitudes of suicidal individuals. *Psychological Reports, 40,* 983–989.

Neuringer, C. (1964). Dichotomous evaluations in suicidal individuals. *Journal of Consulting Psychology, 25,* 445–449.

Neuringer, C. (1961). Rigid thinking in suicidal individuals. *Journal of Consulting and Clinical Psychology, 28,* 54–58.

Newton, R. W. (1988). Psychosocial aspects of pregnancy: The scope for intervention. *Journal of Reproductive and Infant Psychology, 6,* 23–29.

Nisbett, R. E., & Wilson, T. D. (1977). Telling more than we can know: Verbal reports on mental processes. *Psychological Review, 84,* 231–259.

Noble, D. (1951). A study of dreams in schizophrenia and allied states. *American Journal of Psychiatry, 107,* 612–616.

Nolen-Hoeksema, S. (1987). Sex differences in unipolar depression: Evidence and theory. *Psychological Bulletin, 101,* 259–282.

Ogata, S. N., Silk, K. R., Goodrich, S, Lohr, N.E., & Westen, D. (1989). *Childhood sexual and clinical symptoms in borderline patients.* Unpublished manuscript.

O'Leary, K. D., & Wilson, G. T. (1987). *Behavior therapy Application and outcome.* Englewood Cliffs, NJ: Prentice-Hall.

The original Oxford English Dictionary on computer disc (version 4.10) [Computer File]. (1987). Fort Washington, PA: Tri Star.

Paerregaard, G. (1975). Suicide among attempted suicides: A 10-year-follow-up. *Suicide, and Life-Threatening Behavior, 5*, 140–144.

Paris, J., Brown, R., & Nowlis, D. (1987). Long-term follow-up of borderline patients in a general hospital. *Comparative Psychiatry, 28*, 530–535.

Parkes, C. M. (1964). The effects of bereavement on physical and mental health: A study of the case records of widows. *British Medical Journal, ii*, 274–279.

Parloff, M. B., Waskow, I. E., & Wolfe, B. E. (1978). Research on therapist variables in relation to process and outcome. In S. L. Garfield & A. E. Bergin (Eds.), *Handbook of psychotherapy and behavior change: An empirical analysis* (2nd ed., pp. 233–282). New York: Wiley

Patsiokas, A., Clum, G., & Luscomb, R. (1979). Cognitive characteristics of suicide attempters. *Journal of Consulting and Clinical Psychology, 47*, 478–484.

Patterson, G. R. (1976). The aggressive child: Victim and architect of a coercive system. In E. J. Walsh, L. A. Hamerlynck, & L. C. Handy (Eds.), *Behavior modification and families* (pp. 267–316). New York: Brunner/Mazel.

Patterson, G. R., & Stouthamer-Loeber, M. (1984). The correlation of family management practices and delinquency. *Child Development, 55*, 1299–1307.

Pennebaker, J. W. (1988). Confiding traumatic experiences and health. In S. Fisher & J. Reason (Eds.), *Handbook of Life stress, cognition and health* (pp. 669–682). New York: Wiley.

Perloff, R. (1987). Self-interest and personal responsibility redux. *American Psychologist, 42*, 3–11.

Perry, J. C., & Cooper, S. H. (1985). Psychodynamics, symptoms, and outcome in borderline and antisocial personality disorders and bipolar type II affective disorder. In T. H. McGlashan (Ed.), *The borderline: Current empirical research* (pp. 19–41). Washington, DC: American Psychiatric Press.

Pfeffer, C. R. (1986). *The suicidal child.* New York: Guilford Press.

Phipps, S., & Zinn, A. B. (1986). Psychological response to amniocentesis: II. Effects of coping style. *American Journal of Medical Genetics, 25*, 143–148.

Physicians' Desk Reference. (annual editions). Oradell, NJ: Medical Economics.

Polanyi, M. (1958). *Personal knowledge.* Chicago: University of Chicago Press.

Pope, H. G., Jonas, J. M., Hudson, J. I., Cohen, B. M., & Gunderson, J. G. (1983). The validity of DSM-III borderline personality disorder: A phenomenologic, family history, treatment response, and long term follow-up study. *Archives of General Psychiatry, 40*, 23–30.

Posner, M. I., Walker, J. A., Friedrich, F. J., & Rafal, R. D. (1984). Effects of parietal lobe injury on covert orienting of visual attention. *Journal of Neuroscience, 4*, 1863–1874.

Pratt, M. W., Pancer, M. Hunsberger, B., & Manchester, J. (1990). Reasoning about the self and relationships in maturity: An integrative complexity analysis of individual differences. *Journal of Personality and Social Psychology, 59*, 575–581.

Pretzer, J. (1990). Borderline personality disorder. *Clinical applications of cognitive therapy.* New York: Plenum Press.

Rado, S. (1956). *Psychoanalysis of behavior: Collected papers.* New York: Grune & Stratton.

Rando, T. A. (1984). *Grief, dying, and death: Clinical interventions for caregivers.* Champaign, IL: Research Press.

Rees, W. D. (1975). The bereaved and their hallucinations. In E. Schoenberg, I. Gerber, A. Wiener, A. H. Kutscher, D. Pertz, & A. C. Carr (Eds.), *Bereavement: Its psychological aspects* (pp. 66–71). New York: Columbia University Press.

Reich, J. (1992). Measurement of DSM-III and DSM-III-R Borderline Personality Disorder. In J. F. Clarkin, E. Marziali, & H. Munroe-Blum (eds.), *Borderline personality disorder: Clinical and empirical perspectives* (pp. 116–148). New York: Guilford Press.

Rhodewalt, F., & Comer, R. (1979). Induced compliance attitude change: Once more with feeling. *Journal of Experimental Social Psychology, 15,* 35–47.

Richman, J., & Charles, E. (1976). Patient dissatisfaction and attempted suicide. *Community Mental Health Journal, 12,* 301–305.

Rinsley, D. (1980a). The developmental etiology of borderline and narcissistic disorders. *Bulletin of the Menninger Clinic, 44,* 127–134.

Rinsley, D. (1980b). A thought experiment in psychiatric genetics. *Bulletin of the Menninger Clinic, 44,* 628–638.

Rogers, C. R., & Truax, C. B. (1967). The therapeutic conditions antecedent to change: A theoretical view. In C. R. Rogers (Ed.), *The therapeutic relationship and its impact.* Madison: University of Wisconsin Press.

Rose, Y., & Tryon, W. (1979). Judgments of assertive behavior as a function of speech loudness, latency, content, gestures, infection and sex. *Behavior Modification, 3,* 112–123.

Rosen, G. M. (1974). Therapy set: Its effects on subjects' involvement in systematic desensitization and treatment outcome. *Journal of Abnormal Psychology, 83,* 291–300.

Rosen, S. (Ed.). (1982). *My voice will go with you: The teaching tales of Milton H. Erickson, M.D.* New York: Norton.

Rosenbaum, M. (1980). A schedule for assessing self-control behaviors: Preliminary findings. *Behavior Therapy, 11,* 109–121.

Ross, C. A. (1989). *Multiple personality disorder: Diagnosis, clinical features and treatment.* New York: Wiley.

Rothbart, M. K., & Derryberry, D. (1981). Development of individual differences in temperament. In M. E. Lamb & A. L. Brown (Eds.), *Advances in developmental psychology* (pp. 37–86). Hillsdale, NJ: Erlbaum.

Russell, J. A., Lewicka, M., & Niit, T. (1989). A cross-cultural study of a circumplex model of affect. *Journal of Personality and Social Psychology, 57,* 848–856.

Sacks, C. H., & Bugental, D. B. (1987). Attributions as moderators of affective and behavioral responses to social failure. *Journal of Personality and Social Psychology, 53,* 939–947.

Safran, J. D., & Segal, Z. V. (1990). *Interpersonal process in cognitive therapy.* New York: Basic Books.

Sameroff, A. J. (1975). Early influences on development: "Fact or fancy?" *Merrill–Palmer Quarterly, 20,* 275–301.

Sampson, E. E. (1977). Psychology and the American ideal. *Journal of Personality and Social Psychology, 35,* 767–782.

Sampson, E. E. (1988). The debate on individualism: Indigenous psychologies of the individual and their role in personal and societal functioning. *American Psychologist, 43* 15–22.

Saposnek, D. T. (1980). Aikido: A model for brief strategic therapy. *Family Process, 19,* 227–238.

Sarason, I. G., Sarason, B. R., & Shearin, E. N. (1986). Social support as an individual difference variable: Its stability, origins and relational aspects. *Journal of Personality and Social Psychology, 50,* 845–855.

Scarr, S., & McCartney, K. (1983). How people make their own environments: A theory of genotype–environmental effects. *Child Development, 54,* 424–435.

Schachter, S., & Singer, J. (1962). Cognitive, social, and physiological determinants of emotional state. *Psychological Review, 65,* 379–399.

Schaffer, N. D. (1986). The borderline patient and affirmative interpretation. *Bulletin of the Menninger Clinic, 50,* 148–162.

Schmideberg, M. (1947). The treatment of psychopaths and borderline patients. *American Journal of Psychotherapy, 1,* 45–55.

Schotte, D. E., & Clum, G. A. (1982). Suicide ideation in a college population: A test of a model. *Journal of Consulting and Clinical Psychology, 50,* 690–696.

Schroyer, T. (1972). *The Critique of domination.* New York: George Braziller.

Schulz, P., Schulz, S., Goldberg, S., Ettigi, P. Resnick, R., & Hamer, R. (1986). Diagnoses of the relatives of schizotypal outpatients. *Journal of Nervous and Mental Disease, 174,* 457–463.

Schutz, B. M. (1982). *Legal liability in psychotherapy.* San Francisco: Jossey-Bass.

Schwartz, G. E. (1982). Psychophysiological patterning of emotion revisited: A systems perspective. In C. E. Izard (Ed.), *Measuring emotions in infants and children* (pp. 67–93). Cambridge, England: Cambridge University Press.

Sederer, L. I., & Thorbeck, J. (1986). First do no harm: Short-term inpatient psychotherapy of the borderline patient. *Hospital and Community Psychiatry, 37,* 692–697.

Seltzer, L. F. (1986). *Paradoxical strategies in psychotherapy: A comprehensive overview and guidebook.* New York: Wiley.

Selye, H. (1956). *The stress of life.* New York: McGraw-Hill.

Shaver, P., Schwartz, J., Kirson, D., & O'Connor, C. (1987). Emotion knowledge: Further exploration of a prototype approach. *Journal of Personality and Social Psychology, 52,* 1061–1086.

Shearer, S. L., Peters, C. P., Quaytman, M. S., & Ogden, R. L. (1990). Frequency and correlates of childhood sexual and physical abuse histories in adult female borderline inpatients. *American Journal of Psychiatry, 147,* 214–216.

Shearin, E. N., & Linehan, M. M. (1989). Dialectics and behavior therapy: A meta-paradoxical approach to the treatment of borderline personality disorder. In L. M. Ascher (Ed.), *Therapeutic paradox: A behavioral model for implementation and change* (pp. 255–288). New York: Guilford Press.

Shelton, J. L., & Levy, R. L. (1981). *Behavioral assignments and treatment compliance: A handbook of clinical strategies.* Campaign, Il: Research Press.

Sherman, M. H. (1961). Siding with the resistance in paradigmatic psychotherapy. *Psychoanalysis and the Psychoanalytic Review, 48,* 43–59.

Shneidman, E. S. (1984). Aphorisms of suicide and some implications for psychotherapy. *American Journal of Psychotherapy, 38*(3), 319–328.

Shneidman, E. S. (1992). A conspectus of the suicidal scenario. In R. W. Maris, A. L. Berman, J. T. Maltsberger, & R. I. Yufit (Ed.), *Assessment and prediction of suicide* (pp. 50–64). New York: Guilford Press.

Shneidman, E. S., Farberow, N. L., & Litman, R. E. (1970). *The psychology of suicide.* New York: Science House.

Showers, C., & Cantor, N. (1985). Social cognition: A look at motivated strategies. *Annual Review of Psychology, 36,* 275–305.

Silverman, J. Siever, L. Coccaro, E., Klar, H., Greenwald, S., & Rubinstein, K. (1987), December). Risk for affective disorders in relatives of personality disordered patients. Poster presented at the annual meeting of the American College of Neuropsychopharmacology, San Juan, Puerto Rico.

Simon, H. E. (1990). Invariants of human behavior. *Annual Review of Psychology, 41*, 1–20.

Sipe, R. B. (1986). Dialectics and method: Restructuring radical therapy. *Journal of Humanistic Psychology, 26*, 52–79.

Slater, J., & Depue, R. A. (1981). The contribution of environmental events and social support to serious suicide attempts in primary depressive disorder. *Journal of Abnormal Psychology, 90*, 275–285.

Smith, K., Conroy, R. W. & Ehler, B. D. (1984). Lethality of Suicide Attempt Rating Scale. *Suicide and Life-Threatening Behavior, 14* (4), 215–242.

Snyder, S., & Pitts, W. M. (1984). Electroencephalography of DSM-III borderline personality disorder. *Acta Psychiatrica Scandinavica, 69*, 129.

Soloff, P. H., & Millward, J. (1983). Psychiatric disorders in the families of borderline patients. *Archives of General Psychiatry, 40*, 37–44.

Spitzer, R. L., & Williams, J. B. W. (1990). *Structured Clinical Interview for DSM-III-R Personality Disorders.* New York: Biometrics Research Department, New York State Psychiatric Institute.

Stern, A. (1938). Psychoanalytic investigation and therapy in the borderline group of neuroses. *Psychoanalytic Quarterly, 7*, 467–489.

Stone, M. H. (1980). *The borderline syndromes: Constitution, personality, and adaptation.* New York: McGraw-Hill.

Stone, M. H. (1981). Psychiatrically ill relatives of borderline patients: A family study. *Psychiatric Quarterly, 58*, 71–83.

Stone, M. H. (1987). Constitution and temperament in borderline conditions: Biological and genetic explanatory formulations. In J. S. Grotstein, M. F. Solomon, & J. A. Lang (Eds.), *The borderline patient: Emerging concepts in diagnosis, psychodynamics, and treatment* (pp. 253–287). Hillsdale, NJ: The Analytic Press.

Stone, M. H. (1989). The course of borderline personality disorder. In A. Tasman, R. E. Hales, & A. J. Frances (Eds.), *Review of psychiatry* (Vol. 8, pp. 103–122). Washington, DC: American Psychiatric Press.

Stone, M. H., Hurt, S., & Stone, D. (1987a). The PI 500: Long-term follow-up of borderline inpatients meeting DSM-III criteria. I: Global outcome. *Journal of Personality Disorders, 1*, 291–298.

Stone, M. H., Stone, D. K., & Hurt, S. W. (1987b). Natural history of borderline patients treated by intensive hospitalization. *Psychiatric Clinics of North America, 10*, 185–206.

Strongman, K. T. (1987). Theories of emotion. In K. T. Strongman (Ed.), *The psychology of emotion* (pp. 14–55). New York: Wiley.

Strelau, J., Farley, F. H., & Gale, A. (Ed.). (1986). *The biological bases of personality and behavior: Vol. 2. Psychophysiology: Performance and applications.* Washington, DC: Hemisphere.

Suler, J. R. (1989). Paradox in psychological transformations: The Zen koan and psychotherapy. *Psychologia, 32*, 221–229.

Taylor, E. A., & Stansfeld, S. A. (1984). Children who poison themselves: I. A clinical comparison with psychiatric controls. *British Journal of Psychiatry, 145*, 127–135.

Tellegen, A., Lykken, D. T., Bouchard, T. J., Jr., Wilcox, K. J., Segal, N. L., & Rich, S. (1988). Personality similarity in twins reared apart and together. *Journal of Personality and Social Psychology, 54,* 1031–1039.

Thomas, A., & Chess, S. (1977). *Temperament and development.* New York: Brunner/Mazel.

Thomas, A., & Chess, S. (1985). The behavioral study if temperament. In J. Strelau, F. H. Farley, & A. Gale (Eds.), *The biological bases of personality and behavior: Vol. 1. Theories, measurement techniques and development* (pp. 213–235). Washington, DC: Hemisphere.

Tomkins, S. S. (1982). Affect theory. In P. Ekman (Ed.), *Emotion in the human face* (pp. 353–395). Cambridge, England: Cambridge University Press.

Torgersen, S. (1984). Genetic and nosologic aspects of schizotypal and borderline personality disorders: A twin study. *Archives of General Psychiatry, 41,* 546–554.

Tsai, M. & Wagner, N. N. (1978). Therapy groups for woman sexually molested as children. *Archives of Sexual Behavior, 7,* 417–427.

Tuckman, J., & Youngman, W. (1968). Assessment of suicide risk in attempted suicides. In H. L. P. Resnick (Ed.), *Suicide behaviors.* Boston: Little Brown.

Turkat, I. D. (1990). *The personality disorders: A psychological approach to clinical management.* Elsmford, NY: Pergamon Press.

Turkat, I. D., & Brantley, P. J. (1981). On the therapeutic relationship in behavior therapy. *The Behavior Therapist, 47,* 16–17.

Turner, R. M. (1992, November). *An empirical investigation of the utility of psychodynamic technique in the practice of cognitive behavior therapy.* Paper presented at the 26th annual meeting of the Association for the Advancement of Behavior Therapy, Boston, MA.

Van Egmond, M. & Diekstra, R. F. W. (1989). The predictability of suicidal behavior. In R. F. W. Diekstra, R. Maris, S., Platt, *The role of attitude and imitations.* Leiden, The Netherlands: E. J. Brill.

Vinoda, K. S. (1966). Personality characteristics of attempted suicides. *British Journal of Psychiatry, 112,* 1143–1150.

Volkan, V. D. (1983). Complicated mourning and the syndrome of established pathological mourning. In S. Akhtar (Ed.), *New psychiatric syndromes.* New York: Aronson.

Wagner, A. W., Linehan, M. M., & Wasson, E. J. (1989). *Parasuicide: Characteristics and relationship to childhood sexual abuse.* Poster presented at the annual meeting of the Association for Advancement of Behavior Therapy, Washington, DC.

Wang, T. H., & Katsev, R. D. (1990). Group commitment and resource conservation: Two field experiments on promoting recycling. *Journal of Applied Psychology, 20,* 265–275.

Watts, A. W. (1961). *Psychotherapy East and West.* New York: Pantheon.

Watts, F. N. (1990). *The emotions: Theory and therapy.* Paper presented at British Psychology Society Conference, London.

Watzlawick, P. (1978). *The language of change: Elements of therapeutic interaction.* New York: Basic Books.

Weissman, M. M. (1974). The epidemiology of suicide attempts 1960 to 1974. *Archives of General Psychiatry, 30,* 737–746.

Weissman, M. M., Fox, K., & Klerman, G. L. (1973). Hostility and depression associated with suicide attempts. *American Journal of Psychiatry, 130,* 450–455.

Wender, P., & Klein, D. F. (1981). *Mind, mood, and medicine: A guide to the new biopsychiatry.* New York: Farrar, Strauss, Giroux.

Westen, D., Ludolph, P., Misle, B., Ruffins, S., & Block, J. (1990). Physical and sexual abuse in adolescent girls with borderline personality disorder. *American Journal of Orthopsychiatry, 55*–66.

Whitaker, C. A. (1975). Psychotherapy of the absurd: With a special emphasis on the psychotherapy of aggression. *Family Process, 14,* 1–16.

Whitaker, C. A., Felder, R. E., and Malone, T. P., & Warkentin, J. (1982). First-stage techniques in the experiential psychotherapy of chronic schizophrenic patients. In J. R. Neill & D. P. Kniskern (Eds.), *From psyche to system: The evolving therapy of Carl Whitaker* (pp. 90–104). New York: Guilford Press. (Original work published 1962).

Widiger, T. A., & Frances, A. J. (1989). Epidemiology, diagnosis, and comorbidity of borderline personality disorder. In A. Tasman, R. E. Hales, & A. J. Frances (Eds.), *Review of psychiatry* (Vol. 8, pp.8–24). Washington, DC: American Psychiatric Press.

Widiger, T. A., & Settle, S. A. (1987). Broverman et al. revisited: An artifactual sex bias. *Journal of Personality and Social Psychology, 53,* 463–469.

Williams, J. M. G. (1991). Autobiographical memory and emotional disorders. In S. A. Christianson (Ed.), *Handbook of emotion and memory.* Hillsdale, NJ: Erlbaum.

Williams J. M. G. (1993). *The psychological treatment of depression: A guide to the theory and practice of cognitive behavior therapy.* 2nd Ed. New York: Free Press.

Wilson, G. T. (1987). Clinical issues and strategies in the practice of behavior therapy. G. T. Wilson, C. M. Franks, P. C. Kendall, & J. P. Foreyt (Eds.), *Review of behavior therapy: Theory and practice* (Vol. 11, pp. 288–317). New York: Guilford Press.

Woolfolk, R. L., & Messer, S. B. (1988). Introduction to hermeneutics. In S. B. Messer, L. A. Sass, & R. L. Woolfolk (Eds.), *Hermeneutics and psychological theory* (pp. 2–26). New Brunswick, NJ: Rutgers University Press.

Woollcott, P., Jr. (1985). Prognostic indicators in the psychotherapy of borderline patients. *American Journal of Psychotherapy, 39,* 17–29.

Worden, J. W. (1982). *Grief counselling and grief therapy.* London: Tavistock.

Wortman, C. B. & Silver, R. C. (1989). The myths of coping with loss. *Journal of Consulting and Clinical Psychology, 57,* 349–357.

Young, J. (1987). *Schema-focused cognitive therapy for personality disorders.* Unpublished manuscript, Cognitive Therapy Center of New York.

Young, J. (1988). *Schema-focused cognitive therapy for personality disorders.* Paper presented at the Society for the Exploration of Psychotherapy Integration, Cambridge, MA, April.

Young, J. & Swift, W. (1988). Schema-focused cognitive therapy for personality disorders: Part I. *International Cognitive Therapy Newsletter, 4,* 13–14.

Zajonc, R. B. (1965). Social facilitation. *Science, 149,* 269–274.

Zanarini, M. C., Gunderson, J. G., Frankenburg, F. R., & Chauncey, D. L. (1989). The Revised Diagnostic Interview for Borderlines: Discriminating BPD from other Axis II disorders. *Journal of Personality Disorders, 3, 10–18.*

Zanarini, M. C., Gunderson, J. G., Marino, M. F., Schwartz, E. O., & Frankenburg, F. R. (1988). DSM-III disorders in the families of borderline outpatients. *Journal of Personality Disorders, 2,* 291–302.

Zuckerman, M. Klorman, R., Larrance, D. & Spiegel, N. (1981). facial, autonomic, and subjective components of emotion: The facial feedback hypothesis versus the externalizer–internalizer distinction. *Journal of Personality and Social Psychology, 41,* 929–944.

Index

Abilities assessment, 331–333
Acceptance
  balance with change, 20, 98, 99,
    202–204
  imbalance with change, 139
  in therapeutic relationship, 515–517
  therapist skills, 109, 110
Acceptance skills, 148
Action tendencies, 354–356
Active passivity, 78–80
  dialectical dilemma for patient, 84
  dialectical dilemma for therapist, 84,
    85
  versus learned helplessness, 78
  learning of, 79
  temperamental predisposition, 79
  as therapy target, 162, 163
  in women, 80
Activity scheduling, 46
Affect (*see* Emotions)
Affect tolerance, 467
"Affective instability," 15
Aggression (*see also* Anger)
  attributions by men, 70
Agreements (*see* Patient agreements;
  (Therapist agreements)
Alienation, 36
"Anchoring heuristic," 368
Ancillary treatment strategies, 504–514
Anger, 70–72
  blocking of action tendencies, 355,
    356
  cognitive–neoassociationistic model,
    71
  exposure techniques for, 349, 350
  male attributions of, 70
  parasuicidal patients, 14, 16
  theories of, 70
  toward therapist, 425
  treatment effectiveness, 23
  underexpression of, 356
Anger expression, 356

  training in, 355
  in women, 71
Anticonvulsants, 47
Antithesis, in dialectics, 33, 34
"Apparent competence," 80–84
  dialectical dilemma, 84, 85
  and situation–specific learning,
    81, 82
Arousal
  and attention, 44
  modulation of, 46
  and vulnerability, 68
Assertive behavior, 71, 280
Assessment, 438–440
"Attached" patients, 130, 316, 317
Attacks on therapist, 76, 77
Attendance agreements, 114
Attention
  and arousal, 44
  regulation of, temperament, 46,
    47
Attention focusing, 47
Attention shifting, 47
Attributions of blame, 63
Audiotape monitoring strategy, 339,
    340, 444, 455
Autobiographical memory, 36
Autonomic reactivity, 79
"Availability heuristic," 368
Aversion techniques, 306–314
  consultation team use, 313
  correction–overcorrection in, 308,
    309
  guidelines, 306–314
  versus reinforcement, rationale, 294,
    295
  side effects, 313, 314
  termination as last resort, 312, 313
  and vacations from therapy, 307–312
Avoidance behavior
  blocking of, 354, 355
  reaction to therapy, 76

Balanced lifestyle, 124
Behavior deficit model, 280
Behavior therapy (see
    Cognitive–behavior therapy)
Behavioral analyses, 100, 181,
    254–265
  chain analyses in, 258–264
  change procedures relationship, 293
  and contingency clarification, 362,
    363
  as exposure technique, 352, 353
  goal of, 261
  versus insight strategies, 254, 255,
    266
  patient cooperation in, 262
  and problem solving, 253–265
  of suicidal behavior, 372, 373
Behavioral case formulation, 256
Behavioral patterns, 10, 11
Behavioral perspective, 33, 34
Behavioral rehearsal
  in vivo assignments, 340–342
  in skills training, 335, 336
Behavioral skills training (see Skills
    training)
Benzodiazepines, 509
Biasing tendencies, 367, 368
Biofeedback, 335
Biological factors, 12, 47–49
Biosocial theory, 10, 12
  emotion regulation system, 43–49
  implications for therapy, 62–64
  overview, 42, 43
"Blackmail therapy," 98
"Blaming the victim," 425
  iatrogenic effects, 64
  as invalidating environment, 62–64
Blocking action tendencies, 354–356
"Booster sessions," 459
Boundary setting, 135, 136 (see also
    Observing limits)
Brainstorming, 278, 279
Burnout, 133–137
"Butterfly" patients, 130, 316, 317

Carbamazepine, 47
Case conferences, 419, 426–428 (see
    also Consultation-to-the patient)
Case management strategies, 399–434
Catharsis, 46
Chain analysis, 254–264
  of antecedent emotional behaviors,
    265
  in contingency clarification, 362, 363

emotional pain analysis, 265
  goal of, 261
  patient cooperation in, 262
  suicidal behaviors, 474
  of therapy–interfering behaviors,
    495, 496
Change, 292–368
  balance with acceptance, 20, 98, 99,
    202–204
  in dialectics, 33, 34
  natural occurrence of, 217, 218
  persuasion in, 34, 35
  procedures, 292–370
  and self–management skills, 152,
    153
  therapist's skill, 109, 110
"Chaotic" families, 56
Cheerleading strategies, 242–249, 429,
    430
  and commitment, 290, 291
  end of session use, 566
  and invalidation, 243, 244
  strategies for, 242–249, 566
Child abuse, 52–54
Choice, 327, 328
Client–centered therapy, 34
Closure, 454
Cluster analysis, 12, 13
Coaching, in skills training, 336, 337
Co–counseling relationship, 392
Coercive behaviors, 58
Cognitive–behavior therapy
  behavior modes in, 37
  dialectical behavior therapy
    comparison, 20–22, 37, 123,
    124
  invalidation of patient, 77
  targets, 123, 124
  and therapy–interfering behaviors,
    130, 131
Cognitive dysregulation
  cognitive theory, 38
  parasuicidal patients, 13, 15
Cognitive modification, 358–370
  behavioral analysis relationship, 293
  commitment to, 284
  orientation to, 360, 361
  and skills training, 368, 369
  types of, 360
  validation in, 359, 360
Cognitive restructuring, 364–370
  checklist, 365
  contingency clarification
    relationship, 360

and devil's advocate technique, 212
dialectical thinking in, 366
procedures, 364–370
self–observation in, 364, 365
Cognitive theories, 12
Cognitive validation, 239–242
Collaborative behavior, 132, 133
Commitment strategies, 284–291
cheerleading in, 290, 291
levels of, 284, 285
overview, 284–291
and shaping, 290
in treatment structure, 444, 445
Competence (*see* "Apparent
competence")
Complex partial seizures, 47
Confidentiality
in consultation discussions, 434
and suicide threats, 490
therapist's agreement, 116
"Confirmation bias," 368
Confrontation technique, 267, 396
guidelines for use, 307, 308
versus reciprocal communication
style, 371
Consistency agreement, 117–118
Constructive thinking, 121
Consultation-to-the patient
agreement in, 117
arguments against, 421–423
and case conferences, 419
checklist, 410, 411
crisis calls in, 418, 419
and families, 419–421
and handling other professionals,
411–419
inpatient treatment settings, 512, 513
and medical model problems, 421,
422
orientation, 409–411
pharmacotherapy issues, 508, 509
rationale, 407, 408
role of, 400
and skills training, 339, 341, 342
social network role, 419–421
Consultant-to-the therapist, 423
agreements in, 116, 117, 428, 429
and aversion techniques, 313
checklist, 427
confidentiality, 434
need for, 425–427
role of, 400
and staff splitting, 431–433
and suicidal patients, 494

and therapist self-disclosure, 382
and unethical behavior, 433
Contextual perspective, 31, 32
Contextual psychotherapy, 21
Contingency clarification, 361–364
chain analysis use, 362, 363
cognitive restructuring relationship,
360
procedures, 361–364
in reciprocal communication, 363
and therapist self-disclosure, 377,
378
use in therapeutic situation, 363,
368
Contingency management
as exposure technique, 353
versus observing limits, 295, 296
orientation to principles of, 297–301
procedures, 297–319
and skills training, 153
and therapist self-disclosure, 376,
378
Contingency procedures, 292–328
behavioral analysis relationship, 293
commitment to, 284
as exposure technique, 353
observing limits in, 295, 296
procedures, 292–328
rationale, 294, 295
and therapeutic relationship, 296,
297
Continuous change principle, 33, 34
Contracts (*see* Patient agreements;
Treatment contracts)
Controlling environments, 58, 59
Correction-overcorrection, 308–310
Countertransference, 130
Couples sessions, 343
Court-ordered treatment, 438
Covert exposure, 351
Covert response practice, 335
Crisis planning sheets, 479–483, 490
Crises, 85–87
affect tolerance, 467
checklist of management strategies,
463
emotions in, 463, 467
group treatment advantage, 87
precipitants, 464
problem-solving in, 465–467
and rumination, 88
and skills training, 147, 148
stress response, 86
task of therapist, 107, 108, 125, 126

Crises (*cont*)
  and telephone calls, 500, 501
  treatment planning effect, 87
  treatment strategies, 462–468
Cultural effects
  family environments, 57, 58
  ideals for women, 54, 55
Cutting behavior, 60, 490
"Cycloid personality," 10

Daily log, 263, 264 (*see also*
    Diary cards)
Day treatment, 493
Decision-making skills, 162
Denial, 158, 159
Dependency, 61
  and active passivity, 80
  conflict with cultural values, 54, 55
  dialectical dilemma of, 84
Dependent personality disorder, 52
Depression
  parasuicidal patients, 15, 16
  rumination in, women, 47
Description skills, 145
Devil's advocate technique
  and increasing commitment, 286,
    287
  as therapeutic strategy, 212, 213
*Diagnostic and Statistical Manual of
    Mental Disorders-IV*, 8, 9, 16, 18
Diagnostic assessment, 438–440
Diagnostic criteria, 11–13
Diagnostic Interview for Borderlines-
    Revised, 9, 13
  in assessment process, 438
  pejorative terminology, 16, 18
Dialectic dilemmas
  for borderline patients, 74–76, 84,
    93
  for therapist, 76–78, 84, 85, 93
Dialectical behavior therapy
  agreements in, 98
  behavioral targets, 124–129, 165–196
  central tension in, 98, 99
  cognitive-behavior therapy compar-
    ison, 20–22, 37, 123, 124
  core strategies, 99, 100
  effectiveness of, 22
  goal setting, 97, 98
  insight strategies, 265–272
  interfering behaviors, 129–141
  modes of, 101–105
  overview, 19, 20, 97–118, 165–196
  primary targets, hierarchy, 167

problem solving, 250–291
  stages of, 168–173
  strategies, 199–220
  therapeutic relationship in, 21, 98,
    514, 515
  and therapist consultations, 430,
    431
  turf conflicts, 194, 195
  validation in, 221–249
Dialectical thinking/behavior
  encouragement of in cognitive
    restructuring, 366
  as goal of therapy, 120–123
  versus relativistic thinking, 120–122
  teaching of, 204, 205
  as therapy target, 166
Diary cards, 184–186
  behavior monitoring function, 263,
    264
  importance of, 263, 264
  parasuicidal acts record, 184–186
  review of, 452
  and therapy targets, 184–186
  in treatment structure, 452
"Diathesis-stress model," 39, 40
Dichotomous thinking, 15 (*see also*
    Splitting)
Didactic strategies, 272–275
"Difficult child," 49, 57
Direct exposure, 351
Distress tolerance skills, 147, 148
"Door-in-the-face" technique, 288, 289
Dropouts, 76
  criterion, 113
  dialectical behavior therapy effect, 23
  pretreatment orientation effect, 169
Drug abuse
  and exclusion from therapy, 440
  of prescribed medications, 509, 510
Drug overdose, 479–481, 490, 510
DSM-IV, 8, 9, 16, 18
Dysthymia, 16

"Eclectic-descriptive" approach, 8, 12
Electroencephalographic abnormalities,
    47, 48
Emergency room setting, 423, 490
"Emotion-focused coping," 78
Emotional expression
  blocking, 356, 357
  and exposure techniques, 346,
    347
  invalidation of, 72, 73
  learning effects on, 72

modulation of, 346, 347
providing opportunities for, 228–230
validation, 226–235
Emotional inhibition (*see* Inhibited affect)
Emotional pain, 265
Emotional vulnerability
  characteristics, 67–69
  communication of, 82
  effect of therapist's power, 372, 373
  and emotional dysregulation, 43–45
  reduction of, skills, 150
Emotions
  biosocial theory, 43
  and borderline behaviors, 59–61
  chain analysis, 265
  child abuse effects, 53
  in crises, 463
  and exposure techniques, 346, 347
  and identity disturbance, 61
  and impulsive behavior, 60, 61
  inhibition of, 45, 46, 61, 226–235
  invalidating environment effects on, 51, 52, 58, 59, 71–74
  labeling of, 149, 230, 231
  modulation of, 45–47, 346, 347
  in parasuicidal patients, 13–16
  regulation skills, 148–151
  systems view, 38
  as therapy target, 161–163
  validation of, 226–235
  and vulnerability, 43–45
Empathy, 131
Empowerment, 390
"Ensembled individualism," 32
Environment-person system, 40, 41
Environmental control techniques, 153, 154
Environmental intervention, 401–406
  checklist, 405
  mandating conditions, 402–404
  role of, 400
Escape-learning paradigm, 45, 46
Ethics, 433
Ex-therapist role, 460
Exposure techniques
  anger reduction, 349, 350
  behavioral analysis relationship, 293
  checklist, 348, 349
  commitment to, 284, 345–347
  control of, 357
  criteria, 347–350
  guilt reduction, 349

length of, 352
matching in, 350, 351
modulation of emotion, 46
orientation to, 345–347
posttraumatic stress treatment, 171, 172, 344
rationale, 345, 346
response inhibition model, 280
structured form, 358
Expressed emotion, 50
"Extending," 213, 214, 396
Extinction procedure, 302–306
  versus aversion techniques, 306
  explanation of to patient, 300
  paradoxical effect, 304
  versus reinforcement, rationale, 294, 295
  soothing in, 305, 306
  strategies, 305, 304

Facial expression, 346
  and inhibition of emotion, 72
  relaxation procedure, 356
Fading, 343
Fallibility agreement, 118
Family
  consultation, 419–421
  invalidating environments, 56–58
  and suicidal patients, 494
  vicious cycles in, 58, 59
Family history studies, 48
Family sessions
  and consultation, 420, 421
  and skills generalization, 343
Fear, blocking of avoidance response, 354, 355
Fear of abandonment, 70
Fear of praise, 69
Feedback, in skills training, 336, 337
Femininity, and bias, 55, 56
Feminism, 31, 32
Feminist therapy, 390
Focusing skills, 146, 147
"Foot-in-the-door" technique, 288, 289
  and contingency management, 300
Friends, consultation with, 419–421
"Functional analytic psychotherapy," 132

Gender differences (*see* Women)
Generalization of skills, 337–344
  checklist, 338
  family and couples sessions, 343
  inpatient milieu therapy, 193, 194

Generalization of skills (*cont.*)
  inpatient milieu therapy, 193, 194
  natural reinforcement benefits, 318
  procedures, 337–344
  programming, 338, 339
  telephone consultation as aid, 188, 189
  and therapy relationship, 519
Genetic factors, 48
Gestalt techniques, 22
Goal setting
  in dialectical behavior therapy, 97, 98 276–278
  dialectical tension, 277
  freedom to choose, 289, 290
  skills in, 153
  treatment stage, 172, 173, 179
Good-bye hugs, 387, 388
Grief, 88–93
  in borderline patients, 90–92
  dialectical dilemmas in, 93
  inhibition of, 88, 89
  normal responses, 89, 90
  therapist's task, 91, 92
Group treatment
  crisis management advantage, 87
  effectiveness, 25
  hierarchy of target behaviors, 186, 187
  hostile group members, 438, 439
  overview, 103, 104
  parasuicidal behavior responsibility, 192, 492, 493
  psychoeducational format, 103
  structure of, 178
  support function, 103, 104, 187, 192, 492
Guilt, 73
  blocking of repairing response, 355
  and exposure use, 349

"Heart-to-heart" strategy, 378–380
Hiding, 355
"Hindsight bias," 368
Holistic view, 31
Home visits, 485, 486
Homeodynamic model, 39, 40
Homework, 454, 455
  commitment to, 291
  in structured skills training, 341
Hospitalization, 510–514
  dialectical therapy application, 193, 194
  parasuicidal patients, 491

primary therapist's role, 511
  protocol, 510–514
  and suicidal behavior, 487–489
Hostility, 70–72 (*see also* Anger)
  handicap in group therapy, 438
  parasuicidal patients, 14, 15
"How" skills, 146, 147, 371
"Hugging," 387, 388
Hypothesis generation, 264, 265

I–thou relationship, 389
Iatrogenic behaviors, 176
Identity disturbance, 36, 61
"If-then" relationships, 362, 363
Imagined exposure, 351
"Imagined outcome bias," 368
Imitation, 54
Immediate reinforcement, 301, 302
Implicit learning, 261
Impulsive behavior, 60, 61
In vivo behavioral rehearsal, 340–342
Incest (*see* Sexual abuse)
Incubation of distress response, 91
Independence value, 54, 55
Individuated self, 31, 32
Inhibited affect
  and emotions, 45, 46
  identity disturbance, 61
  validation of, 226–235
Inhibited grieving, 88–92
  as therapy target, 162
Inpatient treatment (*see* Hospitalization)
Insight strategies, 265–272
  versus behavioral analysis, 254, 255, 266
  in contingency clarification, 362, 363
  highlighting in, 270
  interpretation in, 266–270
Insomnia, 150
Intent, 327, 328, 441
Intermittent reinforcement, 261
International Classification of Diseases, 26n
Interpersonal needs
  gender differences, 54, 55
  set point theory, 316
Interpersonal relationships
  contingencies, 316, 317
  and emotion, 61, 62
  ingredient in feelings of competence, 83
  parasuicidal patients, 13, 15

Interpersonal relationships (*cont.*)
  premature termination of, 152
  set point theory, 316, 317
  training in, 151, 152
Interpretation
  guidelines, 266–270
  timing, 270
Intimacy, 54
Intrauterine environment, 48
Intrusive thoughts, 158, 159
Intuition, 214
Invalidating environments
  and blaming of victim by therapist,
    62–64
  characteristics, 49–51
  and cheerleading, 248
  consequences of, 51, 52, 71–74
  family types, 56–58
  and poorness of fit, 49
  sexism as contributor, 52–56
  sexual abuse effect, 52–54
  in therapy, 76–78, 222
Involuntary hospitalization, 487–489,
    511
  parasuicidal patients, 491
  and suicidal behavior, 487–489
Involuntary patients, 438
"Irreverent" communications, 100, 101,
    393–398, 409

Judgmental heuristics, 367, 368

Koans, 205, 206

Labeling affect, 149, 230, 231
Learned helplessness
  versus active passivity, 78
  and family environment, 59
Legal liability, 494
Length of sessions, 102
Length of treatment, 112, 113
Lethality of suicidal behavior, 519–523
Liability, and suicide, 494
Limbic system, 47, 53
Limit-setting (*see* Observing limits)
Lying, 17

Manipulative behavior
  explanation to patient, 441
  label in diagnostic manuals, 16–18
  and parasuicide definition, 14
  as pejorative descriptor, 16–18, 61
Masking emotions, 346, 347, 356
Mastery, 150

Medical consultation, 481
Medical model, 421
Medication protocol, 507–510
Meditation
  dialectical behavior therapy basis, 20
  training in, 144
Memory
  affective state influence, 44
  and diary cards, 263
  effect of dialectics, 263
Metaphor, 209–212
Milieu therapy, 193, 194
Mindfulness skills, 144–147
  in crisis management, 466
  as exposure technique, 354
  overview, 144–147
Modeling
  in skills training, 334
  therapist self-disclosure in, 381
Monitoring, 263, 264
"Mood bias," 368
Mood-dependent behavior, 163
Mores of psychotherapy, 421, 422
Motivation, 106, 107
Mourning (*see* Grief)

Napalkov phenomenon, 91
"Needy" behavior, 18
Negative feedback, 337
Noncompliance (*see* Patient
    compliance)
Nonjudgmental stance, 146
Normative validation, 234
Nurturing, 111, 112, 139

Observational skills, 145
Observing limits, 319–328
  in case management, 401
  combination with soothing/
    validation, 326
  contingency management difference,
    295, 296
  honesty in, 324
  monitoring, 322, 323
  prevention of therapist rage, 385,
    386
  rationale, 320, 321
  and therapist self-disclosure, 378,
    384, 391
  and therapist vulnerability, 391
  violations of, 135, 136
Operant suicidal behavior, 486–488
Orientation
  as pretreatment stage, 169

Orientation (*cont.*)
  strategies, 281–283
  in treatment structure, 442, 443
Overt behavioral rehearsal, 335

Paradoxical approaches
  and dialectics, 29, 30, 208
  extinction procedures effect, 304
  and *koans,* 205
  as strategy, 202–209
  tensions in, 208
Parasuicidal behavior
  active passivity pattern, 79, 80
  assessment, 473, 474, 477–481
  behavioral analysis, 472
  and childhood sexual abuse, 53
  concept of, 13–15
  diary cards, 18, 186
  as emotional regulation, 60, 61
  environment-person model, 40, 41
  extinction procedures, 302–305
  interpretation, 268, 269
  metaphors, 210
  operant aspects, 486–488, 490, 491
  patient agreement, 114
  primary therapist's responsibility,
    192, 194
  resistance to problem solving, 182
  solution analysis, 472
  support group responsibility, 192
  and telephone calls, 498–500
  therapist's protocol, 490–495
  as therapy target, 126–128
  treatment effects, 24
  treatment priority, 174
  treatment strategies, 468–495
  validation of, 476
Passivity (*see* Active passivity)
Patient advocacy, 404
Patient agreement
  length of treatment, 112, 113
  in treatment structure, 438, 444
Patient compliance
  in cognitive-behavior therapy, 131
  as treatment goal, 133
Payment, patient agreement, 115
Peer consultation meetings, 426–428
"Perfect" family, 56, 57
Pharmacotherapy, 507–510
Phenomenological empathy agreement,
    118
Physical abuse, 53
Physical touch guidelines, 386–388
Polarity principle, 32, 33

"Poorness of fit," 49
Posttraumatic stress syndrome
  "abuse dichotomy" in, 159
  characteristic symptoms, 156, 157
  denial and intrusive phases, 158,
    159
  exposure techniques, 171, 172, 344
  reduction of, 170–172, 179
  related behaviors 155–159
  stage of treatment, 170–172
Postural expression, 72, 346
  training in, 356
Postvention, 494, 495
Power
  patient's vulnerability, 372
  in therapeutic relationship, 372,
    373, 390
  and therapist invulnerability, 390
Praise
  fear of, 314, 315
  as reinforcer, 314–316
  set point application, 317
Prescription medications, 507–510
Pretreatment orientation, 169
Primary emotions, 227
  blocking of, 356, 357
  definition, 227
  validation of, 234
Primary therapist (*see also* Therapist)
  responsibilities, 168, 192, 193
  role in hospitalization, 511
  suicidal behaviors response, 471–492
Problem solving, 250–291
  behavioral analysis in, 254–265
  combination with observing limits,
    326
  as core strategy, 99, 91
  in crises, 465–467
  levels of, 250, 251
  and mood, 251–253
  overview of strategies, 253, 254
  parasuicidal patients, 15
  resistance to, 182
  and therapist self-disclosure, 377,
    380
  of therapy-interfering behaviors,
    496, 497
  as therapy target, 162, 163
Psychoanalysis, 5–8, 12, 266
Psychodynamics, and dialectics, 33, 34
Psychoeducational therapy
  crisis intervention, 87
  and skills training, 103
Psychosis, 440

Psychotropic medications, 507–510
Punishment, 306–314
  consultation team in, 313
  explanation of principles of, 300, 301
  versus extinction, 306
  guidelines, 306–314
  preference for, 73, 74
  and problem behavior, 261
  versus reinforcement, rationale, 294, 295
  side effects, 313, 314

Rage at patient, 384–386
Reactivity
  and active passivity, 79
  therapy target, 161
  validation, 226
Reading emotions, 231–234
Reading materials, 274
Recall ability, 263
Reciprocal communications, 100, 101, 371–392
  checklist, 374, 375
  and contingency clarification, 363
  contrast with confrontational style, 371
  and power differential in therapy, 372, 373
  self-disclosure in, 376–383, 390–392
  strategies, 372–392
  suicidal behavior response, 475
  therapist errors, 140
  and therapist vulnerability, 390–392
  in transactional model, 39, 40
Reciprocal vulnerability, 390–392
Referrals (see also Consultation-to-the patient)
  for medication, 509
  suicidal patients, 492
  and treatment termination, 460
Reframing, 394, 395
Regression, 176
Reinforcement
  natural versus arbitrary, 317, 318
  orientation to principles of, 297–301
  praise as, 314–316
  and problem behavior, 261
  versus punishment, preferences, 73
  rationale for, 294, 295
  scheduling, 302
  in skills training, 336
  and suicidal behavior, 475

  therapeutic relationship use, 296, 297
  timing of, 301, 302
  use of validation, 302
Relapse prevention, 154
Relational self, 31, 32
Relativistic thinking, 120–122
Renewable treatment agreement, 112, 113
"Representativeness heuristic," 368
Research, patient agreement, 115
Resistance, 129, 181–182, 183
  and blaming the victim, 62-64
  parasuicidal patients, 182
  to problem solving, 182
  rating scale, 131
  reduction of, 129
  in therapist, 183, 184
Response communication style, 373, 375, 376
"Response generalization," 338
Response inhibition model, 280
Role induction, 282
Role playing, 334, 336
Role reversal relationship, 392
Rumination
  crisis response, 88
  gender differences, 47

Secondary emotions, 227
  blocking of, 356, 357
  definition, 227
  validation of, 234
Self-actualization, 34
Self-blame, 157–158
Self-control
  and family environment, 57
  presentation of rationale, 441, 442
Self-disclosure (see Therapist self-disclosure)
Self-image, 13
Self-injurious acts (see also Parasuicidal behavior)
  association with borderline diagnosis, 3, 4
  gender differences, 4
  and parasuicide definition, 14
  therapist's protocol, 490
  as therapy target, 126, 127
Self-management skills, 152, 153
Self-mutilation
  and parasuicide, 14
  relief from negative affect, 60
  as therapy target, 126, 127

Self-observation, 364, 365
Self-regulation, 42
 and family environment, 57
 in skills training, 342, 343
Self-talk, 334
Self-validation, 161
Set point theory, 316, 317
Sexism, 52–56
Sexual abuse
 "abuse dichotomy" in, 159
 association with physical abuse, 53
 as invalidating experience, 52–54
 related behaviors, 155–159
 sequelae, 157
 and shame, 54
 treatment stage, 170–172
Sexual contact, 388
Shame
 blocking of hiding response, 355
 exposure use, 349
 invalidating environment effect, 72,
  73
 result of social environment, 42
 and sexual abuse, 54
 treatment stage, 173
Shaping
 and commitment, 290
 difficulty with borderlines, 73
 in families, errors, 59
 principles of, 318, 319
 in skills training, 337, 342
"Shoulds"
 countering of, 237, 238
 identification of, 237
Silence, use by therapist, 396, 397
Situation-specific learning, 81
Skills trainers
 consultation-to-the patient, 413, 414
 need for staff consultation, 415, 416,
  418
 telephone calls to, 189, 190
Skills training, 329–344
 acquisition procedures, 331–334
 assessment in, 331–333
 behavioral analysis relationship, 293
 behavioral deficit model, 280
 and cognitive modification, 368, 369
 commitment to, 284
 core mindfulness skills, 144–147
 effectiveness, 24
 as exposure technique, 353
 generalization, 337–344
 goals of, 144
 group format, 103
 hierarchy of targets, 186

modeling, 334
 orientation to, 330, 331, 441, 442
 overview, 103, 144–155
 and parasuicidal behavior, 492, 493
 patient agreement, 115
 presentation of rationale, 441, 442
 reinforcement in, 336
 and skills strengthening, 334–337
 and solution to crises, 465, 466
 structure, 177, 178
 and telephone calls, 500, 501
 and therapist self-disclosure, 377, 371
Social network
 consultation, 419–421
 orientation to treatment, 443
 and treatment termination, 458, 459
Social self, 31, 32
Social support
 and competence feelings, 83
 importance in treatment termination,
  458, 459
 and well-being in women, 54
Socratic reasoning, 441
Solution analysis
 strategies, 275–281
 suicidal behavior, 472
 target behaviors, 181
Soothing, 305, 306, 326, 546, 547
Splitting
 in borderline personality, 35, 36
 child abuse effect, 159
 in staff members, 431–433
"Staff splitting," 431–433
Stigmatization, 157
Stimulus avoidance, 154
"Stimulus generalization," 339
Stimulus narrowing, 154
Storytelling, 209–212
Stress, 86 (see also Posttraumatic
  stress syndrome)
Structural strategies, 437–461
Structuralism, 121
Structured Clinical Interview for
  DSM-III-R, 438
Structured life style, 143
Substance abuse (see Drug abuse)
Suicidal behavior, 468–495 (see also
  Parasuicidal behavior)
 assessment, 473, 474
 behavioral analysis, 472
 chain analysis, 474
 collateral therapist's protocol,
  492–495
 extinction procedures, 302–305
 inpatient settings, 194

Suicidal behavior (*cont.*)
  interpretation, 268, 269
  lethality assessment, 519–523
  metaphors, 210
  negative effects, 475
  observing limits, 327
  operant aspects, 486–488
  patient agreements, 114
  primary therapist's responsibility,
    192, 193
  resistance to problem solving, 182
  solution analysis, 472
  and telephone calls, 498–500
  therapist's response, 469, 471–492
  as therapy target, 124–129
  treatment priority, 173, 174
  treatment strategies, 468–495
  validation of, 476
Suicidal ideation
  assessment, 473, 474
  therapist response to, 473
  as therapy target, 127
Suicide attempts (*see also* Parasuicidal
    behavior)
  association with borderline
    diagnosis, 3, 4
  and childhood sexual abuse, 53
  emotional regulation function, 60,
    61
Suicide rates, 4
Suicide risk assessment, 468, 477–481
Suicide threats
  assessment, 477–481
  operant aspects, 486–488
  therapist's protocol, 476–495
Supervision (*see* Consultation-to-the
    therapist)
Supportive relationships, 83
Supportive therapy
  group format, 103, 104
  hierarchy of treatment targets, 187
  parasuicidal behavior responsibility,
    192, 492, 493
Synthesis, in dialectics, 33, 34
Systematic desensitization, 351

Tape recordings, 339, 340, 444, 455
Teeter-totter image, 30, 207, 208
Telephone calls
  to ancillary therapists, 190
  checklist of strategies, 499
  hierarchy of target behaviors,
    188–191
  management of, 503, 504
  observing limits, 326, 327

  overview, 104
  to primary therapist, 188
  scheduling of, 502
  strategies, 497–504
  and suicidal behavior, 498–500
  in treatment structure, 444
  24-hour rule, 498–500
Temperament
  in active passivity, 79
  and attention control, 47
  family environment fit, 57, 58
  and "poorness of fit," 49
Termination, 143, 457–460
  agreements, 113, 114
  and "booster sessions," 459
  as last resort, 312, 313
  social network role, 458, 459
  strategies checklist, 458
  versus vacation from therapy, 311
Therapeutic relationship, 514–519
  acceptance in, 515–517
  balancing strategies, 201–204
  belief in, 247
  contingency use, 296, 297
  development of, 446, 447
  dialectics in, 514, 515
  generalization, 519
  importance of, 21, 98, 514–519
  interpretation of behaviors in, 268
  power in, 372, 373, 390
  strategies checklist, 516
  and telephone calls, 404, 502
  and therapist vulnerability, 390, 391
Therapist
  agreements, 115–119, 428, 429
  attacks on, 76, 77
  blaming the victim, 62–64
  burnout, 133–137
  case consultation, 104, 105, 116,
    117
  characteristics of, 108–112
  communication style factors,
    371–398
  credibility of, 446, 447
  dialectical dilemma, 76–78, 84, 85,
    93
  genuineness, 398–390
  iatrogenic behaviors, 176
  invulnerability of, 390–392
  liability for suicide, 494
  limit-setting, 319–328
  physical touch guidelines, 386–388
  rage at patient, 384–386
  resistance in, 183, 184
  role in hospitalization, 511

Therapist (*cont.*)
  role reversal, 392
  self-disclosure, 376–382
  skills, 108–112
  suicidal behaviors, 469, 471
  therapy interfering behaviors, 131,
    138–141, 183–184
  tolerance of therapy-interfering
    behaviors, 175–176
  treatment of, 101
  warm engagement style, 383–388
Therapist agreements, 115–119
  importance of, 428, 429
  keeping of, 428, 429
  observing-limits in, 118
  in treatment structure, 444
Therapist-patient relationship (*see*
    Therapeutic relationship)
Therapist self-disclosure, 376–382
  forms of, 376
  as modeling, 381
  orientation to, 377
  personal information in, 382
  in skills training, 381
  and validation, 381
  and vulnerability, 390, 391
Thesis and antithesis, 33, 34
Time-limited contracts, 468
Time-limited therapy, 112, 113
Touch
  and good-bye hugs, 387
  guidelines, 386–388
Transactional model
  family environments, 58, 59
  overview, 39, 40
  psychopathology, 39, 40
"Transference," 266, 389
Traumatic stress (*see* Posttraumatic
    stress syndrome)
Treatment contracts, 438–448
  caveats, 447, 448
  in crisis management, 468
  strategies checklist, 439, 440
Treatment failure, 108
Treatment team
  consultation-to-the patient, 408,
    409
  consultation-to-the therapist,
    426–428
Turf conflicts, 194, 195
24-hour rule, 492, 493, 498–500

Twin study, 48
"Typical" families, 57, 58

Unconditional positive regard, 134
"Uncovering approach," 170
Unstable self-image, 18

Vacations from therapy, 310–312
Validation, 221–249
  active observing in, 223
  balance with change, 222
  of behavior, 235–239
  borderline personality difficulties,
    71–74
  and cheerleading, 248
  of cognition, 239–242
  in cognitive modification, 359, 360
  combination with observing limits,
    326
  as core strategy, 99, 221–249
  definition, 222–225
  of emotions, 226–235
  importance by therapist, 76–78
  reasons for, 225, 226
  reflection in, 224
  as reinforcement, 302
  self-disclosure in, 376, 377, 381
  strategies, 225
  of suicidal behavior, 476
  types of, 99
Validation-change quotient, 225
Vicious cycles, 58, 59
Voluntary patients, 438
Vulnerability (*see* Emotional
    vulnerability)

Western culture, 57
"What" skills, 144–146
Willingness, 148
"Wise mind," 214-216, 242
Women
  active passivity pattern, 80
  attributions of blame towards, 63
  conflict in cultural ideals, 54, 55
  femininity bias, 55, 56
  interpersonal needs, 54, 55
  rumination, 47
  self-injurious behavior,

"Yes, but . . ." syndrome, 279

Zen meditation (*see* Meditation)